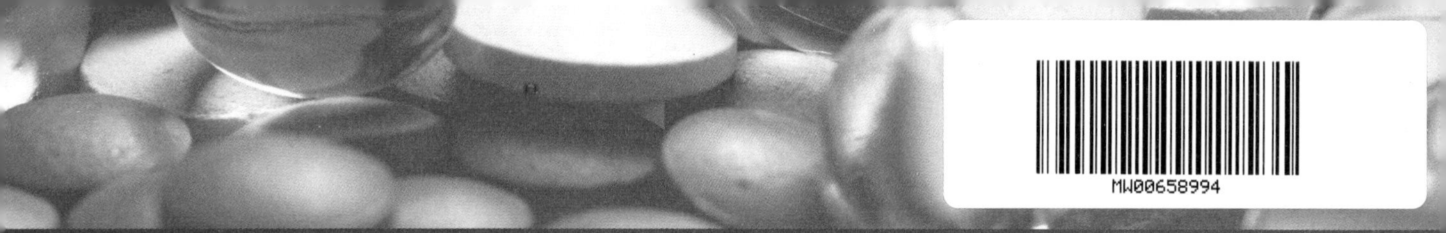

McCarthy's INTRODUCTION TO HEALTH CARE DELIVERY

A Primer for Pharmacists

SIXTH EDITION

KIMBERLY S. PLAKE, PhD

Associate Professor
Department of Pharmacy Practice
Purdue University, College of Pharmacy

KENNETH W. SCHAFERMEYER, PhD

Professor and Director
Office of International Programs
St. Louis College of Pharmacy

ROBERT L. McCARTHY, PhD

Professor and Dean *Emeritus*
School of Pharmacy
University of Connecticut

JONES & BARTLETT
LEARNING

World Headquarters
Jones & Bartlett Learning
5 Wall Street
Burlington, MA 01803
978-443-5000
info@jblearning.com
www.jblearning.com

Jones & Bartlett Learning books and products are available through most bookstores and online booksellers. To contact Jones & Bartlett Learning directly, call 800-832-0034, fax 978-443-8000, or visit our website, www.jblearning.com.

Substantial discounts on bulk quantities of Jones & Bartlett Learning publications are available to corporations, professional associations, and other qualified organizations. For details and specific discount information, contact the special sales department at Jones & Bartlett Learning via the above contact information or send an email to specialsales@jblearning.com.

09842-6

Production Credits
VP, Executive Publisher: David D. Cella
Publisher: Cathy L. Esperti
Editorial Assistant: Carter McAlister
Production Manager: Tina Chen
Director of Marketing: Andrea DeFronzo
VP, Manufacturing and Inventory Control: Therese Connell
Composition: Cenveo® Publisher Services
Cover Design: Kristin E. Parker
Rights & Media Specialist: Jamey O'Quinn
Media Development Editor: Shannon Sheehan
Cover Image: Assortment of multicolored pills: © Peter Topp Enge Jonasen/iStockPhoto; hundred dollar bills: © isak55/Shutterstock; U.S. Supreme Court building: © Orhan Cam/Shutterstock; male pharmacist © racorn/Shutterstock
Printing and Binding: Edwards Brothers Malloy
Cover Printing: Edwards Brothers Malloy

Library of Congress Cataloging-in-Publication Data
Names: Plake, Kimberly S., editor. | Schafermeyer, Kenneth W., editor. | McCarthy, Robert L., editor.
Title: McCarthy's introduction to health care delivery : a primer for pharmacists / [edited by] Kimberly S. Plake, Kenneth W. Schafermeyer ; founding editor, Robert L. McCarthy.
Other titles: Introduction to health care delivery. | Introduction to health care delivery
Description: Sixth edition. | Sudbury, MA : Jones & Bartlett Learning, [2017] | Preceded by: Introduction to health care delivery. 5th ed. c2012. | Includes bibliographical references and index.
Identifiers: LCCN 2016027014 | ISBN 9781284094107 (pbk. : alk. paper)
Subjects: | MESH: Delivery of Health Care | Pharmaceutical Services | Drug Industry | Economics, Pharmaceutical | United States
Classification: LCC RA395.A3 | NLM W 84 AA1 | DDC 362.10973—dc23 LC record available at https://lccn.loc.gov/2016027014

6048

Printed in the United States of America
20 19 18 17 16   10 9 8 7 6 5 4 3 2 1

To my parents, Ralph and Joyce Illingworth,
who instilled in me a love for learning.

—Kimberly S. Plake

To my wife, Donna, and my daughters, Julia and Valerie.

—Kenneth W. Schafermeyer

For my grandchildren, Patrick, Cole, Ellie,
Oliver, Sawyer, and Charlie.

—Robert L. McCarthy

Contents

Preface

When the *First Edition* was published in 1998, Professor McCarthy hoped to meet a textbook need he felt was not adequately met. As an instructor who taught healthcare delivery, systems, and policy, he had long sought a book that provided an introduction to this rapidly evolving area, but that would do so from the perspective of pharmacy. In subsequent editions, we believe that we have been true to his original intent. Over the years, as we developed new editions, we tried to be responsive to the needs of our colleagues by adding, subtracting, and changing subject matter; by providing active learning exercises; and by developing online resources for instructors and students. Given the rapidly changing nature of healthcare delivery, we have also been committed to an aggressive revision schedule; this *Sixth Edition* is being published just 18 years after the *First Edition*.

The *Sixth Edition* includes several major revisions and chapter restructures to reflect the myriad changes that have occurred since the last edition 5 years ago. Chapter 7, *Quality Improvement and Patient Safety*, was added to reflect the growing importance in pharmacists' work in this area. A new author has joined us and completely rewritten Chapter 13, *Government Involvement in Health Care*, using his many years of governmental relations experience to provide the reader a comprehensive, yet easy to follow, overview of how government impacts health care delivery in the United States each day, especially as we enter the sixth year of *The Patient Protection and Affordable Care Act*. Chapter 20, *International Healthcare Services*, again offers an opportunity for the reader to compare the wide array of health care delivery systems around the world, even as the United States opens a new chapter in its relationship with Cuba. We hope you will find the *Sixth Edition* of *Introduction to Health Care Delivery: A Primer for Pharmacists* achieves the goals of its forebears, but also enables instructors and students of healthcare delivery to consider, more fully, how healthcare services in general—and pharmacy services in particular—are delivered. Moreover, we hope that the text and its supplementary materials—including those provided online—will facilitate thoughtful discussions among students, faculty, and practitioners about not only how health care is delivered, but how the system might be improved for all those seeking care.

Kimberly S. Plake, West Lafayette, Indiana

Kenneth W. Schafermeyer, St. Louis, Missouri

Robert L. McCarthy, Storrs, Connecticut

2016

What's New to this Edition

The sixth edition of *McCarthy's Introduction to Health Care Delivery: A Primer for Pharmacists* includes new and updated information to reflect recent changes since the previous edition was published. This edition incorporates important updated material relating to the Affordable Care Act, Medicare and Medicaid, as well as an expanded section on pharmacist roles in public health, including immunizations, bioterrorism, and community health clinics. It includes information on post-graduate education, resources, and credentialing as well as scope of practice and related legislation and information on fellowships.

Information on improving patient safety, drug safety, and pharmaceutical industry and drug development is included in the new Chapter 7, *Quality Improvement and Patient Safety.* This chapter also covers new information on medication use processes including prescribing, monitoring, medication errors, and error prone drug products.

Chapter 13, *Government Involvement in Health Care,* was greatly rewritten to provide new information focusing on government's perspective on the role of pharmacists and specific examples of state health insurance programs, including challenges of the Veterans Health Administration system. Information on global health care and developing countries was also added to this edition.

Recent developments and changes to online healthcare availability led to new information on E-commerce, internet pharmacy, and other technologies used in the health care field today. This edition also discusses electronic prescribing and electronic health records as well as Patient Safety and Clinical Pharmacy Services Collaborative (PSPC). Information on technologies used to improve safety and efficiency is included.

New resources were also added to Chapter 17, *Managed Health Care,* to discuss details on formularies, and drug utilization review, DUR, in greater detail.

New information to Chapter 19, *Pharmacoeconomics* was added to discuss consumer-driven healthcare and pharmacy reimbursement. This chapter also contains additional resources such as documents concerning a consolidated health economic evaluation reporting standards checklist, comparative effectiveness research, information on health technology assessment, and health-related quality of life.

Additionally, updated and new information was added about basic policy issues affecting health care today, pharmacy benefit managers, basic epidemiology, including discussion of incidence, prevalence, and risk, and information on the distribution process including wholesalers and prevention of counterfeits. New information on therapies used at home, as well as new funding for community health centers, patient-centered medical homes, and ambulatory care data was also added to this edition.

NEW TO THE SIXTH EDITION

Updated and enhanced content relating to:

- Expanded section regarding pharmacist roles
- Post-graduate education/resources
- Credentialing/resources
- Affordable Care Act
- Medicare and Medicaid
- Contrasting views of health policy
- Government's perspective on role of pharmacists (provider status)
- Examples of state health insurance programs
- Challenges of the VHA system
- E-commerce, internet pharmacy, and other technologies
- Interdisciplinary models of care
- Scope of practice and related legislation
- Sources of patient information
- Health and illness behavior
- Culture, health literacy, health behavior change and motivational interviewing
- Role of quality improvement in patient safety
- Drug safety
- Pharmaceutical industry and drug development
- Electronic prescribing and electronic health records
- Patient Safety and Clinical Pharmacy Services Collaborative (PSPC)
- Pharmacy benefit managers
- Basic policy issues affecting health care
- Connections between medication use systems and health care delivery models
- Demographics, including compression of morbidity
- Basic epidemiology, including discussions of incidence, prevalence, risk, etc.
- Distribution process, e.g., wholesalers
- Counterfeits and efforts to prevent occurrence
- Internet pharmacy
- DTC advertising
- E-Commerce
- Health care disparities
- Examples of pharmacist roles in public health (immunizations, bioterrorism, community health clinics, etc.)
- Continuous quality improvement
- Measures of quality
- Root cause analysis
- E-prescribing
- Technologies to improve safety and efficiencies
- Reimbursement
- The Joint Commission
- Multihospital systems, horizontal/vertical integration
- Fellowships
- Ambulatory care data
- LTC statistics
- New funding for community health centers
- New therapies used at home
- Economic principles affecting health care
- The uninsured
- Prescription drug plans
- Difference between private pay and Medicaid
- Expand discussion on HEDIS
- Supply-side and demand-side controls
- Consumer-driven healthcare
- PBMS, pharmacy reimbursement
- Details on formularies
- DUR
- Specialty pharmacies
- Cognitive reimbursement and MTM
- Transitions of Care
- Formulary review for expensive biotech drugs
- Health technology assessment
- Pharmacoeconomic methods
- Quality of life and health outcomes measurement
- Health education
- Developing countries
- Accountable care organizations (ACOS)
- Patient-centered medical homes (PCMS)
- Consumer driven health care

Contributors

Thomas E. Buckley, MPH, RPh
Associate Clinical Professor
University of Connecticut, School of Pharmacy
Storrs, Connecticut

Suvapun Bunniran, PhD
Principal Researcher
Comprehensive-Health-Insights | Humana
Louisville, Kentucky

Aleda M. H. Chen, PharmD, MS, PhD
Assistant Professor of Pharmacy Practice and Vice Chair, Pharmacy Practice/Social Sciences
Cedarville University, School of Pharmacy
Cedarville, Ohio

Craig I. Coleman, PharmD
Professor
University of Connecticut, School of Pharmacy
Storrs, Connecticut

Gregory A. Garcia, PharmD
PGY1 Pharmacy Resident
Alameda Health System Highland Hospital
Oakland, California

Louis P. Garrison Jr, PhD
Professor for Pharmaceutical Outcomes, Research, and Policy Program
Department of Pharmacy
Adjunct Professor
Departments of Global Health and Health Services
University of Washington, School of Pharmacy
Seattle, Washington

Scott K. Griggs, PharmD, PhD
Assistant Professor of Pharmacy Administration
St. Louis College of Pharmacy
St. Louis, Missouri

Ardis Hanson, PhD, MLS
Social and Behavioral Researcher; Research Coordinator
Dean's Office
College of Behavioral and Community Sciences
University of South Florida
Tampa, Florida

John B. Hertig, PharmD, MS, CPPS
Associate Director
Center for Medication Safety Advancement
Purdue University College of Pharmacy
Fishers, Indiana

Erin R. Holmes, PharmD, PhD
Associate Professor of Pharmacy Administration
University of Mississippi
University, Mississippi

Kyle E. Hultgren, PharmD
Director
Center for Medication Safety Advancement
Purdue University College of Pharmacy
Fishers, Indiana

Peter D. Hurd, PhD
Professor, Pharmacy Administration and Chair
Department of Pharmaceutical and Administrative Sciences
Saint Louis College of Pharmacy
St. Louis, Missouri

William G. Lang IV, MPH
Senior Policy Advisor
American Association of Colleges of Pharmacy
Alexandria, Virginia

Emily M. Laswell, PharmD, BCPS
Assistant Professor of Pharmacy Practice, School of Pharmacy
Cedarville University
Cedarville, Ohio

Bruce Lubotsky Levin, DrPH, MPH
Associate Professor and Head
Behavioral Health Concentration
Department of Community and Family Health
College of Public Health
Associate Professor and Director
MS Degree in Child & Adolescent Behavioral Health
College of Behavioral and Community Sciences
University of South Florida
Tampa, Florida

David J. McCaffrey III, BS, MS, PhD
Assistant Dean for Student Affairs
St. John Fisher College
School of Pharmacy
Rochester, New York

William W. McCloskey, BA, BS, PharmD
Professor of Pharmacy Practice
Massachusetts College of Pharmacy and Health Sciences
Boston, Massachusetts

Carol A. Ott, PharmD, BCPP
Clinical Associate Professor of Pharmacy Practice
Clinical Pharmacy Specialist, Psychiatry
Eskenazi Health/Midtown Community Mental Health
Purdue University College of Pharmacy
West Lafayette, Indiana

Catherine N. Otto, PhD, MBA
Dean
Health Occupations, Physical Education and Business
Shoreline Community College
Shoreline, Washington

Taehwan Park, PhD
Assistant Professor of Pharmacy Administration
St. Louis College of Pharmacy
St. Louis, Missouri

Ana C. Quiñones-Boex, PhD, MS
Associate Professor of Pharmacy Administration
Midwestern University, Chicago College of Pharmacy
Downers Grove, Illinois

Kyle D. Ross, PhD
Assistant Professor of Economics
Department of Economics
Kansas State University
Manhattan, Kansas

David M. Scott, MPH, PhD
Professor of Pharmacy Practice and Public Health
North Dakota State University, College of Health Professions
Fargo, North Dakota

Jennifer L. Tebbe-Grossman, PhD
Professor of Political Science and American Studies
Massachusetts College of Pharmacy and Health Sciences
Boston, Massachusetts

Reviewers

Susan dosReis, PhD
Associate Professor
Department of Pharmaceutical Health Services Research
University of Maryland School of Pharmacy
Baltimore, Maryland

David Gettman, BS Pharm, MBA, PhD
Professor
D'Youville College School of Pharmacy
Buffalo, New York

Laura Happe, PharmD, MPH
Director of Research and Publications, Humana
Editor in Chief, Journal of Managed Care & Specialty Pharmacy
Louisville, Kentucky

Andrea Kjos, PharmD, PhD
Assistant Professor
Drake University College of Pharmacy and Health Sciences
Des Moines, Iowa

Isaac D. Montoya, PhD
Professor
University of Texas, Houston
Houston, Texas

Kam Nola, PharmD, MS
Vice-Chair, Pharmacy Practice and Associate Professor
Lipscomb University College of Pharmacy
Nashville, Tennessee

Roland A. Patry, DrPH
Professor and Chair
Department of Pharmacy Practice
Texas Tech School of Pharmacy
Amarillo, Texas

Tatjana Petrova, PhD
Assistant Professor
Chicago State University College of Pharmacy
Chicago, Illinois

John M. Polimeni, PhD
Associate Professor
Albany College of Pharmacy and Health Sciences
Albany, New York

Crescent Rowell, PharmD, PhD
Assistant Professor
Lipscomb University College of Pharmacy
Nashville, Tennessee

Justin Scholl, PharmD
Assistant Professor
Lake Erie College of Osteopathic Medicine School of Pharmacy
Erie, Pennsylvania

Patricia Shane, PhD, MPH
Professor
Touro University
Vallejo, California

Charles D. Shivley, PhD, RPh
Associate Professor, Pharmaceutical Sciences and Pharmacist-in-Charge, PC Community Care Pharmacies
Presbyterian College School of Pharmacy
Clinton, South Carolina

Walter Siganga, PhD
Professor
Southern Illinois University Edwardsville School of Pharmacy
Edwardsville, Illinois

Karen L. Smith, MS, PhD, RPh
Assistant Professor
Regis University School of Pharmacy
Denver, Colorado

Michael A. Veronin, PhD, RPh
Associate Professor
Texas A&M University Health Science Center Rangel College of Pharmacy
Kingsville, Texas

Tatiana Yero, PharmD, BCPP
Assistant Professor
Lake Erie College of Osteopathic Medicine School of Pharmacy
Bradenton, Florida

PART

I

SOCIAL ASPECTS OF HEALTHCARE DELIVERY

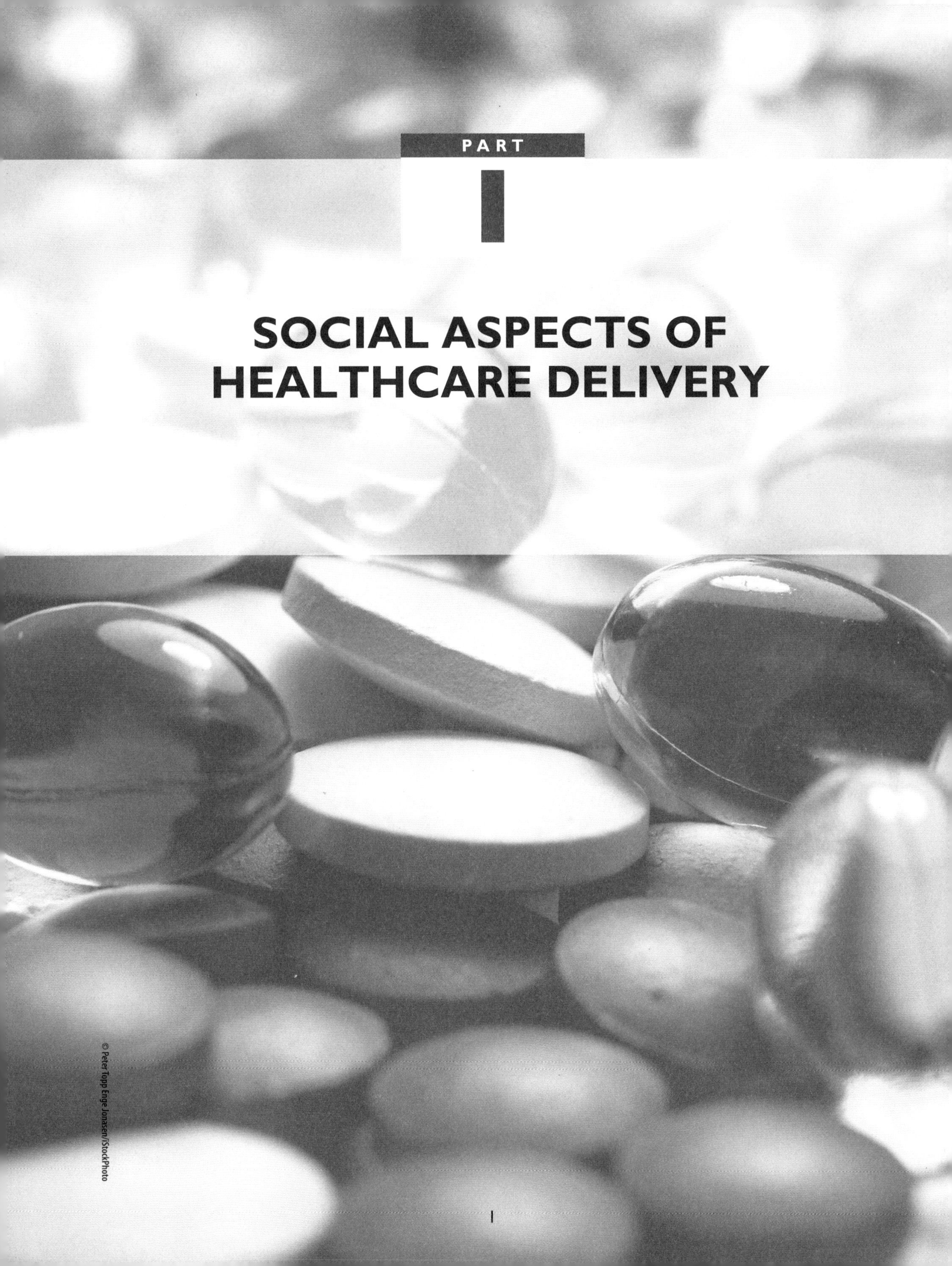

© Peter Topp Enge Jonasen/iStockPhoto

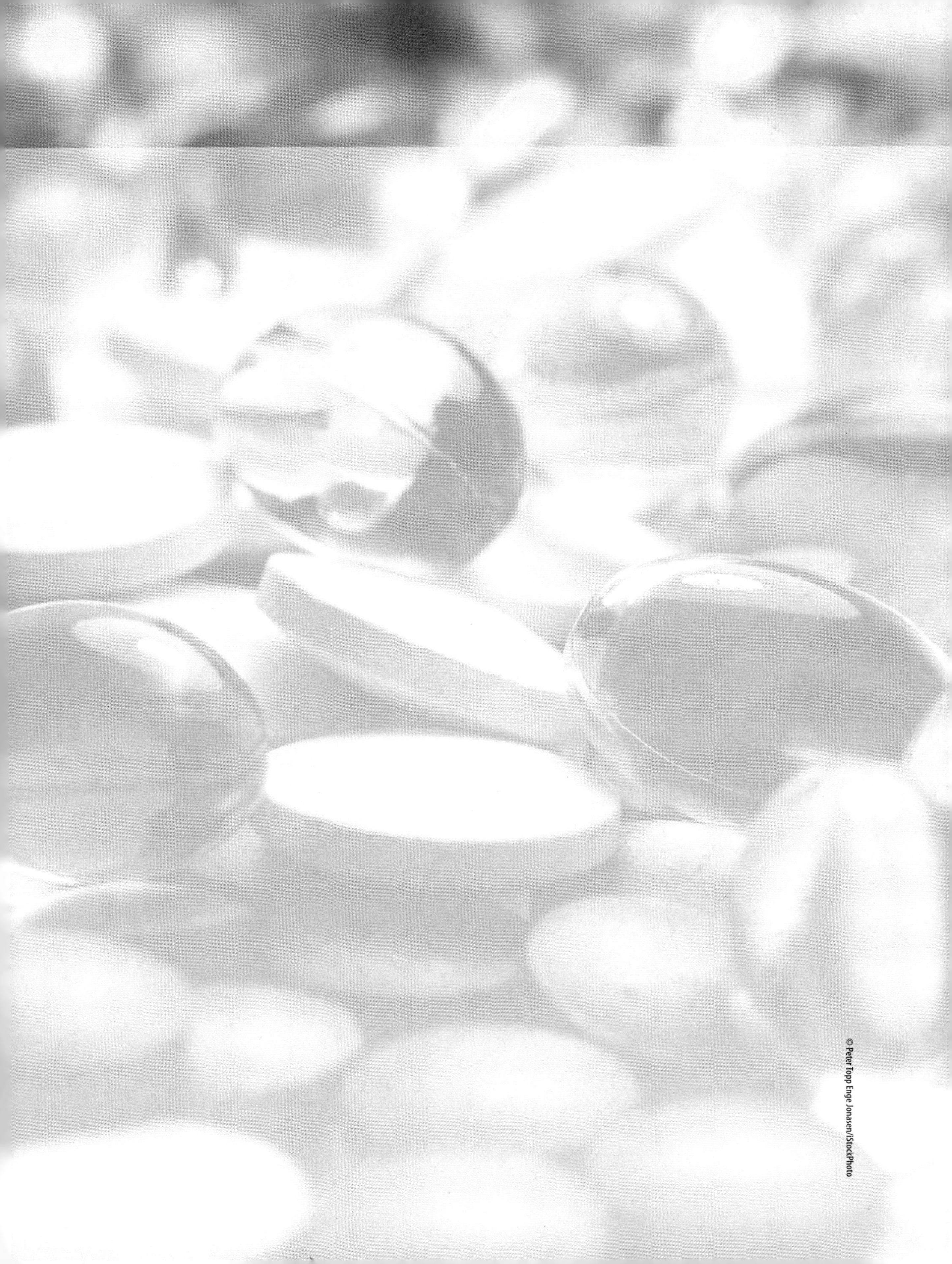

© Peter Topp Enge Jonasen/iStockPhoto

CHAPTER

1

Healthcare Delivery in America: Historical and Policy Perspectives

Jennifer L. Tebbe-Grossman

Case Scenario

The Palmers, a large, extended family, immigrated to New England in the early 1700s. In the 18th and early 19th centuries, the family and their descendants lived on farms in New England. They prospered through farming and some occasional work in small factories in nearby towns. Around 1860, family members moved to the growing cities. A number took jobs in factories; others were fortunate enough to go to high school and even college and found positions in the new professions of teaching, business, and health care. In the 20th century, some family members thrived, especially in the period of rapid economic growth after World War II. Others were barely able to make ends meet, relying at times on government programs and private charities.

One constant in the extended Palmer family is that from the time of their arrival in New England in 1740, various family members kept journals and wrote letters (and later emails or Facebook entries) recording information about their extended family members' daily lives. Suppose that in the 21st century, you have found some of these records spanning several centuries. As a future health professional, you learn about the health and disease history of the Palmer family members: what they thought caused disease and what their philosophies of health and disease were when they made their choices to seek health services, what kinds of diseases family members confronted, the differences public health improvements and technological changes made in their lives, how their health services were paid for, from whom and where they got or didn't get their health services, and why and what they thought about different healthcare policies presented by politicians and branches of government as these policies changed over time in the United States. The written or electronic record covers much of what appears in this chapter.

Based on the material in this chapter, what might you find out about the health experiences and beliefs of the Palmer family members, given their differing socioeconomic backgrounds over time? What might you think about how much or how little healthcare services and their models of delivery have improved over time for American populations?

LEARNING OBJECTIVES

Upon completion of this chapter, the student shall be able to:

- Explain paradoxes of the U.S. healthcare system.
- Explain health conditions in 18th- and 19th-century America in relation to disease patterns and causation theories.
- Explain types of health practices and practitioners and factors explaining access to health care in 19th-century America.
- Explain the various roles of government in healthcare delivery in 18th- and 19th-century America.
- Explain the differences between orthodox and sectarian practitioners and their patients in relation to their perspectives on therapeutics and the delivery of health care.
- Explain changes in the character, organization, and purposes of hospitals as health delivery sites from the early 19th century through the early 21st century.
- Describe reforms in medical education at the turn of the 20th century and the consequences of the Flexner Report of 1910.
- Identify the golden age of medicine and describe what replaced it in the late 20th and early 21st centuries.
- Explain the ways in which medicine and pharmacy pursued professionalization in the late 19th and 20th centuries and how these professions define themselves in the 21st century.
- Explain how the factors of public health, lifestyle (diet, housing, personal hygiene), and medical practice influenced the decline of infectious diseases and increase in life expectancy at the turn of the 20th century.
- Discuss the occurrences of infectious and chronic diseases in the 21st century.
- Discuss the types of government policy that affected healthcare delivery in the 20th and early 21st centuries, particularly in relation to the implementation of public and private health insurance.
- Discuss the implementation of Medicare and Medicaid in the 1960s, the 1973 Health Maintenance Organization (HMO) Act, the 1996 Health Insurance Portability and Accountability Act, the 1997 Children's Health Insurance Program, and the 2010 Patient Protection and Affordable Care Act (PPACA).
- Explain the benefits and costs of the Medicare Part D Drug Plan.
- Explain problems associated with incremental healthcare reform.
- Discuss the major components and the significance of the PPACA.

CHAPTER QUESTIONS

1. What kinds of health beliefs did Americans hold in the 18th and 19th centuries?
2. What factors account for the decline in mortality rates and increases in life expectancy at the turn of the 20th century?
3. What were the benefits and drawbacks of the reforms in education that pharmacists and physicians implemented in the early 20th century as part of the professionalization process?
4. Who provided healthcare services for Americans and in what kinds of settings during the 18th, 19th, 20th, and 21st centuries?
5. What kinds of changes in private and public health insurance plans were considered by Americans in the past?
6. What is the potential for improved healthcare delivery in implementing patient-centered care, interdisciplinary care, and the medical home model of care?
7. How is the 2010 PPACA characteristic of incremental healthcare reform?
8. What are the two most important meanings of the 2012 U.S. Supreme Court ruling in the *National Federation of Independent Business v. Sebelius* regarding the PPACA?
9. What is the meaning of the 2015 U.S. Supreme Court ruling in the *King v. Burwell* case regarding the PPACA?

INTRODUCTION

This chapter examines the historical evolution of health care and health services in the United States. Emphasis is placed on the changes in social spaces where Americans experience healthcare services—from the home, physician's office, neighborhood dispensary, or hospital—to the outpatient clinic, multigroup specialty practice, community pharmacy, or federally qualified community health center. Patterns of health and illness in the United States are examined in the context of mortality and life expectancy and the occurrence of infectious and chronic diseases. The changing social meanings of health and disease, the roles of health professionals, such as pharmacists and physicians, and the expectations of citizens as patients and consumers in an increasingly complex healthcare delivery environment are explored. Of particular concern is the context of changes in attitudes and practice toward individual and social responsibility in the delivery of healthcare services.

PARADOXES OF THE U.S. HEALTHCARE SYSTEM

The U.S. healthcare system is characterized by paradoxes. The United States has the best, most advanced technology available—yet we have a very high rate of medical errors. There are gaps in who has access to health care with different groups of Americans living with "persistent and increasing disparities in health status" (Health Policy Brief: Health Gaps, 2013). Compared to other industrialized nations, the United States has one of the most expensive healthcare systems, especially in terms of administrative costs. The U.S. healthcare system is also fragmented in terms of how it is financed and how healthcare services are organized and delivered. The following overview highlights the paradoxes of health in America, some key components influencing the continuing crisis, as well as reforms that have addressed some U.S. health system problems contained in the PPACA.

Health Expenditures and Technology

The United States easily surpasses all other countries in spending based on data taken from such sources as the Organization for Economic Cooperation and Development, which conducts cross-country analysis of spending, prices, and utilization of health services. The United States spent $9,086 per person on health care in 2013, or 17.1% of GDP, even though this represents a decrease in national expenditures generally attributed to the global financial crisis that occurred between 2007 and 2009. Health spending in the United States is likely to rise to $5.4 trillion and in the context of GDP to 19.6% by 2024. In 2013, it was twice as much as France's expenditures, the next highest spending country compared to the United States with 11.6% of GDP. The United States spends a far greater amount on technology and has higher prices in administrative costs and for pharmaceuticals than other high-income countries. In addition, high healthcare spending in the United States outweighs what is spent on the provision of social services in comparison to other countries that spend more on these areas and have better health outcomes (Keehan et al., 2015; Squires & Anderson, 2015).

To examine one paradox of health spending, magnetic resonance imaging systems, new diagnostics, transplant surgeries, biotechnology-based products, genetic engineering, telemedicine, new reproductive technologies, and health information technology are just a few of the rapid technologic advances that have emerged in recent years in the United States. These developments offer hope for improved quality of life, quicker diagnoses and better treatments, and increased life expectancy. However, reliance on technologic innovation also creates problems. Most Americans expect to receive only the best technical care available, which often leads to overuse of technologic advances. New technologies tend to be updated quickly, often without sufficient examination of cost, effectiveness, or patient safety threat issues. While the meaningful use of electronic health records (EHRs) offers opportunities for cost savings, reduction in medical errors, and improved patient access and outcomes, health professionals raise concerns that in implementing electronic medical records they may lose focus on the interaction between the sick and the healer, thereby leading them to "suspend thinking, blindly accept diagnoses, and fail to talk to patients in a way that allows deep, independent probing" (Hartzband & Groopman, 2008; Ralston, Coleman, Reid, Handley, & Larson, 2010). While many Americans regard access to medical imaging as a sign of the superiority of the U.S. healthcare system, recent health research has focused on the avoidable public health threat that arises from investing so many resources in performing so many procedures as well as the dangers of radiation overdoses in single procedures (Bogdanich, 2010; Lauer, 2009). Finally, technology's benefits are not equally distributed among patient populations, including such preventive measures as breast cancer screening (2014 National Healthcare Quality & Disparities Report, 2015).

Health Insurance

In 2007, the Commonwealth Fund estimated that nearly 25 million Americans had insurance policies in 2007, but were underinsured, meaning their policies often didn't cover important aspects of care, including such items as preventive care health practitioner visits, prescription drug, medical tests, surgery or other medical procedures, or catastrophic medical conditions, and/or policies required significant out-of-pocket payments for services (Gabel, McDevitt, Lore, Pickreign, & Whitmore, 2009). In a 2009 Centers for Disease Control and Prevention National Health Interview survey, 46.3 million Americans of all ages were without health insurance. Between 2008 and 2009, there was an increase in the percentage of adults (18–64 years) lacking health insurance coverage from 19.7% to 21.1%. The survey also indicated 10.9% of the 46.3 million had been without health insurance for more than 1 year (Cohen, Martinez, & Ward, 2010).With the passage of the PPACA in 2010 and successive provisions that have gone into effect since then, there has been a significant increase in the numbers of American who have health insurance. In the early months of 2015, the rate of uninsured Americans was predicted to be 10.7% and the U.S. Department of Health and Human Services anticipated that over 11 million Americans would be enrolled in PPACA plans by the end of 2016 with 4 million of these under the age of 35. This decrease in the numbers of those without health insurance is attributed to more Americans being able to obtain insurance through employers (since the rate of employment had risen) and increased number of individuals able to obtain Medicaid eligibility and to have access to coverage through Health Insurance Marketplaces in the new PPACA. Despite the substantial reform of the PPACA, many low-income working families still lack health insurance because of costs they cannot afford, and people of color are at especially at a higher risk of being uninsured (Humer, Reuters, 2016; Kaiser Family Foundation, 2015; National Center for Health Statistics, 2015).

Health Standards

While health care in the United States is the most expensive across the globe, inadequate, improper, and even dangerous care is all too prevalent. In reports on the performance of healthcare systems internationally, the Commonwealth Fund has found that the United States "consistently underperforms on most dimensions of performance" including in areas of "access, patient safety, coordination, efficiency, and equity" (Bodenheimer, Chen, & Bennett, 2009). Major problems for U.S. patients occur in health worker shortages and the ratio of healthcare clinicians to patients, especially in regard to physicians, nurses (including nurse practitioners), physician assistants, pharmacists, and community health and public health workers providing primary care services in rural and underrepresented areas. With increasing numbers of Americans needing primary care for chronic care services, researchers have called for such new national workforce policies as those fostering interdisciplinary and multidisciplinary care delivered in primary care settings, new financial payment systems for primary care practices and clinics, and increased education of health professionals from underrepresented population groups (Davis, Schoen, & Stremikis, 2010).

In 1999, the Institute of Medicine issued a major report, *To Err Is Human: Building a Safer Health System,* presenting data that showed 44,000 to 98,000 people die each year from medical errors, a higher number than those dying from breast cancer or auto accidents. The report outlined ways to reduce medical errors and urged Congress to create a national patient safety center. In 2005, the federal government enacted the Patient Safety and Quality Improvement Act to continue the effort to foster safety cultures in healthcare institutions. A study commissioned by the Society of Actuaries based on insurance claims data reported that medical errors and the problems that ensued from them resulted in costs of $19.5 billion to the U.S. economy in 2008 (Hobson, 2010). For the same year, the Henry K. Kaiser Foundation stated that "serious medication errors occur in the cases of five to 10 percent of patients admitted to hospitals" (Woo, Ranji, & Salganicoff, 2008).

Those studying patient safety disagree on what progress has been made. Some argue that progress has been made in developing new adverse event reporting systems with the introduction of health information technology systems, advancing national data collection and accreditation standards, and promoting new patient safety initiatives supported by such groups as the Joint Commission and the Institute for Healthcare Improvement. Others, including Donald Berwick, an author of *To Err Is Human* and the new director of the Center for Medicare and Medicaid Services, have seen a change in awareness of medical safety but not fundamental change in the nature of the American healthcare industry (Beresford, 2009; Bosk, Dixon-Woods, Goeschel, & Pronovost, 2009; Furukawa, Raghu, Spaulding, & Vinze, 2008; Gawande, 2010; National Healthcare Quality Report, 2009; Wachter, 2010). Berwick wanted safety responsibility relocated in "the offices and work of leaders of healthcare institutions" and "new safety initiatives ... fostered by teams working at unprecedented levels of collaboration, reaching across traditional boundaries" (Berwick quoted in Beresford, 2010). Government agencies and private foundations studying healthcare quality standards in U.S. health facilities agree that much more work is necessary to ensure safe care for the American population.

Despite many new efforts to reduce medical errors, numbers have risen. As an example, the authors of a study published in 2014 found that "on any given day approximately 1 of every 25 inpatients in U.S. acute care hospitals has at least one health-associated infection" (Magill et al., 2014). In recognizing these problems, the PPACA contains provisions that include naming targets for reducing hospital-associated health infections. The Hospital-Acquired Condition Reduction Program went into effect in October 2014 and requires Medicare payment reductions for some hospitals with the worst performance records (Center for Medicare & Medicaid Services, 2015; Emanuel, 2014).

Health Outcomes

Health professionals and ordinary Americans have consistently been preoccupied with the state of American health through the examination of various outcomes. A study published in 2006 comparing health outcomes in populations with diabetes, hypertension, heart disease, myocardial infarction, strokes, lung disease, and cancer in the United States and the United Kingdom concluded that "based on self-reported illnesses and biological markers of disease, U.S. residents are much less healthy than their English counterparts" (Banks, Marmot, Oldfield, & Smith, 2006). In this study, differences existed at all levels of socioeconomic status, although health disparities were largest for those with the least education and income. The paradox: The United States spends far more on medical care than the United Kingdom does on a per capita basis (Banks et al., 2006).

An often-cited statistic is that the United States ranks lower than many other nations—especially such industrialized nations as Germany, Sweden, and Canada—in terms of infant mortality rates while spending more to prevent infant deaths. In 2010, the United States ranking in reference to infant mortality rates among Organization for Economic Co-operation and Development countries was 26th, with 6.1 deaths per 1,000 live births (MacDorman, Matthews, Mohangoo, & Zeitlin, September 24, 2014). There are a number of reasons to account for the United States' relatively low standing among other nations. For instance, the United States still has significant disparities in infant mortality rates based on race and ethnicity due to such factors as less access to prenatal care, including receiving no prenatal care or not receiving any until the third trimester. In 2013, according to the U.S. Department of Health and Human Services Office of Minority Health, African Americans have 2.2 times the infant mortality rate as non-Hispanic whites (CDC, 2015; Mathews, MacDorman, & Thoma, 2015).

Government programs and corporate-sponsored programs such as "Every Child Succeeds" (ESC) in Cincinnati, Ohio, have achieved success in improving infant mortality rates. In 2006, in seven counties in the Cincinnati area, 8.3 of every 1,000 infants died before the age of 1 year, but for those in the "Every Child Succeeds" program, the infant mortality rate was 2.8, which is a rate that is lower than those reported in every industrialized country. Although the program enrolled 1,800 mothers, its funding allowed only one fifth of the needy women in the Cincinnati area to participate (Naik, 2006). In testimony delivered to the Senate Medicaid Committee in June of 2015, a representative from "Every Child Succeeds" reported that a major goal of the ESC program continued to be the prevention of infant mortality. They noted that infant mortality rates within their program continued to be significantly lower, 4.7/1,000 births, than for the county in which ESC worked—Hamilton Country—8.9/1,000 births, and in Ohio in general, 7.6/1,000 live births (Ammerman, June 3, 2015).

Comparisons of life expectancy show similar race-based disparities. In 1900, the life expectancy in the United States for women was 51.1 years, and for men it was 48.3 years. In 2013, life expectancy for all Americans was 77.8 years—81.2 years for women and 76.4 years for men. In comparing race-based data for 2013, life expectancy for African Americans was 75.5 and 79.1 years for white Americans. Many factors account for disparities in life expectancy, including differences in the quality of neighborhood living environments and access to preventive care services (Epstein, 2003; Kinsella, 1992; National Center for Health Statistics, Revised June 2015; U.S. Census Bureau, 2010).

According to the 2014 *National Healthcare Quality & Disparities Report*, racial, ethnic, and socio-economic disparities have continued in the United States since the report was first issued in 2003. The 2014 report indicated that "disparities in quality and outcomes by income and race and ethnicity are large and persistent, and were not, through 2012, improving substantially"(2014 National Healthcare Quality & Disparities Report, 2015).

Based on outcomes as measures of healthcare risks in the United States, several major concerns were highlighted in the first decade of the 21st century. In examining targets that the Department of Health and Human Services set in *Healthy People 2010*, the incidence of smoking among adults decreased between 1998 (24%) and 2008 (21%), but did not reach the 12% target decrease that had been set in 2000. In addition, the small progress made was threatened with recent decreases in funding for prevention efforts (Koh, 2010, pp. 2475-2576).

Nearly one third of Americans 20 years or older have been identified as obese in 2010. In connecting this obesity statistic to understanding the importance of decreasing the incidence of diabetes, *Healthy People* focused on this disease state and identified a baseline in 1997 of 40 cases of clinically diagnosed diabetes per 1,000 population. Unfortunately, in 2008, the rate of cases increased to 59 per 1,000 population. The *Healthy People* target of 25 cases per 1,000 population for reducing diabetes prevalence in the United States was obviously not achieved, and increased evidence-based diabetes interventions will need to be made by multidisciplinary health professionals in a variety of healthcare settings to assist in caring for these individuals. Thus, the *Healthy People 2020* plan has included the addition of the following two new goals: first, "promoting quality of life, healthy development, and healthy behaviors across life stages; and second, creating social and physical environments that promote good health" (Koh, 2010, p. 1656).

All these existing paradoxes in the U.S. healthcare system are important to consider when reviewing the evolution of health care and the delivery of healthcare services in a variety of settings within American communities over time.

HEALTH, DISEASE, AND HEALTH PRACTITIONERS IN COLONIAL AMERICA

As different groups of European settlers arrived in the Americas in the 16th and 17th centuries, they found a variety of societies and cultures. Some of the indigenous inhabitants of North America only hunted and gathered. Other groups occupied more permanent settlements and subsisted through both agricultural production and hunting and gathering. Contrary to the belief of many Europeans that the Americas promised a new Eden of good health, Native Americans endured significantly high mortality rates. Malnutrition, violence, accidents, fungal infections, anthrax, tapeworms, tuberculosis, and syphilis were common causes of death. European settlers brought influenza—which may not have been seen previously in the Americas—and other new illnesses—including yellow fever, malaria, smallpox, and measles—against which Native Americans had no immunity. Thus, as the historian of medicine, Gerald Grob, notes, the result of early contact between Europeans and Native Americans "was a catastrophe of monumental proportions that resulted in the destruction of a large majority of the indigenous population and facilitated European domination of the Americas" (2002, p. 27).

Arriving debilitated from sea travel, settlers of England's North American colonies did not encounter an Edenic or a utopian environment. Rather, in the early years, many fell victim to malnutrition and dysentery—the consequences of poor food and insufficient clean water supplies. The colonists suffered from a wide range of endemic and epidemic infectious diseases such as yellow fever, measles, smallpox, and malaria. The British government did not implement broad public policies to address problems of health and illness or encourage the establishment of health practitioners or institutions (Cassedy, 1991). Colonial officials addressed such public health problems as garbage disposal, street maintenance, and the regulation of water supply and sanitation occasionally, and with little success in enforcement. Partially because of health emergencies (especially such epidemic outbreaks as smallpox or measles), towns and cities did become accustomed to governments enacting more extensive public health regulations. Examples included quarantines of ships arriving from areas affected by epidemic diseases, setting up isolation or pest houses, and fumigating houses where victims of smallpox or other infectious diseases had lived. Still, the medical historian James Cassedy argued that the application of these public health benefits was "so irregular, tentative, and inconsistent that the benefit to the public health must have been negligible" (1991, pp. 13,14).

When colonists became sick, they depended on various members of the community for access to the healing arts, looking as much for simple human and religious comforts as for therapeutic services. Although physicians, apothecaries, midwives, clergy, and public officials responded to individual or community health needs, it was just as common for family members or neighbors, often the females in the household, to diagnose, make medicines, and physically support the sick.

Until at least 1825, women commonly depended on their female friends and relatives, and midwives when they were available, to attend to them in childbirth in their homes (Bogdan, 1992). European physicians did not look to the colonies, which had small and widely scattered populations, as locations that offered great professional or economic opportunity. Few physicians emigrated, and since medical education in the North American colonies was not considered a priority of government or private agencies, only a minority of physicians or apothecaries completed formal training. Physicians often compounded and dispensed medicines in shops next door to their medical practices. Apothecaries appeared only in small numbers as compounders, dispensers, or sometimes manufacturers and wholesalers of medicines.

In the growing colonies, all these practitioners of the healing arts shared health beliefs that relied on a combination of folklore; mineral, plant, and vegetable herbal remedies; and magic as well as improvisation based on what they found in their environments. The colonists used health practices and medications that were common in Europe and England, such as mercury and opium preparations. They also adopted such Native American health remedies as cinchona bark, which contained quinine (Christianson, 1987; Duffy, 1993; Tannenbaum, 2002).

AMERICA IN THE 19TH CENTURY: THE HEALTHCARE ENVIRONMENT

As the nation expanded westward and its population grew in the early 19th century, Americans exhibited a local outlook on health care that was similar to their attitudes toward economic and political life. A person's health experience as a resident of a town or city on the eastern seaboard was different from the health experience of a farmer in the rural southern or Midwestern areas or of an immigrant traveling west into the new territories.

Rural and Urban Health

Self-reliance was a necessity for farmers and travelers. Poverty, loneliness, exhaustion, accidents, exposure to the elements, and dangerous plant and animal life took their toll. Family members and midwives, who also functioned as social healers within communities, played the most important roles in caring for ordinary people in times of illness. From the era of the American Revolution, the number of physicians who practiced medicine in their own homes and traveled to make house calls in the homes of their patients increased significantly in the 19th century in rural areas and small towns. Both midwives, or social healers, and physicians treated entire families—men, women, and children—and juggled the responsibilities of their health practices with their domestic and community responsibilities. Payment for services was in cash and often in kind, or what families produced by their labor. Many patients could not pay, however, so midwives and physicians needed to rely on other sources of income. Rural and small-town residents could request compounded and proprietary medicines through both physicians and apothecaries. They could also purchase proprietary medicines in the general store and from itinerant healers or medicine men who regularly traveled from town to town (Cassedy, 1991; Leavitt, 1995, p. 4; Ulrich, 1990; Young, 1992).

In urban areas, in the 19th century, social class largely affected a person's quality of life and access to health care. The wealthy and growing upper middle class, including those members of the Palmer family (introduced in the case scenario at the beginning of the chapter) who were well off, had servants, lived in neighborhoods that provided clean air and water, gardens and parks, and health practitioners of their choice. The lower middle classes—including skilled workers, clerks, tradesmen, and widows—could afford food and housing and occasional visits to public parks. They tried to keep their domestic spaces clean despite the unsanitary living conditions offered by tenement landlords. They could pay minimal amounts for self-dosing remedies, medicines, or doctor bills. Most major towns and cities began to provide dispensaries that offered such services as the writing of prescriptions, minor surgeries for fractures, and vaccinations for workers who could pay little or nothing at all (Rosenberg, 1974).

The working classes shared problems with the poor, including lack of such basic municipal services as garbage and sewage removal. As part of the Industrial Revolution, members of the working classes breathed air polluted by coal dust from the factories and railroads that were next to their residences. Congestion, noise, the frenetic pace of commercial life, and the accelerated influx of new waves of immigrants led to a rapid accumulation of new and old health problems, especially rising mortality rates due to infectious diseases. In addition, African Americans confronted even higher degrees of difficulty in relation to quality of life indicators because of slavery and discrimination. They experienced lack of access to health education, health facilities, and basic public health services (Byrd & Clayton, 2000; Cassedy, 1991; Hoy, 1995).

Health Values, Therapeutics, and Practitioners

Health practitioners and the general public have long disagreed about theories regarding the causes of disease and the public policies needed to address them. Some believed that supernatural forces inflicted disease because of human sin. Some believed in contagion or environmental (miasmic) theories of disease. Still others believed that the individual who did not take precautions to lead a healthful life was responsible for disease (Tesh, 1988).

Regardless of their beliefs about disease causation, most Americans generally shared the same values when it came to health, disease, and the body—that is, they looked to Galen's second-century concept of humoralism. The body was an interconnected whole with a natural balance (Warner, 1997, p. 87). As Charles Rosenberg (1985) noted, "every part of the body was related inevitably and inextricably with every other. In health, the body's system was in balance; in disease, the body lost its balance and suffered disequilibrium. If health practitioners were to treat disease effectively, they needed to know about individual patients and their body's system of 'intake and outgo'" (p. 40). What could be observed empirically happening to the patient's body was therapeutically important.

Orthodox physicians (also referred to as allopathic, regular, or mainstream physicians), who had some didactic medical education or at least an apprenticeship under a practicing physician, offered their mostly middle- and upper-class patients heroic medical therapy. They adopted mostly depletive measures, whereas members of the lay public—drawing upon popular domestic medical texts and almanacs—more often employed both depletive and strengthening measures (tonics and astringents) (Horrocks, 2003). Orthodox physicians assumed an active, aggressive role whereby the patient and the family could see very visible changes in secretions and excretions in the body as a result of the physician's interventions. Using leeches, medical instruments, and a variety of drug therapies, orthodox physicians bled, purged, puked, and sweated their patients. Because cures were not often the result of a physician's care during serious illnesses, patients and families could at least share in the knowledge that they had observed the physician's efforts to do something. Rosenberg has noted the ways in which depletive drugs were used in this system:

> Drugs had to be seen as adjusting the body's internal equilibrium; in addition, the drug's action had, if possible, to alter these visible products of the body's otherwise inscrutable internal state. Logically enough, drugs were not ordinarily viewed as specifics for particular disease entities; materiamedica texts were generally arranged not by drug or disease, but in categories reflecting the drug's physiological effects: diuretics, cathartics, narcotics, emetics, diaphoretics (1985, p. 41).

Orthodox physicians competed with sectarians (also called irregulars), who offered a variety of alternative practices, cures, and remedies that were less heroic, including folk medicines, strengthening tonics, and astringents sold by both itinerant quacks and druggists. Sectarians advocated temperance from alcohol; homeopathy, the infinitesimal dose therapeutic that differed significantly from the usually higher levels of medicines required by heroic dosing (Kaufman, 1971); and regimens of fresh air, exercise, and water cures (hydropathy) taken in what Susan E. Cayleff has referred to as comfortable "cure establishments," situated in "natural surroundings" in "country settings" (1987, p. 77). In his popular *Thomson's Almanac*, Samuel Thomson vigorously attacked the orthodox physician's primary reliance on what he deemed excessive depletive measures and advocated his own medical philosophy primarily emphasizing self-treatment through the use of his regimen of herbal medicines, sweating baths, emetics, and purgatives (Haller, 2000; Horrocks, 2003, p. 120). Sylvester Graham worried about the sexual passions and advocated a vegetarian and high-fiber diet and exercise regimen that forbade spices, alcohol, tea, and coffee, in an effort to control those passions (Nissenbaum, 1980).

The commercial manufacture of proprietary medicines developed rapidly during the first half of the 19th century, replacing the functions of the domestic practitioner who formulated the family's home remedies over the hearth fire. Physicians dispensed drugs in their offices and on home visits while "pharmacists began to open stores in towns and cities to fill prescriptions for patients of physicians and to compound drugs requested by their customers" (Cowen & Kent, 1997; Rothstein, 1996a, p. 376). Gregory Higby has observed that pharmacists, as part of a shift of "allegiance from physicians to their customers," also began counter prescribing—that is, "refilling prescriptions without physician authorization, and diagnosing and treating customers" (1992, p. 5). By 1860, many Americans could buy relatively cheap commodities called patent medicines, which were manufactured in small factories, advertised in newspapers, and delivered to any town or city through improved transportation systems. As the 19th century progressed, pharmacists "sold bottles of their own or physicians' concoctions" and became retailers of the prepared drugs (Rothstein, 1996a, p. 376).

At the same time, social reformers and public officials sought to label the production and distribution of patent medicines as "quackery" and warned the consuming public that patent medicine products were dangerous and fraudulent in their claims. Reformers were unsuccessful in their efforts to pass national legislation regulating the industry until the enactment of the Pure Food and Drug Act (1906), which addressed accurate labeling. Nevertheless, such patent medicines as Lydia Pinkham's Vegetable Compound remained popular among middle-class women as a treatment for female complaints because it was seen as an "alternative to orthodox treatments they believed to be unsafe" (Cayleff, 1992, p. 317).

Americans sought out a variety of alternative therapies because they often viewed orthodox (regular) physicians as elitist practitioners who sought to monopolize health care. Many Americans accepted the egalitarian view that a variety of philosophies of healthcare practice should be available to all people. Thus, healthcare services were most commonly delivered in the home, physician's office, drugstore, and cure establishment for the middle and upper classes. The working classes and the poor did not participate in the world of these healthcare services on a regular basis because of the necessity to pay out of pocket at the moment of receiving services. Instead, when most ordinary Americans became sick, they first sought treatment from someone in their own household. They often dosed themselves with self-help remedies that they could afford in an attempt to avoid the cost of treatment from an orthodox physician or one of the many sectarian physicians (Stage, 1979).

The Rise and Transformation of the Hospital: 19th to 21st Centuries

The early 19th-century hospital had its origins in the almshouse or poorhouse, identifying it as an institution with charitable and welfare functions. Most Americans saw the almshouse and hospital as a place that protected the community from those taken in and as a place where patients usually died. Aseptic practices were not commonplace. Generally, admittance for care could be gained only if a prominent member of the community was willing to vouch for the prospective patient's moral character. Patients entering the hospital throughout most of the 19th century were those with the least resources—the "deserving" poor, with so few ties to family or community that no one could care for them. Often they were recent immigrants; however, charitable hospitals sometimes refused certain immigrant populations, particularly the Irish in eastern seaboard cities, and categorically denied admission to African Americans (Vogel, 1979).

Male and female custodial caretakers of the sick were former patients who worked for room and board or local wage-earning residents from the community who had no formal training. Distinguished members of the community served as trustees who financed the institutions, and physicians from upper-class families provided free care to patients, developing new knowledge from the treatment of the very sick (Rosenberg, 1987; Vogel, 1979).

Charitable dispensaries were used by the poor and lower classes, including the poorer members of the Palmer family mentioned in this chapter's case scenario, far more than hospitals from the late 18th century until around 1920. These autonomous, freestanding institutions were located primarily in urban, often new, immigrant neighborhoods and provided such outpatient services as prescribing medication therapies, dental work, and minor surgery. There were few employees: a steward, a house physician, and sometimes a druggist, although the house physician might also act as druggist. Later in the 19th century, established consulting physicians volunteered from the local community (Rosenberg, 1985; Starr, 1991).

Over a 50-year period after the Civil War, the number of U.S. hospitals grew from fewer than 100 to more than 6,000 general and specialty institutions including mental facilities, children's hospitals, and tuberculosis sanitariums. The new hospitals were sponsored and financed by such disparate groups as religious organizations, ethnic associations, women's groups, physician groups (including African American physician associations), and such medical sectarians as homeopathists and eclectics.

As the 19th century drew to a close, the chiefly welfare or charitable nature of the hospital declined. Orthodox physicians and trustees sought private, paying patients from the middle and upper classes. Physicians grew to reject Galen's system of therapeutics with its heroic remedies, replacing it with an increasing acceptance of the germ theory of disease (whereby specific microorganisms were believed to be responsible for the spread of disease). Hospitals introduced new approaches to care, including the enforcement of new aseptic and antiseptic techniques; new technologic methods, including regular anesthetization in surgery and the initial medical application of X-rays; and applied nursing methods patterned on the model developed by Florence Nightingale in England (Kevles, 1997; Pernick, 1985; Reverby, 1987). Architectural designs of hospitals were planned to provide personal service in a pleasant, clean decor with comfortable furnishings.

General practitioners, as well as elite physicians, sought to admit patients to these hospitals to enhance the growth of their private medical practices. Hospitals continued to take charity patients, but the numbers decreased and these individuals received a lesser level of care. By the end of the 19th century, hospitals were well on their way in a journey from charitable guest houses to biomedical showcases, with the wealthier members of the Palmer family having the greatest access to the new technological miracles (Ludmerer, 1999; Risse, 1999, p. 4; Rosenberg, 1987, p. 47; Rosner, 1979, p. 127).

The growth of the modern hospital as an indispensable element in American health care was ensured by the 1946 National Hospital Survey and Construction Act (Hill-Burton Act) and subsequent amendments, which provided federal funding for planning and assisting in the construction of new hospitals and public health centers (Rosenberg, 1987, p. 343). While the Hill-Burton Act led to an overabundance of hospital beds with funds disproportionately going to middle-income communities, Rosenberg noted that technological innovation, increasing application of business management policies, and establishment of the principles of local initiative, state review, and federal support sharing provided for some degree of planning on a state level. Hospitals in the post–World War II era organized the financing and delivery of care around an acute disease model.

While the operation of hospitals and the conduct of medical education and research were more dependent on federal government funding, the government became more interested in pursuing service programs from the 1970s through much of the 1990s. This was particularly connected to the federal funding of Medicare and Medicaid programs beginning in the 1960s. A new emphasis also was placed on encouraging preventive health and pursuing cost-cutting and efficiency measures at the same time that hospitals struggled with the possibility of fulfilling the role of exemplary social institutions to the local community (Fox, 1993, p. 17; Litman, 1997, p. 3; Starr, 1982; Stevens, 1989, p. 364).

In the 1990s, some community hospital mergers and nonprofit to for-profit hospital conversions resulted in the maintenance of clear social missions to local communities, while others led to the closing of many community hospitals that had previously treated the poor and less well off (Bell, 1996; Blumenthal & Weissman, 2000; Cahill, 1997; Lukas & Young, 2000; Opdycke, 1999; Young, Dasai, & Lukas, 1997). In the context of thinking of the patient as a consumer, the hospital as a part of an industry sought to attract the sufficiently insured through "a patient-centered care scheme designed to achieve customer satisfaction by striving to make hospitals more pleasant, comfortable, and user friendly" (Essoyan, 2000, p. A19; La Ferla, 2000, p. 4; Risse, 1999, p. 681). Hospitals were redesigned to streamline healthcare delivery, enhancing efficiency and cost savings by using such strategies as placing patients in focused settings with a satellite pharmacy, a laboratory, and radiologic facilities, and employing "cross-trained multidisciplinary caregiving teams" (Risse, 1999, pp. 682, 683).

At the turn of the 21st century, the lay public and healthcare professionals, including the physician, had confronted identity dilemmas with the use of new language in healthcare settings. When someone is sick or seeks wellness care, is he or she a client, patient, or consumer, and what is the connotation of the word *consumer*? Are physicians, nurses, or pharmacists health professionals, caregivers, or mere health providers (Risse, 1999, p. 682; Tomes, 2006, p. 84)? Finally, given the increasing focus on financial incentives and customer orientation, scholars, journalists, the public, health professionals, and government officials have expressed concerns about the meaning of healing and the 21st-century hospital as a "a place of repairing and damaging, birthing and dying—and red tape and budgets and stress—but also a community struggling with the thorny social forces changing the world around it" (Gordon, 2010; Risse, 1999; Salamon, 2010, p. 9).

Major changes in the early 21st century in the hospital are in process. Among them are electronic record keeping and interprofessional education in the academic hospital setting as methods to improve health quality and efficiency and to reduce medical errors (including adverse drug events). In addition, the roles of primary care physicians, specialists, and hospitalists are evolving in provision of coordinated care in healthcare delivery between inpatient and outpatient settings. Concerns revolving around these changes include potential workforce shortages, the future of medical mecca academic health centers, competing specialized health facilities in the community, and financial imperatives related to private health plan and government hospital reimbursements (Berenson, Ginsburg, & May, 2006; Blue, Mitcham, Smith, Raymond, & Greenberg, 2010; Buring et al., 2009; Casalino, November, Berenson, & Pham, 2008; Crossen & Tollen, 2010; DesRoches et al., 2010; Hamel, Drazen, & Epstein, 2009; Mechanic, 2003).

One of the most discussed changes has been the effort to implement patient-centered care. This term was first introduced in 2001 as a goal for quality care in the Institute of Medicine's report,

Crossing the Quality Chasm. In this report, patient-centered care is defined as "respectful of and responsive to individual patient preferences, needs, and values, and ensuring that patient values guide all clinical decisions" (Institute of Medicine, 2001, p. 3). Various hospitals initiated efforts to institute aspects of patient-centered care, including approaches that involved family members. In 1996, Dana Farber Cancer Institute and Brigham and Women's Hospital began a joint venture to change their paradigm of care to a patient-centered model to involve all parts of the hospital organization including "high-performing teams in which communication, collaboration, transparency, and joint decision-making" (Ponte et al., 2003, p. 84) with hospital executive leadership playing a lead role (Ponte et al., 2003).

In 2006, the American Hospital Association and the Institute for Family-Centered Care developed a tool kit that comprised a video with discussion and resource guides and self-assessment tools that could be used by patients, families, and health practitioners to improve patient care in hospitals through partnerships among the above constituencies (American Hospital Association and Institute for Family-Centered Care Resource Guide, 2006). Late in the first decade of the 21st century, critics of patient-centered care argued for bolder meanings. Donald Berwick, president and chief executive officer of the Institute for Healthcare Improvement and appointed by President Barack Obama in 2010 as administrator of the Centers for Medicare and Medicaid Services, proposed a model for hospitals that included patient and family member participation in rounds, patient decision making on food and clothing (as allowed by health status), and patient ownership of medical records with clinicians needing to have permission to gain access to them (Berwick, 2009, p. w561). Implementation of patient-centered care has been identified as a way to prevent a fragmented healthcare experience that often occurs for patients, especially those with serious or chronic illnesses, as they need care in hospitals, other health organizations, and their homes (Epstein, Fiscella, Lesser, & Stange, 2010).

One area of concern related to incorporating more patient-centered care has been whether the use of the EHR has helped or hindered. The major reasons for using EHRs relate to how they might improve the availability of patient information and patient safety (especially in reference to drug safety use). Some critics of the increasing use of the EHR have pointed to how the record has also been used as a "key instrument for measuring the duration and standardizing the content of patient-doctor interactions in pursuit of 'the one-best way.'" In emphasizing this as a key goal in using the EHR and limiting patient visits in some hospital settings to 15 to 20 minutes, "open-ended interviews, vital for obtaining accurate clinical information and understanding patients' mindsets" have been seen as "almost impossible" to obtain (Hartzband & Groopman, 2016).

Other research shows that progress has been made in relation to reducing the ethnic and racial disparities in the treatment of patients in hospitals. One study looked at three "common medical conditions"—pneumonia, acute myocardial infarction, and heart failure and showed that improving "performance on quality measures" for black, Hispanic, and white adult patients resulted in "increased racial and ethnic equity in performance rates both within and among U.S. hospitals." Efforts to incorporate true patient-centered care into the hospital and to pursue care equity in hospital performance rates clearly reflect the idea of hospitals as exemplary social institutions (Trivedi et al., 2014).

CONTINUITY AND CHANGE IN HEALTH INSTITUTIONS AND PROFESSIONS

As part of a continuing process during the early years of the 20th century, medicine and pharmacy instituted important changes in their pursuit of modern, credential-based professionalization. As self-defined members of individual professions, physicians and pharmacists sought to strengthen their positions in society by employing a variety of strategies. These professions placed new emphasis on their special expertise within their own field of study and practice: increasing the authority and purview of professional organizations, licensing and self-regulation standards; the pursuit of rigorous educational reform and professional autonomy; and a commitment to altruism that placed their clientele above any commercial concern for profit.

Medicine

Beginning in 1908, at the urging of the American Medical Association (AMA), Abraham Flexner conducted a study of medical schools sponsored by the Carnegie Foundation. He published *Medical Education in the United States and Canada* in 1910, recommending numerous changes in the focus, education, and practice of medicine in the 20th century (Flexner, 1910). The Flexner Report paved the way for effectively making allopathic medicine the legally sanctioned form of practice and abandoning the apprenticeship model of medical education and the primarily commercial financing of medical schools by physician-entrepreneurs. In the early 1900s, medical educators and leaders had already reached some consensus on the direction of change as proposed in the Flexner Report, and by 1930, many reforms were in place. Chiefly, these reforms included most states' acceptance that medical schools would be accredited under the control of the AMA; the graduation of fewer students; and the closing of weaker medical schools with the remaining stronger institutions obtaining funding from such sources as state governments and philanthropists to pursue further discoveries in bacteriology and other biomedical sciences and to produce trained clinicians and specialists in such areas as obstetrics, cardiology, and surgery. These reforms also resulted in the reduction of the number of students admitted from the lower classes, ethnic minorities, and women. Their numbers did not reappear in any strength until the 1970s and 1980s, when the number of African Americans and women admitted to medical schools began to increase (Ludmerer, 1985; Markowitz & Rosner, 1979; Morantz-Sanchez, 1992; More, 1999; Starr, 1982). Still, in the early 21st century, "[t]he complexion of the health professions in the United States little resembles the nation's ethnic and racial composition" (Grumbach & Mendoza, 2008, p. 413) despite business arguments that there are "customer service and competitive advantages to the health industry of having a workforce that is culturally and linguistically attuned to the increasing diversity of the nation's health care consumers" (Grumbach & Mendoza, 2008, p. 414). Women have made significant inroads in the early 21st century in relation to increased admissions to medical schools, generally approaching half of students admitted annually. However, concerns have remained in relation to career advancement, sexual harassment and discrimination, fears expressed about the feminization of medicine, and the concentration of women physicians in only a few lower-income medical specialty areas (Boulis, Jacobs, & Veloski, 2001; McGuire, Bergen, & Polan, 2004; Sullivan & Mittman, 2010).

Nonetheless, the medical reform of the early 20th century ushered in what John C. Burnham has termed a *golden age* in which "American physicians enjoyed social esteem and prestige along with an admiration for their work that was unprecedented in any age" (Burnham, 1982, p. 284). In post–World War II America, the biomedical model predominated in research and in areas of clinical care. An emphasis was placed on the "subcellular and molecular level, and life processes were increasingly understood in physical and chemical terms" (Ludmerer, 1999, p. 148). This golden age did not begin to be seriously challenged until the 1960s, when questions were raised both from within the profession and by the public about the physician's priestly pretension and technical performance (Burnham, 1982, p. 291).

From the 1970s through the 1990s, medical education and academic health centers came under increasing duress. Some social inequities were addressed as increasing numbers of women and minorities were admitted to medical schools and such new pedagogies as problem-based learning were widely introduced in medical school curricula to improve clinical skills. At the same time, the new managed care practice made inroads against the pursuit of academic research and the provision of "the importance to the physician's work of having sufficient time with patients" (Ludmerer, 1999, p. 383).

As the 20th century ended, physicians continued to express concern about their roles in managed care systems. They showed a willingness to treat patients in new ways; including group visits where patients with chronic illnesses, such diseases as diabetes, hypertension, and arthritis; and attend seminars led by physicians (Martinez, 2000). They also raised concerns about whether the quality of patient care and their decision-making autonomy were unduly threatened by managed care's increased emphasis on linking the number of patients whom physicians treat to their fees and salaries (Kowalczyk, 2000). Deborah A. Stone argued that the "doctor has been reconceived as an entrepreneur who is now in the business of insuring patients as well as caring for them" (1997, p. 534).

In the early 21st century, many medical schools have been making changes in the education of students to respond to some evidence that show American populations, including socially disadvantaged ones, benefit from the implementation of accountable care strategies in primary care practices within their communities. In addition, the delivery of improved primary care reduces health spending and responds to the needs of large numbers of patients increasingly living with chronic illnesses. The patient-centered medical home model of primary care has been a major way in which policymakers have supported efforts to expand primary care. In 1967, the concept of a medical home originally was explained by the Academy of Pediatrics and demonstrated as more effective in the delivery of good health care to children with special needs. In the intervening years, a "movement" to implement the medical home developed. By 2007, healthcare professional organizations, national health plans, labor unions, consumer organizations, and major corporations expressed support of the medical home model.

While there is not a consensus definition of the patient-centered medical home concept, it incorporates a number of elements. Patients are whole persons rather than disease states. They are active, prepared, knowledgeable participants who work with an interdisciplinary team of caregivers that is led by a primary care physician. The team coordinates patients' preventive, acute, and chronic care across settings in the healthcare system and community. The team draws upon effective information technology, including EHRss, to support communication and quality outcomes (Colwil, 2010; Iglehart, 2008; Larson & Reid, 2010). The hope for the future is that payment will be provided based on the added value that the medical home and its practitioners provided, a combination of "fee-for-service, pay-for performance, and a separate payment for coordination and integration" (Rittenhouse & Shortell, 2009, p. 2039).

A number of demonstration projects have been funded to experiment with the patient-centered medical home model of care for the future (Kilo & Wasson, 2010; Reid et al., 2010). A single-clinic multidisciplinary team practice (including a pharmacist) that is part of a group health cooperative reorganized itself along a medical home model in 2006. A 1-year study of this prototype practice showed that the clinic achieved measurable positive outcomes. In comparison to other clinics in the group health cooperative, the clinic model was able to show 29% fewer patient visits to the emergency room and 6% fewer hospitalizations with cost savings achieved. In addition, patients reported improvement in their experiences of care and in the quality of care they received. Health practitioners noted more job satisfaction and less burnout (Reid et al., 2010). Medical schools have begun to implement curricular changes and to study how medical students are currently exposed to patient-centered approaches to care as they learn in hospital and ambulatory care settings (Morrison, Goldfarb, & Lanken, 2010; Saultz et al., 2010).

Besides emphasizing the medical home setting, many medical schools have emphasized more clinical training in healthcare centers in rural and urban areas that pursue accountable care principles and the recognition of the social determinants of health in the delivery of primary care. Medical schools are emphasizing the need to teach students more about "social medicine" or the social determinants of health—the ability to afford prescription or OTC medications, affording and accessing transportation to health appointments, having adequate housing that does not include dangers that make patients sick (lead, rats, insects, mold) or being able to easily locate, purchase, and cook health foods—within didactic and clinical curricular opportunities. Some medical schools are also pursuing goals and funding for increasing efforts to emphasize the education of students who want to practice primary care in underserved rural and urban areas, including recruitment of potential applicants who come from underserved areas. (Behforouz, Drain, & Rhatigan, 2014; Maxwell, Tobey, & Barron, 2015; Meriweather, 2015).

As the 100th anniversary of the Flexner report was celebrated in 2010, medical education in the United States once again began experiencing significant transformation. Thomas P. Duffy noted in an article surveying the Flexner Report in historical perspective that 21st-century revisions in the medical school curriculum were "reclaiming the rightful eminence of the service component of medicine—the centerpiece of the doctor-patient relationship" (Duffy, 2011).

Pharmacy

As the 20th century began, pharmacists pursued several approaches in an effort to change their practice to modern credential-based professionalization. Challenges to the apprenticeship model of training pharmacists had already occurred in the 1860s and 1870s, when state universities, especially in the Midwest and West, established a pharmacy curriculum based primarily on study in the physical sciences and laboratory instruction. By the turn of the 20th century, there were more than 50 colleges and departments of pharmacy in the United States. Most, however, had minimal standards for admission and length of study, with a combination of the scientific and apprenticeship models too often providing minimal education or training.

In 1900, more than 38,000 U.S. drugstores served a population of 76 million, translating to one store per 2,000 people (Deno, Rowe, & Brodie, 1959). Few practitioners operated in individual establishments devoted exclusively to professional services. Instead, most worked in commercial enterprises—independent, druggist-owned stores or shops—that provided a variety of services and products, including soda fountains, perfumes, telephone booths, magazines, candy, and popular books. Chain drugstores, with the same ownership and the same product lines, began to appear in the early years of the 20th century and quickly expanded regionally and nationally across the United States.

In their effort to professionalize, pharmacists confronted several difficult problems. In 1915, Abraham Flexner asserted that the pharmacist was not a professional in a speech at the National Conference of Charities and Corrections in Baltimore, Maryland. Whereas the physician "thinks, decides, and orders; the pharmacist obeys—obeys of course with discretion, intelligence, and skill—yet in the end obeys and does not originate. Pharmacy, therefore, is an arm added to the medical profession, a special and distinctly higher form of handicraft, not a profession" (Flexner, 1915, p. 158). In addition, the U.S. military decided to train its enlisted soldiers to dispense medications in World War I rather than recruit and appoint pharmacists as officers. The 1922 Code of Ethics established by the American Pharmaceutical Association (currently the American Pharmacists Association, APhA) was unfortunately compatible with Flexner's perspective. Pharmacy's primary object was "the service it can render to the public in safeguarding the handling, sale, compounding and dispensing of medicinal substances" (APA, 1922, p. 728). Ordinary Americans encountered the pharmacist as customers in the neighborhood drugstore, a commercial enterprise identified with a for-profit motive. In the 1920s, hospital pharmacy, although devalued by community druggists and often by the institutional administrations where they were located, was the area where pharmacy thrived as a "bastion of high pharmaceutical technology, art, and science" (Higby with Gallagher, 1992, p. 507).

In response to the aforementioned problems, pharmacy colleges organized their own association, the American Conference of Pharmaceutical Faculties (later renamed the American Association of Colleges of Pharmacy), in the 1920s and struggled to reach their goals of establishing more rigorous standards of education and practice. The American Association of Colleges of Pharmacy instituted the requirement of high school graduation for admission, and by 1932, it mandated 4 years of study for graduation (Deno, Rowe, & Brodie, 1959; Higby with Gallagher, 1992; Higby, 1996; Sonnedecker, 1976). Some practicing pharmacists also saw the value of education in improving their image in the community. For instance, when the consumer market for vitamins increased from $12 million to over $130 million in sales during the 1930s, pharmacists argued that purchases of these OTC products should be made in drugstores rather than grocery stores because of the pharmacist's specialized knowledge and professional training (Apple, 1996).

In World War II, pharmacists were again denied a commission in the U.S. military while these were given to first-year medical students and nurses. Pharmacy organizations responded by contributing funding to a self-study, the 1946 *Pharmaceutical Survey*. This study made recommendations, chief of which was the expansion of the pharmacy curriculum to 6 years. The American Association of Colleges of Pharmacy proposed a 5-year program of study, with a curriculum that continued to focus on the science and technology of pharmaceutical products. Pharmacists in community drugstores in the new age of miracle drugs that followed the discovery of penicillin were relegated to a count and pour role under 1952 federal regulations and the newly promulgated American Pharmaceutical Association's Code of Ethics, which asserted that "the pharmacist does not discuss the therapeutic effects or composition of a prescription with a patient" (American Pharmaceutical Association, 1952, p. 722).

The 1960s have been defined as years of revolution in pharmacy. During this decade, ordinary community and hospital pharmacists began a push for a new identity in clinical pharmacy, where the pharmacist is the drug expert and is responsible for being a therapeutic advisor for patients and other health professionals. In another revision of the APhA Code of Ethics in 1969, the pharmacist was required to "render to each patient the full measure of his ability as an essential health practitioner" (Higby, 1997, p. 12). For the community pharmacist, this would mean a new perception of the people that the pharmacist spoke with across their counters—going from customers to patients. A culminating point in the expression of educational reform was presented in 1975 in *Pharmacists for the Future: The Report of the Study Commission on Pharmacy* (Millis, 1975). This report called for a 6-year curriculum culminating in an entry-level doctor of pharmacy degree that was intended to provide a general education for the whole person, educating pharmacists rather than training them, and to incorporate clinical therapeutics and clerkship opportunities in healthcare workplaces (APhA, 1969; Higby, 1997; Knowlton, 2009; Worthen, 2006).

The underpinning for the new program of study and practice was the concept of *pharmaceutical care*, to be implemented in communities and such institutional settings as hospitals where pharmacists would be equal members of the healthcare team. Hepler and Strand (1990) identified pharmaceutical care as connecting the pharmacist's responsibilities with therapeutic outcomes. While similar to the widely accepted definition, the 2004 construction states that "[P]harmaceutical care is a patient-centered practice in which the practitioner assumes responsibility for a patient's drug-related needs and is held accountable for this commitment" (Cipolle, Strand, & Morley, 2004, p. 26). This concept was a reflection on the Omnibus Budget Reconciliation Act of 1990, which mandated evaluation of drug therapy in the review of patient profiles and established standards of medication counseling for Medicaid patients (Elenbaas & Worthen, 2009; Higby, 1997; McGivney et al., 2007). The 1994 Pharmacist Code of Ethics also emphasized such principles as a "covenantal" relationship between patient and pharmacist; promotion of "the good of every patient in a caring, compassionate, and confidential manner" service to "the individual, community and societal needs"; and the pursuit of "justice in the distribution of health resources" (APhA, 1994, p. 1).

Unfortunately, the bureaucratic and cost-cutting demands of third-party payers and managed care organizations greatly inhibited the ability of pharmacists to actually practice pharmaceutical care in healthcare settings (Navarro, 1999). Despite the presence of more pharmacy technicians and robotics in some cases, pharmacists spent most of their time in dispensing roles and reported dissatisfaction with their general lack of opportunities to more effectively fulfill pharmaceutical care roles. Nonetheless, some community pharmacists became more deeply involved in providing expanded pharmaceutical care services. They documented their care for patients in computerized patient profiles to improve quality of care and to provide evidence of outcomes for compensation for pharmaceutical care services. In a project begun in 1997 in Asheville, North Carolina, for instance, community pharmacists successfully worked with patients with such chronic health problems as diabetes, hypertension, high cholesterol, and asthma, and reported positive clinical and cost-saving outcomes (Brock, Casper, Green, & Pedersen, 2006; Kreling et al., 2006; Smith, Bates, Bodenheimer, & Cleary, 2010). In another case, an owner of an independent drugstore in Augusta, Georgia, explained: "We are not just going to dispense your drugs ... We are going to partner with you to improve your health as well" (Abelson & Singer, 2010, p. A1).

In the first decade of the 21st century, pharmacists along with physicians and other health professionals have also been engaged in determining their roles in the medical home model. As providers of pharmaceutical care, pharmacists had already began to articulate their roles in incorporating medication therapy management services into institutional and community settings in a major way as part of the context of the Medicare Modernization Act of 2003 and Medicare Part D (McGivney et al., 2007). In Chapter 3 of this text, details about the movement away from pharmaceutical care to medication therapy management and its potential for incorporation in medical home models of primary care in the future are discussed.

A number of demonstration projects have also documented the value of including pharmacists in the interdisciplinary care team working in the primary care medical home. A project in six Minnesota ambulatory clinics incorporated employed pharmacists who collaborated with primary care practitioners, resolved patient drug therapy problems, and contributed to reduced costs (Hepler, 2010; Smith et al., 2010).

Pharmacists, physicians, and public health professionals have argued for the place of pharmacists in the medical home of the future because of their expertise in providing services, including comprehensive therapy reviews of prescribed medications and OTC or herbal products, design of adherence programs for patients with asthma, diabetes, or hypertension, personal medication care plans (lists that include actions that patients can take to keep track of managing their own medications), and recommendations for therapies that are cost-effective (American Pharmacists Association & National Association of Chain Drug Stores, 2008; Smith et al., 2010). The 2010 PPACA has embraced the notion of an expanded patient care role for pharmacists in the medical home with the possibility that community pharmacists may obtain funding for new demonstration projects (Traynor, 2010). Finally, pharmacy leaders have been involved in the Patient-Centered Primary Care Collaborative publication of the task force report, *The Patient-Centered Medical Home (PCMH): Integrating Comprehensive Medication Management to Optimize Patient Outcomes*, which supports the pharmacist role. The collaborative involves various healthcare groups, including government officials, insurance companies, and health professionals, who are committed to working together to improve the quality of health care. The report is the third in a series of reports produced by the collaborative that emphasized the need for payment reform for medication management and that "was developed to provide a framework for integrating medication management in the PCMH (patient-centered medical home) as part of the practice redesign that needs to occur when individual and group practices transform into the PCMH" (Patient-Centered Primary Care Collaborative, 2010, p. 4).

Pharmacy has also seen change in the arrival of the retail clinic, which has appeared in chain pharmacies, grocery stores, and superstores that also include pharmacies. These clinics usually offer walk-in visits for convenient, lower-cost care for such acute health problems as sore throat or ear infection symptoms. Staffed by such primary care health professionals as nurse practitioners, there has generally been no formal teaming with pharmacy staff. Community-based pharmacies have also begun to offer vaccinations given by pharmacists who have acquired certification. These innovations offered possibilities for expansion of pharmaceutical care but also raised issues about constructive coordination of health care and confusion over commercial and professional healthcare roles (Farley, Devine, & Hadsall, 2007; Martin, 2010; Pollack, Gidengil, & Mehrotra, 2010).

Pharmacy education in the 21st century has emphasized the importance of providing patient-centered population-based care for patients, especially in the provision of medication therapy management for diseases, whether infectious or chronic. A commitment to being a part of disease prevention and wellness promotion efforts emphasized by their colleagues in other health professions and in public health has been stressed. The pharmacy profession has emphasized the importance of pharmacists playing a greater role in the provision of primary care (especially within the perspective of recent health reform within the PPACA) noting that pharmacists not only dispense medications in community pharmacies but they also play diagnostic, urgent care, and preventive roles. The increasing need for pharmacy to play a greater role in caring for patients has been displayed in such arenas as *Healthy People 2020*, a policy statement from the *American Public Health Association* and a webinar from the *Centers for Disease Control and Prevention*, especially emphasizing the importance of collaborative care on healthcare teams. Changes have been made in pharmacy curricula that have included the addition of public health components in required and elective coursework (APHA, 2014; CDC, 2014; King & Egras, 2015; Offiong, 2011).In particular, pharmacy's role has been noted as essential in improving population health equity. Recent research has noted the need for improved access to community pharmacies in minority neighborhoods and Medically Underserved Areas, which are basically "pharmacy deserts." Recommendations include that pharmacies be placed within community health centers and underserved neighborhoods, as well financial incentives, such as publicly funded programs similar to those that work to improve access to better food (Qato, Daviglus, Wilder, Lee, Qato, & Lambert, 2014).

HEALTH AND SICKNESS PATTERNS IN HISTORICAL PERSPECTIVE

Definitions of Health and Disease

Elliot Mishler notes that broader definitions of health "are neither obsolete, nor of historical and esoteric interest only," (1981, p. 3) when he refers to the World Health Organization's definition of health as a "state of complete physical, mental, and social well-being and not merely the absence of disease or infirmity" (Mishler, 1981, p. 3). In addition, Charles Rosenberg argues for not thinking in narrow constructs:

> Disease is at once a biological event, a generation-specific repertoire of verbal constructs reflecting medicine's intellectual and institutional history, an occasion of and potential legitimization for public policy, an aspect of social role and individual—intrapsychic—identity, a sanction for cultural values, and a structuring element in doctor and patient interactions. In some ways disease does not exist until we have agreed that it does, by perceiving, naming, and responding to it (1992, p. xiii).

In studying healthcare delivery in the United States, how we perceive, name, and respond to health and disease and what we make the primary focus of the healthcare system are major focuses of concern (Brandt, 1997; Tesh, 1988).

Each year the mass media reports statistics from government and research institutions about health and disease levels, mortality and life expectancy, and causes of death both globally and within the United States. Historians have also sought, within biomedical, cultural, social, economic, and political contexts, to account for increases in life expectancy, declines in mortality rates, and changes in causes of death from acute and infectious diseases to, more recently, chronic illnesses.

Health Demographics and Causes of Death

Native Americans and European settlers in the 1600s and 1700s confronted malnutrition daily, making them susceptible to endemic and epidemic infectious illnesses. Such endemic illnesses as dysentery, malaria, and respiratory infections, with occasional epidemics, including smallpox and yellow fever, were prevalent in the 18th century. As the 19th century progressed, people became more concerned with illnesses related to the increasing population that lived in rapidly urbanizing and industrializing cities. Deaths continued to result from dysentery and respiratory infections, but also increasingly from cholera, scarlet fever, whooping cough, measles, diphtheria, smallpox, and—above all—tuberculosis. Improvements in public health could be noted as the 19th century ended. In particular, death rates declined—especially infant mortality rates—and life expectancy increased, as noted earlier in this chapter (Leavitt & Numbers, 1997).

Causes of Death and Disease

In 1900, the leading causes of death were infectious diseases, both epidemic and endemic diseases, including influenza and pneumonia, tuberculosis, gastritis, enteritis, diphtheria, measles, scarlet fever, and whooping cough. Some chronic diseases (noncommunicable diseases or NCDs) such as heart and cerebrovascular disease and cancer also were among the top 10 causes of death in the United States (Lerner & Anderson, 1963, p. 16). The 10 leading causes of death reported in the United States for 2012 were heart disease, cancer, chronic lower respiratory diseases, cerebrovascular diseases, unintentional injuries, Alzheimer's disease, diabetes mellitus, influenza and pneumonia, kidney disease, and suicide (CDC, 2015). In breaking down this list, approximately 87% of deaths in the United States are attributable to the incidence of NCDs with larger numbers of deaths among communities of color (WHO, 2011). This percentage of deaths compares with the figure of 68% of the world's 56 million deaths reported in 2012 as noted in the World Health Organization's 2014 Global Status Report on NCDs (WHO, 2014).

Factors Explaining Health Demographic Change

To understand the meaning of statistics that report declines in infant mortality rates, increases in life expectancy, declines in communicable diseases, and increases in chronic, degenerative illnesses, historians have analyzed the possible factors that account for the changing numbers and have explored public authorities' explanations for these changes. Three factors are generally cited as explanations, which include: (1) changes in standard of living or lifestyle, including improvements in personal hygiene, diet, nutrition, and housing; (2) advances in public health measures; and (3) progress in medical practice, including therapeutic interventions in the treatment of patients.

In examining the evidence, healthcare historians have found that changes in public health measures and lifestyle contributed more to health improvements than therapeutic interventions by physicians in the 19th and early 20th centuries (Leavitt & Numbers, 1997; Rothstein, 1996b). In the latter half of the 19th century, cities recognized the importance of connecting the city's environment and its people's health, including improved sanitation, water supply and delivery, and refuse collection and waste removal (Melosi, 2000). In 1865, New York commissioned a report on public health and later formed a board of health with responsibilities to include enforcing sanitary regulations and controlling epidemics. By 1912, as David Rosner has noted, "garbage collection, meat and milk inspections, pure water, and sewerage systems had been installed throughout the city. Dead animals were now regularly picked up off the streets, and fire safety codes augmented stricter enforcement of housing laws" (1995, p. 15). The Department of Health, in its annual report, attributed "over the course of just forty-five years ... a decrease of over 50 percent" in the death rate to public sanitation measures (1995, p. 15).

William Rothstein emphasizes the importance of educating the public about specific personal behaviors related to standards of living and public health. Until well into the 20th century, millions of Americans drank from metal drinking cups kept next to fountains for all to use, did not sterilize bottles or take other measures necessary for hygienic feeding of infants, let their children sleep in the same bed and play with siblings with contagious diseases like diphtheria and scarlet fever, purchased unrefrigerated and bacteria-laden milk and meat, used polluted wells and water supplies without boiling the water, and took baths in bathtubs after others had used the same water. These and many other similar behaviors declined significantly as the public became more educated about personal hygiene (1996b, pp. 77,78).

At the same time, public health campaigns in the late 19th and early 20th centuries against specific diseases must be seen within the context of how health professionals, public officials, and the general public felt that disease and outsiders threatened the civic order. They often linked epidemics of infectious diseases—including smallpox, tuberculosis, bubonic plague, typhoid, and polio—to new immigrant populations. Some public health efforts focused on isolation, quarantine, and destruction of housing, often using violence to implement these policies. On the other hand, founding of ethnic and religious hospitals; the establishment of visiting and public health nursing, neighborhood clinics, and settlement houses; health advocacy programs to foster individual efforts to improve domestic hygiene; and struggles for effective public health legislation and enforcement were all examples of efforts to assist immigrants in preventive health measures, in improving the living conditions in urban housing, and in occupational safety and health on the job (Kraut, 1994; Leavitt, 1996; Ott, 1996; Tomes, 1998).

Healthcare historians have also discussed the role of clinical medicine and therapeutic or technological intervention in contributing to the decline of mortality rates in infectious diseases at the turn of the 20th century. Very few physician efforts, especially those who employed "heroic" measures, were helpful to patients. Such 19th-century discoveries as anesthesia and X-rays were very important, but general practice physicians could often use these technological improvements in ways that caused more harm than good. The most striking example of therapeutic intervention success did not occur until the mid-20th century with the introduction of antibiotics. Historian John Parascandola has pointed out that "within a decade after penicillin was first made freely available for civilian use in the United States in 1945, antibiotics had become the most important class of drugs in the treatment of infectious disease. In 1948, antibiotics prescriptions accounted for only 1.5% of the total number written in the United States; by 1952, that figure had risen to 13.7%" (1997, pp. 108,109). Parascandola also cited a Federal Trade Commission report from 1958, which indicated a decrease of 56.4% in the total number of deaths from 1945 to 1955 for eight major diseases responsive to antibiotic therapy, versus a decline of only 8.1% for all other causes of death. In the 21st century, major public health efforts have continued to focus on when and how to implement programs using appropriate antibiotic therapy and on how to educate the public about the misuse and overuse of antibiotics, stressing the limitations of wonder drugs (Parascandola, 1997, pp. 109, 110).

Successful public health measures have often been cited to help explain some decline in infant death rates in various U.S. cities in the late 20th century. These measures included better access to stable housing and prenatal care for low-income pregnant women. Conversely, when funding decreased in a community for various programs aimed at healthy mothers and babies, infant mortality rates rose (Steinhauer, 2000). Recommendations from health professionals across disciplines for improving children's health in the beginning of the 21st century continue to include such public health measures as community and school-based clinics and education programs on diverse health populations that are public-health based and present in health professional curricula (Markel & Golden, 2004).

Chronic Illness or Noncommunicable Diseases (NCDs) and Infectious Diseases in the 20th and 21st Centuries

Since the 1920s, government agencies, biomedical health researchers, and health professionals have recognized that chronic disease must be a health policy priority in the United States (Fox, 1988). In discussing how the United States should address the fact that chronic illnesses afflict close to half the population, costing nearly $470 billion in 1990, a number of issues related to public health measures, environmental factors, standard of living, lifestyle, and therapeutic interventions are raised. Medical researchers cite such "diseases of affluence" as sedentary lifestyle, poor diet, smoking, and alcohol abuse as major causes of chronic illness (Knox, 1996, p. A11). Other researchers documented concerns about the lack of good management of chronic disease and people's inability to receive the help they need to live on an everyday basis with chronic health conditions. Dr. Halstad R. Holman, director of an arthritis center at Stanford University, noted, "Our health care system—its structure, practices, education, and even research agendas—was developed for acute disease. We have a profound mismatch between our entire health care system and what it's structured to do and what we need it to do" (Knox, 1996, p. A11). In the early 21st century, the United States faced a crisis in treating chronic illness far more costly than in 1990, with three fourths of the more than $2 trillion spent on health care directed toward the treatment of chronic illnesses, especially those connected to worsening health habits. Thus, the emphasis has been put on health promotion and disease prevention regardless of whether the provision of preventive care is more or less expensive (Goetzl, 2009, p. 41; Maciosek, Coffield, Edwards, Flottemesch, Goodman, & Solberg, 2006).

There are many efforts in the United States to address the problems of NCDs including efforts to address the cancer burden. As an example, the Community Preventive Services Taskforce has noted the adoption of various policies that provide services and programs, including those that address excessive sun exposure and alcohol consumption, promote exercise activities, reduce tobacco consumption, and increase access to preventive services, as part of regular medical care (Community Preventive Services Task Force, 2015). The program *Healthy People 2020* has also focused attention on a number of NCDs, reporting success in reducing children's exposure to secondhand smoke, meeting targets for adults practicing aerobic and muscle-strengthening activities, and improvement in hypertension control and colorectal cancer screening (Healthy People 2020: A Report Card on the Health of the Nation, 2014).

In the 20th and 21st centuries, concerns about infectious diseases continued. Tuberculosis became endemic in many highly industrialized urban areas until the discovery of antibiotics and the use of multidrug therapy and polio outbreaks occurred until vaccination became widely practiced beginning in the mid-1950s. In the late 20th and early 21st centuries, Americans became concerned about epidemics and pandemics in the forms of emerging and reemerging diseases. In terms of reemerging diseases, the appearance of tuberculosis, the arrival of West Nile virus, and alarming new cases of measles in the United States occurred due to such causes as decreased funding in public health infrastructure, changes in the environment and not immunizing enough individuals. In the case of decreased use of immunizations, factors include people not realizing or getting vaccinations on time and those refusing vaccinations based on personal, religious, or philosophical reasons. With increasing globalization as well as continuing problems in sufficient funding for public health infrastructure, Americans have also experienced newly emerging diseases, including HIV/AIDS and Severe Acute Respiratory Syndrome (SARS). Most recently Ebola, Middle East Respiratory Syndrome (MERS), or the Zika virus traveling from other parts of the globe to the United States have generated concerns (Blinder, 2016; CDC, 2016; Sands, Mundaca-Shah, & Dzau, 2016).

HEALTH POLICY OVERVIEW: 1900–1950

New Legislation in the Early 20th Century

The major hallmark of 20th-century health care was the increased role of government policy making at the local, state, and especially the federal level. During the first two decades of the 20th century, the federal government assumed a more vigorous role in public health, symbolized by its renaming of the Marine Hospital Service as the U.S. Public Health Service in 1912. Partially as a consequence of muckraking journalists' exposure of dangerous practices in the food and drug industries, the U.S. Congress enacted the Pure Food and Drug Act in 1906 and then significantly strengthened its oversight of this industry with more comprehensive legislation under the 1938 Federal Food, Drug, and Cosmetic Act. In addressing the plight of America's poor children, many of whom lacked good nutrition and housing and were forced to work in dangerous conditions, Congress established the Children's Bureau in 1912. This legislation was followed in 1921 by the Sheppard-Towner Maternity and Infancy Act, which provided federal funding to support children's health clinics until 1929. In 1930, the National Institutes of Health and the Veterans Administration were established and the National Cancer Act in 1937 helped launch biomedical research (King, 1993; Patterson, 1987; Temin, 1980).

Public and Private Health Insurance

Twentieth-century changes in health insurance can be traced back to at least 1798, when government hospitals were established in some coastal cities to provide care for merchant seamen. In the 19th century, small numbers of Americans obtained some form of insurance against sickness primarily by gaining income protection through such groups as trade unions, fraternal organizations, or their employers (Numbers, 1997, p. 277). Some purchased protection against sickness from commercial insurers. Generally, only mining and lumber companies provided actual medical benefits.

In the early 20th century, progressive reformers and labor unions began to talk about some form of government-sponsored health insurance. In 1914, workers' compensation or compulsory sickness insurance programs appeared. Operating on a state level, they generally provided cash payments for injuries or disease related to the workplace. In later decades, payments were made for medical expenses and death benefits. Employers usually purchased these programs from commercial insurers. In 1912, the American Association for Labor Legislation's Committee on Social Insurance put forward a model bill for state legislatures to consider. Until 1917, many medical leaders and associations expressed support for compulsory health insurance efforts. Opposition developed from physicians concerned about seeing their incomes decrease rather than increase. During World War I, many began to perceive social insurance proposals as un-American since the German enemy had employed compulsory insurance for industrial workers since 1883 (Numbers, 1997, pp. 269–271; Starr, 1982; Stevens, 1971).

Following the significant drops in physician and hospital income that occurred in the wake of the Great Depression, hospitals reconsidered insurance plans. In 1929, Baylor University Hospital enrolled public school teachers in a plan covering hospital costs. The American Hospital Association in 1939 approved Blue Cross insurance to cover costs of care in whichever hospital patients chose to enter. In the same year, the Blue Shield insurance plan was first approved by the California Medical Association to help cover fees physicians charged for their services. These insurance programs, which served as a third-party payment system, presented an attractive alternative to the tradition of patients paying health practitioners directly for health services. The AMA and medical associations such as the State Medical Society of Wisconsin expressed support for implementation of voluntary private insurance plans, rather than "wait for a state controlled compulsory plan" (Numbers, 1997, p. 274).

During the Franklin D. Roosevelt administration, Congress considered the Murray-Wagner-Dingall bill, which proposed to provide health care for the poor primarily through federal grants given to the states. Ultimately, this national health effort was defeated (Numbers, 1997). Private insurance, though greatly fragmented, rapidly expanded in the next two decades with some form of health insurance held by 51% of the civilian population by 1951 and 737 health insurance companies selling some kind of insurance by 1959 (Richmond & Fein, 2005; Stevens, 2008, p. 467).

POST–WORLD WAR II HEALTHCARE CHANGES

In the second half of the 20th century, President Harry Truman spoke forcefully in favor of national health insurance that offered protection to all Americans (Poen, 1979). Nonetheless, legislative proposals failed largely because they evoked strong opposition from the AMA. As part of its effort to defeat the Truman proposal, the AMA undertook a $4.5 million national education campaign, warning that "national health insurance would lead to federal control of health care" (Johnson & Broder, 1996, p. 66). In the Cold War era, which was characterized by a virulent anticommunism movement, the AMA's public relations campaign equated national health insurance with socialized medicine.

In the 1950s, with support from the federal government through tax-deductibility rulings, employers and labor unions increasingly offered U.S. workers healthcare plans as part of their benefits programs. In the 1960s, the federal government established two governmental purchasing programs—Medicare and Medicaid. While a push for these programs began under the John F. Kennedy administration, President Lyndon Johnson was successful in achieving their passage with his landslide victory in the 1964 presidential election and his leadership in advancing Great Society legislation through Congress. Medicare was initially designed in two parts: Part A for hospital insurance coverage and Part B for medical care insurance including physicians and various medical services. In 1972, Medicare insurance was extended to those of any age with proven disabilities or to those with end-stage renal disease to pay for dialysis or transplant costs. Medicaid was established as a joint federal and state program to provide health care for the low-income elderly and other categories of people, including the disabled and families with children (Patel & Rushefsky, 1995; Stevens, 2008, p. 471). See Chapter 18.

Despite these incremental reforms, healthcare costs continued to rise in the 1960s and 1970s, and problems of access to services for the uninsured increased. Once again raising the possibility of a comprehensive national health policy, Senator Edward Kennedy and President Jimmy Carter launched unsuccessful attempts in the 1970s to pass such legislation as Kennedy's Health Security Act, which was designed to provide quality health care for all Americans at affordable prices (Kennedy, 1972). By 1980, the mostly private model of a healthcare system best described how most Americans were covered—that is, by private insurance programs purchased through plans offered by their employers. Coverage of the healthcare costs of only a few needy groups (e.g., veterans, the elderly, and some disabled or low-income families and individuals) was provided through government-sponsored public insurance programs (Patel & Rushefsky, 1995, p. 25).

Prepaid Health Care, Health Maintenance Organizations, and Managed Care

While Congress did not adopt broad health insurance coverage, in 1973 it passed the Health HMO Act. This legislation represented a form of prepaid health coverage. Prepaid health plans were first introduced in the United States in isolated rural areas where workers needed health care in the 19th century. In the building of the Grand Coulee Dam in 1938, the highly successful Kaiser Permanente Medical Care Program initially offered healthcare services to workers employed by Henry F. Kaiser. The prepaid plan expanded its provision of comprehensive health care to workers in his steel mills and shipyards, and eventually to the general public on the West Coast and to a lesser extent in the Midwest. Unlike their strong opposition to compulsory health insurance legislative initiatives, medical organizations did not oppose Kaiser's effort because individual physicians involved in the programs economically benefited. The 1973 HMO Act required every employer with more than 25 employees that offered a health plan to include at least one HMO plan providing comprehensive medical care for a fixed fee to its enrollees. A companion bill "requiring employers to provide a basic minimum package of benefits to all their employees" (Johnson & Broder, 1996, p. 67) failed, with the AMA and the health insurance industry lobbying against the bill (Hendricks, 1993).

Rapid growth of HMOs did not become pronounced until the 1990s and a backlash against the movement developed with the public expressing concerns about access to health care and payment for services provided if a patient became very ill. In 1995, HMOs covered nearly 60 million individuals, and the less structured preferred provider organizations covered an additional 91 million people, including Medicare and Medicaid recipients (Anders, 1996; Blendon et al., 1998; Peterson, 1997). By 1998, 77 million Americans were enrolled in an HMO, and the number of Americans in some form of managed care had reached 135.37 million in 2010 (Managed Care On-Line, 2010; U.S. DHHS, 1999); see Chapter 17.

Renewed Efforts for National Health Insurance

As the 20th century ended, the American public experienced significant social, economic, and political changes that affected both the U.S. healthcare system and the delivery of healthcare services. In 1991, the Democratic presidential candidate, Bill Clinton, made health care a major issue in his presidential campaign, offering a step-by-step plan to achieve healthcare coverage for all Americans through his health security plan. Despite the AMA dropping its opposition to national health insurance, in 1994, Congress defeated proposals for implementing national health insurance, including President Clinton's health security plan, which was successfully lobbied against by the pharmaceutical, hospital, and health insurance industries (Hacker, 1997; White House Domestic Policy Council, 1993).

Incremental Policy Proposals

Later in the decade, however, other pieces of incremental health legislation affecting Americans' access to health care were passed. In 1996, the Health Insurance Portability and Accountability Act specified in its Title I section that employers or insurers of new employees could impose a waiting period of no more than 12 months before covering them under the employer's health plan. Title II of the Health Insurance Portability and Accountability Act addressed issues of healthcare fraud and abuse and set standards for using and disseminating health information (leading to

EHRss) to increase efficiency in the healthcare system. Congress also passed the Children's Health Insurance Program as part of the Balanced Budget Act of 1997 with the intent that it would provide health insurance for at least half of the 11 million children who lacked such coverage. In 2009, the Children's Health Insurance Program was extended by Congress with the passage of the Children's Health Insurance Program Reauthorization Act (Atchinson & Fox, 1997; Castellblanch, 1996; Fairbrother, Carle, Cassedy, & Newacheck, 2010; Goldstein, 1999; Pear, 1997). By 2013, the Centers for Medicare and Medicaid Services announced that 8.1 million children in the U.S. were enrolled in the program. In 2015, Congress and President Barack Obama approved the extension for 2 years of children's health insurance through passage of the Medicare Access and CHIP Reauthorization Act. The legislation also provided funding for additional programs, including the Childhood Obesity Demonstration Project and the Maternal, Infant, and Early Childhood Home Visiting Program (National Conference of State Legislatures, 2015).

At the beginning of the 21st century, Congress considered several bills to reduce drug prices and to expand Medicare coverage by including prescription medications. The *Medicare Prescription Drug, Improvement, and Modernization Act*, the largest revision of Medicare in its 38-year history, was passed in 2003. Its most important provision was Medicare Part D, which provided a voluntary prescription drug benefit program through private insurance plans. Medicare beneficiaries could choose to enroll in the program that took effect on January 1, 2006. Many reported confusion in trying to choose a program and how to join, especially in regard to the Medicare Advantage plans offered. Additional criticisms included a lack of ability for the government to negotiate prescription drug prices, and especially the temporary gap in coverage that occurred, limiting the coverage of drugs in the program. The gap in coverage became widely known as the "doughnut hole."

By June 2006, 22.5 million senior American citizens had enrolled in the program and research soon showed that there was an 18.4% reduction in spending on medications out of pocket and a 12.8% increase in drug utilization as a result of the legislation (Lichtenberg & Sun, 2007; Pear, 2006; Schneeweiss et al., 2009; Yin et al., 2008); see Chapter 18. By 2013 there were over 39 million Americans enrolled in Medicare Part D. The PPACA included aspects that reformed Medicare and this included alleviation of some of the higher cost problems during the "doughnut hole" time period with the provision that the "hole" would be closed by 2020. After 10 years of the program being in place and now considered by many health policy planners as "firmly established," concerns continue, especially in relation to the benefit's design and utilization management strategies. Many elderly recipients do not review the plan they have chosen in order to opt for a more cost-efficient and better quality plan during the annual opportunity period because of the difficulties of how to enroll in new plans. Cost issues remained with a spending growth estimation of $88.6 billion in 2015 from the initial costs of $44.3 billion in 2006 (Hoadley, Cubanski, & Neuman, 2015; Kaiser Family Foundation, 2015).

THE PATIENT PROTECTION AND AFFORDABLE CARE ACT (PPACA)

Despite its outstanding achievements, a majority of Americans have repeatedly reported dissatisfaction with the U.S. healthcare system primarily on the basis of problems with access, cost, and quality issues and "have favored addressing problems in the healthcare system since at least the mid-1980s" (Brodie, Altman, Deane, Buscho, & Hamel, 2010, p. 1127). They have thought about healthcare reform in the context of how it affects the country as a whole and how it relates to their own lives and futures. Many have expressed serious concerns about the number of uninsured or underinsured Americans and called for comprehensive reform of the U.S. healthcare system that would extend health coverage to all Americans. Others have theoretically endorsed universal health insurance yet feared the loss of their own private insurance if a comprehensive plan was established to include those without any health insurance. Many Americans have expressed a lack of trust in the U.S. healthcare system to deliver safe and high-quality care. They have advocated for more primary and preventive care, with transitional and longer-term management of chronic conditions that allow for patient participation in decision making and in personal adherence and management of their health problems (Blendon & Benson, 2009; Davidson, 2010; Hacker, 2008; Johnson & Johnson, 2010; Sered & Fernandopulle, 2005).

Following the 2009 presidential election year where healthcare system reform was a major campaign issue, the U.S. Congress began consideration of new health legislation. With constant and often trenchant media coverage and intense partisan and sometimes volatile conflict among Democrats and Republicans, the PPACA, designed to provide an additional 32 million Americans with some form of health insurance by 2018 (with the establishment of competitive health insurance exchanges in 2014), was enacted into law in March 2010 (Krugman, 2010; Mackey, 2010). President Obama said that the legislation embodied "the core principle that everybody should have some basic security when it comes to their health care" (The White House, 2010, p.1). This new reform represented incremental health reform. The U.S. Congress rejected proposals that would provide universal health coverage such as in many western and northern European countries. It also did not adopt a plan that argued for a low-cost alternative to private health insurance—similar to the existing Medicare model—as a form of national insurance. The PPACA did not provide comprehensive change in the fundamental structure of the U.S. healthcare system. It is not a single-payer system.

The provisions of the PPACA include four key aspects:

- Mandating that Americans obtain at least a minimum amount of health insurance or pay a penalty; health insurance could be obtained with insurance companies through employers or purchased individually, through Medicaid, or for those with incomes too low to purchase insurance through designated federal subsidies.
- Making changes in health insurance performance activities that included such provisions as stopping the practice of imposing refusal to cover, or charging more for, preexisting conditions; ensuring that current insurance plans may be renewed; providing coverage beyond childhood to the age of 26; requiring that insurers justify premium increases of 10% or more before rates can take effect; expansion of designated preventive services.
- Establishing insurance marketplaces or exchanges on a state basis where individuals and small-businesses could purchase health insurance plans. These exchanges were made available through online government websites. States can run the exchanges and if they don't wish to, instead the federal government may run them.
- Expanding the Medicaid program in order to provide the opportunity for more Americans to obtain health insurance.

Other kinds of reforms incorporated in the PPACA were investment in education and training for an expanded health workforce, and the support of pilot projects to reform Medicare and Medicaid healthcare delivery and payment. Implemented through the secretary of Health and Human Services office, various projects also included the fostering of the patient-centered medical home model and community health centers, and the support of expanding EHRs (Collins, Rasmussen, Doty, & Beutel, 2015; HealthCare.gov, 2016; Iglehart, 2010; Kaiser Family Foundation, 2015; Oberlander, 2010). The PPACA reinforced and expanded previous federal government commitments to public health disease and illness prevention programs as well as maintained a focus on pursuing antibiotic resistance and health-associated infection prevention programs (Prevention and Public Health Fund, 2016).

Despite significant ongoing opposition to the PPACA and major problems in inaugurating the Healthcare.gov online website since 2010, the numbers of insured Americans has significantly increased. For instance, the uninsured rate in the United States in 2014 was 12.1% with early data for 2015 indicating that the uninsured rate as the decade began would be 10.7%, which are the lowest rates seen in at least two decades. Persons who gained coverage have included Americans who are in poor and low-income families and who are among various racial and ethnic groups. Studies indicate that the greatest decreases in uninsured rates are among Hispanic and Black Americans. For those who still remain uninsured, many live in states with the least generous Medicaid eligibility requirements, are unaware they are eligible for coverage under the PPACA, find they simply cannot afford any coverage, or are undocumented immigrants. With the third enrollment period for the PPACA ending January 31, 2016, expectations were that over 11 million people would enroll in PPACA health insurance, (Kaiser Family Foundation, 2015; Pear, 2016).

Given the partisan conflict that occurred during the debate over the new legislation, public officials and individuals often supported by various interest groups instituted lawsuits within the courts to fight implementation of the new healthcare law within and beyond the first 6 months after the act's passage. In many ways, the lawsuits reflect the ongoing difficulty in balancing the interests of the individual and those of the community and the concerns of the federal versus state governments, as well as growing efforts to influence negative attitudes against the role of government in American life. Three cases went to the U.S. Supreme Court and two of them had broader meanings. In the 2012 case, *National Federation of Independent Business v. Sebelius,* the PPACA was found to be constitutional with a 5-4 majority vote. The case revolved around several issues, most important of which were whether Congress could enact an individual insurance mandate and if they could not provide Medicaid funding to states that did not wish to expand Medicaid funding. The second case in 2014, *King v. Burwell,* upheld that subsidies to help individuals or small businesses purchase insurance could be obtained through federal or state operated health insurance exchanges or marketplaces. The U.S. Congress also filed a lawsuit against the PPACA, and the body has initiated 62 efforts to repeal the law with 61 of these not going to President Barack Obama for his approval. In January 2016, with Republican Party majorities in the House and Senate, a bill for repeal went to the President and was vetoed. In the 2016 presidential election campaign, some candidates continue to promise to repeal the PPACA while others wish to extend its benefits or to establish full universal health insurance. The debate about whether health care is a human right or a privilege in the United States will continue (Harris, 2016; Jost, 2015; Rosenbaum & Westmoreland, 2012).

Obviously there are ongoing issues that must be addressed in the delivery of health care to Americans and in the implementation of the PPACA. The chief of these is the affordability of the new health plans in terms of premiums, co-pays, and other costs. What will be the responses of private health insurance companies and state and government to this problem (Islam, 2015)?

While there is continued opposition to the PPACA, others have hailed the new law for its potential to make health care available to more Americans, more affordable, and higher in quality (Sack, 2010a, 2010b). In 2010, Jonathan Oberlander, a professor of social medicine, health policy, and management, noted that "[E]ven with all its shortcomings, the Patient Protection and Affordable Care Act is a great leap forward for the American health care system" (Oberlander, 2010, p. 1116). In a "Health Policy Report" published in the *New England Journal of Medicine* in 2015, the authors argued that the enactment of the PPACA "may constitute the most important event of the Obama presidency and could fundamentally affect the future of health care in the United States" (Blumenthal, Abrams, & Nuzum, 2015, p. 2451).

CONCLUSION

In looking at healthcare changes over time, the people of the United States have seen decreases in mortality rates and increases in life expectancy and changes in other health rankings that show improvements and setbacks in access, costs, and quality of healthcare delivery for American citizens. We have also seen that factors accounting for positive and negative changes have involved public policy decisions that have affected public health, housing, diet, hygiene, therapeutic and technologic interventions. Chronic or noncommunicable diseases have become more prevalent, and new and reemerging infectious diseases have become more worrisome in the 21st century than many experts expected following the discovery of miracle drugs in the mid-20th century.

The U.S. government has attempted to improve access, cost, and quality of health care for American citizens chiefly through implementing incremental health reforms (Vladek, 2003). What will be the long-term effects of the most recent efforts at health reform? Will recent healthcare reforms decrease disparities in care among different groups of Americans? Will health outcomes for most Americans improve? The United States faces very hard economic and social choices related to healthcare delivery in national and global contexts. The need for humane health care will increase significantly as the 21st century advances.

QUESTIONS FOR FURTHER DISCUSSION

1. How will the conflict between the entrepreneurial role of health delivery organizations and the health professional's responsibility to serve the community be resolved in the future?
2. Lifestyle improvements, public health measures, and therapeutic interventions all affect health and disease patterns. How much money and effort should be devoted to these areas to address the health problems of Americans? What should the priorities be among the three areas? What roles should private and public institutions play? What roles should health professionals play?
3. To what degree is the healthcare system "in crisis" in the 21st century and how has the PPACA attempted to address the "crisis" concerns?

KEY TOPICS AND TERMS

Blue Cross
Blue Shield
Charitable hospitals
Children's Health Insurance Program (CHIP)
Children's Health Insurance Program Reauthorization Act
Chronic diseases or noncommunicable diseases (NCDs)
Community health centers
Dispensary
Flexner Report
Health Insurance Portability and Accountability Act (HIPAA)
Health Maintenance Organization Act
Heroic medical therapy
Hill-Burton Act (National Hospital Survey and Construction Act)
Humoralism
Incremental healthcare reform
Infectious diseases
King v. Burwell (2015)
Medicaid
Medical home
Medicare
Medicare Part D
Medicare Prescription Drug, Improvement, and Modernization Act
Medication therapy management (MTM)
National Federation of Independent Business v. Sebelius (2012)
Orthodox physicians
Patent medicines
Patient-centered care

Patient Protection and Affordable Care Act (PPACA)
Pharmaceutical care
Quackery
Sectarians
Self-dosing
Social healers

REFERENCES

2914–2015 Annual Report to Congress, Federal Agencies and Stakeholders, including a Special Update on Recommendations to Prevent Cancers (2015). *Community Preventive Services Taskforce 2015, 8*. Retrieved from http://www.thecommunityguide.org/annualreport/2015-congress-report-full.pdf

Abelson, R., & Singer, N. (2010, August 14). In health shift, more patients get pharmacist's appointment. *The New York Times, A1*, A11.

Agency for Healthcare Research and Quality. (2011, October). *Fact sheet: AHRQ projects to prevent healthcare-associated infections, fiscal year 2010*. Retrieved from http://www.ahrq.gov/research/findings/factsheets/errors-safety/haify10/index.html

Agency for Healthcare Research and Quality. (2015, June). *2014 National Healthcare Quality & Disparities Report*. Retrieved from http://www.ahrq.gov/research/findings/nhqrdr/nhqdr14/index.html

American Hospital Association and the Institute for Family-Centered Care Resource Guide. (2006). *Strategies for leadership: Patient and family-centered care*. Washington, DC: American Hospital Association and the Institute for Family-Centered Care. Retrieved from http://www.aha.org/aha/issues/Quality-and-Patient-Safety/strategies-patientcentered.html

American Pharmaceutical Association. (1922). Code of ethics of the American Pharmaceutical Association. *Journal of the American Pharmaceutical Association, 11*(9), 728–729.

American Pharmaceutical Association. (1952). Code of ethics of the American Pharmaceutical Association. *Journal of the American Pharmaceutical Association, 13*(10), 721–723.

American Pharmacists Association. (1994). *Code of ethics for pharmacists*. Retrieved from http://www.pharmacist.com/AM/Template.cfm?Section=Search1&template=/CM/HTMLDisplay.cfm&ContentID=2903

American Pharmacists Association & National Association of Chain Drug Stores. (2008, March). *Medication therapy management in pharmacy practice: Core elements of an MTM service model*. Retrieved from http://www.pharmacist.com/AM/Template.cfm?Section=Home2&TEMPLATE=/CM/ContentDisplay.cfm&CONTENTID=15496

American Public Health Association. (2014). The role of the pharmacist in public health, policy number 200614, American Public Health Association policy statement database. Retrieved from http://www.apha.org/policies-and-advocacy/public-health-policy-statements/policy-database/2014/07/07/13/05/the-role-of-the-pharmacist-in-public-health.

Ammerman, R. T. (2015, June 3). Testimony to Senate Medicaid Committee. Every Child Succeeds.

Anders, G. (1996). *Health against wealth: HMOs and the breakdown of medical trust*. Boston, MA: Houghton Mifflin.

Apple, R. D. (1996). *Vitamania: Vitamins in American culture*. New Brunswick, NJ: Rutgers University Press.

Atchinson, B. K. & Fox, D. M. (1997). From the field: The politics of the Health Insurance Portability and Accountability Act. *Health Affairs, 16*(3), 146–150.

Banks, J., Marmot, M., Oldfield, Z., & Smith, J. P. (2006, May 3). Disease and disadvantage in the United States and in England. *Journal of the American Medical Association, 295*(17), 2037–2045.

Behforouz, H. L., Drain, P. K., & Rhatigan, J. J. (2014). Rethinking the social history. *New England Journal of Medicine, 371*(14), 1277.

Bell, J. E. (1996, May/June). Saving their assets: How to stop plunder at Blue Cross and other nonprofits. *The American Prospect, 26*, 60–66.

Berenson, R. A., Ginsburg, P. B., & May, J. H. (2006, December 5). Hospital-physician relations: Cooperation, competition, or separation? *Health Affairs, 26*(1) [Web exclusive], W31–W42.

Beresford, L. (2009). Medical mistakes, 10 years post-op: HM and renewed emphasis on patient safety grow in tandem. *The Hospitalist, 13*(11). Retrieved from http://www.the-hospitalist.org/details/article/423625/Medical_Mistakes_10_Years_Post-Op.html

Berwick, D. M. (2009, May). What 'patient-centered' should mean: Confessions of an extremist. *Health Affairs, 28*(4), w555–w565.

Blendon, R. J., & Benson, J. M. (2009, August 27). *New England Journal of Medicine, 361*(9), e13(1)–e13(4).

Blendon, R. J., Brodie, M., Benson, J. M., Altman, D. E., Levitt, L., Hoff, T., & Hugick, L. (1998, July/August). Understanding the managed care backlash. *Health Affairs, 17*(4), 80–94.

Blinder, A. (2016, January 17). In rural Alabama, a longtime mistrust of medicine fuels a tuberculosis outbreak. *New York Times*. Retrieved from http://www.nytimes.com/2016/01/18/us/in-rural-alabama-a-longtime-mistrust-of-medicine-fuels-a-tuberculosis-outbreak.html

Blue, A. V., Mitcham, M., Smith, T., Raymond, J., & Greenberg, R. (2010, August). Changing the future of health professions: Embedding interprofessional education within an academic center. *Academic Medicine*, (*85*)8, 1290–1295.

Blumenthal, D., Abrams, M., & Nuzum, R. (2015, June 18). The Affordable Care Act at 5 Years. *New England Journal of Medicine, 372*(25), 2451–2458.

Blumenthal, D., & Weissman, J. (2000). Trends: Selling teaching hospitals to investor-owned hospital chains: Three case studies. *Health Affairs, 19*, 158–166.

Bodenheimer, T., Chen, E., & Bennett, H. D. (2009, January/February). Confronting the growing burden of chronic disease: Can the U.S. health care workforce do the job? *Health Affairs, 28*(1), 64–74.

Bogdan, J. C. (1992). Childbirth in America, 1650–1990. In R. D. Apple (Ed.), *Women, health, and medicine in America: A historical handbook* (pp. 101–120). New Brunswick, NJ: Rutgers University Press.

Bogdanich, W. (2010, August 1). The mark of an overdose: After stroke scans, patients face serious health risks. *The New York Times*, A1, A12.

Bosk, C. L., Dixon-Woods, M., Goeschel, C. A., & Pronovost, P. J. (2009, August 8). Reality check for checklists. *The Lancet, 374* (9688), 444–445.

Boulis, A., Jacobs, J., & Veloski, J. J. (2001, October). Gender segregation by specialty during medical school. *Academic Medicine, 76*(10), S65–S67.

Bradley, E. H. & Taylor, L. A. (2013). *The American health careparadox: Why spending more is getting us less.* New York, NY: Public Affairs.

Brandt, A. M. (1997). The cigarette, risk, and American culture. In W. G. Rothstein (Ed.), *Readings in American health care: Current issues in socio-historical perspective* (pp. 138–150). Madison, WI: University of Wisconsin Press.

Brill, S. (2015). *America's bitter pill: Money, politics, backroom deals, and the fight to fix our broken healthcare system.* New York, NY: Random House.

Brock, K. A., Casper, K. A., Green, T. R., & Pedersen, C. A. (2006). Documentation of patient care services in a community pharmacy setting. *Journal of the American Pharmaceutical Association, 46*(3), 378–384.

Brodie, M., Altman, D., Deane, C., Buscho, S., & Hamel, E. (2010, June). Liking the pieces, not the package: Contradictions in public opinion during health reform. *Health Affairs, 29*(6), 1125–1130.

Buring, S. M., Bhusan, A., Brazeau, G., Conway, S., Hansen, L., & Westberg, S. (2009, August). Keys to successful implementation of interprofessional education: Learning location, faculty development, and curricular themes. *American Journal of Pharmaceutical Education, 73*(4), 1–11.

Burnham, J. C. (1982, March 19). American medicine's golden age: What happened to it? *Science, 245*, 1474–1479.

Byrd, W. M. & Clayton, L. A. (2000). *An American health dilemma: A medical history of African Americans and the problem of race, beginning to 1900* (Vol. 1). New York, NY: Routledge.

Cahill, S. (1997). The Wal-Mart of hospitals. *In These Times, 21*(8), 14–16.

Casalino, L. P., November, E. A., Berenson, R. A., & Pham, H. H. (2008, September/October). Hospital-physician relations: Two tracks and the decline of the voluntary medical staff model. *Health Affairs, 27*(5), 1305–1314.

Cassedy, J. H. (1991). *Medicine in America: A short history.* Baltimore, MD: Johns Hopkins University Press.

Castellblanch, R. (1996). Legislation for sale. *In These Times, 20*, 14–16.

Cayleff, S. E. (1987). *Wash and be healed: The water-cure movement and women's health.* Philadelphia, PA: Temple University Press.

Cayleff, S. E. (1992). Self-help and the patent medicine business. In R. D. Apple (Ed.), *Women, health, and medicine in America: A historical handbook* (pp. 303–328). New Brunswick, NJ: Rutgers University Press.

Centers for Disease Control and Prevention. (2014). How pharmacists can improve our nation's health. Retrieved from http://www.cdc.gov/cdcgrandrounds/archives/2014/oct2014.htm

Centers for Disease Control and Prevention. (2015). Infant mortality statistics from the 2013 period linked birth/infant death data set. Table A. *National vital statistics reports.* Retrieved from http://www.cdc.gov/nchs/data/nvsr/nvsr64/nvsr64_09.pdf

Center for Medicare & Medicaid Services. (2015). Better care, smarter spending, healthier people: Improving our health care delivery system. Fact sheet. Retrieved from https://www.cms.gov/Newsroom/MediaReleaseDatabase/Fact-sheets/2015-Fact-sheets-items/2015-01-26.html

Centers for Disease Control and Prevention. (2016). National Center for Emerging and Zoonotic (NCEZID). Retrieved from http://www.cdc.gov/ncezid/

Central Intelligence Agency. (2009). *The CIA World Factbook, 2010.* New York, NY: Skyhorse Publishing.

Christianson, E. H. (1987). Medicine in New England. In R. L. Numbers (Ed.), *Medicine in the New world: New Spain, New France, and New England* (pp. 101–153). Knoxville, TN: University of Tennessee Press.

Cohen, R. A., Martinez, M. E., & Ward, B. W. (2010, June). *Health insurance coverage: Early release of estimates from the National Interview Survey, 2009.* Atlanta, Georgia: National Center for Health Statistics. Retrieved from http://www.cdc.gov/nchs/data/nhis/earlyrelease/insur201006.htm

Collins, S. R., Rasmussen, P. W., Doty, M. M., & Beutel, S. (2015). The rise in health care coverage and affordability since health reform took effect. Findings from the Commonwealth fund Biennial Health Insurance Survey, 2014. Issue brief. The Commonwealth Fund. Retrieved from http://www.commonwealthfund.org/~/media/files/publications/issue-brief/2015/jan/1800_collins_biennial_survey_brief.pdf

Colwil, J. M. (2010, May). A case of 'medical homelessness.' *Health Affairs, 29*(5), 1067–1070.

Cowen, D. L., & Kent, D. F. (1997). Medical and pharmaceutical practice in 1854. *Pharmacy in History, 39,* 91–100.

Crosson, F. J. & Tollen, L. A. (2010). *Partners in health: How physicians and hospitals can be accountable together.* Hoboken, NJ: Jossey-Bass Publishers.

Davidson, S. M. (2010). *Still broken.* Stanford, CA: Stanford Business Books.

Davidson, S. M. (2013). *A new era in U.S. health care: Critical next steps under the Affordable Care Act.* Stanford, CA: Stanford Briefs, Stanford University Press.

Davis, K., Schoen, C., & Stremikis, K. (2010, June). *Mirror, mirror on the wall: How the performance of the U.S. health care system compares internationally; 2010 update.* Retrieved from http://www.commonwealthfund.org/~/media/Files/Publications/Fund%20Report/2010/Jun/1400_Davis_Mirror_Mirror_on_the_wall_2010.pdf

Delaney, L. R., & Gunderman, R. B. (2008, January). Hand hygiene. *Radiology, 246*(1), 15–19.

Deno, R. A., Rowe, T. D., & Brodie, D. C. (1959). *The profession of pharmacy: An introductory textbook.* Philadelphia, PA: J. B. Lippincott.

DesRoches, C. M., Campbell, E. G., Bogeli, C., Zheng, J., Rao, S. R., Shields, A. E., & Jha, A. K. (2010, April). Electronic health records' limited successes suggest more targeted uses. *Health Affairs, 29*(4), 639–646.

Duffy, J. (1993). *From humors to medical science: A history of American medicine* (2nd ed.). Urbana and Chicago, IL: University of Illinois Press.

Duffy, T. P. (2011). The Flexner Report---100 years later. *Yale Journal of Biology and Medicine, 84,* 276.

Eckholm, E. (2009, November 27). Trying to explain a drop in infant mortality. *The New York Times.* Retrieved from http://www.nytimes.com/2009/11/27/us/27infant.html?ref=infant_mortality

Elenbaas, R. M., & Worthen, D. B. (2009). Transformation of a profession: An overview of the 20th century. *Pharmacy in History, 51*(4), 151–182.

Emanuel, E. J. (2014). *Reinventing American health care: How the Affordable Care Act will improve our terribly complex, blatantly unjust, outrageously expensive, grossly inefficient, error prone system.* New York: NY, Public Affairs.

Epstein, H. (2003, October 12). Enough to make you sick? *New York Times Sunday Magazine.* Retrieved from http://www.nytimes.com/2003/10/12/magazine/ghetto-miasma-enough-to-make-you-sick.html

Epstein, R. M., Fiscella, K., Lesser, C. S., & Stange, K. C. (2010, August). Why the nation needs a policy push on patient-centered health care. *Health Affairs, 29*(8), 1489–1495.

Essoyan, S. (2000, August 13). Hospital mixes high-tech, human touch. *Boston Globe*, p. A19.

Fairbrother, G. L., Carle, A. C., Cassedy, A., & Newacheck, P. W. (2010, July). Impact of parental job loss on children's health insurance coverage. *Health Affairs, 29*(7), 1343–1349.

Farley, J. F., Devine, J. W., & Hadsall, R. S. (2007, May/June). Professional implications of the expansion of pharmacy-based medical clinics. *Journal of the American Pharmacists Association, 47*(3), 410–414.

Fletcher, M. A. (2008, March 24). *The Washington Post*. Retrieved from http://www.washingtonpost.com/wpdyn/content/article/2008/03/23/AR2008032301770_pf.html

Flexner, A. (1910). *Medical education in the United States and Canada* (Bulletin No. 4). New York, NY: Carnegie Foundation for the Advancement of Teaching.

Flexner, A. (1915). Is social work a profession? *Proceedings of the National Conference of Charities and Corrections*. Forty-second annual session, Baltimore, MD, May 12–19, 1915. Reprinted in March 2001 in *Research on Social Work Practice, 11*(2), 152–265.

Fox, D. M. (1988). A historical perspective: Health policy and changing epidemiology in the United States—chronic disease in the twentieth century. In R. C. Maulitz (Ed.), *Unnatural causes: The three leading killer diseases in America* (pp. 11–31). New Brunswick, NJ: Rutgers University Press.

Fox, D. M. (1993). *Power and illness: The failure and future of American health*. Berkeley, CA: University of California Press.

Furukawa, M. F., Raghu, T. S., Spaulding, T. J., & Vinze, A. (2008, May/June). Adoption of health information technology for medication safety in U.S. hospitals, 2006. *Health Affairs, 27*(3), 865–875.

Gabel, J. R., McDevitt, R., Lore, R., Pickreign, J., & Whitmore, H. (2009). Trends in underinsurance and the affordability of employer coverage, 2004–2007. *Health Affairs, 28*(4), w595–w606.

Gawande, A. (2004, March 25). On washing hands. *New England Journal of Medicine, 350*(13), 1283–1286.

Gawande, A. (2010). *The checklist manifesto: How to get things right*. New York, NY: Metropolitan Books.

Goetzl, R. Z. (2009, January/February). Do prevention or treatment services save money? The wrong debate. *Health Affairs, 28*(1), 37–41.

Gordon, S., Ed. (2010). *When chicken soup isn't enough: Stories of nurses standing up for themselves, their patients, and their profession*. Ithaca, NY: ILR Press.

Grob, G. N. (2002). *The deadly truth: A history of disease in America*. Cambridge, MA: Harvard University Press.

Grumbach, K., & Mendoza, R. (2008, March/April). Disparities in human resources: Addressing the lack of diversity in the health professions. *Health Affairs, 27*(2), 413–422.

Hacker, J. S. (1997). *The road to nowhere: The genesis of President Clinton's plan for health security*. Princeton, NJ: Princeton University Press.

Hacker, J. S. (2008). *The great risk shift: The new economic insecurity and the decline of the American dream*. New York, NY: Oxford University Press.

Haller, J. S., Jr. (2000). *The people's doctors: Samuel Thomson and the American botanical movement, 1790–1860*. Carbondale, IL: Southern Illinois University Press.

Hamel, M. B., Drazen, J. M., & Esptein, A. M. (2009, March 12). The growth of hospitalists and the changing face of primary care. *New England Journal of Medicine, 360*(11), 1141–1143.

Hartman, M., Martin, A., Nuccio, O., & Catlin, A. (2010, January). Health spending growth at a historic low in 2008. *Health Affairs, 29*(1), 147–155.

Harris, G. (2016, January 8). Obama vetoes bill to end health law and end planned parenthoodfunding. *New York Times*. Retrieved from http://www.nytimes.com/2016/01/09/us/politics/obama-vetoes-bill-to-repeal-health-law-and-end-planned-parenthood-funding.html

Hartzband, P., & Groopman, J. (2008, April 17). Off the record—avoiding the pitfalls of going electronic. *New England Journal of Medicine, 358*(16), 1656–1658.

Hartzband, P., & Groopman, J. (2016). Medical Taylorism. *New England Journal of Medicine, 374*(2), 107.

HealthCare.gov (2010, June 22). The affordable care act's new patient's bill of rights. Retrieved from http://www.healthcare.gov/news/factsheets/aca_new_patients_bill_of_rights.html

Health Policy Brief: Health Gaps. (2013, August 15). Health Affairs. Retrieved from http://www.healthaffairs.org/healthpolicybriefs/brief.php?brief_id=98

Hendricks, R. (1993). *A model for national health care: The history of Kaiser Permanente*. New Brunswick, NJ: Rutgers University Press.

Hepler, C. D. (2010, August 15). A dream deferred. *American Journal of Health-System Pharmacy, 67*, 1319–1325.

Hepler, C. D., & Strand, L. (1990). Opportunities and responsibilities in pharmaceutical care. *American Journal of Hospital Pharmacy, 47*, 533–543.

Heron, M. (2015, August 31). Deaths: Leading causes for 2012. *National vital statistics reports, 64*(10). Hyattsville, MD: National Center for Health Statistics.

Higby, G. J. (1992). *In service to American pharmacy: The professional life of William Procter, Jr.* Tuscaloosa, AL: University of Alabama Press.

Higby, G. J. (1996). From compounding to caring: An abridged history of American pharmacy. In C. Knowlton & R. Panna (Eds.), *Pharmaceutical care* (pp. 18–45), New York, NY: Chapman and Hall.

Higby, G.J. (1997). American pharmacy in the twentieth century. *American Journal of Health Systems Pharmacy, 54*, 1805–1815.

Higby, G. J., & Gallagher, T. C. (1992). Pharmacists. In R. D. Apple (Ed.), *Women, health, and medicine in America: A historical handbook* (pp. 489–508). New Brunswick, NJ: Rutgers University Press.

Hoadley, J. F., Cubanski, J., & Neuman, P. (2015). Medicare's part D drug benefit at ten years: firmly established but still evolving. *Health Affairs, 34*(10), 1682–1687.

Hobson, K. (2010, August 9). Study puts cost of medical errors at $19.5 billion. *The Wall Street Journal*. Retrieved from http://blogs.wsj.com/health/2010/08/09/study-puts-cost-of-medical-errors-at-195-billion/

Hooper, D. C. (2009). Making strides in hand hygiene compliance: To 90% and beyond. Retrieved from http://www.macoalition.org/Initiatives/docs/MassGeneralHospitalPresentation.pdf

Horrocks, T. A. (2003). Rules, remedies, and regimens: Health advice in early American almanacs. In C. E. Rosenberg (Ed.), *Right living: An Anglo-American tradition of self-help medicine and hygiene* (pp. 112–146). Baltimore, MD: Johns Hopkins University Press.

Hoy, S. (1995). *Chasing dirt: The American pursuit of cleanliness*. New York, NY: Oxford University Press.

Humer, C. (2016, January). U.S. says 11.3 million Americans have signed up for 2016 Obamacare plans. Reuters. Retrieved from http://www.reuters.com/article/us-usa-healthcare-obamacare-idUSKBN0UL2CW20160107

Iglehart, J. K. (2008, September 18). No place like home—testing a new model of care delivery. *New England Journal of Medicine, 359*(12), 2100–2102.

Iglehart, J. K. (2010, May). Entry point. *Health Affairs, 29*(5), 758–759.

Institute of Medicine. (2000). In L. T. Kohn, J. M. Corrigan, & M. S. Donaldson (Eds.), *To err is human: Building a safer health system*. Washington, DC: National Academies Press.

Institute of Medicine. (2001). *Crossing the quality chasm: A new health system for the 21st century*. Washington, DC: National Academies Press.

Islam, I. (2015). Trouble ahead for high deductible health plans. *Health Affairs Blog*. Retrieved from http://healthaffairs.org/blog/2015/10/07/trouble-ahead-for-high-deductible-health-plans/

Johnson, H., & Broder, D. (1996). *The system: The American way of politics at the breaking point*. Boston, MA: Little, Brown.

Johnson, N. J., & Johnson, L. P. (Eds.). (2010). *The care of the uninsured in America*. New York, NY: Springer.

Jost, T. (2015, June 25). Implementing health reform: The Supreme Court upholds tax credits in the federal exchange. *Health Affairs Blog*. Retrieved from http://healthaffairs.org/blog/2015/06/25/implementing-health-reform-the-supreme-court-upholds-tax-credits-in-the-federal-exchange/

Kaiser Family Foundation. (2010, March). Trends in health care costs and spending. Retrieved from http://www.kff.org/insurance/upload/7692_02.pdf

Kaiser Family Foundation. (2015, October 13). The Medicare Part D prescription drug benefit. Retrieved from http://kff.org/medicare/fact-sheet/the-medicare-prescription-drug-benefit-fact-sheet/

Kaufman, M. (1971). *Homeopathy in America: The rise and fall of a medical heresy*. Baltimore, MD: Johns Hopkins University Press.

Keehan, S. P., Cuckler, G. A., Sisko, A.M., Madison, A. J., Smith, S. D., Stone, D. A., ... Lizonitz, J. M. (2015). National health expenditure projections, 2014–2024: Spending growth faster than recent trends. *Health Affairs, 34*(8), 1407–1417. Retrieved from http://content.healthaffairs.org/content/34/8/1407.full.html

Kennedy, E. M. (1972). *In critical condition: The crisis in America's health care*. New York, NY: Simon and Schuster.

Kevles, B. H. (1997). *Medical imaging in the twentieth century*. New Brunswick, NJ: Rutgers University Press.

Kilo, C. M., & Wasson, J. H. (2010). Practice redesign and the patient-centered medical home: History, promises, and challenges. *Health Affairs, 29*(5), 773–778.

King, C. R. (1993). *Children's health in America: A history*. New York, NY: Twayne.

King, A. E., & Egras, A. M. (2015). A required online course with a public health focus for third professional year pharmacy students. *American Journal of Pharmaceutical Education, 79*(5), 1–11.

Kinsella, K. G. (1992). Changes in life expectancy 1900–1990. *American Journal of Clinical Nutrition, 55*(6), 1196S–1202S.

Knowlton, C. H. (2009). Pharmacy practice: Where's the value proposition? *Pharmacy in History, 51*(3), 94–97.

Knox, R. A. (1996, November 13). Widespread chronic illness cited. *Boston Globe*, p. A11.

Koh, H. K. (2010, May 6). A 2020 vision for healthy people. *New England Journal of Medicine, 362*(18), 1653–1656.

Koh, H. K., Blakey, C. R., & Roper, A. Y. (2014). Healthy People 2020: A report card on the health of the nation. *Journal of the Medical Association, 311*(24), 2475–2476.

Kowalczyk, L. (2000). A stretched-thin doctor draws a line. *Boston Globe*, pp. A1, C6.

Kraut, A. M. (1994). *Silent travelers: Germs, genes, and the "immigrant menace."* New York, NY: Basic Books.

Kreling, D. H., Doucette, W. R., Mott, D. A., Gaither, C. A., Pedersen, C. A., & Schommer, J. C. (2006). Community pharmacists' work environments: Evidence from the 2004 national pharmacist workforce study. *Journal of the American Pharmaceutical Association, 46*(3), 331–339.

Krugman, P. (2010, January 22). Do the right thing. *The New York Times*, A21.

La Ferla, R. (2000, August 13). Hospitals are discovering their inner spa. *New York Times*, sect. 9, pp. 1, 4.

Larson, E. B., & Reid, R. (2010, April 28). The patient-centered medical home movement: Why now? *Journal of the American Medical Association, 303*(16), 1644–1645.

Lauer, M. S. (2009, August 27). Elements of danger—the case of medical imaging. *New England Journal of Medicine, 361*(9), 841–843.

Leavitt, J. W. (1995). A worrying profession: The domestic environment of medical practice in mid-19th century America. *Bulletin of the History of Medicine, 69*, 1–29.

Leavitt, J. W. (1996). *Typhoid Mary: Captive to the public's health*. New York, NY: Beacon Press.

Leavitt, J. W., & Numbers, R. L. (1997). Sickness and health: An overview. In J. W. Leavitt & R. L. Numbers (Eds.), *Sickness and health in America: Readings in the history of medicine and public health* (3rd ed., pp. 3–10). Madison, WI: University of Wisconsin Press.

Lerner, M., & Anderson, O. W. (1963). *Health progress in the United States: 1900–1960*. Chicago, IL: University of Chicago Press.

Lichtenberg, F. R., & Sun, S. X. (2007, November/December). The impact of Medicare Part D on prescription drug use by the elderly. *Health Affairs, 26*(6), 1735–1744.

Litman, T. J. (1997). The relationship of government and politics to health and health care—a sociopolitical overview. In T. J. Litman & L. S. Robins (Eds.), *Health politics and policy* (3rd ed., pp. 3–45). New York, NY: Delmar.

Ludmerer, K. M. (1985). *Learning to heal: The development of American medical education*. New York, NY: Basic Books.

Ludmerer, K. M. (1999). *Time to heal: American education from the turn of the century to the era of managed care*. New York, NY: Oxford University Press.

Lukas, C. V., & Young, G. J. (2000, March/April). Trends: Public hospitals, privatization and uncompensated care. *Health Affairs, 19*(2), 1–6.

MacDorman, M. F., Matthews, T. J., Mohangoo, A. D., & Zeitlin, J. (2014). International comparisons of infant mortality and related factors: United States and Europe 2010. *National vital statistics reports, 63*(5). Hyattsville, MD: National Center for Health Statistics.

Maciosek, M. V., Coffield, A. B., Edwards, N. M., Flottemesch, T. J., Goodman, M. J., & Solberg, L. I. (2006). Priorities among effective clinical preventive services: Results of a systematic review and analysis. *American Journal of Preventive Medicine, 20*(10), 1–10.

Mackey, J. (2010, August 11). The whole foods alternative to Obama Care. *The Wall Street Journal*, p. A15.

Magill, S. S., Edwards, J. R., Bamberg, W., Beldavs, Z. G., Dumyati, G., Kainer, M. A., ... Fridkin, S. K. (2014). Multistate point-prevalence survey of health care-associated infections. *New England Journal of Medicine, 370*(13), 1198–1208.

Managed Care On-Line (MCOL). (2010). National HMO enrollment. National statistics. Managed care fact sheets. Retrieved from http://www.mcol.com/

Markel, H. (2004). *When germs travel: Six major epidemics that have invaded America and the fears they have unleashed.* New York, NY: Vintage Books.

Markel, H., & Golden, J. (2004, September/October). Children's public health policy in the United States: How the past can inform the present. *Health Affairs, 23*(5), 147–152.

Markowitz, G. E., & Rosner, D. (1979). Doctors in crisis: Medical education and medical reform during the progressive era, 1895–1915. In S. Reverby & D. Rosner (Eds.), *Health care in America: Essays in social history* (pp. 185–205). Philadelphia, PA: Temple University Press.

Martin, T. W. (2010, August 17). Suntan lotion, flip-flops ... and flu shots. *The Wall Street Journal*, p.B1.

Martinez, B. (2000, August 21). Now it's mass medicine. *Wall Street Journal*, pp. B1, B4.

Mathews, T. J., MacDorman, M. F., & Thoma, M. E. (2015, August 6). Infant mortality statistics from the 2013 period linked birth/infant data set. *National vital statistics reports, 64*(9), 1–29. Hyattsville, MD: National Center for Health Statistics.

Maxwell, J., Tobey, R., & Barron, C. (2015, September 2). Community health center strategies for pursuing accountable care [Web log post]. Retrieved from http://healthaffairs.org/blog/2015/09/02/community-health-center-strategies-for-pursuing-accountable-care/

McGivney, M. S., Meyer, S. M., Duncan-Hewitt, W., Hall, D. L., Goode, J. R., & Smith, R.B. (2007, September/October). Medication therapy management: Its relationship to patient counseling, disease management, and pharmaceutical care. *Journal of the American Pharmacists Association, 47*(5), 620–628.

McGuire, L. K., Bergen, M. R., & Polan, M. L. (2004, April). Career advancement for women faculty in a U.S. school of medicine: Perceived needs. *Academic Medicine, 79*(4), 319–325.

McKenna, M. (2010). *SUPERBUG: The fatal menace of MRSA.* New York, NY: Free Press.

Mechanic, R. E. (2003, November/December). What will become of the medical mecca? Health care spending in Massachusetts. *Health Affairs, 22*(6), 131–141.

Melosi, M. V. (2000). *The sanitary city: Urban infrastructure in America from colonial times to the present.* Baltimore, MD: Johns Hopkins University Press.

Meriweather, K. (2015, July 28). A Perfect combination: The Cleveland neighborhood model for urban health care education [Web log post]. Retrieved from http://healthaffairs.org/blog/2015/07/28/a-perfect-combination-the-cleveland-neighborhood-model-for-urban-health-care-education/

Millis, J. S. (1975). *Pharmacists for the future: The report of the Study Commission on Pharmacy.* Ann Arbor, MI: Health Administration Press.

Mishler, E. G. (1981). Viewpoint: Critical perspectives on the biomedical model. In E. G. Mishler (Ed.), *Social contexts of health, illness, and patient care* (pp. 1–13). New York, NY: Cambridge University Press.

Morantz-Sanchez, R. (1992). Physicians. In R. D. Apple (Ed.), *Women, health, and medicine in America: A historical handbook* (pp. 469–487). New Brunswick, NJ: Rutgers University Press.

More, E. S. (1999). *Restoring the balance: Women physicians and the profession of medicine, 1850–1995.* Cambridge, MA: Harvard University Press.

Morrison, G., Goldfarb, S., & Lanken, P. N. (2010, February). Team training of medical students in the 21st century: Would Flexner approve? *Academic Medicine, 85*(2), 254–259.

Murray, C. J. L., & Lopez, A. D. (Eds.). (1996). *The global burden of disease: A comprehensive assessment of mortality and disability from diseases, injuries, and risk factors in 1990 and projected to 2020.* Cambridge, MA: Harvard University Press.

Naik, G. (2006, June 20). Cincinnati applies a corporate model to saving infants. *Wall Street Journal*, pp. A01, A14.

National Center for Health Statistics. (2014). *Health, United States 2014:* With special feature on adults 55–64. Hyattsville, MD. Revised June 2015.

National Center for Health Statistics. (2009). *Health, United States, 2009: With special feature on medical technology.* Hyattsville, MD: U.S. Government Printing Office.

National Conference of State Legislatures. (2015, April 17). Children's Health Insurance Program Overview. U.S. Department of Health and Human Services. Retrieved from http://www.ncsl.org/research/health/childrens-health-insurance-program-overview.aspx

Navarro, R. P. (1999). *Managed care pharmacy practice*. Gaithersburg, MD: Aspen Publications.

Nissenbaum, S. (1980). *Sex, diet, and debility in Jacksonian America: Sylvester Graham and health reform*. Westport, CT: Greenwood Press.

Numbers, R. L. (1997). The third party: Health insurance in America. In J. W. Leavitt & R. L. Numbers (Eds.), *Sickness and health in America: Readings in the history of medicine and public health* (3rd ed., pp. 269–283). Madison, WI: University of Wisconsin Press.

Oberlander, J. (2010, June). Long time coming: Why health reform finally passed. *Health Affairs, 29*(6), 1112–1116.

Offiong, C. Y., Oji, V. U., Bunyan, W., Lewis, J. A., Moore, C., & Olusanya, O. A. (2011). The role of colleges and schools of pharmacy in the advent of Healthy People 2020. *American Journal of Pharmaceutical Education, 75*(3).

Opdycke, S. (1999). *No one was turned away: The role of public hospitals in New York City since 1900*. New York, NY: Oxford University Press.

Organization for Economic Cooperation and Development. (2009). *Health at a Glance: OECD Indicators*. Washington, DC: OEDC Publishing.

Ott, K. (1996). *Fevered lives: Tuberculosis in American culture since 1870*. Cambridge, MA: Harvard University Press.

Parascandola, J. (1997). The introduction of antibiotics into therapeutics. In J. W. Leavitt & R. L. Numbers (Eds.), *Sickness and health in America: Readings in the history of medicine and public health* (3rd ed., pp. 102–112). Madison, WI: University of Wisconsin Press.

Patel, K., & Rushefsky, M. E. (1995). *Health care politics and policy in America*. Armonk, NY: M. E. Sharpe.

Patient-Centered Primary Care Collaborative. (2010). The patient-centered medical home: Integrating comprehensive medication management to optimize patient outcome. Retrieved from http://www.pcpcc.net/files/medmanagement.pdf

Patterson, J. T. (1987). *The dread disease: Cancer and modern American culture*. Cambridge, MA: Harvard University Press.

Pear, R. (1997, April 2). New health insurance rules spell out rights of workers. *New York Times*, p. A15.

Pear, R. (2006, June 11). In Texas town, patients and providers find new prescription drug plan baffling. *New York Times*, p. 30.

Pernick, M. S. (1985). *A calculus of suffering: Pain, professionalism, and anesthesia in nineteenth-century America*. New York, NY: Columbia University Press.

Peterson, M. A. (1997). Introduction: Health care into the next century. *Journal of Health Politics, Policy and Law, 22*, 291–313.

Pitout, J. D. D. (2010, August 11). The latest threat in the war on antimicrobial resistance. *The Lancet Infectious Diseases, 10*(1016), 1–2.

Poen, M. M. (1979). *Harry S. Truman versus the medical lobby: The genesis of Medicare*. Columbia, MO: University of Missouri Press.

Pollack, C. E., Gidengil, C., & Mehrotra, A. (2010, May). The growth of retail clinics and the medical home: Two trends in concert or in conflict? *Health Affairs, 29*(5), 998–1003.

Ponte, R. P., Conlin, G., Conway, J. B., Grant, S., Medeiros, C., Nies, J.,... Conley, K. (2003, February). Making patient-centered care come alive: Achieving full integration of the patient's perspective. *Journal of Nursing Administration, 33*(2), 82–90.

Prevention and Public Health Fund. (2016, April 11). HHS.gov. Retrieved from http://www.hhs.gov/open/prevention/

Pronovost, P., Needham, D., Berenholtz, S., Sinopoli, D., Chu, H., Cosgrove, S.,...Goeschel, C. (2006, December 28). An intervention to decrease catheter-related bloodstream infections in the ICU. *New England Journal of Medicine, 355*(26), 2725–2732.

Qato, D. M., Daviglus, M. L., Wilder, J., Lee, Qato, D., & Lambert, B. (2014). 'Pharmacy deserts' are prevalent in Chicago's predominantly minority communities, raising medication access concerns. *Health Affairs, 33*(11), 1958–1965.

Ralston, J. D., Coleman, K., Reid, R. J., Handley, M. R., & Larson, E. B. (2010, April). Patient experience should be part of meaningful-use criteria. *Health Affairs, 29*(4), 607–613.

Reid, R. J., Coleman, K., Johnson, E. A., Fishman, P. A., Hsu, C., Soman, M. P.,… Larson, E. B. (2010, May). The group health medical home at year two: Cost savings, higher patient satisfaction, and less burnout for providers. *Health Affairs, 29*(5), 835–843.

Reinhardt, U. E., Hussey, P. S., & Anderson, G. F. (2004, May/June). U.S. health care spending in an international context. *Health Affairs, 2*(3), 10–25.

Reverby, S. M. (1987). *Ordered to care: The dilemma of American nursing, 1850–1945*. New York, NY: Cambridge University Press.

Richmond, J. B., & Fein, R. (2005). *The health care mess: How we got into it and what it will take to get out*. Cambridge, MA: Harvard University Press.

Risse, G. B. (1999). *Mending bodies, saving souls: A history of hospitals*. New York, NY: Oxford University Press.

Rittenhouse, D. R., & Shortell, S. M. (2009, May 20). The patient-centered medical home: Will it stand the test of health reform? *The Journal of the American Medical Association, 301*(19), 2038–2040.

Rosenberg, C. E. (1974). Social class and medical care in 19th century America: The rise and fall of the dispensary. *Journal of the History of Medicine and Allied Sciences, 29*(1), 32–54.

Rosenberg, C. E. (1985). The therapeutic revolution: Medicine, meaning, and social change in 19th-century America. In J. W. Leavitt & R. L. Numbers (Eds.), *Sickness and health in America: Readings in the history of medicine and public health* (2nd ed., pp. 39–52). Madison, WI: University of Wisconsin Press.

Rosenberg, C. E. (1987). *The care of strangers: The rise of America's hospital system*. New York, NY: Basic Books.

Rosenberg, C. E. (1992). Framing disease: Illness, society, and history. In C. E. Rosenberg & J. Golden (Eds.), *Framing disease: Studies in cultural history* (pp. xiii–xxvi). New Brunswick, NJ: Rutgers University Press.

Rosenbaum, S., & Westmoreland, T. M. (2012, August). The Supreme Court's surprising decision on the Medicaid expansion: How will the federal government and states proceed? *Health Affairs, 31*(8), 1663–1672.

Rosner, D. (1979). Business at the bedside: Health care in Brooklyn, 1890–1915. In S. Reverby & D. Rosner (Eds.), *Health care in America: Essays in social history* (pp. 117–131). Philadelphia, PA: Temple University Press.

Rosner, D. (1995). Introduction: Hives of sickness and vice. In D. Rosner (Ed.), *Hives of sickness: Public health and epidemics in New York City* (pp. 1–12). New Brunswick, NJ: Rutgers University Press.

Rothstein, W. G. (1996a). Pharmaceuticals and public policy in America: A history. In W. G. Rothstein (Ed.), *Readings in American health care: Current issues in socio-historical perspective* (pp. 375–391). Madison, WI: University of Wisconsin Press.

Rothstein, W. G. (1996b). Trends in mortality in the twentieth century. In W. G. Rothstein (Ed.), *Readings in American health care: Current issues in socio-historical perspective* (pp. 71–86). Madison, WI: University of Wisconsin Press.

Sack, K. (2010a, October 7). Judge rules health law is constitutional. *The New York Times*. Retrieved from http://www.nytimes.com/2010/10/08/health/policy/08health.html?_r=1&scp=1&sq=health%20care%20reform%20constitutional&st=cse

Sack, K. (2010b, October 15). Challenging health law, suit advances. *The New York Times*. Retrieved from http://www.nytimes.com/2010/10/15/health/policy/15health.html?scp=1&sq=challenging%20health%20law,%20suit%20advances&st=cse

Salamon, J. (2010). *Hospital: Man, woman, birth, death, infinity, plus red tape, bad behavior, money, God, and diversity on steroids*. New York, NY: The Penguin Press.

Sands, P., Mundaca-Shah, C., & Dzau, V. J. (2016, March, 31). The neglected dimension of global security—A framework for countering infectious-disease crises. *New England Journal of Medicine, 374*(13), 1281–1287.

Saultz, J. W., O'Neil, P., Gill, J. M., Biagioli, F. E., Blanchard, S., O'Malley, J. P., … Carney, P. A. (2010, June). Medical student exposure to components of the patient-centered medical home during required ambulatory clerkship rotations: Implications for education. *Academic Medicine, 85*(6), 965–973.

Schneeweiss, S., Patrick, A. R., Pedan, A., Varasteh, L., Levin, R., Liu, N., & Shrank, W. H. (2009, March/April). The effect of Medicare Part D coverage on drug use and cost sharing among seniors without prior drug benefits. *Health Affairs, 28*(2), w305–w316.

Sered, S. S. & Fernandopulle, R. (2005). *Uninsured in America: Life and death in the land of opportunity.* Berkeley, CA: University of California Press.

Smith, M., Bates, D. W., Bodenheimer, T., & Cleary, P. D. (2010, May). Why pharmacists belong in the medical home. *Health Affairs, 29*(5), 906–913.

Sonnedecker, G. (1976). *Kremer's and Urdang's history of pharmacy* (4th ed.). Philadelphia, PA: J. B. Lippincott.

Squires, D., & Anderson, C. (2015, October). U.S. Health care from a global perspective: Spending, use of s ervices, prices, and health in 13 countries. The Commonwealth Fund. Retrieved from http://www.commonwealthfund.org/publications/issue-briefs/2015/oct/us-health-care-from-a-global-perspective

Stage, S. (1979). *Female complaints: Lydia Pinkham and the business of women's medicine.* New York, NY: W. W. Norton.

Starr, P. (1982). *The social transformation of American medicine: The rise of a sovereign profession and the making of a vast industry.* New York, NY: Basic Books.

Starr, P. (1991). *The logic of health care reform (The grand rounds press).* Knoxville, TN: Whittle Direct Books.

Steinhauer, J. (2000, February 29). High infant mortality rates in Brooklyn mystify experts. *New York Times,* pp. A1, A23.

Stevens, R. (1971). *American medicine and the public interest.* New Haven, CT: Yale University Press.

Stevens, R. (1989). *In sickness and in wealth: American hospitals in the twentieth century.* New York, NY: Basic Books.

Stevens, R. (2008). History and health policy in the United States: The making of a health care industry, 1948–2008. *Social History of Medicine, 21*(3), 461–483.

Stone, D. A. (1997). The doctor as businessman: The changing politics of a cultural icon. *The American Prospect, 22*(2), 533–556.

Sullivan, L. W., & Mittman, I. S. (2010, February). The state of diversity in the health professions a century after Flexner. *Academic Medicine, 85*(2), 246–253.

Tannenbaum, R. (2002). *The healer's calling: Women and medicine in early New England.* Ithaca, NY: Cornell University Press.

Temin, P. (1980). *Taking your medicine: Drug regulation in the United States.* Cambridge, MA: Harvard University Press.

Tesh, S. N. (1988). *Hidden arguments: Political ideology and disease prevention policy.* New Brunswick, NJ: Rutgers University Press.

Tomes, N. (1998). *The gospel of germs: Men, women, and the microbe in American life.* Cambridge, MA: Harvard University Press.

Tomes, N. (2006). Patients or health-care consumers? Why the history of contested terms matters. In Stevens, R. A., Rosenberg, C. E., & Burns, L. R. (Eds.), *History and health policy in the United States.* New Brunswick, NJ: Rutgers University Press.

Traynor, K. (2010, September 1). Pharmacy makes inroads in medical home movement. *American Journal of Health Systems Pharmacy, 67,* 1402, 1404.

Trivedi, A. N., Wato, N., Hausmann, L. R. M., Lee, J. S., Ma, A., Bratzler, D. W., ... Fine, M. J. (2014). *New England Journal of Medicine, 371*(4), 2298, 2307.

Ulrich, L. T. (1990). *A midwife's tale: The life of Martha Ballard, based on her diary, 1785–1812.* New York, NY: Alfred A. Knopf.

U.S. Census Bureau. (2010). *Statistical abstract of the United States.* Washington, DC: Government Printing Office.

U.S. Department of Health and Human Services. (1999). *Health: United States 1999.* Washington, DC: Government Printing Office.

Vladek, B. (2003, January). Universal health insurance in the United States: Reflections on the past, the present, and the future. *American Journal of Public Health, 93*(1), 16–19.

Vogel, M. J. (1979). The transformation of the American hospital, 1850–1920. In S. Reverby & D. Rosner (Eds.), *Health care in America: Essays in social history* (pp. 105–116). Philadelphia, PA: Temple University Press.

Wachter, R. M. (2010, January). Patient safety at ten: Unmistakable progress, troubling gaps. *Health Affairs, 29*(1), 165–173.

Warner, J. H. (1997). From specificity to universalism in medical therapeutics: Transformation in the 19th-century United States. In J. W. Leavitt & R. Numbers (Eds.), *Sickness and health in America: Readings in the history of medicine and public health* (3rd ed., pp. 87–101). Madison, WI: University of Wisconsin Press.

Weiss, G. L., & Lonnquist, L. E. (2006). *The sociology of health, healing, and illness* (5th ed.). Upper Saddle River, NJ: Pearson Prentice Hall.

The White House. (2010, March 23). Remarks by the president and vice president at signing of the health insurance reform bill. Retrieved from http://www.whitehouse.gov/the-press-office/remarks-president-and-vice-president-signing-health-insurance-reform-bill

White House Domestic Policy Council. (1993). *The president's health security plan*. New York, NY: Times Books.

Woo, A., Ranji, U., & Salganicoff, A. (2008, May). Reducing medical errors. *Kaiser EDU.org*. Retrieved from http://www.kaiseredu.org/topics_im.asp?id=137&parentID=70&imID=1

World Health Organization. (2014). Global Status Report on noncommunicable diseases 2014. Retrieved from https://cspinet.org/new/pdf/who-global-status-report-on-ncds-2014__1_.pdf

World Health Organization. (2011). Noncommunicable diseases country profiles 2011. WHO global report. Retrieved from http://apps.who.int/iris/bitstream/10665/44704/1/9789241502283_eng.pdf

World Health Organization. (2009). WHO guidelines in hand hygiene in health care: First global patient safety challenge; clean care is safer care. Geneva, Switzerland: WHO Press.

Worthen, D. B. (Ed.). (2006). *The Millis study commission on pharmacy: A road map to a profession's future*. Binghamton, NY: The Haworth Press.

Yin, W., Basu, A., Zhang, J. X., Rabbani, A., Meltzer, D. O., & Alexander, G. C. (2008, February 5). The effect of the Medicare Part D prescription benefit on drug utilization and expenditures. *The Annals of Internal Medicine, 148*, 169–177.

Young, G., Dasai, K., & Lucas, C. V. (1997). Does the sale of nonprofit hospitals threaten health care for the poor? *Health Affairs, 16*(1), 137–141.

Young, J. H. (1992). *American health quackery: Collected essays*. Princeton, NJ: Princeton University Press.

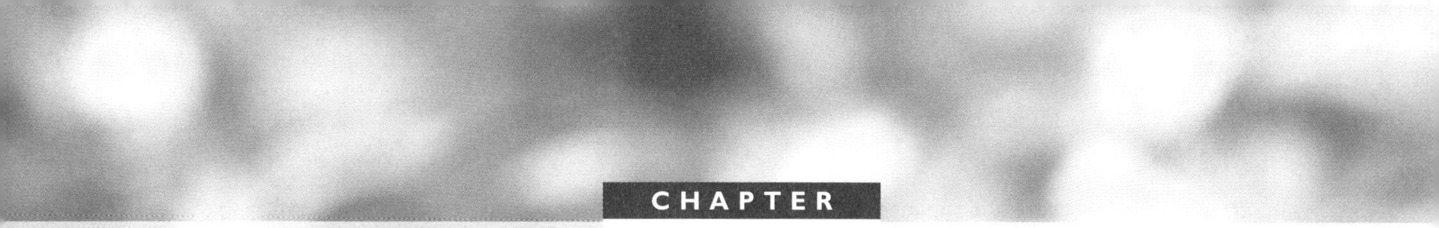

CHAPTER

2

Healthcare Professionals and Interdisciplinary Care

Suvapun Bunniran and David J. McCaffrey III*

Case Scenario

Bob Jones has been a patient of WeCare Pharmacy for almost 20 years. Bob has multiple chronic conditions, including hypertension, diabetes, coronary artery disease, and osteoarthritis and is on 10 different medications. Bob uses a nurse practitioner for his overall care, but sees a specialist for his cardiac condition. Bob struggles with managing his medications, as well as adhering to the dietary recommendations that his providers give him. His wife, Anne, visits the pharmacy regularly to collect prescriptions and other healthcare needs for herself and her husband. At her most recent visit, she mentions that she worries about Bob and his health. She comments, "It's just hard to keep track of everything with his medications. I know I should be helping him with his diet, but it's just so overwhelming." The pharmacist empathizes with Mrs. Jones and suggests she and Bob come to the pharmacy for a medication therapy management appointment. During the appointment, the pharmacist reviews Bob's medication list with him, as well as suggests some changes. When contacting the nurse practitioner regarding the medication changes, she relays Anne's concerns regarding Bob's diet. Two days later, someone from the nurse practitioner's office contacts Bob about a referral to a dietician to help him with dietary changes. All the providers involved in Bob's care provide documentation to one another, as well as share suggestions with one another.

LEARNING OBJECTIVES

Upon completion of this chapter, the student shall be able to:

- Discuss the characteristics of a profession and how professions are distinguished from other occupations.
- Describe the education/training, scope of practice, and availability of various healthcare professions.
- Compare and contrast multidisciplinary care and interdisciplinary care.
- Recognize the various stages of the pharmacist–physician collaborative working relationship and identify strategies available to the pharmacist to establish these cooperative arrangements with physicians.

*With acknowledgment to Alice M. Sapienza.

- Describe continuity of care and the medical home and the role that a pharmacist can and should play in this process.
- Define quality and describe the role of interdisciplinary care in the quality movement.
- Describe the three ways that healthcare quality is reported and how interested parties might use this information.
- Describe how continuous quality improvement efforts influence the manner in which healthcare professionals practice.
- Explain the positive and negative attributes of pay for performance.
- Describe how technology would influence interdisciplinary care.
- Identify quality measurements and organizations involved in collecting and disseminating this information.

CHAPTER QUESTIONS

1. How it is that professions and occupations differ? Does health care constitute a special case of a profession?
2. What are the primary similarities shared between pharmacy and the other healthcare professions? Major differences?
3. How would you explain to a patient the benefits of interdisciplinary care over multidisciplinary care?
4. What are the challenges that pharmacists face when attempting to establish collaborative practice agreements with other healthcare providers?
5. How is it that a medical home affects continuity of care?
6. What is healthcare quality to a patient, to a healthcare provider, and to a payer?
7. How might the technologies that are currently being developed change the landscape of pharmacy practice?

INTRODUCTION

Health care requires the interaction among many different providers of care and ancillary personnel. Pharmacists can and do play an important role in connecting these different providers; pharmacists also fulfill this role well because of the opportunity for interaction with the patient (e.g., the community pharmacist may see a patient as often as once per month or even more). Moreover, pharmacists have opportunities to influence the health and well-being of patients through the provision of patient-centered services (e.g., medication therapy management); however, these services rarely are provided without the pharmacist's direct interaction with other healthcare providers. As such, this chapter will present an overview about how pharmacists may work with different healthcare occupations while providing patient care. Moreover, information about many of the principle healthcare occupations with which pharmacy will interact will be presented. While this number potentially is great, the space available in the chapter is not, and as a result, the chapter will focus on the healthcare-related occupations with which pharmacy has the greatest interaction. The authors suggest that readers interested in other healthcare-related occupations visit the *Occupational Outlook Handbook* produced by the Bureau of Labor Statistics for an overview of these occupations (www.bls.gov) as well as an annual update on the healthcare occupations presented herein. The chapter will conclude with a discussion of a variety of issues affecting pharmacy and the healthcare system currently and in the immediate future.

PROFESSIONS

While the term *professional* is used almost without thought, defining a professional in exacting terms can be quite difficult. In health care, do all providers deserve the title, "professional?" Over the years, various healthcare occupations have been considered just that—an occupation without professional status; pharmacy was one of those healthcare occupations. But exactly what are the characteristics that allow an occupation to be elevated to the level of a profession? Research as to what constitutes a profession has largely revolved around evaluating the qualities of recognized professions (e.g., law, medicine, and clergy) (Klass, 1961). While it was generally recognized that there was no one test for an occupation being a profession, occupations that were considered professions shared certain characteristics. These shared attributes have come to define which occupations society considers as professions.

While it is recognized generally that professions exist to serve society, merely providing services that the public needs and demands does not define a profession. The literature reveals five characteristics that are common to occupations considered professions; these include systematic theory and body of knowledge, professional authority and special privileges, community sanction and social utility, ethical codes and internal control, and professional culture and organizations (Buerki & Vottero, 1996). *Systematic theory and body of knowledge* is an important first distinction between the profession and the public whom it serves (Mrtek & Catizone, 1989). It results from the didactic education received in the various professional schools and continues throughout the life of the professional as he or she is required to maintain competence through continuing education. Members of professions are expected to have extensive theoretical knowledge and to use that knowledge (and the associated skill) when they provide service to society.

Professional authority and special privileges refer to the professional's ability to practice in his or her area of expertise as well as being afforded the opportunity to provide services to the public, services that the members of the public cannot presumably perform for themselves (Buerki & Vottero, 1996). The client surrenders a portion of his or her autonomy to the professional, because the client acknowledges the superior competence of the professional to do the job that the client cannot do. The client trusts the professional's judgment about which course of action will best meet the client's needs.

It is believed that professions serve a socially necessary function (*social utility*) and provide a service that is of great importance to society. As such, the function of a profession is sanctioned (*community sanction*) by society in a number of different ways. The most widely recognized sanctioning is the system of licensure (Buerki & Vottero, 1996). Licenses for professions are granted by various professional boards, and these boards exist to protect society. That being said, most boards include members of society in addition to members of the profession. Another recognized community sanction is the restriction on the use of a professional title.

While society is beholden to the laws that govern the land, a profession has *ethical codes and internal control*. The professional accepts responsibility and is accountable through not only the law but also his or her profession. This is accomplished through formal and informal internal controls (e.g., codes of ethics). A profession accepts the responsibility to maintain a standard of conduct beyond the law. Despite the obvious importance of ethical codes and internal control to the value of a profession, the most difficult part about codes of ethics is enforcement. Thus the inclusion of a code of ethics as an attribute of a profession is probably the weakest part of attribute theory of professions. This is surprising somewhat given that the most effective technique for avoiding public (external) control over the profession is for the profession to maintain strong control over its members (Goode, 1957). Members of professions enjoy relative freedom from direct on-the-job supervision and from direct public scrutiny. However, when supervision does exist, the supervisor of a professional typically is a member of the same profession.

The *professional culture* is made up of values, norms, and symbols. Values are the central beliefs of a profession; the values of a profession usually include a belief in the importance and merit to society of the profession's unique expertise and a belief that the service cannot be better provided by another occupation. Another belief underlying the profession's value system is the belief that the service provided is essential, in that society would suffer if the service was withdrawn. Values are the central beliefs of a profession, and norms are the accepted ways of social behavior within the profession. Symbols are often used to identify the calling of the profession. Symbols include a specific insignia, vocabulary, and dress (e.g., white lab coat).

Professions also rely upon a network of *organizations* that promote the profession and serve a number of other functions. These organizations may assist with licensure, provide continuing education, and promote a sense of collegiality. Professional organizations perform an important function for society, connecting members of the profession to one another and to other important groups, such as other professions, educational institutions, government bodies, and consumer groups. Without professional organizations, communication would be very difficult, if not impossible. Professional organizations are involved in activities that promote the interests of the profession.

Lastly, it is believed that a profession is required to render an individualized, unstandardized service directly to clients (Buerki & Vottero, 1996). Efforts made by the various healthcare professions to improve the quality of the services provided through standardization do not mean that healthcare providers do not meet this criterion. Many of the current efforts surrounding patient safety revolve around creating processes such that errors may be reduced or eliminated. This is a laudable goal; however, patients present with an almost infinite number of signs, symptoms, and personal characteristics that require that these processes be executed with the patient's best interest in mind. That best interest can only be determined by a thorough understanding of the patient's needs and wants and requires flexibility on the part of the provider to change as the patient's needs and/or wants change. The nature of health care makes the requirement of providing individualized and unstandardized service to clients seem logical; however, it may be said that healthcare providers sometimes fail to treat the patient as an individual.

Pharmacists

The profession of pharmacy has experienced a marked transformation over the past 50 years. Today's pharmacists complete more years of formal education and are much more likely to complete postgraduate training and as a result, have abilities that many do not realize and many would have never imagined would be possible. Pharmacy practice is evolving from a profession whose primary responsibility was supervising the distribution of medications to one where its members are providing medication therapy management services and advising patients on disease prevention and management (Paolini & Rouse, 2010). A complete discussion of the historical development of the profession of pharmacy as well as the current practice philosophies, roles, and responsibilities will be presented in detail in Chapter 3; however, an appreciation of the nature of collaborative relationships between healthcare providers must begin with a rudimentary understanding of the background and characteristics of one's own profession—in this case, pharmacy.

Educational Requirements

Pharmacy education has experienced many changes since its inception. Early pharmacy practitioners in the United States were trained as apprentices of experienced apothecaries. After a few years of service in these types of arrangements, the apprentice graduated and was able to practice pharmacy (Sonnedecker, 1976).

Formal university-granting education in the pharmaceutical sciences began in the late 19th century; however, at the time, no state required a pharmacy degree to practice pharmacy. In 1910, the state of New York began requiring a diploma from a recognized pharmacy school, and as a result, several states followed suit (Mrtek, 1976). At that time, formal pharmacy education consisted of at least 2 years of university-based education resulting in a PhG degree (Higby, 1996). While most pharmacy schools provided the required 2 years of education, several more offered programs of 3 or even 4 years of length despite no legal or regulatory mandate to do so. A 3-year degree in pharmacy became the standard in 1925, the 4-year degree in 1932, and the 5-year degree in 1960 (Higby, 1996).

Today, a doctor of pharmacy (PharmD) is the minimum requirement for pharmacy licensure in all states. PharmD programs vary in length and structure among the various colleges/schools of pharmacy. While two years of preprofessional work is the minimum, some programs require three years of preprofessional education while others require a baccalaureate degree. Regardless of the length of the prepharmacy requirement, the final 4 years of education (or its equivalent) must be attained in a college/school of pharmacy (ACPE, 2014). Pharmacy education is a mix of didactic and experiential learning. Students spend the majority of their time in the earliest part of the curriculum in a classroom setting with some experiential learning interspersed. The later part of pharmacy curricula (typically the last year of the PharmD program) involves advanced pharmacy practice experiences exclusively. As of July 2015, there were 132 U.S.-based colleges and schools of pharmacy with accredited (full or candidate status) professional degree programs and an additional three schools with precandidate status (AACP, 2015).

To practice pharmacy in the United States, the District of Columbia, Guam, Puerto Rico or the U.S. Virgin Islands, one must possess a pharmacy license. Pharmacy licensure is predicated on the successful completion of the North American Pharmacist Licensure Examination (NAPLEX). The NAPLEX assesses whether a prospective pharmacist can identify practice standards for safe and effective pharmacotherapy and optimize therapeutic outcomes in patients, can identify and determine safe and accurate methods to prepare and dispense medications, and can provide and apply health care information to promote optimal health care (NABP, 2015d). In order to sit for this exam, one must have graduated from an accredited college/school of pharmacy, or, in the case of graduates from foreign schools of pharmacy, achieve a suitable score on the Foreign Pharmacy Equivalency Examination (FPGEE) (NABP, 2015a). In addition to the NAPLEX, new pharmacists must successfully complete the Multistate Pharmacy Jurisprudence Exam (MPJE) or a state-level equivalent law examination. The MPJE combines federal- and state-specific questions to test the pharmacy jurisprudence knowledge of prospective pharmacists (NABP, 2015b).

Postgraduate residencies and fellowships are available for pharmacists. A pharmacy residency is defined as "an organized, directed, postgraduate training program in a defined area of pharmacy practice"(ASHP, 1987, p. 1142) and lasts 12 months or longer. A fellowship "is a directed, highly individualized, postgraduate program designed to prepare the participant to become an independent researcher (ASHP, 1987, p. 1142). While residencies are available in both the first and second postgraduate years, a fellowship is usually sought by individuals with master's or doctoral degrees in a health science discipline (ACCP, 2004). Additionally, it is expected that the fellowship possess practice skills relevant to the fellowship; these skills may be garnered through a residency or through prior practice experience (ACCP, 2004; Kane-Gill, Reddy, Gupta, & Bakst, 2008). The match program associated with pharmacy residencies are handled by the American Society of Health-System Pharmacists (ASHP). Postgraduate year 1 (PGY1) residencies are designed to enhance the general competencies of the resident in managing medication-use systems, and as such it supports optimal medication therapy outcomes for patients with a broad range of disease states (ASHP, 2012a). Residencies usually are housed in hospitals; however, the number of PGY1 residencies in other areas of pharmacy practice (e.g., community pharmacies, home care and long-term care facilities, ambulatory care settings, managed care facilities, and others) has increased significantly over the last decade. The number of pharmacists seeking PGY1 residencies has increased steadily over the past few years (ASHP, 2015). Postgraduate year 2 (PGY2) residencies are available for those who have completed a PGY1 residency and are available in ambulatory care, cardiology, critical care, drug information, emergency medicine, geriatric pharmacy, health-system pharmacy administration, infectious diseases, informatics, internal medicine, medication-use safety, nuclear medicine, nutrition support pharmacy, oncology pharmacy, pain management and palliative care, pediatric pharmacy, pharmacotherapy, psychiatric pharmacy, and solid organ transplant (ASHP, 2012b).

Like medicine, there are varieties of specialties available for pharmacy practitioners; however, pharmacy is unique in that specialization is achieved after one is eligible to practice, not before. In pharmacy, practitioners have the ability to advance their abilities such that they can seek recognition of that training through specialization. The Board of Pharmacy Specialties (BPS) recognizes eight areas of pharmacy specialization, which are ambulatory care pharmacy, critical care pharmacy, nuclear pharmacy, nutrition support pharmacy, oncology pharmacy, pediatric pharmacy, psychiatric pharmacy, and pharmacotherapy (Board of Pharmacy Specialties, 2015a); the latter is available as a stand-alone specialty as well as with an added qualification in cardiology and infectious diseases (Board of Pharmacy Specialties, 2015b).

Practice Environment

In spite of many advances in pharmacy practice, pharmacists continue to have the distribution of medications to patients as a primary responsibility. Along with this responsibility, pharmacists serve as a valuable source of medication-related information for patients and healthcare providers. Overall, pharmacists spend nearly half (49%) of their time in medication dispensing, 21% in patient care services, 13% in business/organization management, 7% in education, 4% in research, and 6% in other activities (Midwest Pharmacy Workforce Research Consortium, 2015). These proportions vary significantly based on practice setting. Pharmacists in community pharmacies can be expected to spend at least 68% of their time in dispensing-related activities. Hospital pharmacists and those reported to be engaged in other patient care roles can expect to spend less than half (43%) of their time to medication dispensing. Both hospital pharmacists and pharmacists who described their setting as other patient care reported spending one-third and just over one-quarter of their time respectively on direct patient care activities (Midwest Pharmacy Workforce Research Consortium, 2015).

The number of licensed pharmacists has grown steadily over the last 10 years (**Figure 2-1**). In 2012, there were 286,400 licensed pharmacists working in the United States (U.S. BLS, 2014b). Pharmacists are employed in a variety of settings including community-based practice as well as institutional-based practice. The proportion of actively practicing pharmacists working in traditional community pharmacy practice settings (independent, chain, mass merchandiser, and supermarket pharmacies) decreased to 44.1% after being relatively stable since 2000 (~54%). (Midwest Pharmacy Workforce Research Consortium, 2015). About 82.3% of working pharmacists are reported to be working full-time (40+ hours per week) with an average of just over 44 hours per week (44.2 hours) (Midwest Pharmacy Workforce Research Consortium, 2015). The rate of part-time employment among active pharmacists decreased in 2014 (17.7%) after experiencing growth over the period between 2000 and 2009. The proportion of pharmacists employed part time was 18.7% for females and 16.4% for males.

In 1990, just under one third of all practicing pharmacists were women. Currently, women represent 57.1% of the pharmacy practitioners in the United States (Midwest Pharmacy Workforce Research Consortium, 2015). Minorities continue to be underrepresented in the pharmacy workforce. Census estimates in 2008 indicated that 25% of the U.S. population identified with a racial minority group; however, only 18% of pharmacists are reported to be a member of a racial minority

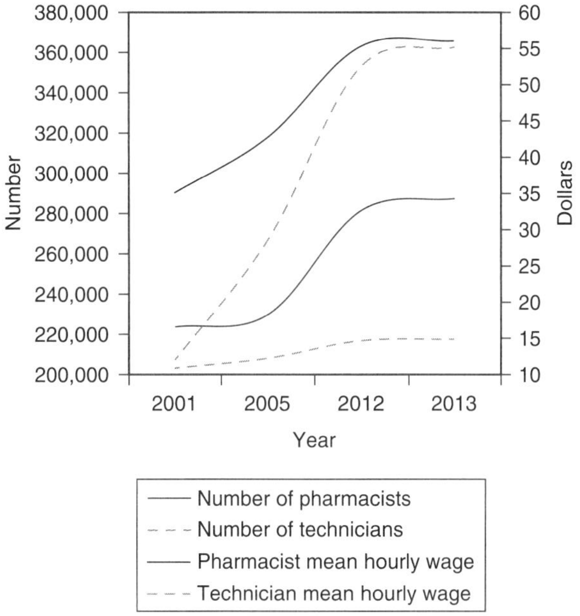

Figure 2-1 Pharmacy Staff and Mean Hourly Wage.

Source: National Center for Health Statistics. (2010). *Health, United States, 2009: With special feature on medical technology*. Hyattsville, MD: National Center for Health Statistics.

group (HRSA Bureau of Health Professions, 2008). This difference is even more dramatic when one considers Hispanic or Latino population. While the U.S. population is over 15% Hispanic or Latino, only 3.2% of the U.S. pharmacist population is Hispanic or Latino (HRSA, 2008).

The supply of pharmacists is expected to be adequate to meet the demand for the foreseeable future. Despite an expected increase in demand for pharmaceuticals due in part to growth in the elderly population, the passage and implementation of the Affordable Care Act, and increases in science such that new therapies are available, it is expected that the pharmacist supply will keep pace and even exceed demand by 2025 (HRSA, 2012).

Pharmacy Technicians

The presence of pharmacy technicians is commonplace in institutional and retail pharmacy settings. In fact, as pharmacy continues its progress toward more involvement in direct patient care, pharmacy technicians will play an important role by freeing the pharmacist from some of his or her distributive tasks in favor of contemporary pharmacy practice roles (ASHP, 2003). The modern-day pharmacy technician in the United States grew out of the efforts of the U.S. Army to develop pharmacy specialists who could assist pharmacists with the preparation and distribution of medications to soldiers (Council on Credentialing in Pharmacy, 2003). The focus on pharmacy technicians increased in the late 1960s partly due to a call by the federal government for the development of a pharmacist aide curriculum in junior colleges and other educational institutions (Council on Credentialing in Pharmacy, 2003). Today, pharmacy technicians "help licensed pharmacists prepare prescription medications, provide customer service, and perform administrative duties within a variety of practice settings, including community, health-system, and federal pharmacy. They are generally responsible for receiving prescription requests, counting tablets, labeling bottles, maintaining patient profiles, preparing insurance claim forms, and performing administrative functions such as answering phones, stocking shelves, and operating cash registers (Pharmacy Technician Certification Board, 2014).

Educational Requirements

State level requirements for pharmacy technicians vary greatly. Some states have established age minimums, as well as educational minimums, such as a high school diploma or its equivalent (U.S. BLS, 2014c), while others have instituted training requirements for pharmacy technicians. Currently, 45 states regulate pharmacy technicians in some manner (certification, licensure, or registration) (PTCB, 2015a). Of the 50 states, the District of Columbia, Puerto Rico, and Guam, 37 government bodies have established technician training requirements (NABP, 2014); however, it is generally recognized that there is little uniformity among states regarding pharmacy technician education and training requirements (NABP, 2014). In addition to initial training and education, some states (21) are requiring pharmacy technicians earn continuing education credits (NABP, 2014). This requirement varies greatly in number of hours and to whom the requirement applies. While it may be true that some states do not require technician training, it is not appropriate to conclude that pharmacy technicians in these states do not seek or receive training; it is common that pharmacy technicians receive, at least, on-the-job training (U.S. BLS, 2014c).

National certification examinations are available from the Pharmacy Technician Certification Board and the Institute for the Certification of Pharmacy Technicians. Each of these bodies requires that candidates have a high school diploma or equivalent and no felony convictions or previous revocation of state certification or licensure (pharmacy or from another healthcare board). The certification examinations cover a broad range of topics related to aspects of pharmacy technician practice. For example, the Pharmacy Technician Certification Examination (PTCE) covers nine knowledge domains. These domains and the percentage of content on the PTCE are pharmacology for technicians (13.75%), pharmacy law and regulations (12.50%), sterile and nonsterile compounding (8.75%), medication safety (12.50%), pharmacy quality assurance (7.50%), medication order entry and fill process (17.50%), pharmacy inventory management (8.75%), pharmacy billing and reimbursement (8.75%), and pharmacy information systems usage and application (10.00%)(PTCB, 2015b).

Practice Environment

The number of pharmacy technicians has increased dramatically since 1999 (Figure 2-1). It is estimated that in 2012, there were 355,300 active pharmacy technicians (U.S. BLS, 2010c). Pharmacy technicians work in a variety of settings (e.g., community pharmacies, hospitals, branches of the military, and mail order pharmacies); however, most (~72%) are employed by retail pharmacies (U.S. BLS, 2014c).

Pharmacy technicians assist pharmacists in the preparation of prescription medications (e.g., computer entry, counting medications, and labeling prescription bottles), assisting customers, and performing administrative duties within the pharmacy (e.g., record keeping, insurance claims, and prescription inventory control). Activities that explicitly would be prohibited include at a minimum, drug regimen review, clinical conflict resolution, prescriber contact concerning prescription drug order clarification or therapy modification, patient counseling, dispensing process validation, prescription transfer, and the receipt of new prescription drug orders (NABP, 2015c).

While there exists a general understanding of the nature and scope of pharmacy technician practice, the specific duties that are able to be performed by pharmacy technicians vary by state and practice setting (e.g., retail versus institutional practice) (NABP, 2014). Each of the aforementioned duties of the pharmacy technician is performed under the direct supervision of a licensed pharmacist.

Physicians

Physicians have been the professional exemplar in health care. Physicians are concerned primarily with maintaining or restoring the health of their patients through the diagnosis and treatment of disease or injury. For pharmacy, the physician holds an important position. The physician is the healthcare provider who prescribes the most and as such, creates a great deal of demand for pharmacy products and services.

Educational Requirements

Prior to the start of the 20th century, physician education was varied. The earliest medical practitioners in what would become the United States attended informal classes and demonstrations (primarily anatomy) (Flexner, 1910). Formal medical education began in 1765, when it was proposed that a professorship in the theory and practice of medicine be established at the College of Philadelphia (Flexner, 1910). This early education focused on didactic training; however, the realization that medical education required practicum came very quickly. In fact, the earliest formal medical education resembles modern-day medical education, namely a combination of didactic and experiential learning. Over the course of some 150 years, medical education evolved such that physicians were being trained in one of three ways, an apprenticeship system, a proprietary schools system, or a university system (Beck, 2004). As a result, many of the turn-of-the-20th-century physicians were ill equipped to provide patient care.

A major turning point in medical education in the United States was the publication of the Flexner report. In 1908, at the request of the American Medical Association (AMA), a survey of medical education was undertaken; the result of this effort was the Flexner report. The report served as a major indictment of the so-called proprietary schools. Flexner, like the AMA, believed that these schools operated more for profit than for education. The report found that these schools had loose admission standards, inadequate faculty, insufficient laboratory experiences, and poor apprenticeship programs. This report made recommendations that included minimum educational standards for admission to medical schools, a minimum length of medical school education of 4 years, and the closure (or combination with universities) of the proprietary medical schools that existed at the time (Flexner, 1910).

As a result, many medical schools closed their doors, and those that remained changed such that they met these new standards. It is interesting to find that many aspects of the present-day American medical profession and its educational processes are a direct result of the publication of the Flexner report. There is no one premedical curriculum for aspiring doctors. Medical school admissions policies should encourage "potential applicants to the medical education program to acquire a broad undergraduate education that includes the study of the humanities, natural sciences, and social sciences, and confines its specific premedical course requirements to those deemed essential preparation for successful completion of its medical curriculum" (LCME, 2015). Today, medical education in the United States is a postbaccalaureate program that begins with 2 years of didactic study (M1 & M2) in the sciences (experiential learning is present to a lesser degree in the first 2 years of medical education) in an accredited medical school (preclinical education). During this didactic phase, it is expected that medical curricula will include biomedical, behavioral, and social sciences, organ systems/life cycle/primary care/prevention/wellness/symptoms/signs/differential diagnosis, treatment planning, impact of behavioral and social factors, scientific method/clinical /translational research, critical judgment/problem-solving skills, societal problems, cultural competence and health-care disparities, medical ethics, communication skills, and interprofessional collaborative skills (LCME, 2015). Following their didactic education, medical students (M3 & M4) begin their clerkship training. Clerkship training during these clinical years of education includes required rotations (e.g., internal medicine, surgery, pediatrics, psychiatry, obstetrics and gynecology, family medicine, and neurology) and elective rotations. With few exceptions, these 4 years of medical school are similar for all physicians. In 2015, there were 145 accredited, medical doctorate- (MD-) granting medical schools in the United States (AAMC, 2015).

An alternative educational opportunity for those interested in practicing medicine is the doctor of osteopathic medicine (DO) degree. In the United States, osteopathic medical schools have curricula that are similar to allopathic (MD-granting) medical schools. Unlike allopathic medical schools, osteopathic medical education emphasizes hands-on diagnosis and treatment through a system of therapy known as osteopathic manipulative medicine (AACOM, 2015b). Additionally, advocates of osteopathic medicine point to a focus on health promotion and disease prevention in their curricula, although this is also part of allopathic medical education as well. Currently, there are 31 osteopathic medical schools in the United States (AACOM, 2015a).

Regardless of one's type of medical degree, medical licensure in the United States involves a three-step examination process (NBOME, 2015, USMLE, 2015). Medical students and graduates complete the United States Medical Licensing Examination (USMLE) and students and graduates of osteopathic medicine schools complete the Comprehensive Osteopathic Medical Licensing Examination (COMLEX). The step 1 (level 1) examination is taken typically during the second year of medical school. It assesses a student's understanding of and ability to apply scientific concepts to the practice of medicine. Specifically, areas covered on the exam include anatomy, behavioral sciences, biochemistry, microbiology, pathology, pharmacology, and physiology. The COMLEX also includes osteopathic principles. Step 2 (level 2) exams are divided into two parts. The first part of the exam assesses clinical knowledge while the second part of the exam assesses clinical skill. The clinical knowledge examination assesses internal medicine, obstetrics and gynecology, pediatrics, preventive medicine, psychiatry, and surgery. The examination also includes emergency medicine, family medicine, and osteopathic principles. Interestingly, the assessment of clinical skills is accomplished through the use of standardized patients. Because of this fact, sites for the clinical skills exams are limited; there are five testing centers for the USMLE (Atlanta, Chicago, Houston, Los Angeles, and Philadelphia) and one for the COMLEX (Conshohocken, Pennsylvania). The step 3 (level 3) exam is taken typically at the end of the first year of residency and is designed to assess a graduate's (resident's) suitability for unsupervised medical practice.

While some states allow medical school graduates to become fully licensed after a 1-year postgraduate internship, most seek a residency (FSMB, 2015). A residency is a stage of graduate medical training that allows the resident to practice medicine for a prescribed period of time under the supervision of fully licensed physicians. Most residencies require three years of training (general surgery is five years) (AMA, 2015b). Residents may enter a residency following the completion of an internship, or the internship might be incorporated into the residency program. Fellowship positions in subspecialties are available for physicians having already completed a residency.

Medical students begin the process of deciding their career direction during the M4 year. In addition to selecting their preferred sites for residency, medical students are selecting their preference for specialization. The process for selecting medical residencies is similar to that for pharmacy residencies; the student will list preferred sites and the residency sites will rank their preference for students (along with the number of residents they can house). If the process works as it is intended, students will be placed in residencies where they were a desired candidate. This process is referred to as matching. The National Resident Matching Program handles this process for residencies and fellowships (NRMP, 2015).

Medical specialty certification in the United States is a voluntary process. While medical licensure continues to be the minimum requirement to be a physician in the United States, the licensure examination is not specialty specific. Board certification signifies that a physician possesses expertise in a specialty and/or subspecialty of medical practice. The American Board of Medical Specialties is the umbrella organization of 24 member boards that offer certification in more than 150 specialties and subspecialties (ABMS, 2015). In addition to the American Board of Medical Specialties, the American Board of Physician Specialties oversees 12 medical specialty boards of certification representing 18 medical specialties (ABPS, 2015). The American Osteopathic Association Bureau of Osteopathic Specialists offers certification in any of 18 specialty areas to doctors of osteopathic medicine (AOA, 2015).

Continuing medical education is required by 57 of 62 medical boards (AMA, 2014). The number of hours needed varies by state with the majority requiring between 20 and 50 hours per year (AMA, 2014). Additionally, some states require specific continuing medical education content each license cycle (e.g., error prevention, infection control) while some states accept certificates/awards (e.g., those from the American Osteopathic Association and the American Board of Medical Specialties) as documentation of continued competence (AMA, 2014).

Practice Environment

There has been a steady increase over the years in the number of physicians practicing in the United States (**Figure 2-2**).

Despite this increase, there continues to be fears that the rate of increase has not kept pace with the rate of increase in the U.S. population. Additionally, there are concerns that because of population aging and population growth (as well as the estimated expansion of health insurance coverage as a result of the full implementation of the Affordable Care Act), there may be an even greater shortage (hyper-demand) of physicians; this increased demand is estimated to be 18% by 2020 over 2010 (HRSA, 2013). This concern applies especially to primary care (**Figure 2-3**). While the number of primary care providers has increased dramatically, the largest increases in primary care providers was seen in nurse practitioners and physician assistants. The increase in the number of physicians in primary care is the result of foreign medical graduates (GAO, 2008). Specialists and subspecialists can and do provide primary care to their patients; however, the trend toward more specialists

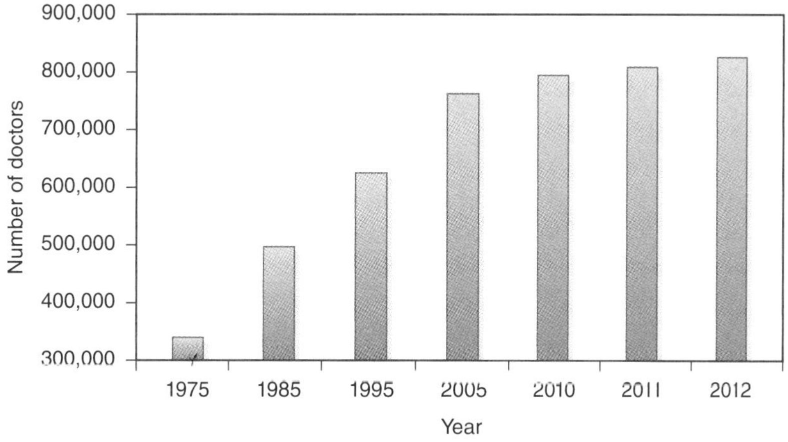

Figure 2-2 Active Doctors of Medicine.

Source: National Center for Health Statistics. (2010). *Health, United States, 2009: With special feature on medical technology*. Hyattsville, MD: National Center for Health Statistics.

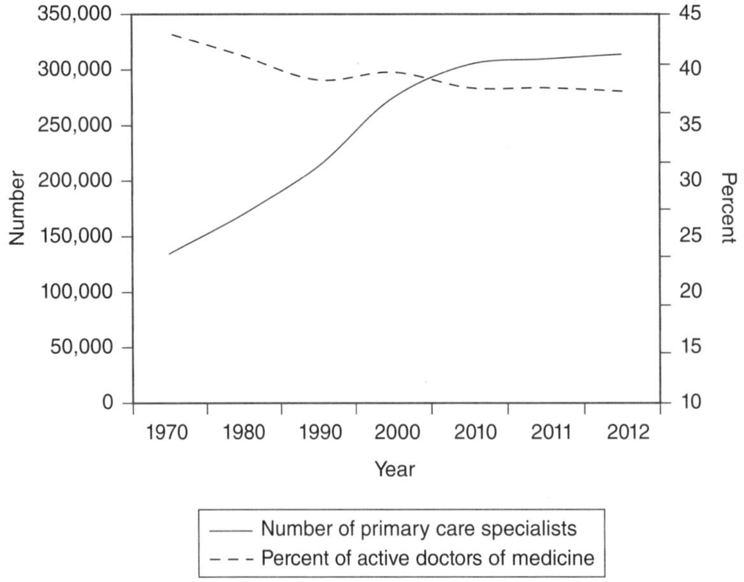

Figure 2-3 Doctors of Medicine in General Primary Care.

Source: National Center for Health Statistics. (2010). *Health, United States, 2009: With special feature on medical technology*. Hyattsville, MD: National Center for Health Statistics.

and less primary care does have implications for the future of the practice of pharmacy. As a result of increased demand for primary care, pharmacists may have an increased role in meeting the needs of patients by fulfilling their responsibilities to provide patient-centered care and, in states where it is allowed, through their expanded responsibilities in collaborative drug therapy management (ASHP, 1999).

Representation of females among the physician ranks continues to increase. In 1990, women represented only 16.9% of the physician workforce; in 2013, women accounted for 31.9% of the total physician population (AMA, 2015a). Census estimates in 2010 indicated that just under 25% of the U.S. population identified with a racial minority group (US Census Bureau, 2010); however, just over 20.6% of physicians are reported to be a member of a racial minority group (AAMC, 2014). Of that percentage, 4.1% were Black or African American, 4.4% were Hispanic or Latino, 0.4% were American Indian or Alaska Native, and 11.7% were Asian (AAMC, 2014).

Nurses

Nursing represents the largest of all of the healthcare occupations. According to the American Nursing Association, nursing is "the protection, promotion, and optimization of health and abilities, prevention of illness and injury, alleviation of suffering through the diagnosis and treatment of human response, and advocacy in the care of individuals, families, communities, and populations" (ANA, 2015a). As this definition would imply, currently, there are many different types of nurses. The two different entry-level types of nurses are the registered nurse (RN) and licensed vocational/practical nurse (LPN). The RN is the more advanced of the two nursing designations owing to the requirements for more education. As a result, the scope of practice for the RN is broader than that for the LPN. Oftentimes, the LPN works under the supervision of a RN. In addition to the LPN and RN, nurses have the opportunities for advanced practice roles. The nurse practitioner, clinical nurse specialist, certified RN anesthetist, and certified nurse midwife are all designations used by advanced practice nurses (APNs). These practitioners have at least a master's degree and clinical practice requirements beyond that required of all RNs (ANA, 2015b). Moreover, these APNs have prescriptive authority in most jurisdictions, and in some jurisdictions, APNs may practice independently without physician collaboration or supervision.

Educational Requirements

The educational requirements for the RN and LPN differ in scope and length. Becoming an LPN usually requires 1 year of study resulting in the issue of a diploma or certificate. The requisite education for RNs is as diverse as the career opportunities in nursing. There are three recognized educational pathways for those interested in being RNs; these are a bachelor's degree, an associate's degree, or a diploma from an approved nursing program. Nurses most commonly enter the occupation by completing an associate degree or bachelor's degree program. Prior to entering practice, graduate nurses must successfully complete the National Council Licensure Examination (NCLEX). The NCLEX is recognized by boards of nursing in all 50 states and U.S. territories. The NCLEX is divided into two separate exams; the NCLEX-RN is for RNs and the NCLEX-PN for vocational/practical nurses. While there are different examinations for RNs and for vocational/practical nurses, there is not a separate NCLEX-RN examination or passing standard for associate degree, baccalaureate degree, or diploma nursing school graduates (NCSBN, 2015b). Similar to other health professions, nurses have the opportunities to specialize in any of a number of areas of nursing practice. Certification programs are available for RNs in over 20 different areas, such as ambulatory care nursing, general nursing practice, pediatric nursing, and psychiatric-mental health nursing (ANCC, 2015).

APN designations require additional education above and beyond that required for licensure as an RN. APNs have at least 2 years of graduate education (e.g., master's degree); however, a new standard for qualification as an APN, the doctor of nursing practice was advocated for and is appearing as an educational option in 264 programs in 48 states and territories (AACN, 2015). The doctor of nursing practice is an advanced-level practice degree that focuses on the clinical aspects of nursing (e.g., evidence-based practice, quality improvement, and systems leadership) rather than academic research (contrast PhD in nursing) (AACN, 2015). APNs are licensed through their respective state boards of nursing separate from RNs and LPNs. In addition to being licensed as RNs, APNs are required in some states to submit evidence of advanced education as well as evidence of certification through organizations such as the American Nurses Credentialing Center, the American Academy of Nurse Practitioners, or others (NCSBN, 2015a).

The requirements for evidence of continued competence differs across states and across nurse type. Currently, 77% of states and jurisdictions require continuing competence for nurses (NCSBN, 2015c). The continued competence requirements include but are not limited to continuing education, minimal practice hours, peer review, periodic refresher courses, continued competency assessment, and competency examinations. Currently, the majority of states require some type of continued competence for APNs. The requirements vary by state and APN designation, but can include recertification, continuing education beyond that required for the basic RN license, practice requirements, and pharmacology course work (or pharmacology continuing education credits) (NCSBN, 2015b).

Practice Environment

There were estimated to be 738,400 LPNs in the United Stated in 2012 (U.S. BLS, 2014a). LPNs work nights, weekends, and holidays depending on the setting in which they are employed. LPNs often assist patients with activities of daily living. As such, LPNs are often employed by nursing homes, home health care, and hospice, as well as office-based practices of physicians and hospitals. The roles that LPNs can fulfill vary by state. In 2012, there were estimated to be between 2.7 and 2.9 million licensed RNs in the United States (HRSA Bureau of Health Professions, 2014; U.S. BLS, 2014e). The percentage of RNs whose initial nursing education was an associate's degree was 45.4, that of a baccalaureate degree was 34.2, and a diploma in nursing, 20.4. Nurses with advanced degrees comprised 13.2% of all licensed RNs (HRSA, 2010). The majority of nurses (62.2%) work in the hospital setting (HRSA, 2010). Other notable employment opportunities for RNs exist within ambulatory care (10.5%) and public health (7.8%). Currently, minorities are underrepresented in the nursing population. Approximately 17% of RNs are reported to be a member of a minority group. While Asians are slightly overrepresented, blacks, Hispanics, and American Indians/Alaska Natives are underrepresented in comparison to population statistics. Nursing continues to be a female-dominated profession, with only 6% of RNs reported to be male. APNs work in a variety of healthcare settings. The level of practice independence and prescriptive authority differs by state (independent practice, collaborative agreements/protocols, or practice under physician supervision) and APN designation (e.g., nurse practitioner, clinical nurse specialist, certified nurse midwife, and certified nurse anesthetist) (NCSBN, 2015a).

Physician Assistants

Physician assistants' (PA) role in the health system is unique in that these providers practice medicine in a team environment under the direction of a physician. As part of their comprehensive responsibilities, PAs take medical histories, conduct physical exams, diagnose and treat illnesses, order and interpret tests, develop treatment plans, counsel on preventive health care, assist in surgery, prescribe medications, and make rounds in hospital and skilled nursing facilities (AAPA, 2015). However, the specific duties of PAs are determined by the supervising physician and by state law (U.S. BLS, 2014d).

Educational Requirements

PA programs began in the 1960s as an effort to address the need for assistants for physicians who would work only with physician supervision. The first program devoted to the education of PAs was located at the Duke University School of Medicine (Jones, 2007). As other programs have developed, each has adhered to the basic tenets that a PA would not have independent authority and the curriculum would be competency based (Jones, 2007). Today, PAs are educated in programs that are accredited by the Accreditation Review Commission on Education for the Physician Assistant (ARC-PA). These programs are housed in community colleges as well as 4-year colleges and universities (Jones, 2007). Regardless of its location, the PA curriculum averages 26 months. PAs are trained to diagnose and treat medical problems. As such, the PA curriculum consists of didactic instruction in the basic medical and behavioral sciences as well as experiential learning. Clinical rotations are used in the later portions of PA education. Currently, there are 200 accredited PA programs in the United States (ARC-PA, 2015). Like many other healthcare workers, PAs are required to complete continuing medical education (100 hours every 2 years). Additionally, PAs are retested on their clinical skills on a regular basis (every 6 years) (NCCPA, 2010).

Practice Environment

In 2012, there were over 86,000 PAs in the United States (U.S. BLS, 2014d). The largest percentage of clinically practicing PAs work in primary care (32%), followed by surgical subspecialties (27.0%), emergency medicine (11.0%), and internal medicine subspecialties (10.0%) (AAPA, 2014). The greatest percentage of PAs report being employed in a group medical practice (27.9 %).

Almost one-quarter of all clinically practicing PAs are employed in hospitals, and 11.6% in solo physician practices. The majority of PAs (65%) are female and a predominant percentage (88.9%) is white. Minorities are underrepresented among the ranks of PAs with 3.9% Asian, 2.9% black, 3.6% Hispanic/Latino, and 0.6% American Indian/Alaska Native (AAPA, 2014).

Other Allied Health Professionals

Table 2-1 provides a list of additional healthcare professionals pharmacists may interact with in their patient care activities.

Table 2-1 Other Allied Health Professionals

Occupation	Education	Degree(s)	Roles
Optometrists	7–9 yrs	OD	Optometrists are the primary providers of vision care. They examine eyes to diagnose vision problems, and prescribe eyeglasses and contact lenses. They diagnose diseases of the eye (e.g., glaucoma) and may have limited prescriptive authority.
Social workers	4–6 yrs	BSW, MSW	Social workers assist people by helping them cope with and solve issues in their everyday lives, such as family and personal problems and dealing with relationships. Some social workers help clients who face a disability, life-threatening disease, or a social problem, such as inadequate housing, unemployment, or substance abuse. Social workers also assist families that have serious domestic conflicts, sometimes involving child or spousal abuse.
Podiatrists	9 yrs	DPM	Podiatrists diagnose and treat disorders, diseases, and injuries of the foot and lower leg. They may prescribe medications, perform physical therapy, fit orthotics, set fractures, and perform surgery.

(Continues)

Table 2-1 Other Allied Health Professionals (continued)

Occupation	Education	Degree(s)	Roles
Dentists	6–10 yrs	DDS, DMD	Dentists diagnose and treat problems with teeth and tissues in the mouth. They may prescribe medications, perform surgery, and extract teeth.
Psychologists	6+ yrs	Specialist, MS, PhD, PsyD	Psychologists assess, diagnose, treat, and prevent mental disorders. They advise people on how to deal with problems of everyday living, including problems in the home, place of work, or community, to help improve their quality of life.
Dieticians/ nutritionists	4 yrs	BS, MS	Dietitians and nutritionists plan food and nutrition programs, supervise meal preparation, and oversee the serving of meals. Illness prevention activities occur by promoting healthy eating habits and recommending dietary modifications.
Occupational therapists	4–6 yrs	MS	Occupational therapists help patients improve their ability to perform tasks in living and working environments. They work with individuals who suffer from a mentally, physically, developmentally, or emotionally disabling condition. The goal is to help clients have independent, productive, and satisfying lives.
Recreational therapists	4 years	BS	Recreational therapists provide activities (arts and crafts, interaction with animals, sports, games, dance and movement, drama, music, and community outings) for individuals with disabilities or illnesses to improve and maintain their physical, mental, and emotional well-being.

Table 2-1 Other Allied Health Professionals (continued)

Occupation	Education	Degree(s)	Roles
Physical therapists	4+ yrs	MS, DPT	Physical therapists work with patients who have limitations in their ability to move and perform functional activities. They examine patients and develop a plan using treatment techniques designed to promote the ability to move, reduce pain, restore function, and prevent disability.

Source: Data from U.S. Bureau of Labor Statistics. (2014). *Occupational Outlook Handbook* (2014–2015 ed.). Retrieved from http://www.bls.gov/oco/

COLLABORATION WITH HEALTHCARE PROVIDERS

The primary role of the pharmacist is largely focused around medication consumption (e.g., to screen for contraindications and drug–drug interactions, to serve as the physician's resource for information about medical therapies, and to provide patient education about medications) (Peterson et al., 2008). For high-risk disease states, pharmacists can play an ever more important role as a part of the medication management team. For example, the inclusion of a pharmacist on the multidisciplinary cardiovascular team was found to decrease medication-related errors dramatically. One research study demonstrated that when a pharmacist rounded with the intensive care unit team, there was a 66% decrease in the rate of preventable adverse drug events (Leape et al., 1999). Translated into dollars, another study found that the inclusion of pharmacists in surgical wards resulted in $7.00 of savings for every $1.00 invested (Nevelle et al., 2014). The role of a pharmacist on a team was further cemented when LaPointe and Jollis (2003) found that over a 5-year period, a clinical pharmacist on the cardiology ward identified and corrected a significant number of medication errors (24 errors per 100 admissions). This same study also found the most common point of error occurred in the transition from the outpatient to the inpatient setting, underlining the importance for continuity of care and communication between practitioners within different organizations. Furthermore, pharmacy-led interventions have been shown to improve medication compliance in hospitalized, heart failure and postmyocardial infarction patients (Bouvy et al., 2003). Reductions in all-cause hospitalizations and medical costs as well as improved survival rates have been observed when a multidisciplinary team is engaged in patient care (Peterson et al., 2008).

In today's healthcare environment, there exists a call to increase both the safety and quality of services provided; this call expressly includes medication therapy. The complexity of the healthcare system makes it very difficult for one provider to be all things to all patients; in fact, many of the discussions surrounding patient safety and healthcare quality specifically mention the use of teams of healthcare providers (IOM, 1990). In order for a pharmacist to participate effectively as a team member, he or she needs to have a fundamental understanding of his or her healthcare colleagues as well as the nuances of collaborating with other healthcare providers.

Interdisciplinary Care versus Multidisciplinary Care

The various healthcare professionals bring much expertise to the service of the patient. However, an important distinction must be made between the types of relationships that may exist between the different healthcare providers, such as between multidisciplinary care and interdisciplinary care (Jessup, 2007). *Multidisciplinary care* refers to many different professionals working for the good of the patient, albeit somewhat independently. The typical model of health care in the United States is replete with examples of multidisciplinary care. For example, a patient visiting a physician's office for an illness will likely interact with a nurse who may collect information about the patient's condition, a physician who may diagnose a disease and prescribe a treatment, and after a trip to the pharmacy, a pharmacist who will dispense the medication and educate the patient on its appropriate use. While this model of care is generally recognized to lead to an improvement in outcomes, it does not take full advantage of the talents of the healthcare system. It is, at worst, a sum of the inputs from the various healthcare professionals. *Interdisciplinary care* means that the many different professionals working together for the patient's good also communicate effectively among themselves and with the patient. Teams with greater cohesiveness are associated with better communication, improved outcomes, decreased length of stay, and improved patient (and staff) satisfaction (Epstein, 2014).

While the importance of collaboration should not be underestimated, neither should the challenges that one faces when trying to establish collaborative relationships. Common barriers to the establishment of collaborative working relationships include boundary concerns, poor communication, power concerns, lack of trust of the other party, and poor proximity. Some of these barriers are as a result of teaching health professional students in "silos" and their limited knowledge of other professionals' skills, as well as interaction with them during the formative stages of their careers, more specifically, interaction during their formal professional education. To encourage the incorporation of interprofessional education in health profession education, the Interprofessional Education Collaborative (IPEC) was formed (Interprofessional Education Collaborative Expert Panel, 2011; Josiah Macy Foundation, ABIM Foundation, & Robert Wood Johnson Foundation, 2011). IPEC consists of representatives from the American Association of Schools of Nursing, American Association of Colleges of Osteopathic Medicine, American Association of Colleges of Pharmacy, American Dental Education Association, Association of American Medical Colleges, and Association of Schools of Public Health. This group developed a core set of competencies to ensure students had the requisite skills needed to participate effectively in team-based care. These competencies include:

1. Values/ethics of interprofessional practice
   - Act with honesty and integrity in relationships with patients, families, and other team members
   - Respect the dignity and privacy of patients while maintaining confidentiality in the delivery of team-based care
2. Roles/responsibilities for collaborative practice
   - Communicate one's role and responsibilities clearly to patients, families, and other professions
   - Explain the role and responsibilities of other care providers and how the team works together to provide care
3. Interprofessional communication
   - Choose effective communication tools and techniques, including information systems and communication technologies, for facilitating discussions and interactions that enhance team function
   - Give timely, sensitive, instructive feedback to others about their performance on the team and respond respectfully as a team member to feedback from others

4. Interprofessional teamwork and team-based care
   - Engage other health professions—appropriate to the specific care situation—in shared patient-centered problem solving
   - Reflect on both individual and team performance improvement (Macy Foundation, et al., 2011)

The collaborative working relationship model (McDonough & Doucette, 2001) describes the process by which pharmacists can establish effective and productive working relationships (**Figure 2-4**). This stage model posits that pharmacists' and physicians' relationships mature as the trust, shared decision making, and interdependence between the two providers develops.

Stage 0, *professional awareness,* would best be described as the traditional pharmacist–physician working relationship. At this stage, exchanges between the pharmacist and physician are discrete and minimal. For example, a stage 0 relationship would be characterized by the pharmacist seeking refill authorization, alerting the physician to a potential or actual drug-related problem (e.g., drug–drug interaction), or discussing some other pharmacotherapy-related issue that revealed itself during dispensing. According to the model, these interactions are short in duration with no attempt to change the existing relationship. Moreover, stage 0 interactions "are considered professionally safe, routine, and defined by well-established expectations" (Brock & Doucette, 2004, p. 359).

Stage 1, *professional recognition,* involves exclusively the pharmacist's effort to establish a relationship with the physician. In stage 1, the pharmacist informs the physician of the services that

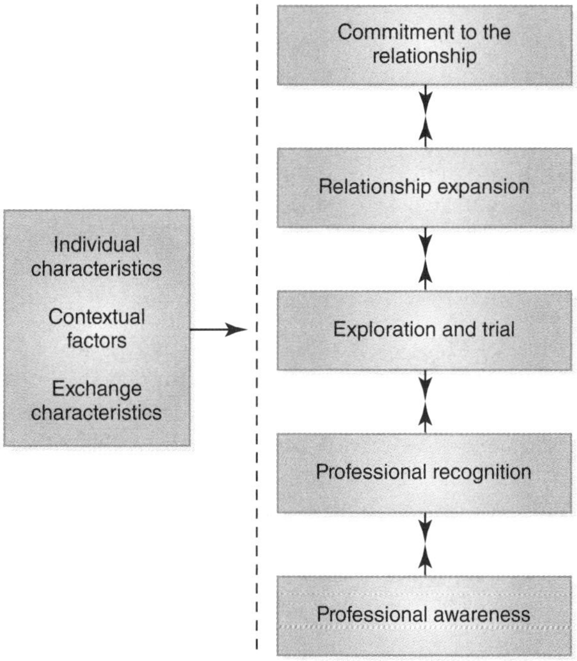

Figure 2-4 Model of Pharmacist Collaborative Working Relationships.

Source: Data from Brock, K. A., & Doucette, W. R. (2004). Collaborative working relationships between pharmacists and physicians: An exploratory study. *Journal of the American Pharmaceutical Association, 44*(3), 358–365.

the pharmacist can provide. This is an important step in the establishment of the collaborative relationship because the pharmacist's role definitions and role boundaries have been established by past experiences that the physician has had with pharmacists, including the one attempting to establish a collaborative working relationship (stage 0). The goal of this state in the model would be trust. Pharmacists are working to enhance their own attractiveness or usefulness to the physician during stage 1 interactions (Brock & Doucette, 2004). A thorough understanding of the pharmacist role on the healthcare team is imperative to its success. When the pharmacist's role is clear and understood by other members of the healthcare team, the pharmacist will feel engaged in patient care and team activities; when the pharmacist's role was unclear, unknown, misunderstood, or not valued, the pharmacist and other healthcare team members may experience challenges (Makowsky et al., 2009).

Stage 2, *exploration and trial,* requires some low level of commitment on the part of the physician above and beyond what has been demonstrated in the first two stages; however, the pharmacist remains the primary initiator of interaction. The trial may involve the physician referring a patient or a few patients so that he or she can assess the pharmacist's ability to deliver both the quantity of services as well as the quality of the services as promised and the risks and benefits associated with being involved in the collaborative relationship.

Stage 3, *professional relationship expansion,* is the natural progression of activities undertaken in stages 1 and 2. In stage 3, the pharmacist can expect that the physician initiates the exchange; however, the pharmacist can expect that the exchange efforts remain unbalanced (the pharmacist still has more responsibility as an initiator). The content of pharmacist-initiated communication continues to center on the benefits derived from the pharmacist's services as well as seeking feedback on past performance. This give-and-take exchange represents some level of commitment on the part of the physician toward the collaborative relationship; however, the pharmacist can and should expect that professional conflict will occur in this fine-tuning of the relationship.

Stage 4, *commitment to a collaborative working relationship,* is achieved when the physician is convinced that the benefits of the collaborative relationship outweigh any risks. For commitment in a relationship to exist, at the very least, the relationship needs to be relatively lengthy, consistent, and should involve a high level of input from all parties (Brock & Doucette, 2004). Commitment is most likely to be reached if there is equity in effort toward maintaining the relationship. Additionally, once commitment is achieved, work remains to be done. Failure to attend to the relationship by both parties may lead to its demise. In other words, a collaborative working relationship is a relationship in every sense of the word. Unlike earlier stages of the model, the pharmacist cannot be the sole source of relationship effort; the physician must also attend to the relationship's needs.

The success of efforts or the rapidity with which relationships are established will depend on the individuals involved. Factors found to positively influence the development of the pharmacist–physician collaboration were trustworthiness, role specification, relationship initiation, and professional interactions (Doucette, Nevins, & McDonough, 2005; Zillich, McDonough, Carter, & Doucette, 2004). As such, pharmacists must provide services that are valued by the physician and deliver on all promises made. Moreover, both parties must recognize the complementary roles of the pharmacist and physician that may result in interdependence. Lastly, frequent and meaningful interactions are important to sustain the collaborative working relationship. If the pharmacist is out of sight (or out of touch), he or she is out of mind, and there is no collaboration.

Continuity of Care

Consistent with the ideals of interdisciplinary care and collaborative work relationships is continuity of care. The days are long gone when one doctor, with the help of a nurse, provided all the health care a person needed. Now, it is not uncommon for patients to see several healthcare practitioners. They may receive care from doctors, nurses, nurse practitioners, physician assistants, pharmacists, dietitians, physical or occupational therapists, social workers, and nurse's aides. They may have several doctors, each specializing in one organ system or disease. To complicate matters, as people age they are also likely to move from one place of care to another. They may receive care in a doctor's office, hospital, rehabilitation facility, board-and-care facility, an assisted living facility, nursing home, or at home. At the end of life, they may receive hospice care. Ideally, all people involved in a person's health care, including the person receiving care, communicate and work with each other to coordinate the health care. Additionally, all interested parties (at least patient and providers) should agree on and understand the goals for health care. Then, changes in practitioners and places of care could occur smoothly, lessening the impact of care disruption. Two core concepts or aspirations of continuity are revealed by the preceding definitions. First, continuity is about the care of a single patient. As such, continuity is *not* an attribute of providers or organizations (Haggerty et al., 2003). The second element is that care is provided over time. When taken together these core elements represent a continuous care relationship, a laudable goal in health care.

Whether continuity of care represents a process or outcome remains unsettled (Christakis, 2003). Perhaps it is both, a means to an end and an end itself that can then be used similar to other intermediate outcomes in determining quality of care. However, regardless of the type of study, three types of continuity are recognized: (1) informational continuity, (2) management continuity, and (3) relational continuity. Informational continuity is considered by some to be the *sine qua non* in continuity of care; "it is the common thread linking care from one provider to another and from one healthcare event to another" (Haggerty et al., 2003, p. 1220). Information tends to center on the medical condition (disease focused), but also can include information about the patient's values and preferences (patient focused). It is believed that the importance of patient preferences increases across separate care events.

Management continuity is the consistent and coherent approach to the management of a health condition that is responsive to a patient's changing needs (Haggerty et al., 2003). In other words, it is the need for an established plan of care that meets the needs of the patient. This is believed to be particularly important in instances when a patient's case is complex or the patient suffers from chronic disease (Haggerty et al., 2003). Management continuity is achieved when care is provided in a complementary and timely manner. The use of protocols and shared management plans are evidence of management continuity of care and provide comfort to both provider and patient (Haggerty et al., 2003).

Relational continuity is also referred to as interpersonal continuity. Relational continuity represents an ongoing therapeutic relationship between a patient and one or more providers. This personal relationship between the patient and clinician is characterized by personal trust and responsibility (Saultz, 2003). As one can imagine, interpersonal continuity is believed to foster improved communication, trust, and a sustained sense of responsibility, and is associated with higher levels of satisfaction with care (Saultz & Albedaiwi, 2004). It is important to understand that strong interpersonal continuity of care is associated with improved use of preventative services, reduced hospitalizations, and lower costs of care (Saultz & Lochner, 2005, Hussey, et al., 2014).

THE PATIENT CENTERED MEDICAL HOME (PCMH)

Reflecting the concepts of interdisciplinary care, collaborative work relationships, and continuity of care, the patient centered medical home (PCMH) refers to a partnership approach in the provision of primary health care that encompasses five functions and attributes: comprehensive care, patient-centered, coordinated care, accessible services, and quality and safety (Higgins, et al., 2015). As such, a PCMH is primary health care implemented to improve the patient's health across a continuum of referrals and services (Sia, Tonniges, Osterhus, & Taba, 2004). It is based on a relationship between the patient and physician, formed to improve the patient's health via open communication within a team care framework. The primary focus is to have one central clearinghouse in which all patient medication records are kept up to date, embracing the idea for shared information among healthcare professionals and thus facilitating continuity of care.

Whereas the term was used originally to describe a place—a single source of all medical information about a patient—and introduced in 1967 by the American Academy of Pediatrics, it is now a concept adopted by the numerous medical associations because it is associated with improved quality, reduced errors, and increased satisfaction (both patient and provider) (Jackson, et al., 2013; Crabtree, et al., 2010). Medical homes have been linked with better health, lower overall costs of care, and reductions in disparities in health. Primary care organizations, including the American Board of Family Medicine, have promoted the concept as an answer to government agencies seeking political solutions for making quality health care affordable and accessible to all Americans (Sia, Tonniges, Osterhus, & Taba, 2004).

Pharmacists can have a role in the patient-centered medical home model because it is another model requiring a team-based approach to patient care. While most conceptualizations of the medical home recognize the physician only as the primary healthcare provider, it is evident that this initiative requires a multidisciplinary approach from the entire healthcare team, including nurses, pharmacists, physicians, therapists, and other health professionals. Pharmacists should and can have a role in medication therapy management in the medical home model, as well as open shared communication with physicians. Pharmacists have been typically underused in this role, yet have great potential to demonstrate professional expertise in this model of care.

Demonstration projects have documented the value of having pharmacists as care team members by their involvement in clinical decision making, such as medication evaluations to assess medication-related problems or the failure to achieve desirable outcomes (Smith et al., 2010). Pharmacists can play important roles in optimizing therapeutic outcomes and promoting safe, cost-effective medication use for patients in medical homes, especially patients with chronic conditions (Smith et al., 2010). Barriers to medical home implementation are similar to any other model that requires change in behavior. This involves developing relationships with other professionals who are willing to work collaboratively, communicating expectations with team members, finding a patient population interested in utilizing a medical home concept, and changing reimbursement and payment policies such that it will incentivize providers to adopt a change in practice.

While the healthcare practitioners who affect the role of the pharmacist will be varied, one consistency remains the responsibility to evaluate the manner in which care is delivered and to change what is necessary to provide improved outcomes for patients. The impetus for team-based approaches to care has often been less than desired/expected outcomes associated with care. As such, it is important to understand the concept of quality in health care and the measures that interested parties use to identify quality.

DEFINING QUALITY

Quality means different things to different people and can be based on involvement, need, price, and experience. In other words, quality may mean the availability of appointment times in a physician's office; to others, it means how friendly and accommodating the staff at the organization is to the patient. Quality also may be evaluated on the basis of the diagnosis or the medication providing a cure for the patient. The Institute of Medicine (IOM) has defined *quality* as "the degree to which health services for individuals and populations increase the likelihood of desired health outcomes and are consistent with current professional knowledge" (IOM, 1990, p. 21). Another prominent definition of quality has been offered by the Agency for Healthcare Research and Quality (AHRQ), who has defined quality as "doing the right thing for the right patient, at the right time, in the right way, to achieve the best possible results" (AHRQ, 2005, p. 3).

While both definitions provide a clear picture of good quality health care, based on scientific and medical evidence, the so-called quality movement has attempted to take the specific details of a patient's life into consideration in order to improve the health and life of the patient being treated. As such, there are believed to be six components of healthcare quality (**Table 2-2**). Each of these components of quality can be influenced by every member of the healthcare team. As a result, organizations and professionals should focus their efforts to provide care that meets all of these standards in an interdisciplinary effort to achieve desired health outcomes. Unfortunately, the current state of the healthcare system frequently results in one or more of these components being unmet, so patients often struggle with inadequate quality in health care.

The six components of healthcare quality suggest the need for an interdisciplinary approach to care because it would be quite challenging for any one healthcare provider to satisfy all these quality elements for every patient under his or her care.

How Is Quality Assessed?

Although it is understood generally what quality is, how quality in health care is assessed is much less understood by healthcare providers, including pharmacists. The measures used to assess

Table 2-2 Components of Healthcare Quality

Effective	Providing services based on scientific knowledge to all who could benefit and refraining from providing services to those not likely to benefit.
Safe	Avoiding injuries to patients from the care that is intended to help them.
Timely	Reducing wait times and harmful delays for both those who receive and those who give care.
Patient centered	Providing care that is respectful of and responsive to individual patient preferences, needs, and values and ensuring that patient values guide all clinical decisions.
Equitable	Providing care that does not vary in quality because of personal characteristics such as gender, ethnicity, geographic location, and socioeconomic status.
Efficient	Avoiding waste, including waste of equipment, supplies, ideas, and energy.

Source: Data from Agency for Healthcare Research and Quality (AHRQ). (2009, March). 2008 National healthcare quality & disparities reports (AHRQ Publication No. 09-0001). Available at http://archive.ahrq.gov/research/findings/nhqrdr/nhqr08/nhqr08.pdf

healthcare quality are used to benchmark performance. These can include structure, process, outcome, and patient experience-related measures. More specifically, healthcare quality may be measured in any of a number of ways including: (1) clinical performance measures of how well providers deliver specific services needed by specific patients (e.g., children receiving recommended immunizations); (2) assessments by patients of how well providers meet healthcare needs from the patient's perspective (e.g., do providers communicate clearly?); and (3) outcome measures (e.g., mortality rates from cancers preventable by screening) that may be affected by the quality of health care received. (AHRQ, 2009; AHRQ, 2010).

Clinical performance measures are those that are most valued from the clinician's perspective, as it is those measures that most directly influence the clinical outcomes of the patient (Kozma, Reeder, & Schultz, 1993). An example of a clinical performance measure is following standard procedures after the patient is admitted to the hospital for an acute myocardial infarction (e.g., administration of an aspirin within 24 hours of arrival). The patient's assessment of care, probably the most important to the patient as it relates to how he or she perceives his or her treatment to be, is often measured with patient report cards of quality. Lastly, the outcomes of quality measures are of particular interest to researchers, policy makers, and administrators because these measures can be used to objectively review trends over time or typically take a macro perspective of how the end result was affected by some type of intervention or objectively reviewed trends over time. Varying aspects of the healthcare delivery are valuable for different reasons to different parties, depending on their perspective and the role in which they play in the patient care process. There is an abundance of quality information available and is reported in one of three ways: accreditation, report cards, and consumer ratings.

Accreditation

Healthcare organizations seek accreditation from a variety of agencies. Accreditation is the process by which certification of competency, authority, or credibility is presented to an organization. This information is used by the Centers for Medicare and Medicaid Services (CMS), third-party administrators, employers, and consumers as one component of value assessment. Medicare payments to hospitals and other facilities are contingent, among other things, on the facility meeting standards set by the Joint Commission. The Joint Commission was formed in 1952 (formerly the Joint Commission on the Accreditation of Healthcare Organizations) under the aegis of the American Hospital Association and the AMA. It not only serves as the standard accrediting body for hospitals, long-term care facilities, and other healthcare organizations, but it also participates in developing performance standards for healthcare organizations.

Much like the Good Housekeeping seal for consumer products, these performance measures serve as an indicator of quality to those unfamiliar with the healthcare organization. Possessing accreditation means that the healthcare organization has met national standards, including clinical performance measures. The Joint Commission presides over a growing, national, comparative performance measurement database that can inform its members of internal healthcare organization quality improvement activities, external accountability, pay-for-performance programs, and advance research.

Report Cards

While accreditation status is an important quality indicator, there are other quality initiatives in which organizations participate. One such effort involves the development of quality indicators and measures and providing audiences with report cards of the assessment of the organization, healthcare plan, or healthcare provider. These summary reports of key indicators are used by a variety of audiences including but not limited to consumers and employers. The National

Committee for Quality Assurance (NCQA) is an entity that produces report cards for clinicians, healthcare plans, and other healthcare organizations. Their mission is "to improve the quality of health care" (NCQA, 2015). NCQA hopes to accomplish this laudable goal by transforming healthcare quality through measurement, transparency, and accountability (NCQA, 2015).

Managed care organizations may seek NCQA accreditation by sharing with patients and potential clients the report cards indicating that they meet agreed-upon standards of quality. Although accreditation is voluntary, plans usually promote themselves on the basis of their grades. For example, the NCQA has developed and provides Health Care Effectiveness Data and Information Set (HEDIS) measures which are used by more than 90% of America's health plans to measure performance on important dimensions of care and service. **Table 2-3** contains a sample list of organizations that offer some type of accreditation and/or provide quality measures specific to the type of organization.

Patient Ratings

Not only do organizations evaluate themselves using the measures that indicate quality care, but patients also evaluate these organizations. Many quality initiatives have developed surveys for patients to complete in order to rate these organizations. Many of these surveys are available on paper or on the Internet; patients rate their experience with a provider or healthcare organization. This aggregate information is subsequently published for others to see and use in evaluating potential providers and organizations. Although patient participation in this type of evaluation is not widespread, organizations continue to work to increase awareness of the patient information in the quality initiative. These websites allow for comparisons between different organizations on certain dimensions of quality of care, such as those discussed earlier. It is believed that patients will use these resources when making choices about providers or to report on their experiences with a provider. It is expected that these resources would be used as a resource for decision making much like a consumer would use product reviews on websites to evaluate product quality.

Table 2-3 A Sample of Organizations Providing Quality Information

Organization type	Example of quality initiative
Managed care organizations	National Committee for Quality Assurance (NCQA)
Medicare	Medicare Health Outcomes Survey (HOS)
Inpatient setting	CMS Hospital Compare CMS Nursing Home Quality Initiative
Outpatient setting	Accreditation Association for Ambulatory Health Care
Physicians	Ambulatory Care Quality Alliance (AQA) National Committee for Quality Assurance (NCQA)
Pharmacies	Pharmacy Quality Alliance (PQA)

Patients candidly sharing quality information about provider services are supplemented by payers finding ways to compensate these providers for good, cost-efficient care. **Table 2-4** contains a sample of organizations that collect information by patients for patient use.

The manner in which these organizations collect this type of information is through surveys, primarily. These surveys allow patients to rate their provider's performance, or the organization may examine protocols within the practice organization to determine if they meet the benchmarked standards of each item of interest. For example, the consumer assessment of healthcare providers and systems (CAHPS) program presents survey items for ambulatory-level care and facility-level care, including items related to provider communication such as "doctor respected patient's comments" and "doctor spent enough time with patient." Patients respond to the survey items and item responses are aggregated and presented in summary in the form of reports.

Table 2-4 Sample Quality Organizations Collecting Information for Patients

Organization name	Website	Description
Agency for Healthcare Research and Quality's Consumer Assessment of Healthcare Providers and Systems	https://www.cahps.ahrq.gov	Develop standardized surveys of patients' experiences with ambulatory and facility-level care
CMS's Hospital Compare	https://www.medicare.gov/hospitalcompare/search.html	Allows patients to search for information on quality care at hospitals
CMS's Nursing Home Compare	https://www.medicare.gov/nursinghomecompare/search.html	Allows consumers to search for information on quality care for Medicare and Medicaid-certified nursing homes
Joint Commission's Quality Check	http://www.qualitycheck.org/consumer/searchQCR.aspx	Allows patients to search for accredited hospitals and other healthcare organizations
National Committee for Quality Assurance	http://www.ncqa.org/ReportCards.aspx	Provides information on report cards for choosing quality health care
U.S. News & World Report	http://health.usnews.com/	Publishes annual rankings of America's best health plans and best hospitals

IMPORTANT TRENDS AFFECTING HEALTHCARE PROFESSIONALS

Healthcare quality is a major area of focus currently within the healthcare system and requires the insight and initiative of all practitioners involved. There are five related areas that continue to receive attention and will affect the various healthcare professionals as this quality paradigm becomes the standard of practice. These areas are patient-focused care, critical pathways, continuous quality improvement (CQI), pay for performance, and technological advances.

Patient-Focused Care

Patient-focused care in a healthcare facility is characterized by decentralization of services, cross-training of personnel from different departments to provide basic care, interdisciplinary collaboration, various degrees of organizational restructuring, simplification and redesign of work to eliminate steps and save time, and an increased involvement of patients in their own care (Vogel, 1993, p. 2321).

In patient-focused care, objectives include (1) improving patients' perceptions of the quality of care and staff members' job satisfaction and (2) using nonclinical and clinical staff more effectively and efficiently (Vogel, 1993).

Patient-focused care attempts to improve patient care by organizationally and physically moving selected service functions, such as basic laboratory, pharmacy, admitting/discharge, medical records, housekeeping, and material support services to patient care areas, thus effecting an organizational restructuring (Wakefield et al., 1994). In providing such care, health professionals work in teams to increase and improve communication among themselves and with the patient. In an institutional setting, it would appear that this type of care could be facilitated by organizational changes; however, in the ambulatory setting, the shift to patient-focused care will require extraordinary effort on the part of individual practitioners to collaborate with other professionals. In other words, differences in organizational relationships, locations, and technologies, between different providers in the ambulatory care setting make the establishment of collaborative working relationships more challenging and thus the establishment of the patient-centered medical home more challenging.

However, the overall theme remains the same in any setting: improving patient care and, as a result, improving outcomes requires a partnership between pharmacy professionals, doctors, patients, and payers.

Patient-focused care is a systematic and comprehensive team approach composed of multiskilled or cross-trained individuals capable of providing more of the services directly to patients. Pharmacists can be and should be key members of a multidisciplinary team who have the opportunity to assume shared responsibility for drug therapy management and patient outcomes. Pharmacists are now being trained as clinical pharmacotherapy specialists and have extensive medication-related knowledge to contribute to a team-based approach to care.

Meeting quality standards requires a culture of quality. In order to ensure quality care, a redesign of the system to support a team approach is required. Quality improvement organizations, such as NCQA, have developed tools and resources to assist in creating an interdisciplinary work environment in order to influence patient outcomes. One of these tools, Team Strategies and Tools to Enhance Performance and Patient Safety (TeamSTEPPS) is a comprehensive set of ready-to-use materials and a training curriculum to integrate teamwork principles into any healthcare system (AHRQ, 2015a). Developed by the Department of Defense, in collaboration with the Agency for Healthcare Research and Quality (AHRQ), this program has been implemented in many different healthcare organizations and is now on Version 2.0 (AHRQ, 2015b).

Facilitating patient-focused care requires reengineering of healthcare systems. Reengineering has been defined as the fundamental re-thinking and radical redesign of business processes to achieve dramatic improvements in critical, contemporary measures of performance, such as quality, cost, service, and speed (Hammer and Champy, 1993). The purpose of reengineering is to achieve improved efficiencies and quality. Reengineering seeks to combine multiple jobs into one, empower workers and make them more accountable, sequence the elements of work more naturally, create greater flexibility, and blur or move organizational boundaries (Al-Shaqha & Zairi, 2000). The goals of reengineering can be met by increasing efficiency, decreasing redundancy, and eliminating waste. Extensive redesign of the basic work processes as proposed by patient-focused care advocates may result in significant changes in employee job scope, task responsibilities, professional autonomy, and reporting relationships. From the employee's perspective, such changes may be neither warranted nor welcomed. Therefore, obtaining employee buy-in and establishing appropriate incentive structures to facilitate desired changes is critical in implementing patient-focused care (Wakefield et al., 1994).

Critical Pathways

One of the ways to implement reengineering in pharmacy is to use the critical pathway process as a guide to reengineering procedures related specifically to the management of a patient's care. Critical pathways represent comprehensive management plans that aim to optimize and streamline patient care (Kirk et al., 1996). Critical pathways have been referred to in the medical literature by a number of different terms, including care path, care map, clinical pathway, critical path of care, case management plan, multidisciplinary action plan, collaborative care track, plan of care, clinical care plan, and care guide (Lumsdon & Hagland, 1993). These plans define key steps in the management of the patient not only to improve the quality of health care, but also to reduce resource utilization (Shane, 1995). Critical pathways are similar in many ways to clinical practice guidelines; however, critical pathways are considered an "optimal sequencing and timing of interventions by healthcare professionals for a particular diagnosis or procedure, designed to minimize delays and resource utilization and maximize the quality of care" (Coffey et al., 1992, p.45).

Some of the specific goals of critical pathways include providing continuous quality improvement, decreasing service fragmentation (increasing continuity of care), optimizing cost-effectiveness of healthcare delivery, guiding the patient and family through expected treatment and progress, and increasing satisfaction of patients, families, staff, physicians, and third-party payers (Shane, 1995). Critical pathways create targeted patient outcomes and quality end points, which form a foundation for common expectations, shared responsibility, regular communication, and early problem detection and intervention among all members of the healthcare team (Coffey et al., 1992). Further, they identify specific time frames and desired outcomes associated with each care step, with the goals of minimizing delays and maximizing resource utilization (Shane, 1995). Both decreased length of stay and lower overall hospital costs have been found following implementation of critical pathways as well as improved patient outcomes through coordinated and less fragmented care (Rotter et al., 2010).

Project managers in the construction and engineering fields have used critical pathways for many years. As in these other fields, critical pathways in health care are developed usually for high-volume, high-risk, or high-cost procedures. Because of increasing competition within health care, "managers have embraced critical pathways as a method to reduce variation in care, decrease resource utilization, and potentially improve healthcare quality" (Every, Hochman, Becker, Kopecky, & Cannon, 2000, p. 461). Critical pathways require organizational change such that they facilitate interdisciplinary teamwork. For example, reductions in all-cause hospitalizations and medical costs as well as improved survival rates have been observed with multidisciplinary teams (Peterson et al., 2008). The teams document pharmacologic as well as nonpharmacologic therapies, interventions, and outcomes throughout the entire course of care from admission to discharge.

Critical pathways require coordinated care from everyone on the healthcare team and delineate which treatments should be done on each day of the patient's stay. Critical pathways have been shown to reduce variations in the care provided, facilitate achieving expected outcomes, decrease delays, and improve cost-effectiveness (Coffey et al., 1992).

Continuous Quality Improvement

Continuous quality improvement (CQI), also called total quality management and total quality improvement, is another mechanism in which interdisciplinary involvement is crucial. W. Edwards Deming, a statistician, introduced methods of CQI with the premise that improved quality will decrease costs because of less rework, fewer mistakes, fewer delays, and better use of people and materials. The Deming method has been incorporated into the day-to-day activities of many major companies (Gitlow & Melby, 1991). CQI enables a cross-functional, interdisciplinary team to examine processes that could or should be improved. It brings together a team of healthcare workers who know a particular procedure well and takes advantage of the fact that employees generally are more receptive to change when they are active participants in the change process.

CQI can also be viewed as a method of performance appraisal in which structures, processes, and outcomes are assessed to determine specific areas where improvement is needed. It typically follows the FOCUS-PDCA cycle (Graham, 1995):

Find a process to improve.
Organize a team that knows the process.
Clarify current knowledge of the process.
Understand sources of process variation.
Select the process improvement.

Plan the improvement.
Do the improvement, collect data, and analyze data.
Check and study the results.
Act to hold the gain and to improve the process further.

The PDCA cycle is used in the daily management of CQI and to determine the actions necessary to maintain, improve, or innovate standard methods to achieve measurable benchmarks. Inherent within CQI is the belief that it is wiser to maximize efforts to design a product or process to be right the first time and to minimize resources devoted to inspection and repair caused by poor processes (Wakefield et al., 1994). Patient-focused care builds upon previous CQI healthcare efforts by focusing on ways to improve continuity of care and by examining what, if any, changes in underlying structures and processes may be required. In a patient-focused care organization, CQI functions as a methodology for examining and improving the process of care and patient-care outcomes, regardless of internal departmental or profession-based organizational boundaries.

Pay for Performance

Pay for performance (P4P) in health care is a topic of wide discussion, especially among managed care executives, for its ability to contain costs, to improve health outcomes, and to raise the overall quality of health services. P4P has emerged as a new model built on defined measures, data collection, and public reporting that includes payment incentives aimed at quality, efficiency, and patient satisfaction (ASHP, 2009). The focus of P4P is on value, which takes into account the relationship between quality and cost. While P4P is not a new concept, it has arrived in health care due to a convergence of events including increasing cost of care, provision of patient-centered care, the progression of evidence-based medicine, the patient safety movement, and the use of electronic data systems and the Internet.

In order to incentivize providers to provide quality care, providers are rewarded in P4P. P4P has been defined by the CMS as "quality based purchasing ... the use of payment methods and other incentives to encourage high quality and patient-focused, high value care" (CMS, 2006, p. 1). An effective P4P program should incorporate clinical quality, efficiency, and patient satisfaction. CMS and other payers are believed to be moving toward this model, as it has been demonstrated to improve quality in a cost-effective manner. P4P programs increasingly are focusing their efforts on outcome and cost-efficiency measures, rather than clinical process measures alone. The use of specific measure sets have increased drastically for outcomes, information technology, and cost efficiency, while measures for patient satisfaction and processes have maintained a similar proportion over the years. Challenges associated with adopting P4P include overcoming physician resistance, determining the necessary size of incentive pools to capture the provider's attention, and finding the resources necessary to continue funding the program (Rosenthal & Dudley, 2007).

There is evidence that P4P programs have an effect on quality (Werner et al., 2011). Measurement provides physicians with a new perspective on their practice and encourages change in their processes and delivery systems in order to meet program standards. Adoption of process changes (in order to meet the benchmarked standards) has shown that some organizations have difficulty in achieving national standards, specifically small organizations and large organizations. However, the use of national standards helps rewards programs get started (O'Kane, 2007) in order to incentivize providers to meet these standards of care. The development of national standards that are accepted widely, and consistent requirements to meet the standards, are key in the implementation of CQI to achieve them.

Healthcare Services and Technological Advances

Both healthcare services and the professions providing care are influenced by the introduction of new technologies. Health information technology has been shown to improve quality by increasing adherence to guidelines, enhancing disease surveillance, and decreasing medication errors (Chaudhry et al., 2006). Technological advances have made many new procedures and methods possible; for example, robotic devices automate many of the tasks associated with medication dispensing. In addition, tablets and similar handheld devices provide physicians and pharmacists with updated drug information. Moreover, the exchange of information between healthcare practitioners and the information acquisition by patients has changed exponentially when compared to past decades. The movement toward quality health care is believed also to involve the creation of interoperable transparent systems with an ultimate goal of developing an electronic health record for each patient to be used by all involved in the healthcare system.

The fragmented nature of the U.S. healthcare system includes thousands of hospitals, many thousands of healthcare professionals (e.g., physicians, nurses, and pharmacists), and many more thousands of facilities and other interested parties. This environment creates an ideal situation and incentive to incorporate technologies that can span different sites and caregivers in order to help integrate services. With the large volume of transactions in the system and the need to integrate new scientific evidence into practice and other complex information management activities, the limitations of paper-based information management are obvious (Chaudhry et al., 2006). Evidence supports the use of clinical decision support and computerized provider order entry as a means to affect quality (Jones et al., 2014).

There is the potential for many of the key players to resist the adoption of new technologies, such as electronic health records (EHRs). While the benefits of health information technologies are clear, adapting new information systems to health care has proven difficult and rates of use have been limited. In fact, most technology applications have been created for administrative and financial transactions rather than for delivering clinical care (Chaudhry et al., 2006). Reforming the system such that incentives are provided to patients and providers is considered to be a first step toward engaging and implementing a healthcare system for all health professionals to provide better patient care. An example of incentivizing the adoption of technology-based practice changes would be e-prescribing. CMS established an incentive-disincentive program to speed the adoption of e-prescribing by Medicare providers. Beginning in 2009, CMS provided incentives for the adoption of e-prescribing for 3 years; however, beginning in 2012, CMS added financial penalties for providers who failed to adopt e-prescribing (CMS, 2010).

In order to ensure safe medication and procedure delivery within hospitals, organizations have implemented the use of technology such as bar codes on patient admission bracelets, requiring these scans to match electronic records prior to completing procedures and medication dispensing. Electronic health records and electronic medical records have been cited as a method to increase communication between healthcare professionals and allow for continuity of care. While all these structure and process changes within the system are made to affect positively patient health outcomes, it remains the responsibility of the *professionals* in healthcare to develop and maintain methods to sustain quality health care, as it is what we have committed to when becoming professionals. It appears that today's version of interdisciplinary collaboration requires electronic systems to facilitate communication. While health information technology is one method in making this a possibility, electronic health records will only work if they are utilized to their fullest extent. Overcoming adoption barriers and utilizing the new systems to their capability are imperative to creating a fully functional system.

CONCLUSION

Interdisciplinary care is becoming more important as providing quality care becomes the gold standard for practitioners. There are a number of factors that will help ensure good quality health care (NCQA, 2007), which are:

1. Effectively utilize the best available medical research.
2. Ensure complete information exchange regarding a patient's health to other practitioners.
3. Coordinate care among multiple professionals.
4. Provide comprehensive, continuous care.
5. Pay for quality instead of volume.
6. Engage patients in their care.

Understanding the role and function of others in the healthcare system is the first step to providing collaborative interdisciplinary care. It is important to note that people are not the focus of quality; rather it is achieved through refinement of an organization's standard methods (best practices) through the use of CQI. CQI occurs through modifying standard methods as well as via system changes of structure and processes. While most of the system changes are not visible to the patient, these changes are made to provide better care.

QUESTIONS FOR FURTHER DISCUSSION

1. Consider the characteristics of a profession; in light of those characteristics, discuss pharmacy. For each of the characteristics where pharmacy does not possess or partially possesses the requirement, what remedies do you recommend?
2. Are the characteristics that have been applied historically to occupations for the purpose of defining professions relevant today? Why or why not?
3. How is it that your pharmacy education will prepare you to practice as part of a multidisciplinary team? An interdisciplinary team?
4. What are the potential benefits of engaging in collaborative practice agreements? What are the risks?
5. Collaborative practice agreements refer to the practice where healthcare providers (e.g., physicians) authorize pharmacists to perform specific activities to help patients achieve better health outcomes. In which areas of pharmacy practice would you expect most to have a collaborative practice agreement, and why?
6. People are not the focus of change; rather it is believed that developing systems that require people to provide a high quality of care through refinement of an organization's standard methods should be our focus to bring about needed change. What types of healthcare *system* changes can be made to facilitate establishing continuity of care and the medical home as the typical standard of care?
7. Critical pathways include providing continuous quality improvement, decreasing service fragmentation (increasing continuity of care), optimizing cost-effectiveness of healthcare delivery, guiding the patient and family through expected treatment and progress, and increasing satisfaction of patients, families, staff, physicians, and third-party payers. These pathways are typically implemented for high-volume, high-risk, or high-cost procedures. Many of the studies have demonstrated the utility of critical pathways in an institutional setting. How might this concept be applied to a community pharmacy setting?
8. Technology and the possibility of electronic health records have been repeatedly touted as the solution to eliminating the fragmentation of the healthcare system. Most of this chapter has discussed how these changes will influence practitioners. How do you think these changes will influence patients' interactions with healthcare professionals? What are the pros and cons from the patient perspective?
9. Suppose you were asked by a national pharmacy organization to increase utilization of patient-reported quality measures. Describe how you would get patients to use these services and how you would get practitioners and payers to use the results from these patient-reported measures. What influence will increased utilization of patient-reported measures have on practice?

KEY TOPICS AND TERMS

Collaborative working relationships
Continuity of care
Continuous quality improvement
Critical pathways
Health information technology
Interdisciplinary care
Medical home
Multidisciplinary care
Patient-focused care
Pay for performance (P4P)
Profession
Professional
Quality of care

REFERENCES

Accreditation Council for Pharmacy Education. (2014). *Accreditation standards and key elements for the professional program in pharmacy leading to the doctor of pharmacy degree.* Chicago, IL: Accreditation Council for Pharmacy Education.

Accreditation Review Commission on the Education for the Physician Assistant (ARC-PA). (2015). *Accredited PA programs.* Retrieved from http://www.arc-pa.org/acc_programs/

Agency for Healthcare Research and Quality (AHRQ). (2005, September). *Guide to health care quality: How to know it when you see it* (AHRQ Publication No. 05-0088). Rockville, MD.

Agency for Healthcare Research and Quality (AHRQ). (2015, August). *About TeamSTEPPS.* Retrieved from http://www.ahrq.gov/professionals/education/curriculum-tools/teamstepps/about-teamstepps/index.html

Agency for Healthcare Research and Quality (AHRQ). (2015, September). *TeamSTEPPS 2.0.* Retrieved from http://www.ahrq.gov/professionals/education/curriculum-tools/teamstepps/instructor/index.html

Al-Shaqha, W. M., & Zairi, M. (2000). Reengineering pharmaceutical care: Towards a patient-focused approach. *International Journal of Health Care Quality Assurance, 13*(5), 208–217.

American Academy of Physician Assistants (AAPA). (2014). *2013 AAPA Annual Survey Report.* Retrieved from https://www.aapa.org/WorkArea/DownloadAsset.aspx?id=2902

American Academy of Physician Assistants (AAPA). (2015). *What is a PA?* Retrieved from https://www.aapa.org/what-is-a-pa/

American Association of Colleges of Nursing (AACN). (2015). *The Doctor of Nursing Practice (DNP).* Retrieved from http://www.aacn.nche.edu/media-relations/fact-sheets/dnp

American Association of Colleges of Osteopathic Medicine (AACOM). (2015a). *Osteopathic Medical College information book: Entering class 2016.* Retrieved from http://www.aacom.org/news-and-events/publications/cib

American Association of Colleges of Osteopathic Medicine (AACOM). (2015b). *What is osteopathic medicine?* Retrieved from http://www.aacom.org/become-a-doctor/about-om

American Association of Colleges of Pharmacy. (2015). *Academic pharmacy's vital statistics.* Retrieved from http://www.aacp.org/about/Pages/Vitalstats.aspx

American Board of Medical Specialties (ABMS). (2015). *Frequently asked questions.* Retrieved from http://www.abms.org/about-abms/faqs/

American Board of Physician Specialties (ABPS). (2015). *What is the ABPS?* Retrieved from http://www.abpsus.org/abps

American College of Clinical Pharmacy (ACCP). (2004). *ACCP guidelines for clinical research fellowship training programs.* Lenexa, KS: American College of Clinical Pharmacy.

American Medical Association (AMA). (2015a). *Physician characteristics and distribution in the U.S.* Chicago, IL: American Medical Association.

American Medical Association (AMA). (2015b). *Requirements for becoming a physician.* Retrieved from http://www.ama-assn.org/ama/pub/education-careers/becoming-physician.page

American Medical Association (AMA). (2014). *State medical licensure requirements and statistics, 2014.* Chicago, IL: American Medical Association.

American Nurses Association (ANA). (2015a). *What is nursing?* Retrieved from http://www.nursingworld.org/especiallyforyou/what-is-nursing

American Nurses Association (ANA). (2015b). *What nurses do?* Retrieved from http://www.nursingworld.org/EspeciallyForYou/What-is-Nursing/Tools-You-Need/RNsAPNs.html

American Nurses Credentialing Center (ANCC). (2015). *ANCC certification center.* Retrieved from http://www.nursecredentialing.org/Certification

American Osteopathic Association (AOA). (2015). *AOA board certification.* Retrieved from http://www.osteopathic.org/inside-aoa/development/aoa-board-certification/Pages/default.aspx

American Society of Health-System Pharmacists (ASHP). (1999). ASHP statement on the pharmacist's role in primary care. *American Journal of Health-System Pharmacy, 56*, 1665–1667.

American Society of Health-System Pharmacists (ASHP). (2003). White paper on pharmacy technicians 2002: Needed changes can no longer wait. *American Journal of Health-System Pharmacy, 60*(1), 37–51.

American Society of Health-System Pharmacists (ASHP). (2009). *Pay-for-performance (P4P): Evaluating current and future implications: Issues for pharmacy.* Retrieved from http://www.ashp.org/doclibrary/policy/qii/pay-for-performance.aspx

American Society of Health-System Pharmacists (ASHP). (2012a). *ASHP accreditation standard for postgraduate year one (PGY1) pharmacy residency programs.* Retrieved from http://www.ashp.org/doclibrary/accreditation/asd-pgy1-standard.aspx

American Society of Health-System Pharmacists (ASHP). (2012b). *ASHP accreditation standard for postgraduate year two (PGY2) pharmacy residency programs.* Retrieved from https://www.ashp.org/DocLibrary/Accreditation/ASD-PGY2-Standard.aspx

American Society of Health-System Pharmacists (ASHP). (2015). *Pharmacy residency match day results show continued growth.* Retrieved from http://www.ashp.org/menu/News/NewsCapsules/Article.aspx?id=1567#sthash.qO5slTu9.dpuf.

American Society of Hospital Pharmacists (ASHP). (1987). Definitions of pharmacy residencies and fellowships. *American Journal of Hospital Pharmacy, 44,* 1142–1144.

Association of American Medical Colleges (AAMC). (2014). *Diversity of the physician workforce: Facts & figures 2014.* Retrieved from http://aamcdiversityfactsandfigures.org/section-ii-current-status-of-us-physician-workforce/

Association of American Medical Colleges (AAMC). (2015). *Medical Schools.* Retrieved from https://www.aamc.org/about/membership/378788/medicalschools.html

Beck, A. H. (2004). The Flexner report and the standardization of medical education. *Journal of the American Medical Association, 291*(17), 2139–2140.

Board of Pharmacy Specialties (BPS). (2015a). *Specialties.* Retrieved from http://www.bpsweb.org/specialties/specialties.cfm

Board of Pharmacy Specialties (BPS). (2015b). *Specialties: Added qualifications.* Retrieved from http://www.bpsweb.org/specialties/qualification.cfm

Bouvy, M. L., Heerdink, E. R., Urquhart, J., Grobbee, D. E., Hoes, E. W., & Leufkens, H. G. (2003). Effect of a pharmacist-led intervention on diuretic compliance in heart failure patients: A randomized controlled study. *Journal of Cardiac Failure, 9,* 404–411.

Brock, K. A., & Doucette, W. R. (2004). Collaborative working relationships between pharmacists and physicians: An exploratory study. *Journal of the American Pharmaceutical Association, 44*(3), 358–365.

Buerki, R. A, & Vottero, L. D. (1996). The purposes of professions in society. In C. H. Knowlton, R. P. Penna (Eds.), *Pharmaceutical care* (pp. 3–17). New York, NY: Chapman and Hall.

Centers for Medicare and Medicaid Services (CMS). (2006). State Medicaid Director Letter #06-003, dated April 6, 2006.

Centers for Medicare and Medicaid Services (CMS). (2010). *Electronic prescribing (eRx) incentive program.* Retrieved from http://www.cms.gov/ERxIncentive/

Chaudhry, B., Wang, J., Wu, S., Maglione, M., Mojica, W., Roth, E., ... Shekelle, P. G. (2006). Systematic review: Impact of health information technology on quality, efficiency, and costs of medical care. *Annals of Internal Medicine, 144,* E-12–E-22.

Christikis, D. A. (2003). Continuity of care: Process or outcome? *Annals of Family Medicine, 1*(3), 131–133.

Coffey, R. J., Richards, J. S., Remmert, C. S., LeRoy, S. S., Schoville, R. R., & Baldwin, P. J. (1992). An introduction to critical paths. *Quality Management in Health Care, 1*(1), 45–54.

Council on Credentialing in Pharmacy. (2003). Sesquicentennial Stepping Stone Summits—Summit two: Pharmacy technicians. *Journal of the American Pharmacists Association. 43*(1), 84–92.

Council on Credentialing in Pharmacy. (2009). *Scope of contemporary pharmacy practice: Roles, responsibilities, and functions of pharmacists and pharmacy technicians.* Available at http://www.pharmacycredentialing.org/ccp/Contemporary_Pharmacy_Practice.pdf

Crabtree, B. F., Nutting, P. A., Miller, W. L., Stange, K. C., Stewart, E. E., & Jaen C. R. (2010) Summary of the national demonstration project and recommendations for the patient-centered medical home. *Annals of Family Medicine, 8*(Supp. 1), s80–s90.

Doucette, W. R., Nevins, J., & McDonough, R. P. (2005). Factors affecting collaborative care between pharmacists and physicians. *Research in Social and Administrative Pharmacy, 1*(4), 565–578.

Every, N. R., Hochman J., Becker, R., Kopecky, S., & Cannon, C. P. (2000). Critical pathways: A review. *Circulation, 101,* 431–435.

Federation of State Medical Boards (FSMB). (2015). *State-Specific Requirements for Initial Medical Licensure*. Retrieved from http://www.fsmb.org/policy/public-resources/state_specific

Flexner, A. (1910). *Medical education in the United States and Canada*. New York, NY: Carnegie Foundation.

Gitlow, H. S., & Melby, M. J. (1991). Framework for continuous quality improvement in the provision of pharmaceutical care. *American Journal of Hospital Pharmacy, 48*, 1917–1925.

Goode, W. J. (1957). Community within a community: The professions. *American Sociological Review, 22*(2), 194–200.

Government Accounting Office (GAO). (2008). *Primary care professionals: Recent supply trends, projects, and valuation of services*. Available at http://www.gao.gov/new.items/d08472t.pdf

Graham, N. O. (1995). *Quality in health care: Theory, application, and evolution*. Gaithersburg, MD: Aspen Publications.

Grumbach, K., Bodenheimer, T. (2004). Can health care teams improve primary care practice? *Journal of the American Medical Association, 291*, 1246–1251.

Haggerty, J. L., Reid, R. J., Freeman, G. K., Starfield, B. H., Adair, C. E., & McKenfry, R. (2003). Continuity of care: A multidisciplinary review. *British Medical Journal, 327*, 1219–1221.

Hammer, D., & Champy, J. (1993). *Reengineering the corporation*. New York, NY: Harper Business.

Health Resources & Services Administration (HRSA). (2010). *The registered nurse population: Findings from the 2008 national sample survey of registered nurses*. Retrieved from http://bhpr.hrsa.gov/healthworkforce/rnsurveys/rnsurveyfinal.pdf

Health Resources & Services Administration (HRSA). (2012). *Health workforce projections: Pharmacists*. Retrieved from http://bhpr.hrsa.gov/healthworkforce/supplydemand/usworkforce/projections/pharmacists.pdf

Health Resources & Services Administration (HRSA). Bureau of Health Professions. (2008). *The adequacy of pharmacist supply: 2004–2030*. Retrieved from ftp://ftp.hrsa.gov/bhpr/workforce/pharmacy.pdf

Health Resources & Services Administration (HRSA). Bureau of Health Professions. (2013). *Projecting the supply and demand for primary care practitioners through 2020*. Retrieved from http://bhpr.hrsa.gov/healthworkforce/supplydemand/usworkforce/primarycare/projectingprimarycare.pdf

Health Resources & Services Administration (HRSA). Bureau of Health Professions. (2014). *The future of the nursing workforce: National and state-level projections, 2012–2025*. Retrieved from http://bhpr.hrsa.gov/healthworkforce/supplydemand/nursing/workforceprojections/nursingprojections.pdf

Higby, G. J. (1996). From compounding to caring: An abridged history of American pharmacy. In C. H. Knowlton & R. P. Penna (Eds.), *Pharmaceutical care* (pp. 3–17). New York, NY: Chapman and Hall.

Higgins T. C., Schottenfeld L., & Crosson J. (2015). *Primary care practice facilitation curriculum* (Module 25; AHRQ Publication No. 15-0060-EF). Rockville, MD: Agency for Healthcare Research and Quality.

Hussey, P. S., Schneider, E. C., Rudin, R. S., Fox, S., Lai, J., & Pollack, C. E. (2014). Continuity and the costs of care for chronic disease. *Journal of the American Medical Association Internal Medicine, 174*(5), 742–748.

Interprofessional Education Collaborative Expert Panel. (2011). *Core competencies for interprofessional collaborative practice: Report of an expert panel*. Washington, DC: Interprofessional Education Collaborative.

Institute of Medicine. (1990). IOM. *Medicare: A strategy for quality assurance*. K.N. Lohr (Ed.). Washington, DC: National Academies Press.

Jackson, G. L., Power, B. J., Chatterjee, R., PrvuBettger, J., Kemper, A. R., Hasselblad, V., Dolor, R. J., Irvine, R. J., Heidenfelder, B. L., Kendrick, A. S., Gray, R., & Williams Jr., J. W. (2013). The patient-centered medical home: A systematic review. *Annuals of Internal Medicine, 158*(3), 169–178.

Jessup, R. L. (2007). Interdisciplinary versus multidisciplinary care teams: Do we understand the difference? *Australian Health Review, 31*(3), 330–331.

Jones, P. E. (2007). Physician assistant education in the United States. *Academic Medicine, 82*(9), 882–887.

Jones, S. S., Rudin, R. S., Perry, T., & Shekelle, P. G. (2014). Health information technology: an updated systematic review with a focus on meaningful use. *Annals of Internal Medicine, 160*, 48–54.

Kane-Gill, S., Reddy, P., Gupta, S. R., & Bakst, A. W. (2008). Guidelines for pharmacoeconomic and outcomes research fellowship training programs. *Pharmacotherapy, 28*(10), 269e–276e.

Kirk, J. K., Michael, K. A., Markowsky, S. J., Restino, M. R., & Zarowitz, B. J. (1996). Critical pathways: The time is here for pharmacist involvement. *Pharmacotherapy, 16*, 723–733.

Klass, A. A. (1961). What is a profession? *Canadian Medical Association Journal, 85*, 698–701.

Kozma, C. M., Reeder, C. E., & Schultz, R. M. (1993). Economic, clinical, and humanistic outcomes: A planning model for pharmacoeconomic research. *Clinical Therapeutics, 15*(6), 1121–1132.

LaPointe, N. M., & Jollis, J. G. (2003). Medication errors in hospitalized cardiovascular patients. *Archives of Internal Medicine, 163,* 1461–1466.

Leape, L., Cullen, D. J., Dempsey, C. M., Burdick, E., Demanaco, H. J., Ives, E. J., & Bates, D. W. (1999). Pharmacist participation on physician rounds and adverse drug events in the intensive care unit. *Journal of the American Medication Association, 282,* 267–270.

Liaison Committee on Medical Education. (2010). *Standards for Accreditation of Medical Education Programs Leading to the M.D. Degree.* Retrieved from http://www.lcme.org/publications/2016-17-functions-and-structure.doc

Lumsdon L., & Hagland M. (1993). Mapping care. *Hospital & Health Networks, 67,* 34–40.

Makowsky, M. L., Schindel, T. J., Rosenthal, M., Campbell, K. Tsuyuki, R. T., & Madill, H. M. (2009). Collaboration between pharmacists, physicians and nurse practitioners: A qualitative investigation of working relationships in the inpatient medical setting. *Journal of Interprofessional Care, 23*(2), 169–184.

McDonough, R. P., & Doucette, W. R. (2001). A conceptual framework for collaborative working relationships between pharmacists and physicians. *Journal of the American Pharmaceutical Association, 41,* 682–692.

Midwest Pharmacy Workforce Research Consortium. (2015). *Final report of the 2014 national sample survey of the pharmacist workforce to determine contemporary demographic and practice characteristics and quality of work-life.* Alexandria, VA: American Association of Colleges of Pharmacy.

Mrtek, R. G. (1976). Pharmaceutical education in these United States—An interpretive historical essay of the twentieth century. *American Journal of Pharmaceutical Education, 40*(4), 339–365.

Mrtek, R. G., & Catizone, C. (1989). Pharmacy and the professions. In A. I. Wertheimer, M. C. Smith (Eds.), *Pharmacy practice: Social and behavioral aspects* (pp. 23–57). Baltimore, MD: Williams and Wilkins.

National Association of Boards of Pharmacy (NABP). (2014). *2015 survey of pharmacy law.* Mount Prospect, IL: National Association of Boards of Pharmacy.

National Association of Boards of Pharmacy (NABP). (2015a). *Foreign pharmacy graduate equivalency examination.* Retrieved from http://www.nabp.net/programs/examination/fpgee/#FPGEE

National Association of Boards of Pharmacy (NABP). (2015b). *MJPE.* Retrieved from http://www.nabp.net/programs/examination/mpje

National Association of Boards of Pharmacy (NABP). (2015c). *Model State Pharmacy Act and model rules of the National Association of Boards of Pharmacy.* Mount Prospect, IL: National Association of Boards of Pharmacy.

National Association of Boards of Pharmacy (NABP). (2015d). *NAPLEX.* Retrieved from http://www.nabp.net/programs/examination/naplex

National Board of Osteopathic Medical Examiners (NBOME). (2015). *Comprehensive Osteopathic Medical Licensing Examination.* Retrieved from http://www.nbome.org/exams-comlex.asp?m=serv

National Center for Health Statistics (NCHS). (2015). *Health, United States, 2014: With special feature on adults aged 55–64.* Hyattsville, MD: National Center for Health Statistics.

National Commission on Certification of Physician Assistants (NCCPA). (2010). *Certification process overview.* Retrieved from http://www.nccpa.net/CertificationProcess.aspx

National Committee for Quality Assurance (NCQA). (2007). *The essential guide to health care quality.* Washington DC: National Committee for Quality Assurance.

National Committee for Quality Assurance (NCQA). (2015). *About NCQA.* Retrieved from http://www.ncqa.org/AboutNCQA.aspx

National Council of State Boards of Nursing (NCSBN). (2015a). *Advanced practice member board profile 2014.* Chicago, IL: National Council of State Boards of Nursing.

National Council of State Boards of Nursing (NCSBN). (2015b). *Frequently asked questions about general NCLEX information.* Retrieved from https://www.ncsbn.org/General_FAQ.pdf

National Council of State Boards of Nursing (NCSBN). (2015c). *Licensure member board profile 2014.* Chicago, IL: National Council of State Boards of Nursing.

National Resident Matching Program (NRMP). (2015). *How a match works.* Retrieved from http://www.nrmp.org/match-process/

Nevelle, H. L., Chevalier B., Daley, C, Nodell, L., Harding, C., Hiltz, A., MacDonald T., Skedge, C., MacKinnon, N. J., & Slayter, K. (2014). Clinical benefits and economic impact of post-surgical care provided by pharmacists in a Canadian hospital. *International Journal of Pharmacy Practice, 22*(3), 216–222.

O'Kane, M. E. (2007). Performance-based measures: The early results are in. *Journal of Managed Care Pharmacy, 13*(2 Suppl B): S3–S6.

Paolini, N., & Rouse, M. J. (2010). Scope of contemporary pharmacy practice: Roles, responsibilities, and functions of pharmacists and pharmacy technicians—Executive summary. *American Journal of Health-System Pharmacy, 67*, 1030–1031.

Peterson, E. D., Albert, N. M., Amin, A., Patterson, J. H., & Fonarow, G. C. (2008). Implementing critical pathways and a multidisciplinary team approach to cardiovascular disease management. *The American Journal of Cardiology, 102* (suppl), 47G–56G.

Pharmacy Technician Certification Board. (2014). *Career Outlook—Role in Pharmacy.* Retrieved from http://www.ptcb.org/resources/career-outlook#.VjeCBCvGrHq

Pharmacy Technician Certification Board. (2015). *Pharmacy Technician State Regulations.* Retrieved from http://www.ptcb.org/resources/cpht-toolkit/state-regulations#.VjeI7CvGrHo

Pharmacy Technician Certification Board. (2015b). *Prepare for the Pharmacy Technician Certification Exam.* Retrieved from http://www.ptcb.org/get-certified/prepare#.VjjcZivGrHo

Rosenthal, M. B., & Dudley, R. A. (2007). Pay-for-performance: Will the latest payment trend improve care? *Journal of the American Medical Association, 297*(7), 740–744.

Rotter, T., Kinsman, L., James, E. L., Machotta, A., Gothe, H., Willis, J., Snow, P., & Kugler, J. Clinical pathways: effects on professional practice, patient outcomes, length of stay and hospital costs. *Cochrane Database of Systematic Reviews* 2010, Issue 3. Art. No.: CD006632.

Saultz, J. W. (2003). Defining and measuring interpersonal continuity of care. *Annals of Family Medicine, 1*(3), 134–143.

Saultz, J. W., & Albedaiwi, W. (2004). Interpersonal continuity of care and patient satisfaction: A critical review. *Annals of Family Medicine, 2*(5), 445–451.

Saultz, J. W., & Lochner, J. (2005). Interpersonal continuity of care and care outcomes: A critical review. *Annals of Family Medicine, 3*(2), 159–166.

Shane, R. (1995). Take the first step on the critical pathway. *American Journal of Health-System Pharmacy, 52*, 1051–1053.

Sia, C., Tonniges, T. F., Osterhus, E., & Taba, S. (2004). History of the medical home concept. *Pediatrics, 113*(5), 1473–1478.

Smith, M., Bates, D. W., Bodenheimer, T., & Cleary, P. D. (2010). Why pharmacists belong in the medical home. *Health Affairs, 29*(5), 906–913.

Sonnedecker, G., (Ed.). (1976). *Kremers and Urdang's history of pharmacy* (4th ed.). Philadelphia, PA: Lippincott.

U.S. Bureau of Labor Statistics (U.S. BLS). (2014a). Licensed practical and licensed vocational nurses. *Occupational outlook handbook* (2014–15 ed.). Retrieved from http://www.bls.gov/ooh/Healthcare/Licensed-practical-and-licensed-vocational-nurses.htm

U.S. Bureau of Labor Statistics (U.S. BLS). (2014b). Pharmacists. *Occupational outlook handbook* (2014–15 ed.). Retrieved from http://www.bls.gov/ooh/healthcare/pharmacists.htm

U.S. Bureau of Labor Statistics (U.S. BLS). (2014c). Pharmacy technicians and aides. *Occupational outlook handbook* (2014–15 ed.). Retrieved from http://www.bls.gov/ooh/healthcare/pharmacy-technicians.htm#tab-1

U.S. Bureau of Labor Statistics (U.S. BLS). (2014d). Physician assistants. *Occupational outlook handbook* (2014–15 ed.). Retrieved from http://www.bls.gov/ooh/Healthcare/Physician-assistants.htm

U.S. Bureau of Labor Statistics (U.S. BLS). (2014e). Registered nurses. *Occupational outlook handbook*, (2014–15 ed.). Retrieved from http://www.bls.gov/ooh/Healthcare/Registered-nurses.htm

U.S. Medical Licensing Examination (USMLE). (2015). *Bulletin of information.* Retrieved from http://www.usmle.org/pdfs/bulletin/2015bulletin.pdf

Vogel D. P. (1993). Patient-focused care. *American Journal of Hospital Pharmacists, 50*, 2321–2329.

Wakefield, D. S., Cyphert, S. T., Murray, J. F., Uden-Holman, T., Hendryx, M. S., Wakefield, B. J., & Helms, C. M. (1994). Understanding patient-centered care in the context of total quality management and continuous quality improvement. *The Joint Commission Journal on Quality Improvement, 20*(3), 152–161.

Werner, R. M., Kolstad, J. T., Stuart, E. A. & Polsky, D. (2011). The effect of pay-for-performance in hospitals: lessons for quality improvement. *Health Affairs, 30*(4), 690–698.

Zillich, A. J., McDonough, R. P., Carter, B. L., & Doucette, W. R. (2004). Influential characteristics of physician/pharmacist collaborative relationships. *Annals of Pharmacotherapy, 38*, 764–769.

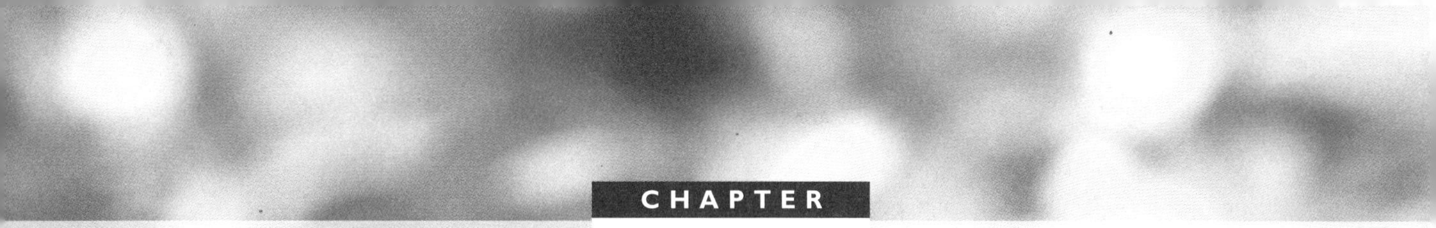

CHAPTER

3

The Pharmacist and the Pharmacy Profession

Erin R. Holmes*

Case Scenario

It is your first day working as a pharmacist at WeCare pharmacy, the same community pharmacy that you've worked at as a pharmacy student. The phone rings, and just as you have done hundreds of times before, you answer the phone, "WeCare pharmacy, intern speaking…uh…I mean, pharmacist speaking." It isn't until then that it finally hits you. You are the pharmacist now. *You* verify prescriptions. *You* counsel patients. *You* manage technicians. *You* are in charge of controlled substances.

You then verify the *first* prescription you've ever verified as a pharmacist. It is a simple prescription for Ativan 0.5 mg, but you know you've verified it at least 10 times. After all, it is *your* pharmacist license on the line now. The day is still young, however. It is the first of the month, and your pharmacy is due to dispense at least 600 prescriptions today. The technician, who was supposed to put in the inventory order, did not show up today. In the back of your mind, you are thinking about the new medication synchronization program you are about to start in response to health insurance plans wanting to improve quality indicators in your pharmacy, such as medication adherence. You try to counsel patients when they pick up their prescriptions, but there hardly seems like there is time. Then it hits you—a pharmacy student will be starting her rotation, and her preceptor is not here today, so you need to get her started on her first day here.

You have a moment of panic until you take a deep breath and say to yourself, "I've got this." This might be your first day as a pharmacist, but you've trained with the best pharmacists and have already learned how to manage all of these issues. You know there's a lot to juggle as a pharmacist, but you love it and are ready for the challenge.

LEARNING OBJECTIVES

Upon completion of this chapter, the student shall be able to:

- Identify three eras in pharmacy practice and education during the 20th century. Describe the principal forces that shaped the profession.
- Describe ways in which pharmacists' professional roles have expanded over the years. Identify barriers to pharmacists' role expansions and describe where the profession stands in its implementation.

*With acknowledgement to Shane P. Desselle

- Identify postgraduate educational opportunities for pharmacists.
- Compare and contrast licensure and certification.
- Discuss opportunities for pharmacists to obtain certification.
- Describe the roles played by professional pharmacy organizations. Identify benefits for pharmacists who join professional pharmacy organizations. Describe the mission and goals of several key professional pharmacy organizations.
- Describe the roles and functions of pharmacy technicians. Discuss the trend toward technician certification and professionalization and explain what these will mean to pharmacy practice.
- Describe how the Internet and other technological, financial, and political forces have affected pharmacy practice. Discuss advantages of and possible threats to patient safety from Internet pharmacy practice. Identify other technologies affecting contemporary pharmacy practice.
- Discuss the implications of the pharmacist workforce for practice and education. Describe factors that affect the pharmacist labor supply. Discuss estimates of the pharmacy workforce for the coming decades.

CHAPTER QUESTIONS

1. How have pharmacists' education and training and the roles they play in society evolved throughout the 20th century?
2. What is *pharmaceutical care*? What are its goals? Why did the pharmacy profession embrace it as a mission? How has pharmaceutical care evolved into the concept of medication therapy management (MTM)? Which barriers might prevent pharmacists from providing optimal level of care guided by these two concepts and how might these be overcome?
3. What are the subdisciplines that constitute pharmacy education and practice? What are some of the postgraduate educational and career options in these areas?
4. What is the difference between certification and licensure? What are some areas in which pharmacists may obtain board certification?
5. What purposes do professional pharmacy organizations serve? What are some of the key organizations that shape pharmacists' practice?
6. What are some trends concerning the roles of pharmacy technicians in practice?
7. What are the advantages and disadvantages of using Internet pharmacies from a patient's perspective? What are some of the public health concerns regarding the proliferation of Internet pharmacies?
8. What types of various technologies are shaping the way that health care and MTM services are being delivered and how?
9. Why is the pharmacy workforce such a critical issue to the profession? What do estimates of pharmacists' labor supply suggest?

INTRODUCTION

Chapter 2 introduced the concepts of professionalism and interdisciplinary care while briefly describing the training, expertise, and professional roles of pharmacists and some of the many healthcare professionals with whom pharmacists interact on a regular basis. This chapter examines in greater detail those same aspects of the pharmacy profession, its pharmacist members, and pharmacy education; it is divided into seven major sections.

The first section of this chapter is an abridged history of the profession and the evolution of current medication use systems. This appropriately leads into the second section, a discussion of pharmacy's mission and philosophy of practice, termed pharmaceutical care, and its evolution into MTM. The third section discusses current and expected future trends in practice, emphasizing pharmacist specialization and examining the various settings in which pharmacists practice.

A multitude of professional organizations represent pharmacists in each of these settings, as discussed in the fourth section. The fifth section describes the roles of pharmacy technicians, now pharmacists' most important adjuncts in providing pharmaceutical care.

The sixth section examines the influence of technology on the pharmacy profession. Other trends affecting the future of our practice are examined as well, including the projected increase in the number of prescriptions written and dispensed in the United States in the coming decades. This provides a nice segue into the seventh, very critical section of this chapter—the discussion of workforce issues. The labor supply has important implications for the future of pharmacy, including pharmacist education and training; pharmacy laws, rules, and regulations; policy regarding the use of ancillary personnel; pharmacist salaries; and, most importantly, the therapeutic outcomes of patients.

EVOLUTION OF THE PROFESSION AND MEDICATION USE SYSTEMS

Historians of pharmacy have used a variety of methods to categorize the evolution of pharmacy within the context of either waves or shifts in educational and industrial forces (Hepler, 1987), stages of professional identity (Hepler & Strand, 1990), or political shifts in the promulgation of our healthcare delivery system (Broeseker & Janke, 1998). Fortunately, there are a number of commonalities in their descriptions of the forces that have shaped our current method of practice and management of medication use systems. The approach taken here is simply to describe pharmacy practice, pharmacy education, and medication use within three distinct periods of the American 20th century leading up to today.

Before the 1940s

Pharmacy practice in the United States dates back to shortly after the country's founding. However, aside from the formation of professional associations and the first colleges of pharmacy during the 1800s, the predominant forces shaping pharmacy and medication use today took effect largely during the 20th century. Before this time, pharmacy was primarily an occupation for which its practitioners were trained via apprenticeship, much like participants in other trades. Pharmacy was considered an art that did not require theoretical knowledge and could best be learned "by daily handling and preparing the remedies in common use" (Sonnedecker, 1963, p. 204).

Without any credible standards or enforceable laws regarding the safety of therapeutic agents, the use of patent medicines was the norm. Pharmacists or apothecaries often were engaged in the wholesale manufacture and distribution of such products. The public had to rely on them to ensure that the compounds they sold were pure and unadulterated. Pharmacists came under considerable scrutiny, especially from physicians, when their increasingly profitable trade bred unscrupulous and unknowledgeable practitioners. Many of the patent medicines sold at the time were inefficacious, mislabeled, and even unsafe for consumption.

The first major piece of legislation to affect medication use in the 20th century was the Pure Food and Drug Act of 1906. Because the food and drug product industries were considered to be engaging in interstate commerce, the federal government passed this law to enable authorities to enforce penalties for certain types of misbranding and adulteration. The original statute was not particularly comprehensive or well written, so manufacturers, prescribers, and dispensers found many loopholes through which they could evade prosecution. Moreover, the Pure Food and Drug Act of 1906 did little to address the issue of efficacy in drug products.

Pressure continued to mount on the federal government to strengthen the food and drug laws, but unfortunately, it took a tragedy before more comprehensive measures were taken. During 1937, at least 73 deaths were attributed to ingestion of the toxic elixir sulfanilamide (Sonnedecker, 1963, p. 200). This scandal provided the necessary impetus for passage of the Food, Drug, and Cosmetic Act of 1938. This act afforded greater authority to the Food and Drug Administration (FDA), the federal agency charged with enforcing it, and with approving new drugs and new indications of drugs before they could be marketed in the United States. The statutes within the act and subsequent regulations issued by the FDA make it easier to enforce standards of safety and efficacy of drug products.

During the early part of the 20th century, pharmacists continued to engage in their roles as drug curators and dispensers. Interestingly, no formal legislation addressed the categorization of drugs into nonprescription and prescription products. Persons typically did not have to visit a physician if they desired a remedy for an ailment. Without such formal restrictions on dispensing, it could be argued that the pharmacist indirectly had some prescribing authority. Additionally, the pharmacist was relied on to provide advice to consumers on compounds he or she prescribed and dispensed (Hepler, 1987). Anecdotally, since pharmacists were—and still are—very accessible and visited frequently by customers, they were often the first source of entry into the healthcare system, particularly in rural areas that may have been underserved by physicians. They continued to fill this role despite a report published in 1910 by Abraham Flexner, who was appointed to study medical education, in which he contended that pharmacy was not a profession because its only responsibility was to carry out orders given by physicians. In response to this and other reports questioning the standing of pharmacy among other occupations, the American Association of Colleges of Pharmacy (AACP) commissioned a study directed by W.W. Charters. The study ultimately served as the basis for the AACP to require a 4-year baccalaureate degree program to be established by all colleges of pharmacy (Hepler, 1987).

The 1940s to the Early 1970s

The relatively brief period from the 1940s to the early 1970s brought significant changes in how health care was organized, delivered, and financed. This period has previously been described as the "era of expansion" (Relman, 1988, p. 1221). The Hospital Survey and Construction (Hill-Burton) Act of 1946 provided considerable grant monies for the renovation and expansion of existing hospitals, as well as the construction of new ones, primarily in underserved inner-city and rural areas (Torrens, 1993; see Chapter 8). Continuous mounting pressure from the growing number of persons who were unable to access the healthcare system led to the passage in 1965 of the Titles XVIII and XIX amendments to the 1935 Social Security Act, which established the Medicare and Medicaid programs. The result was a significant increase in the number of persons with some type of health coverage and a dramatic rise in the utilization of medical care goods and services. The Medicaid program, in particular, resulted in a dramatic shift in the use of pharmaceuticals and significantly increased the number of prescriptions dispensed (see Chapter 18).

In contrast with the trend of expanding roles for other allied healthcare professionals during this period, pharmacists began to see their roles in medication use management diminish. Several forces were at play in bringing about these changes. First, large, wholesale apothecaries were eventually transformed into large-scale manufacturers of pharmaceutical products. Previously, the majority of products dispensed by pharmacists were the result of their compounding bulk agents. Technological advances in industrial manufacturing and pharmaceutics, coupled with the increasing number of available compounds and societal demand that medicinal products become more uniform in their composition, resulted in the ability of and desire by manufacturers to prefabricate drugs in standardized dosage forms such as elixirs, syrups, tablets, and capsules.

The most influential piece of legislation that affected the medication use process in the United States was passed in 1951. The Durham-Humphrey amendment to the Food, Drug, and Cosmetic Act created the prescription or "legend" drug, whose label was required to carry the warning, "Caution: Federal law prohibits dispensing without a prescription." The result was an entirely new class of products that pharmacists did not have the ability to dispense without written orders from a licensed prescriber. At the same time, the profession's code of ethics as derived by the American Pharmaceutical (now Pharmacists) Association stated that "The pharmacist does not discuss the therapeutic effects or composition of a prescription with a patient. When such questions are asked, he suggests that the qualified practitioner is the proper person with whom such matters should be discussed" (Buerki & Vottero, 1994, p. 93). These forces relegated the pharmacist largely to a dispenser of presynthesized drug products.

The 1940s to early 1970s period also ushered in tremendous changes in pharmacy curricula throughout the United States. As part of this reform, many baccalaureate pharmacy programs were expanded to include a fifth year. Many of the extra didactic credit hours in these curricula were devoted to the further inclusion of scientific courses. Hepler (1987) contends that the primary objective of pharmaceutical education was to legitimize faculties, curricula, and, ultimately, the profession itself. He argues that the pharmaceutical industry encouraged research at pharmacy schools that was oriented toward the drug product. Courses in pharmacognosy gave way to natural products and medicinal chemistry; zoology was transformed into physiology; and galenical pharmacy evolved into pharmaceutics. In addition, new disciplines, such as pharmacology, biopharmaceutics, and pharmacokinetics, were born from the melding and application of other basic sciences. An argument for inclusion of these courses into curricula is that with the proliferation of new drug discoveries, practitioners required a scientific background to interpret literature and understand the proper use of drug products that would continue to enter the market throughout the pharmacist's career.

Nevertheless, it was argued that pharmacists became "overeducated and underutilized" during this period (Hepler, 1987, p. 537). Brodie (1967) wondered if the profession had lost the mainstream of its practice. A pioneer in pharmacy, he coined the term *drug use control*, a mantle suggesting pharmacists use their education to promote patient welfare in the form of drug safety. He defined this term as "that system of knowledge, understanding, judgments, procedures, skills, controls and ethics that assures optimal safety in the distribution and use of medication" (Brodie, 1967, p. 65).

The Early 1970s to the Present

The 1970s ushered in considerable concern over skyrocketing healthcare costs that were consuming an increasingly larger portion of the U.S. gross national product. The previous era in health care had resulted in the rapid perfusion of expensive new medications and technologies, professionalization and specialization of healthcare occupations, and proliferation of medical diagnoses for conditions not previously linked to biomedical origins (medicalization), such as alcoholism. Moreover, the structure of most insurance plans unintentionally provided incentives for medical care providers and patients to overuse healthcare services, often resulting in duplication and a loss of continuity in the care provided.

In recent years, several measures have been taken to counter these trends. Although they had existed before that time, the Health Maintenance Organization Act of 1973 paved the way for managed care organizations to garner a larger share of the health insurance market. Perhaps even more critical was the implementation of a prospective payment system of diagnosis-related groups by the Health Care Financing Administration (now the Centers for Medicare and Medicaid Services [CMS]) for Medicare patients (Pink, 1991). Diagnosis-related groups, commonly referred to as DRGs, are used to create a taxonomy of disease states and conditions for which patients may be admitted into a hospital. Reimbursement to hospitals for treating Medicare patients was set prospectively according to their diagnosis, regardless of the length and intensity of care. This system provided an incentive for hospitals to discharge patients quicker and sicker into other less intensive and expensive healthcare settings.

This period for pharmacy began with two reports that raised concerns among the entire profession. First, the Dichter Institute study, a survey commissioned by the American Pharmaceutical Association (APhA, now the American Pharmacists Association) in 1973 found that more respondents saw pharmacists as businesspeople than as healthcare providers (Maine & Penna, 1996). With the rapid expansion of large, full-service chain pharmacies that sold many products besides medicines, along with a lack of knowledge of pharmacists' training and expertise, study respondents viewed pharmacists more as extensions of pharmaceutical manufacturers and wholesalers.

The second study that generated some alarm was the Millis Commission's report in 1975, *Pharmacists for the Future: The Report of the Study Commission on Pharmacy* (Millis, 1975). Authors of this report suggested that pharmacists found themselves inadequately prepared in systems analysis, management skills, and communication skills. A subsequent report suggested including more of the behavioral and social sciences into pharmacy curricula and encouraged faculty participation in practice settings and research related to practice (Millis, 1976).

Before the release of these reports, the American Society of Hospital (now Health-Systems) Pharmacists published *Mirror to Hospital Pharmacy*, which stated bluntly that pharmacy had lost its way in producing professionals, and noted that practitioner frustration and dissatisfaction were beginning to affect students (Hepler, 1987). The clinical pharmacy movement was created to capture the essence of the drug use control concept put forth by Brodie and to promote the pharmacist's role as therapeutic advisor. This movement brought about changes in pharmacy education and practice.

In the late 1960s, the 6-year PharmD degree was introduced, with the additional year being devoted mostly to therapeutics courses and experiential education. Throughout the 1970s, 1980s, and into the early 1990s, an increasing number of colleges of pharmacy began offering the PharmD degree, but primarily as a postbaccalaureate program. Pharmacists who completed such programs secured jobs as clinical pharmacists, primarily in hospitals where they performed fewer dispensing functions and provided more services such as pharmacokinetic dosing, therapeutic monitoring, and drug information. Eventually, colleges of pharmacy began phasing out their baccalaureate programs. In 1995, the Argus Commission of the AACP recommended the 6-year PharmD as the entry-level degree into the profession (American Association of Colleges of Pharmacy, 1996).

EXPANDING THE PHARMACIST'S ROLE

Pharmaceutical Care

Despite the strides made by the profession during the 1970s and 1980s, questions existed about pharmacy's place in society (Penna, 1990). It was argued that clinical pharmacy, in itself, maintained its focus on products and services and not on the patient. It was also becoming increasingly apparent that medicalization and the increasing use of medications had repercussions in addition to benefits. Studies indicating dramatic rises in adverse drug reactions, hospitalizations, and even deaths from drug misadventuring grew more common (Manasse, 1989a, p. 936; 1989b, p. 1148).

Patient nonadherence to medications also was pervasive (Boyd, Covington, Stanaszek, & Coussons, 1974), which affected patient outcomes (Col, Fanale, & Kronholm, 1990).

Linda Strand and her colleagues identified eight categories of drug-related problems that could arise and result in poorer health outcomes and drug-related morbidity and mortality of patients. These categories are (1) untreated indications, (2) improper drug selection, (3) subtherapeutic dosage, (4) failure to receive drugs, (5) overdosage, (6) adverse drug reactions, (7) drug interactions, and (8) drug use without indications (Strand, Cippole, Morley, Ramsey, & Lamsam, 1990). Hepler and Strand then proposed that many of these problems could be reduced or prevented by pharmacists—that pharmacy's mission should be to serve society by maximizing the benefits and minimizing the negative effects of drug therapy for patients (Hepler & Strand, 1990).

This recognition operationally defined pharmacy's mandate for the 21st century: pharmaceutical care as: "the responsible provision of drug therapy for the purpose of achieving definite outcomes that improve a patient's quality of life. These outcomes are (1) cure of a disease, (2) elimination or reduction of a patient's symptomatology, (3) arresting or slowing of a disease process, or (4) preventing a disease or symptomatology" (Hepler & Strand, 1990, p. 539).

Hepler and Strand further delineated this concept to describe it as a process in which the pharmacist establishes a covenantal relationship with the patient in a mutually beneficial exchange. The pharmacist cooperates with the patient and other professionals in designing, implementing, and monitoring a therapeutic plan that will produce specific outcomes, thereby performing three basic functions: (1) identifying potential and actual drug-related problems, (2) resolving actual drug-related problems, and (3) preventing potential drug-related problems (Hepler & Strand, 1990).

By the mid-1990s, pharmaceutical care became a unifying mission for leaders in practice, professional organizations, and academia. Changing the mission and practice philosophy of an entire profession, however, is not easy, particularly when many barriers exist. Some of these barriers included:

1. Drug product focus: Pharmacists have historically been focused on dispensing drug products.
2. Service focus: Some services provided by pharmacists are not visible to the patient and may be performed without regard to the resultant outcomes to the recipient (e.g., pharmacokinetic dosing calculations).
3. Other healthcare professionals: Some physicians, nurses, and other allied healthcare professionals viewed pharmaceutical care as an infringement on their turf.
4. Lack of incentives: Methods for paying and rewarding pharmacists centered on dispensing volume, not on the care provided.
5. Logistical barriers: Many pharmacies were not designed and equipped properly to provide private consultation, disease monitoring, and dissemination of information—all key to the pharmaceutical care process.
6. Pharmacy ignorance and inertia: "The greatest barrier to pharmaceutical care is ourselves. The success of an idea requires the dedication of people who believe in it and who pledge themselves to its general acceptance and implementation" (Penna, 1990, p. 547).

The last barrier was especially significant because the term *pharmaceutical care* generated ambivalence among many pharmacists. It is difficult to blame individual practitioners for their failure to embrace this notion. For years, a considerable amount of ambiguity surrounded the concept. Pharmaceutical care represents an entire philosophy of practice; therefore, identification of the steps involved in preparing and following up on care plans, while useful, is not enough to guide pharmacists in this mission. Pharmacists' interactions with patients are just one component of implementing an effective practice. Other things must be considered, including adequate human, financial, and technical resources, in addition to management, marketing, and legal issues. **Table 3-1** presents a more contemporary view of pharmacy care that includes these and other domains. Pharmacists must be competent in each of these areas to maximize their ability to provide effective patient-oriented services.

Table 3-1 Pharmaceutical Care Practice Domains

I. Risk management
• Devise system of data collection
• Perform prospective drug utilization review
• Document therapeutic interventions and activities
• Obtain over-the-counter medication history
• Calculate dosages for drugs with a narrow therapeutic index
• Report adverse drug events to FDA
• Triage patients' needs for proper referral
• Remain abreast of newly uncovered adverse effects and drug—drug interactions
II. Patient advocacy
• Serve as patient advocate with respect to social, economic, and psychological barriers to drug therapy
• Attempt to change patients' medication orders when barriers to compliance exist
• Counsel patients on new and refill medications as necessary
• Promote patient wellness
• Maintain caring, friendly relationship with patients
• Telephone patients to obtain medication orders called in and not picked up
III. Disease management
• Provide information to patients on how to manage their disease state/condition
• Monitor patients' progress resulting from pharmacotherapy
• Carry inventory of products necessary for patients to execute a therapeutic plan (e.g., inhalers, nebulizers, glucose monitors)
• Supply patients with information on support and educational groups (e.g., American Diabetes Association, Multiple Sclerosis Society)
IV. Pharmaceutical care services marketing
• Meet prominent prescribers in the local area of practice
• Be an active member of professional associations that support the concept of pharmaceutical care
• Make available an area for private consultation services for patients as necessary
• Identify software that facilitates pharmacists' patient care-related activities
V. Business management
• Utilize technicians and other staff to free up the pharmacist's time
• Ensure adequate work flow for efficiency in operations

Source: Copyright © 2009 by the McGraw-Hill Companies. Originally published in Desselle, S.P. (2009). Pharmaceutical care as a management movement. In S.P. Desselle and D.P. Zgarrick, 2nd ed. (Eds.), *Pharmacy management: Essentials for all settings* (pp. 3–17). New York: McGraw-Hill.

Medication Therapy Management

While the pharmaceutical care movement made an indelible mark on the profession, its terminology is being replaced with more contemporary language that reflects pharmacists' growing roles in the provision of public health services (Desselle and Zgarrick, 2009, p. 3). In recognizing the morbidity and mortality resulting from medication errors as a public health problem, pharmaceutical care has evolved into the concept of medication therapy management (MTM). MTM represents a comprehensive and proactive approach to help patients maximize the benefits from drug therapy and includes services aimed at facilitating or improving patient adherence to drug therapy, educating entire populations of persons, conducting wellness programs, and becoming more intimately involved in disease management and monitoring. Eleven professional pharmacy organizations came together to produce a white paper on the core elements of an MTM service model. The model is designed to improve collaboration among pharmacists, physicians, and other healthcare professionals; enhance communication between patients and their healthcare team; and optimize medication use for improved patient outcomes. The core elements of an MTM service model include medication therapy review, a personal medication record, a medication-related action plan, intervention and/or referral, and documentation and follow-up. **Figure 3-1** illustrates the MTM core elements service model. First the pharmacist, with assistance from properly trained staff, interviews the patient and creates a database with appropriate information, reviews the patient's medication regimen, identifies any medication-related problems, prioritizes them, and creates a plan for the patient. This may be accomplished with the assistance of other healthcare professionals to whom pharmacists may triage the patient should the need arise. The pharmacist implements a plan by creating and communicating the personal medication record and medication-related action plan while documenting all actions taken and following up with the patient.

Pharmaceutical care and MTM do not differ much in their basic tenets and core elements, that is, becoming more proactive and taking greater responsibility for patients' medication therapy-related

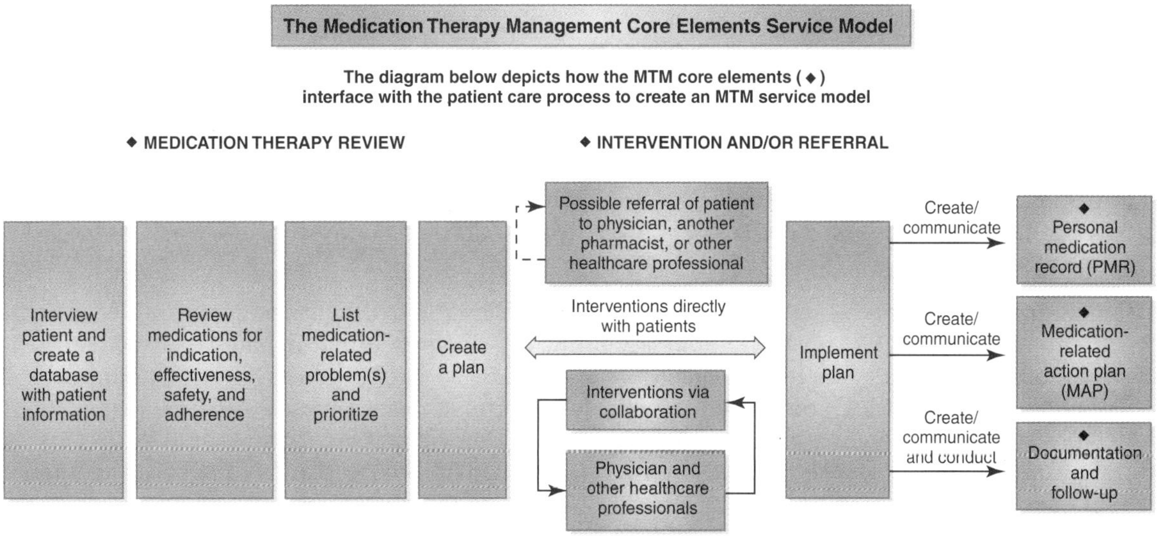

Figure 3-1 Flow Chart of a Medication Therapy Management Service Model.

 MTM = medication therapy management.

outcomes. The shift from pharmaceutical care to MTM reflects a more collaborative approach between the pharmacist and other healthcare providers, facilitating greater likelihood in collaborative working relationships and enhancing the likelihood of reimbursement for services. Moreover, the concept of pharmaceutical care might be criticized as pharmacy taking an overly insular individualistic approach to advancing the profession and treating patients. The MTM movement was strengthened by language in the Medicare Prescription Drug, Improvement and Modernization Act (MMA) of 2003 (public law number 108-173), which mandates payment for MTM services and includes pharmacists as viable health professionals, or providers, who may offer such services.

Reimbursement and Provider Status

The profession has made strides to address many barriers toward advancing pharmacy practice and MTM services, but still has further to go in having pharmacists formally recognized as providers and educators who should be reimbursed for providing patient-related services. Pharmacists have long had opportunities to become certified as experts in pharmacotherapy, but recognition of those achievements outside the pharmacy profession has been problematic. In the 1990s and early 21st century, state governments aided this quest by beginning to pass legislation expanding pharmacists' scope of practice to include broader pharmacotherapeutic decision making, implementation of home healthcare services, and provision of immunizations.

Many leaders in pharmacy hailed the passage of MMA. While there have been concerns about some of its provisions, the MMA was comprehensive federal legislation that recognized the need for MTM services in ambulatory care. The MMA does not strictly govern face-to-face encounters or mandate that such services be provided by a pharmacist, but its language does position pharmacy as a choice to fulfill a role in reducing drug-related morbidity and educating older adults on the proper pharmacologic and nonpharmacologic management of comorbid diseases. To date, MMA appeared to be a mixed bag for both pharmacy and patients, with additional persons being afforded drug coverage at relatively stable premiums, but with more rapid inflationary costs of prescription drugs and limited, albeit important strides made toward reimbursement of pharmacists for direct MTM involvement. Health plans often have filled the niche for MTM services to qualified beneficiaries through the use of telephone and mail services often implemented by nurses and other healthcare professionals.

Since the passage of MMA, technologies have been developed to facilitate pharmacist MTM and subsequent reimbursement. Companies like Mirixa (www.mirixa.com), OutcomesMTM (www.outcomesmtm.com), and PharmMD (www.pharmmd.com) use Internet-based platforms and other innovative technologies to facilitate pharmacist MTM and subsequent reimbursement. These companies provide a platform to pharmacists to document their services. In some cases, they provide additional services to their members, such as policies and procedures, quality assurance, and resources.

Some progress also is being made in the private sector. The Asheville project featured a long-term effort supported by employers to reimburse pharmacists for providing diabetes management services to their employees. The results suggested that pharmacists could help patients in improving both short-term (Cranor & Christensen, 2003) and long-term (Cranor, Bunting, & Christensen, 2003) outcomes, while saving employers money from averted medical costs. To that end, it appears as though some patients may be willing to pay for pharmacists' services out of pocket if necessary (MacKinnon & Mahrous, 2002).

The pharmacy profession's fight for *provider status* gained significant ground in 2013. Being recognized by the federal government as providers would allow pharmacy services to be eligible for reimbursement under Medicare Part B. Currently, the exclusion of pharmacists as providers under Medicare Part B limits Medicare beneficiaries' access to pharmacy services. Currently Medicare Part B providers include physicians, physician assistants, certified nurse practitioners, qualified psychologists, clinical social workers, certified nurse midwives, and certified nurse anesthetists. In addition, omission as providers from Medicare Part B is often cited by private health plans as a reason for the lack of coverage and reimbursement for pharmacists' services (American Pharmacists Association, 2013).

The American Pharmacist Association, along with the support of other pharmacy organizations, actively lobbies for provider status. On the federal level, the Pharmacy and Medically Underserved Areas Enhancement Act was introduced into Congress in January 2015. Thirty-eight states have legislated provider/practitioner status for pharmacists, with additional states introducing legislation (American Pharmacists Association, 2015). In addition, 10 states pay for pharmacists' services through their Medicaid programs. Several other states have legislation regarding payment for services and scope of practice.

Pharmacy Quality Measures

In 2007, CMS introduced the Star Ratings System, which uses a scale from 1 to 5 stars where 5 is the highest star rating. This system evaluates health plans on their performance, much like customers rate products that they purchase from Amazon. In 2012, the Affordable Care Act authorized Medicare Advantage plans and Medicare Advantage plans with Part D with the highest ratings to receive incentives in the form of quality bonus payments (QBPs). A significant part of how health plans are rated comes from a number of pharmacy measures developed by the Pharmacy Quality Alliance (PQA, http://www.pqaalliance.org). Some of these measures include adherence to diabetes, cholesterol, and hypertension medications, which are measures that pharmacists can influence through the provision of patient care. Pharmacies are rated based on the percentage of patients adhering to prescribed therapies. Thus, pharmacies are receiving pressure from health plans to perform well on these pharmacy measures, so that the plans in turn perform well and are more likely to receive bonus payments.

In order to improve performance on adherence measures, pharmacists have developed innovative programs that go beyond dispensing to improve patient outcomes. One of these programs is medication synchronization, which started gaining traction in 2008. The premise of medication synchronization is that all of a patient's chronic medications are synchronized so that they are refilled one day each month, not multiple times each month. Thus, synchronization programs are ideal for patients (particularly the elderly) who may take multiple medications. When the medications are refilled, only the amount the patient needs is provided, not the entire amount (of say, 30 or 90 days) to prevent stockpiling and waste. An important aspect of medication synchronization is patient contact with the pharmacist, in order to monitor and address medication adherence and other medication-related problems. Synchronization programs not only improve patient outcomes but they also build efficiencies into a pharmacy's workflow by reducing walk-in traffic. Research studies are beginning to demonstrate improved medication adherence from medication synchronization (APhA Foundation, 2013; Ateb, 2013; Holdford & Inocencio, 2013). Pharmacy care becomes proactive rather than reactive. Many medication synchronization programs exist, and a growing number of software programs are also becoming available to assist pharmacists in implementing these programs.

PHARMACY EDUCATION AND TRAINING

Pharmacy education and training has evolved over the years with notable trends. First, the PharmD has replaced the baccalaureate (bachelor of science) degree as the entry-level degree in the pharmacy field. Another trend in pharmacy education is the continued efforts by colleges of pharmacy to incorporate more of the social and administrative sciences into their curricula. Colleges of pharmacy were initially slow to respond to the changes proposed by the Millis Commission. The AACP refocused its efforts to encourage a more liberal education for pharmacy students in the 1990s with its Commission to Implement Change in Pharmaceutical Education (1993; American Association of Colleges of Pharmacy, 1996). Among the issues addressed by the commission were the incorporation of specific courses and concepts related to health policy organization, communication, economic analysis, and the understanding of cultural diversity throughout the curriculum. The commission also addressed how courses should be taught, stressing multidisciplinary, problem- or service-based approaches to delivering course content to encourage problem-solving and critical-thinking skills in future practitioners.

Other trends related to pharmacy practice concern the proliferation of new and exciting areas of practice, the emergence of collaborative working relationships, expanded scope of practice agreements legislated by a number of states, the use of automated technology and technicians for dispensing functions, and shifts in the pharmacist labor supply. Accreditation standards for schools/colleges of pharmacy are evolving based on the role of practitioners in current practice settings and in the future. In the most recent standards, Standards 16, there is an increased emphasis on interprofessional education, as well as personal and professional development (e.g., leadership, innovation and entrepreneurship, and professionalism) (https://www.acpe-accredit.org/pdf/Standards2016FINAL.pdf).

Licensure Requirements

Pharmacy continues to be one of the more rewarding professions with respect to the starting salaries of its members following completion of the entry-level degree and licensure. In addition to completing the PharmD degree, prospective pharmacists must log a certain number of hours as an intern practicing under the supervision of a licensed preceptor pharmacist; the number of hours required varies across states. The graduate must also successfully complete the North American Pharmacist Licensure Examination (NAPLEX) and his or her respective state's MPJE (Multistate Pharmacy Jurisprudence Exam) or equivalent jurisprudence examination. When the requirements for licensure within a state have been completed, the candidate is qualified to become a registered pharmacist (RPh) who is licensed to practice in that particular state. Once registered, pharmacists can apply for licensure in other states through a process called reciprocation. The process to reciprocate varies by individual state. To learn about individual requirements, visit the State Board of Pharmacy website.

Postgraduate Educational Opportunities

A choice of exciting careers awaits the pharmacy graduate. Some career paths, however, require the student to pursue postgraduate education. Master's and Ph.D. degree programs are offered at many colleges of pharmacy in the general areas of medicinal chemistry, pharmaceutics, pharmacology/toxicology, and social and administrative sciences, with each college tailoring its specific programs in each of these areas to student needs and faculty interests and backgrounds. Pursuing one of these degrees is ideal for the student who is interested in a career in academia, the pharmaceutical industry, government, or another setting requiring research expertise. Individuals who are interested in advancing their careers in the practice arena may seek one of any number of residencies and fellowships offered through universities, hospitals, and other healthcare providers throughout the United States. Depending on the student's ultimate career path, other degrees such as a master's degree in business administration (MBA), Juris Doctor (JD), and master's degree in public health (MPH) can serve to complement their clinical training.

Specialization Through Certification

Other opportunities are available to pharmacists through the process of certification. Certification is recognition by a nongovernment association or agency that an individual has completed predetermined qualifications in a field of specialized knowledge. Pharmacists may become board certified in any of the following eight specialties through programs administered by the Board of Pharmacy Specialties (BPS):

1. *Oncology pharmacy.* Addresses medication therapy needs of patients with cancer. Specialists are closely involved in recognition, management, and prevention of unique morbidities associated with cancer and cancer treatment and recognition of the balance between improved survival and quality of life as primary outcome indicators.
2. *Psychiatric pharmacy.* Addresses the often complex medication therapy regimens and concomitant somatic comorbidities of patients with psychiatric disorders. The specialist is responsible for optimizing drug treatment and patient care by conducting patient assessments, recommending treatment plans, monitoring patient response, and recognizing drug-induced problems.
3. *Nutrition support pharmacy.* Addresses the care of patients who receive specialized nutrition support, including parenteral and enteral nutrition. The specialist has responsibility for promoting maintenance and/or restoration of optimal nutritional status and designing and modifying treatment needs. He or she often functions as a member of a multidisciplinary nutrition support team.
4. *Nuclear pharmacy.* Seeks to improve and promote public health through the safe and effective use of radioactive drugs for diagnosis and therapy. A nuclear pharmacist specializes in procurement, compounding, quality assurance, dispensing, distribution, and development of radiopharmaceuticals.
5. *Pharmacotherapy.* Assumes responsibility for ensuring the safe, appropriate, and economical use of drugs in patient care. The specialist often has responsibility for direct patient care, may conduct clinical research, and serves as a primary source of drug information for other healthcare professionals.
6. *Ambulatory care pharmacy.* Addresses care necessary for patients in outpatient settings with a particular focus on chronic disease management. The ambulatory care pharmacist must understand and apply skills related to pharmacists' roles in public health, develop rapport with ambulatory patients, prioritize patients' drug-related problems, apply pharmacoeconomic principles when designing a treatment plan, perform health screening, and conduct physical assessment procedures, as appropriate.
7. *Critical care pharmacy.* Ensures the safe and effective use of medications in critically ill patients as an integral member of an interprofessional team. The critical care pharmacist makes rapid decisions using pharmacodynamic, pharmacokinetic, and other data for patients whose clinical situation is rapidly changing.
8. *Pediatric pharmacy.* Specializes in safe and effective medication use in children ranging from pediatrics to adolescents. Pediatric pharmacists provide direct care for pediatric patients through interdisciplinary teams as well as serve as educators and advocates for children and their families (BPS, 2015).

These programs are rigorous and require extensive work and study. Pharmacists may also complete other certification programs in a wide variety of areas—most notably in the management of certain disease states/conditions, such as diabetes, hypertension, and pain management. Other potential areas of focus include geriatrics, pediatrics, managed care, and management/marketing. These programs are administered by professional or health organizations, such as the American Diabetes Association, and they are often approved by the American Council on Pharmaceutical Education, though they do not indicate board certification.

Unlike licensure, certification does not give the recipient any legal privileges; however, it does offer the recipient many advantages. Aside from the implicit value of the knowledge and expertise gained, some job descriptions posted by medical care institutions require certification. In addition, third-party payers may be more likely to reimburse a board-certified specialist or reimburse such a professional for the same services at a higher rate. Board certification also represents a marketing tool that specialists can use to advocate their services. As of 2014, 21,560 pharmacists are certified through the Board of Pharmacy Specialties, with close to 16,000 of those certifications in pharmacotherapy (BPS, 2015).

PROFESSIONAL PHARMACY ORGANIZATIONS

A Brief History

The diversity of pharmacists' practice settings is reflected in the large number of professional pharmacy organizations. The first professional pharmacy organization, the APhA, was founded in 1852 for the purpose of establishing national standards of quality for drugs and chemicals. Its founding came in response to criticism of the pharmacy trade by physicians who threatened to regulate the profession. Shortly thereafter, the APhA developed a code of ethics for its member practitioners. During the 1900s, other professional associations developed. Some of them were offshoots from within various sections of the APhA. The number of professional organizations continues to grow as the interests and work environments of pharmacists expand.

The Purpose and Functions of Pharmacy Organizations

Professional pharmacy organizations represent a few of the tens of thousands of national associations in the United States, not including state and local associations. The primary reason that these organizations exist is to serve the interests of their members. They publish position papers as well as lobby governments, other professional organizations, and private businesses on behalf of their members. Examples of issues targeted for lobbying efforts include the crafting of specific language beneficial to pharmacists in regulations proposed by federal agencies, reimbursement for pharmacy services, and expansion of the scope of pharmacy practice.

Specific benefits and services that professional pharmacy organizations provide include the following:

- *Information dissemination.* Publishing of journals and newsletters to disseminate the results of pertinent studies and updates on professional practice and legal issues. Associations often provide daily or weekly updates by email or on their websites.
- *Maintenance of practitioners' competency.* Establishing codes of ethics and standards of practice, as well as providing free continuing education and professional meetings.
- *Career planning assistance.* Posting of jobs in related fields, placement of advertisements in journals by employers, and sponsorship of workshops for career advancement.

- *Financial benefits.* Providing discount rates on items such as resource materials, credit cards, liability coverage, and insurance policies.
- *Participation in governance.* Providing an opportunity for members to help create and revise organization policies at professional meetings and serve on committees.

Professional Organizations With Pharmacist Membership

Individual pharmacists may enroll as members of some of the organizations that directly or indirectly serve the profession.

Arguably the most diverse pharmacy-related organization in terms of its membership, *American Pharmacists Association* (APhA, www.pharmacist.com) serves pharmacists in all practice settings. Headquartered in Washington, D.C., it is actively involved in lobbying the government on pharmacists' behalf. Its student organization, the Academy of Student Pharmacists, has more student members than any other professional association. The APhA publishes numerous journals and newsletters, including *Pharmacy Today,* to help students and practitioners keep abreast of current issues, and *Journal of the American Pharmacists Association*, which features research in the administrative, basic, and clinical pharmaceutical sciences. It also publishes monographs, such as those describing the MMA of 2003, which are very helpful to pharmacists.

Formerly the American Society of Hospital Pharmacists, the *American Society of Health-Systems Pharmacists* (ASHP, www.ashp.org) changed its name to reflect the evolution of hospitals into integrated delivery networks. The ASHP is a national accrediting organization for pharmacy residency and pharmacy technician training programs. It publishes numerous educational materials and handbooks, including *American Hospital Formulary System Drug Information.* It also publishes *American Journal of Health-Systems Pharmacy* and produces *International Pharmaceutical Abstracts*, a bimonthly abstracting and indexing service. The ASHP promotes guidelines, standards, and best practices in a number of pharmacy practice arenas. Its annual clinical meeting is the largest gathering of pharmacists worldwide.

Founded as the National Association of Retail Druggists, the mission of the *National Community Pharmacists Association* (NCPA, www.ncpanet.org) is to keep the business of independent pharmacy viable. The NCPA is the voice for America's independent community pharmacists. It provides continuing education through its publication, *America's Pharmacist.* The NCPA's Management Institute serves as a clearinghouse for up-to-date management information. The NCPA administers the National Institute for Pharmacist Care Outcomes program and sponsors the NCPA Foundation, which awards grants intended to promote the profession and pharmacy care outcomes. With the aid of sponsors, the NCPA also publishes *NCPA Digest.* The *NCPA Digest* allows independent community pharmacies to assess and compare their financial and clinical performance with indicators for other pharmacies of similar size.

The *Academy of Managed Care Pharmacy* (www.amcp.org) serves patients and the public through the promotion of wellness and rational drug therapy by the application of managed care principles. Part of its mission is the advancement of pharmacy practice in managed healthcare systems. The Academy of Managed Care Pharmacy publishes *Journal of Managed Care Pharmacy*, which highlights research on administrative issues and on the rational use of drug therapies, including cost-effectiveness and outcomes studies. This organization has been a leader in efforts to standardize formulary submissions and to improve the quality of formulary decisions made by insurers and institutions. It also provides weekly email and fax-on-demand services that keep its members informed about drug therapy and legislative issues from around the United States.

Membership in the *American College of Apothecaries* (www.acainfo.org) is open to pharmacists who own or hold shares in a pharmacy, primarily apothecary-style pharmacies with low levels of front-end merchandise. Among its publications are *Guidelines for Improving Communication in Pharmacy Practice* and *Guidelines for Marketing Your Community Pharmacy Practice.*

Founded to strengthen pharmacy's role in long-term care, in particular the care of elderly patients, the *American Society of Consultant Pharmacists* (www.ascp.com) publishes the journal, *Consultant Pharmacist,* which features articles on the results of drug utilization reviews and clinical studies, drug information, and managerial aspects of consultant pharmacy. Among its other publications is *Drug Regimen Review: A Process Guide for Pharmacists.*

Founded to advance the practice of clinical pharmacy, the *American College of Clinical Pharmacy* (www.accp.com) promotes clinical research, rational drug therapy, and fellowship training. It also publishes educational materials related to pharmacoeconomics and outcomes research. Many faculty members in departments of pharmacy practice are members of the American College of Clinical Pharmacy.

The *National Pharmaceutical Association* (www.nphanet.net) is dedicated to representing the views and ideas of minority pharmacists on critical issues affecting health care and pharmacy as well as advancing the standards of pharmaceutical care among all practitioners.

The *National Council on Patient Information and Education* (www.talkaboutrx.org) is dedicated to improving communication between healthcare professionals and patients. It also makes available the *Talking About Prescriptions Planning Kit* and *Educate Before You Medicate* promotional materials.

Organizations With Corporate Membership

Pharmacists may also be affected by or interact with other organizations of which they are not members. The members of these organizations are corporations, rather than individuals.

Formerly the National Wholesale Druggists Association, the *Healthcare Distribution Management Association* (www.healthcaredistribution.org) is the national association of full-service drug wholesalers. This organization's mission is to strengthen relations between wholesalers, their suppliers, and customers, and to sponsor and disseminate research and information on new technology and management practices for wholesalers. Full-service drug wholesalers are typically large companies involved in myriad aspects of drug distribution, including automated dispensing technologies and storage of specialty compounds.

The *Institute for Safe Medication Practices* (www.ismp.org) is the United States' only nonprofit organization devoted entirely to medication error prevention and safe medication use. It oversees a voluntary medication error-reporting system and promotes error reduction strategies to the healthcare community, policy makers, and the public.

The voice of the chain drug store industry, the *National Association of Chain Drug Stores* (www.nacds.org), is involved in numerous professional activities, including sponsoring student recruitment programs in high schools, conducting visitation programs for faculty and students to chain store headquarters operations, and awarding grant support for studies in management and administration. It posts positions for pharmacists in chain pharmacies throughout the United States on its website and, along with organizations such as the NCPA, supports the SureScripts Electronic Prescribing Network to allow for the electronic exchange of information between prescribers and pharmacies.

The *Pharmaceutical Researchers and Manufacturers of America* (www.pharma.org) is a powerful consortium of manufacturers of brand-name products that is heavily involved in supporting research and development of new drugs and pharmaceutical delivery systems.

Formerly the Nonprescription Drug Manufacturers Association (NDMA), the *Consumer Healthcare Products Association* (www.chpa-info.org) is concerned with issues relevant to makers of over-the-counter medications and encourages responsible self-medication practices by consumers. The Consumer Healthcare Products Association conducts a voluntary labeling review service for members and promotes the readability of over-the-counter product labels.

The *Generic Pharmaceutical Association* (www.gphaonline.org) represents manufacturers and distributors within the generic drug industry. The Generic Pharmaceutical Association is dedicated to the provision of high-quality, cost-effective equivalents to brand-name prescription drugs. It provides lawmakers, government agencies, regulators, prescribers, and pharmacists with information regarding the safety, effectiveness, and therapeutic equivalence of generic medicines.

The *Pharmacy Quality Alliance* (PQA) (www.pqaalliance.org), which was recently established in 2006, is an organization whose mission is to improve medication management and patient health through the development and implementation of pharmacy quality performance measures. The PQA has over 160 member organizations that include academic institutions, health plans, government agencies, and chain pharmacy corporations, among others. The PQA emphasizes a collaborative approach to improving pharmacy quality.

Educational and Regulatory Organizations

Some organizations provide services to pharmacists (who may or may not be members of those groups) and regulate their practice and educational requirements.

Society grants pharmacy the power of self-regulation as long as society can reap the benefits of having highly competent and moral professionals serving its interests. The *National Association of Boards of Pharmacy* (NABP, www.nabp.net) assists state boards of pharmacy in protecting the public by developing, implementing, and enforcing uniform standards. The NABP develops and administers the NAPLEX and oversees reciprocity of licenses across states.

The *Accreditation Council for Pharmacy Education* (www.acpe-accredit.org) is a national agency that provides for the accreditation of professional degree programs in pharmacy and for the approval of providers of continuing pharmaceutical education. The Accreditation Council for Pharmacy Education is an autonomous agency whose board of directors is made up of members of the AACP, APhA, NABP, and American Council on Education.

The *American Association of Colleges of Pharmacy* (AACP) is a national organization representing the interests of pharmaceutical educators. The AACP is committed to excellence in pharmaceutical education. Both individual faculty members and schools of pharmacy constitute its membership. It publishes the *American Journal of Pharmaceutical Education*, with contributions from pharmacy faculty throughout the United States, to disseminate information on course content, curricula, and innovative teaching strategies.

The mission of the *American Foundation for Pharmaceutical Education* (www.afpenet.org) is to advance and support pharmaceutical sciences education at U.S. schools and colleges of pharmacy by awarding scholarships and grants to pharmacy students and faculty.

PHARMACY TECHNICIANS

As the practice of pharmacy evolves, so do the roles of pharmacy technicians. The number of prescriptions dispensed in the United States has increased rapidly in recent years, as has the diversity of settings in which pharmacists practice. To keep up with the rising demand for pharmaceutical products and services, technicians will play a greater role in support of pharmaceutical care. This section examines pharmacy technicians, their expanding roles and responsibilities, and certification and management issues.

The Choice of a Career as a Pharmacy Technician

In 2012, approximately 355,300 pharmacy technicians were practicing in the United States (Bureau of Labor Statistics, 2014–2015) with a median hour wage of $14.10 with exact earnings dependent upon their location, practice setting, experience, and certification status. Technicians receive their training through formal educational programs at vocational or technical schools and community colleges, formal on-the-job training programs sponsored by employers, or informal on-the-job training. An increasing number of nationally accredited technician training programs exist, with the standard for accreditation by the ASHP calling for 600 hours of contact time, extending over at least 15 weeks (American Society of Health-System Pharmacists, 2013).

Pharmacy Technicians' Expanding Roles and Responsibilities

Published in 2009, the Scope of Pharmacy Practice Project revealed that certified pharmacy technicians spent more than 66% of their time assisting pharmacists to serve patients by: receiving prescription/medication orders, collecting and communicating patient-specific data, assessing a prescription/medication order for completeness, accuracy, authenticity, legality, and reimbursement eligibility, processing a prescription/medication order, providing a prescription to the patient/caregiver, and directing the patient/caregiver to the pharmacist for counseling. Certified technicians spent 22% of their time maintaining medication and inventory control systems by identifying drugs and other products to be ordered, removing expired, discontinued, or slow moving inventory or overstock from shelves, and performing and documenting inventories. Finally, certified technicians spend 12% of their time participating in the administration and management of pharmacy practice by coordinating communications in the practice setting, updating and maintaining patient information, using and maintaining automation, and communicating with third-party payers (American Society of Health-System Pharmacists, 2009).

While these data alone suggest that the technician's role is expanding, there is more evidence to suggest that technicians are taking on even more roles, such as in the areas of patient safety and medication-error prevention. They also are assisting pharmacists in monitoring patient outcomes by the collection of patient data. They have expanded supervisory responsibilities that include order-entry verification and preparing medications for final approval of a pharmacist. They perform billing and accounting tasks, evaluate other employees' performance, and participate in the development of policies and procedures (American Society of Health-System Pharmacists, 2009). As the practice of medication synchronization grows, technicians are now commonly overseeing or coordinating these programs for their pharmacies.

Pharmacy Technician Education and Training

Many concerns have been raised about the need for standardization in technician training and education (American Pharmaceutical Association, 2003; Cooksey et al., 2002). In light of the changing environment of pharmacy practice, establishing a minimum knowledge and skills set for pharmacy technicians may be warranted. While most definitions of pharmacy technicians exclude the use of the term, *professional judgment*, a study by Wilson, Kimberlin, and Brushwood (2005) demonstrated that technician practice fits a model of professional expertise and that technicians use reasoning and judgment skills in their tasks. As such, pharmacy practice might be better served with some sort of technician credentialing process to optimize their contributions to pharmacy practice.

Some progress toward improving education and training for technicians has been made. In 2002, the Sesquicentennial Stepping Stones Summits, a consortium of pharmacy leaders and stakeholders, firmly established the need and potential future credential requirements of pharmacy technicians (American Pharmaceutical Association, 2003b). While stronger terminology such as *licensure* was not applied to technicians, it was agreed upon that national registration of technicians and further requirements of standardized education are essential in driving a skilled and knowledgeable workforce of future pharmacists' support personnel. More recently, ASHP began the Pharmacy Technician Initiative to advocate for state laws that require completion of ASHP-accredited pharmacy technician training and for national certification (Desselle, 2005).

Pharmacy Technician Certification

The trend toward expansion of pharmacy technicians' roles is reflected in the movement toward voluntary certification of these professionals. A certified pharmacy technician has completed requirements promulgated by either the Pharmacy Technician Certification Board or the Institute for the Certification of Pharmacy Technicians. Their rigorous examinations include questions on communication, organizational and interpersonal skills, pharmacy operations, pharmacy law, and calculations. The Pharmacy Technician Certification Board was founded jointly by the APhA, the ASHP, the Illinois Council of Health-System Pharmacists, and the Michigan Pharmacists Association. As of December 31, 2014, the Pharmacy Technician Certification Board has granted 555,713 pharmacy technician certifications (PTCB, 2015).

Certification offers advantages to both the technician and the pharmacist. For technicians, certification may result in an increase in pay or a promotion in title. It may also bring greater job security and give the person an edge when seeking a job or changing jobs. It may also result in expanded job functions and responsibilities and—perhaps most importantly—increased satisfaction on the job. The increased confidence and satisfaction from the technician becoming certified may enhance his or her performance, thereby increasing the pharmacy's productivity. It may also decrease training time and lower the cost of on-the-job training.

Pharmacists have historically been reticent to allow technicians to expand their scope of practice, but this reluctance is changing. Today's pharmacists are more secure in their roles and are beginning to see that certified technicians can reduce their workloads and mitigate their stress levels (Mott, Vanderpool, & Smeenk, 1998). One study indicated that pharmacists see certification as valuable toward enhancing technicians' knowledge sets, attitudes, and skills (Schmitt & Desselle, 2009).

In addition to addressing the problem of an acute shortage of pharmacists, technician certification has grown more popular because of the progress made in curricula and in the training of technicians, thanks to the development of the Model Curriculum for Pharmacy Technician Training (American Pharmaceutical Association, 2003a). Also, a majority of states have revised their pharmacy practice acts in areas related to technicians, and a number of states have liberalized their pharmacist-to-technician ratios. Finally, states have begun making certification a requirement for technician registration or licensure.

TECHNOLOGY AND THE PHARMACY PROFESSION

Internet Pharmacy

No formal definition exists for *Internet pharmacy*, also known as *online pharmacy*, *cyberpharmacy*, and *e-pharmacy*. There are basically three types of Internet pharmacies. One type provides legend pharmaceuticals pursuant to a valid prescription order; it is essentially a mail-order pharmacy whose business address is in cyberspace. Upon receipt of a prescription from a physician who is not affiliated with the website, the pharmacist will fill it, mail the product to the patient, and then either bill the patient directly or bill his or her insurance company. The pioneers in this field expanded rapidly to provide many other services.

A second type of Internet pharmacy includes sites that offer free information and counseling for a fee but without the dispensing component. These businesses can be grouped with many other websites that offer health information, with or without a fee, but that are not necessarily pharmacies. While some of these sites are legitimate, such as those operated by various professional groups, others are not.

It is the third type of online pharmacy that has drawn the concern of medical professionals, government, regulatory agencies, and society at large. At these sites, consumers log on and complete a survey or questionnaire about their medical problem or make a direct request for a particular prescription drug product. The consumer may be charged a fee for completing the questionnaire, which may be returned or discounted if the physician does not issue a prescription. At legitimate sites of this kind, a physician reviews the data. Many sites, however, pretend to have licensed prescribers and pharmacists in house. They have obtained the medications illegally and are selling them to consumers at high prices without regard for purchasers' safety.

Illegal pharmacy sites pose a significant health threat to many Americans. The drugs acquired from certain Internet sources may be adulterated or perhaps even not contain the listed active ingredient. Stopping illegal Internet pharmacy operations has been an arduous task for authorities because it is difficult to find their geographic locations. Few enforceable laws govern these types of businesses.

Issues related to Internet pharmacy include reimportation and diversion of pharmaceuticals. As prescription drugs continue to take up a larger portion of the monies spent on health care, many persons are seeking alternatives to traditional means for purchasing prescription drugs. Some, for example, try to purchase medications from pharmacies in Canada and Mexico to save money. In fact, some state governments have formed cooperatives to arrange for purchase of medications from Canadian pharmacies for state employees or for Medicaid beneficiaries. This contradicts FDA regulations; to date, the federal government has not strictly enforced those rules. There is considerable debate about the authenticity of medications acquired from Canadian Internet sites. The acquisition of drugs from legitimate Canadian operations poses little, if any threat, beyond that normally accompanying medication use without face-to-face counseling with a health professional; however, many web-based pharmacy operations use a Canadian name or domain name, but are not legally recognized Canadian pharmacies.

The NABP responded to illegal online sales of prescription drugs quickly by unveiling its Verified Internet Pharmacy Practice Site program in February 1999 (Paulsen, 1999). Verified Internet Pharmacy Practice Site is a voluntary program designed to certify each participating online pharmacy's ability to dispense pharmaceuticals. Certification involves documenting licensure from the appropriate state board of pharmacy, ensuring that the pharmacy meets a rigorous 19-point set of criteria, and conducting an on-site review of the pharmacy's written policies and procedures by an NABP-trained inspection team. Certified pharmacies display the Verified Internet Pharmacy Practice Site seal on the home page of their website. This seal contains a hyperlink to NABP's home page, where visitors can view information about the online pharmacy.

Some states have also taken measures against illegal online prescription sales. For example, the state of Arkansas passed a law that requires any pharmacy shipping prescription drugs to a resident of the state to have at least one pharmacist licensed to practice by Arkansas's state board (Conlan, 1999). Other states have enacted similar legislation. A few state health departments have successfully identified illegal operations and prosecuted those involved.

Perhaps the most effective means to curb patients' acquisition of medications from specious sources is to improve access to drug therapy. The MMA greatly improved many seniors' ability to obtain necessary medications and afforded them the opportunity to receive expanded MTM services. Additionally, manufacturers of branded drug products offer an array of medication assistance programs to qualified patients. These programs also have limitations, such as paperwork for providers and the occasional delay for patients receiving medication, but they provide access to medications for many persons in need, particularly those for whom generic or therapeutic substitution is not an option. These and other government and private sector solutions, such as the Affordable Care Act, attempt to reduce the number of indigent persons without prescription drug access and will undoubtedly reduce the demand for prescription drugs from alternative sources. Pharmacists working in bricks-and-mortar operations can do their part by providing quality service to patients. Although web-based commerce is preferred—and even mandated—by payers for a certain segment of the population, pharmacists may advocate to patients that direct, face-to-face communication is optimal. One study found that information provided via ask-the-pharmacist services on the web was less than optimal, even from trusted sources (Holmes, Desselle, Nath, & Markuss, 2005). Yet another found poor readability and incomplete information for certain drugs on the websites of national chain pharmacies (Ghoshal & Walji, 2006).

Telemedicine

One thing that hardly seems to slow is the rate of technological innovation, and this includes the delivery of health care. Telemedicine is an application of clinical medicine where medical information is transferred through interactive audiovisual media for the purpose of consulting and sometimes for remote medical procedures or examinations. Telemedicine has become increasingly widespread. Breakthroughs in videoconferencing, software facilitating remote access, and electronic medical records technologies are changing the way health care is delivered and facilitating access among previously underserved populations. Just as there have been advances in telemedicine, the same has occurred with telepharmacy. Many of the services currently provided in a community pharmacy can be provided through telepharmacy, including dispensing of medications, patient counseling, and MTM. The use of telepharmacy is beneficial to rural communities where there may be limited access to pharmacy and medical services.

Electronic Prescribing

Electronic prescribing, more commonly known as e-prescribing, has grown since its implementation in 2005. Still, only 56% of prescribers utilized e-prescribing in 2014 for a total of 1.2 billion prescriptions of the over 4 billion total prescriptions written (Surescripts, 2014).

Although e-prescribing of controlled substances is legal in nearly every state, its adoption has been tremendously limited by the number of prescribers enabled to actually prescribe controlled substances electronically. While 73% of pharmacies are enabled to receive controlled substances, only 1.4% of prescribers are enabled to prescribe controlled substances (Surescripts, 2014).

There are numerous benefits that come with e-prescribing. E-prescribing began on the premise that drugs errors could be reduced due to less dependence on interpreting handwritten prescriptions. Additionally, the physician can check for compliance with the patient's insurance formulary and obtain the patient's drug history for drug utilization evaluation messaging, all on the same system, before the prescription is even transmitted. Claims can even be preadjudicated before the prescription reaches the pharmacy. In such a case, the prescription will not require manual entry by pharmacy personnel.

However, the limitations that remain are the training and time that is necessary for prescribers to implement e-prescribing in their offices. Additionally, while e-prescribing has made strides in preventing medication errors, there is still always the possibility that the physician may select the wrong drug or dose from a pull down menu. Finally, there still appears to be challenges when communicating to patients that they have a prescription, especially a new prescription. Primary nonadherence rates (the rate of getting a prescription filled for a newly prescribed medication) for electronic prescriptions have been found to range from 7.4% to 28.3% (Fischer, Stedman, Lii, et al., 2010; Raebel, Carroll, Ellis, et al., 2011; Shin, McCombs, Sanchez, et al., 2012). However, unlike paper prescriptions, pharmacists, and technicians who receive e-prescriptions for patients know whether or not patients are coming in to pick up a prescription for the first time, and can intervene accordingly.

Pharmacy Software

There is an increasing availability of software aimed specifically to help pharmacists and other medical professionals document care and interventions, which may be helpful in increasing quality of care, securing reimbursement for services, and fending off costly litigation. As previously described in this chapter, programs like Mirixa (www.mirixa.com), OutcomesMTM (www.outcomesmtm.com), and PharmMD (www.pharmmd.com) can facilitate efficient processing of MTM in the community pharmacy. Equipp (www.equipp.org) is an online quality improvement platform for pharmacies trying to navigate the CMS star ratings system and quality measures in pharmacy. An increasing number of inventory management programs are available from wholesalers to more efficiently manage pharmacy inventory. Additionally, pharmacy dispensing programs are adding modules and programming that help pharmacists manage medication synchronization, inventory, dispensing automation, and MTM. There is no question that pharmacy software will continue to advance and make it easier for pharmacies to provide better services to their patients.

Dispensing Automation

Advances in robotics technology and automation are helpful to mail-order, health-system, nursing home, and other types of pharmacies dispensing large quantities of prescription orders in order to improve work flow, increase accuracy, and manage systems. However, more recently, there has been a trend in using medication packaging automation that would otherwise be used for nursing home patients for patients seen every day in the community pharmacy, especially for those patients whose medications are synchronized. Through this approach, patients can receive their medication in medication packs, whereby all of their medication doses for a particularly time of day, such as the morning, for example, can all be found in one convenient packet.

Many other technologies will affect pharmacy and medication use systems that are beyond the scope of this chapter. Pharmacists are encouraged to embrace but also be shrewd evaluators of technology and stay abreast of current developments in the field to provide higher quality care and leverage their careers.

PHARMACY WORKFORCE

Implications of Workforce Size for Pharmacy

The final section of this chapter addresses an issue that is intrinsically tied to many of the concepts discussed throughout this text—namely, the number of pharmacists and support personnel available in the United States as measured in terms of the number of full-time equivalent (FTE) employees. Maintaining an adequate supply of pharmacists is critical on several fronts.

First, given that the number of prescriptions dispensed annually has continued to rise, an adequate number of pharmacists must be working in community settings to fulfill society's demand for cost-effective pharmaceuticals that are dispensed promptly and accurately.

Second, an adequate supply of well-trained pharmacists is essential to the provision of pharmacy care and MTM services. If the number of available FTE pharmacists is unable or minimally able to meet society's need for dispensing, it becomes that much more difficult for the profession to continue along its path of maturation from a product- to a patient-centered focus.

Third, an adequate workforce is required to meet the need for public safety. In recent years, medication-related errors and their resultant morbidity and mortality in the hospital setting have come under intense scrutiny. Although pharmacists are not entirely responsible for all of these errors, a number of steps can be taken to mitigate this problem. The lay press has also called attention to the lack of consistency in detecting prescription-related problems in pharmacies across the United States (CNN.com, 2007). Part of the problem is that many pharmacies are understaffed or are staffed consistently with floater pharmacists who do not have a regular site at which to practice.

Pharmacy workforce issues are also important to pharmacy's role in reforming the healthcare system. As greater emphasis is placed on preventive care, pharmacists may be increasingly called upon to provide MTM services, as well as healthy lifestyle counseling, disease management, immunizations, and other public health initiatives, including disaster relief. Additionally, the government continues to grapple with shortages of primary care practitioners in inner-city and rural areas. One study showed that the presence of pharmacists in combination with other healthcare professionals such as nurse practitioners in rural areas suffering from a scarcity of physicians can mitigate the problem of diminished access to health care (Knapp, Paavola, Maine, Sorofman, & Politzer, 1999).

The size of the pharmacy workforce is also a source of concern for state boards of pharmacy and the academic community. State boards of pharmacy enforce regulations that affect the number and use of pharmacy technicians. Some state boards have enacted rules limiting the number of technicians who are allowed to work in direct care settings by specifying a maximum ratio of technicians to pharmacists. For their part, schools of pharmacy have the responsibility for continuing to graduate pharmacists to meet the needs of society while maintaining the quality and integrity of their programs. The AACP, the Accreditation Council for Pharmacy Education, and individual schools must keep abreast of supply trends by region and across the United States.

Factors Affecting Pharmacist Labor Supply

As the profession continues to operate within a dynamic healthcare environment while undergoing comprehensive change, numerous forces appear poised to affect the current and future supply of pharmacists.

First, the demographic composition of pharmacists is shifting toward a greater proportion of female practitioners. Whereas the profession was once virtually all male, the U.S. Census Bureau reported in 2011 that women accounted for 52.6% of all pharmacists (US Census Bureau, 2011). This trend has significant implications because childbearing women often take some time for maternity leave and women are more likely than men to work part-time for child rearing or other reasons.

The effects of other factors on pharmacist labor supply are less certain. Pharmacist specialization, while increasing pharmacists' competency to provide pharmaceutical care, may result in their propensity to work in nontraditional settings and reduce their supply in distributive settings. As of 2014, there were over 21,000 pharmacists who had acquired certification through the Board of Pharmacy Specialties, and this number is expected to grow (BPS, 2015).

Finally, two factors that directly affect the pharmacy labor supply are pharmacy technicians and automation. Certification of technicians can serve to increase their level of competence and allow these individuals to perform roles that had previously been within the pharmacist's scope of practice only. Automation and other technologies can free up time for pharmacists, allowing them to turn their attention toward patient consultative and disease management activities.

Estimates of the Pharmacist Workforce

Although leaders in the profession agree that workforce issues are important, there has been less consensus on how to measure the labor supply and, therefore, where the profession stands. A variety of methods have been used to quantify the pharmacy labor supply, including worker–population ratios, demand versus supply techniques, the relative income of pharmacists, and the internal rate of return for investing in pharmacy education (Sorkin, 1989). Data on pharmacy manpower are generated primarily from the following three sources: (1) the Pew Health Professions Commission, (2) the Bureau of Labor Statistics, and (3) the Bureau of Health Professions (BHP).

The most comprehensive attempt to measure and predict the future pharmacist labor supply has been the combined effort of professional associations and the BHP in creating the Pharmacy Manpower Project census database (Gershon et al., 2000). This model incorporates the change in the entry-level degree, the opening of new pharmacy schools, the influx of international pharmacy graduates, and separation rates (actuarial estimates of retirement, death, and occupational mobility). It projected a workforce of 196,011 active pharmacists in 2000 and predicts a workforce of 249,086 active pharmacists by 2020. It implies further that the ratio of active pharmacists to the general population will increase by 2020 to a level 76.7 pharmacists per 100,000 population, compared with 68.9 pharmacists per 100,000 population in 1995. The model does not consider FTE employees; however, and its primary drawback is that its definition of active pharmacists includes a potentially increasing number of practitioners who are working part-time.

Efforts are being made to track the balance of supply and demand forces of pharmacists longitudinally by making survey-based estimates of the amount of difficulty faced by employers in filling open pharmacist positions (Knapp & Livesey, 2002). As of 2001, there was considerable demand in excess of available supply, with the problem being more acute in certain states. This issue is of particular concern as patients experience a number of unmet needs in medication use (e.g., medication counseling and drug therapy monitoring) (Law, Ray, Knapp, & Balesh, 2003) and a sizable portion of pharmacists' work hours are consumed by activities not directly related to patient care (Schommer, Pedersen, Doucette, Gaither, & Mott, 2002). The projected shortage encouraged a number of new colleges/schools of pharmacy to open across the United States as a response to the unmet need.

The Pharmacy Manpower Project, a consortium of professional pharmacy organizations, has collaborated with researchers to create the Aggregate Demand Index. The Pharmacy Manpower Project seeks to collect, analyze, and disseminate data on the supply of licensed pharmacists in the United States (Aggregate Demand Index, 2015). The Aggregate Demand Index reports an index from 1 to 5 for each state and for various practice settings, wherein 1 indicates a high surplus and 5 indicates a high demand for pharmacists. In July 2015, the aggregate index for the nation was 3.62, indicating a slight demand for pharmacists to fill position in the United States. However, there is considerable variability across the United States based on upon the state.

CONCLUSION

The pharmacy profession has come a long way in a little more than a century. The current pace of change, however, promises more momentous transitions over the next few decades. It is difficult to gauge exactly what pharmacy practice will be like in another century with the profession's renewed focus on patients, the continued specialization of pharmacists in specific disease states, the growing trend of pharmacy technician certification, the rapid diffusion of technology as a facilitator to the provision of care, and a shift in the composition of its workforce. It remains clear, however, that pharmacy will remain an integral part of our healthcare delivery system and an exciting career choice for its practitioners.

QUESTIONS FOR FURTHER DISCUSSION

1. How will pharmacists' roles continue to evolve over the next 10 to 20 years? What will be the status of pharmacy care and MTM service delivery in 20 years?
2. Should the focus on pharmacist credentialing be on general pharmacotherapy or on further specialization to create experts in managing specific disease states?
3. Why are proportionately fewer pharmacists active in professional associations at a national level compared to physicians and other healthcare professionals? How has this hindered pharmacy as a profession?
4. What is the contribution of each subdiscipline within pharmacy toward practice, education, and research?
5. Should certification of pharmacy technicians be mandated? Why or why not?
6. How can pharmacy professionals leverage the Internet and other technologies to improve patient care, enhance reimbursement, and advance our roles on interdisciplinary care teams?
7. What can be done to ensure an adequate supply of pharmacists for the future?

KEY TOPICS AND TERMS

History of pharmacy
Pharmaceutical care
Pharmacy technician
Pharmacy workforce
Professional pharmacy organizations
Technology

REFERENCES

Aggregate Demand Index. (2015). Retrieved from http://www.pharmacymanpower.com/index.jsp

American Association of Colleges of Pharmacy. (1996). Paper from the Commission to Implement Change in Pharmaceutical Education: Maintaining our commitment to change. *American Journal of Pharmaceutical Education, 60*, 378–384.

American Pharmaceutical Association. (2003a). Pharmacy technicians (2002): Needed changes can no longer wait [white paper]. *Journal of the American Pharmaceutical Association, 43*, 93–107.

American Pharmaceutical Association. (2003b). Sesquicentennial Stepping Stone Summits-summit two: Pharmacy technicians. *Journal of the American Pharmaceutical Association, 43*, 84–92.

American Pharmacists Association. (2013). Provider status: What pharmacists need to know now. Retrieved from http://www.pharmacist.com/provider-status-what-pharmacists-need-know-now

American Pharmacists Association. (2015). More states address pharmacists' provider status recognition. Retrieved from https://www.pharmacist.com/node/877933?is_sso_called=1

American Society of Health-System Pharmacists. (2009). Scope of contemporary pharmacy practice: Roles, responsibilities, and functions of pharmacists and pharmacy technicians. Retrieved from https://www.accp.com/docs/positions/misc/CCPwpScope_Pharmacy_Practice_2-2009.pdf

American Society of Health-System Pharmacists. (2013). ASHP Accreditation Standard for Pharmacy Technician Training Programs. Retrieved from http://www.ashp.org/DocLibrary/Accreditation/Regulations-Standards/Pharmacy-Technician-Education-and-Training-Programs.pdf

APhA Foundation. (2013). Pharmacy's appointment based model: A prescription synchronization program that improves adherence. [Online]. Retrieved from http://www.aphafoundation.org/sites/default/files/ckeditor/files/ABMWhitePaper-FINAL-20130923(3).pdf

Ateb, Inc. (2013). Assessing the impact of a community pharmacy-based medication synchronization programon adherence rates. NCPA. [Online]. Retrieved from http://www.ncpanet.org/pdf/survey/2014/ncpa-study-results.pdf

Board of Pharmacy Specialties (BPS). 2014. *Annual Report.* (2015). Retrieved from http://board-of-pharmacy-specialties.epaperflip.com/v/2014-BPS-Annual-Report/#?page=0

Board of Pharmacy Specialties (BPS). (2015). *Specialties.* Retrieved from http://www.bpsweb.org/index.cfm

Boyd, J. R., Covington, T. R., Stanaszek, W. F., & Coussons, R. T. (1974). Drug defaulting, part 2: Analysis of noncompliance patterns. *American Journal of Hospital Pharmacy, 31*, 485–491.

Brodie, D. C. (1967). Drug-use control: Keystone to pharmaceutical service. *Drug Intelligence, 1*, 63–65.

Broeseker, A., & Janke, K. K. (1998). The evolution and revolution of pharmaceutical care. In R. L. McCarthy (Ed.), *Introduction to health care delivery: A primer for pharmacists* (pp. 393–416). Gaithersburg, MD: Aspen.

Buerki, R. A., & Vottero, L. D. (1994). *Ethical responsibility in pharmacy practice.* Madison, WI: American Institute of the History of Pharmacy.

Bureau of Labor Statistics. (2014–2015). *Occupational outlook handbook* (2014–2015 ed.). Retrieved from http://www.bls.gov/ooh/healthcare/pharmacy-technicians.htm

CNN.com. (2007). *Don't be a victim of pharmacy errors.* Retrieved from http://articles. cnn.com/2007-10-25/health/pharmacy.errors_1_pharmacy-prescription-walgreens?_ s=PM:HEALTH

Col, N., Fanale, J. E., & Kronholm, P. (1990). The role of medication noncompliance and adverse drug reactions in hospitalizations in the elderly. *Archives of Internal Medicine, 150*, 841–845.

Commission to Implement Change in Pharmaceutical Education. (1993). Background paper II: Entry-level curricular outcomes, curricular content and educational process. *American Journal of Pharmaceutical Education, 57*, 386–399.

Conlan, M. F. (1999, May 17). It's the law. *Drug Topics, 143*, 72, 74.

Cooksey, J. A., Knapp, K. K., Walton, S. M., & Cultice, J. M. (2002). Challenges to the pharmacist profession from escalating pharmaceutical demand. *Health Affairs, 21*, 182–188.

Cranor, C. W., Bunting, B. A., & Christensen, D. B. (2003). The Asheville project: Long-term clinical and economic outcomes of a community pharmacy diabetes care program. *Journal of the American Pharmaceutical Association, 43*, 173–184.

Cranor, C. W., & Christensen, D. B. (2003). The Asheville project: Short-term outcomes of a community pharmacy diabetes care program. *Journal of the American Pharmaceutical Association, 43*, 149–159.

Desselle, S. P. (2005). Job turnover intentions among certified pharmacy technicians. *Journal of the American Pharmacists Association, 45*, 676–683.

Desselle, S. P., & Zgarrick, D. P. (2009). *Pharmacy management: Essentials for all practice settings* (2nd ed.). New York, NY: McGraw-Hill.

Fischer, M. A., Stedman, M. R., Lii, J., Vogeli, C., Shrank, W. H., & Brookhart, M. A. (2010). Primary medication non-adherence: Analysis of 195,930 electronic prescriptions. *Journal of General Internal Medicine, 25*, 284–290.

Gershon, S. K., Cultice, J. M., & Knapp, K. K. (2000). How many pharmacists are in our future? The Bureau of Health Professions projects supply to 2020. *Journal of Managed Care Pharmacy, 6*, 298–306.

Ghoshal, M., & Walji, M. F. (2006). Quality of information available on retail pharmacy websites. *Research in Social and Administrative Pharmacy, 2*, 479–498.

Hepler, C. D. (1987). The third wave in pharmaceutical education: The clinical movement. *American Journal of Pharmaceutical Education, 51*, 369–385.

Hepler, C. D., & Strand, L. M. (1990). Opportunities and responsibilities in pharmaceutical care. *American Journal of Hospital Pharmacy, 47*, 533–543.

Holdford, D. A., & Inocenico T. J. (2013). Adherence and persistence with an appointment-based medication synchronization program. *Journal of the American Pharmacists Association, 53*(6), 576–583.

Holmes, E. R., Desselle, S. P., Nath, D. M., & Markuss, J. M. (2005). Quality analysis of consumer drug information provided through Internet pharmacies. *Annals of Pharmacotherapy, 39*, 662–667.

Knapp, K. K., & Livesey, J. C. (2002). The aggregate demand index: Measuring the balance between pharmacist supply and demand, 1999–2001. *Journal of the American Pharmaceutical Association, 42*, 391–398.

Knapp, K. K., Paavola, F. G., Maine, L. L., Sorofman, B., & Politzer, R. M. (1999). Availability of primary care providers and pharmacists in the United States. *Journal of the American Pharmaceutical Association, 39*, 127–135.

Law, A. V., Ray, M. D., Knapp, K. K., & Balesh, J. K. (2003). Unmet needs in the medication use process: Perceptions of physicians, pharmacists, and patients. *Journal of the American Pharmaceutical Association, 43*, 394–402.

MacKinnon, G. E., III, & Mahrous, H. (2002). Assessing consumers' interest in health care services offered in community pharmacies. *Journal of the American Pharmaceutical Association, 42*, 512–515.

Maine, L. L., & Penna, R. P. (1996). Pharmaceutical care—An overview. In C. Knowlton & R. Penna (Eds.), *Pharmaceutical care* (pp. 133–154). New York, NY: Chapman and Hall.

Manasse, H. R. (1989a). Medication use in an imperfect world: Drug misadventuring as an issue of public policy, part 1. *American Journal of Hospital Pharmacy, 46*, 929–944.

Manasse, H. R. (1989b). Medication use in an imperfect world: Drug misadventuring as an issue of public policy, part 2. *American Journal of Hospital Pharmacy, 46*, 1141–1152.

Millis, J. S. (1975). *Pharmacists for the future: The report of the Study Commission on Pharmacy.* Ann Arbor, MI: Health Administration Press.

Millis, J. S. (1976). Looking ahead—The report of the Study Commission on Pharmacy. *American Journal of Hospital Pharmacy, 33*, 134–138.

Mott, D. A., Vanderpool, W. H., & Smeenk, D. A. (1998). Attitudes of Ohio hospital pharmacy directors toward national voluntary pharmacy technician certification. *American Journal of Health-Systems Pharmacy, 55*, 1799–1803.

Paulsen, M. (1999). New NABP program combines criteria, inspections to certify online pharmacy quality. *Journal of the American Pharmaceutical Association, 39*, 870.

Penna, R. P. (1990). Pharmaceutical care—pharmacy's mission for the 1990s. *American Journal of Hospital Pharmacy, 47*, 543–549.

Pharmacy Technician Certification Board (PTCB). (2015). CPhT Statistics. Retrieved from http://www.ptcb.org/who-we-serve/pharmacy-technicians/statistics#.VeNXqvlVhBc

Pink, L. A. (1991). Hospitals. In J. E. Fincham & A. I. Wertheimer (Eds.), *Pharmacists and the U. S. healthcare system* (pp. 158–190). Binghamton, NY: Pharmaceutical Products Press.

Raebel, M. A., Carroll, N. M., Ellis, J. L., Schroeder, E. B., & Bayliss, E. A. (2011). Importance of including early nonadherence in estimations of medication adherence. *Annals of Pharmacotherapy, 45*, 1053–1060.

Relman, A. S. (1988). Assessment and accountability: The third revolution in medical care. *New England Journal of Medicine, 319*, 1220–1222.

Schmitt, M. R., & Desselle, S. P. (2009). Pharmacists' attitudes toward technician certification: A qualitative study. *Journal of Pharmacy Technology, 25*, 79–88.

Schommer, J. C., Pedersen, C. A., Doucette, W. R., Gaither, C. A., & Mott, D. A. (2002). Community pharmacists' work activities in the United States during 2000. *Journal of the American Pharmaceutical Association, 42*, 399–406.

Shin, J., McCombs, J. S., Sanchez, R. J., Udall, M., Deminski, M. C., & Cheetham, T. C. (2012). Primary nonadherence to medication in an integrated healthcare setting. *American Journal of Managed Care, 18*, 426–434.

Sonnedecker, G. (1963). *Kremers and Urdang's history of pharmacy.* Philadelphia, PA: J. B. Lippincott.

Sorkin, A. L. (1989). Some economic aspects of pharmacy manpower. *American Journal of Hospital Pharmacy, 46*, 527–533.

Strand, L. M., Cippole, R. J., & Morley, P. C. (1988). Documenting the clinical pharmacist's activities: Back to basics. *Drug Intelligence and Clinical Pharmacy, 22*, 63–66.

Strand, L. M., Cippole, R. J., Morley, P. C., Ramsey, R., & Lamsam, G. D. (1990). Drug-related problems: Their structure and function. *DICP Annals of Pharmacotherapy, 24*, 1093–1097.

Surescripts. (2014). 2014 National Progress Report. Retrieved from http://surescripts.com/docs/default-source/national-progress-reports/surescripts-2014-national-progress-report.pdf

Torrens, P. R. (1993). Historical evolution and overview of health service in the United States. In J. S. Williams & P. R. Torrens (Eds.), *Introduction to health services* (4th ed., pp. 3–28). Albany, NY: Delmar.

US Census Bureau. (2011). America's changing labor force. Retrieved from http://www.census.gov/how/pdf/EEO_infographic_text.pdf

Wilson, D. L., Kimberlin, C. L., & Brushwood, D.B. (2005). Exploring the professional expertise of pharmacy technicians. *Journal of Pharmacy Technology, 21*, 341–347.

CHAPTER

4

The Patient

Kimberly S. Plake*

Case Scenario

Mary is a 67-year-old woman who is greatly concerned about her health. She currently has type 2 diabetes and hypertension, and she knows that she is at least 50 pounds overweight. Lately, Mary has been experiencing symptoms that do not seem to be explained by her current chronic diseases. Because she does not have insurance and has limited access to health services owing to her rural location, she decided to do some research on her symptoms before making an appointment with the physician. Mary became concerned because she found some information on the Internet that indicated that she might have early signs of arthritis. She started taking Tylenol (acetaminophen) when she saw a commercial indicating that it can be used for her symptoms. However, it did not seem to be controlling all of her pain.

Mary decided that she must go to a physician because she could no longer stand the pain. Before meeting with her physician, she talked to her neighbor, Mrs. Johnson, who suffers from arthritis. After learning of Mary's suspicions, Mrs. Johnson gave her an article about arthritis from a women's magazine. A couple of pages after the article, Mary saw an advertisement for glucosamine supplements and planned to talk with her physician about this medication.

At her appointment, Mary asked the physician about the information she obtained from the Internet and about glucosamine. In addition, she brought a list of her current symptoms. The physician, sensing that Mary would like to be an active participant in her health care, answered her questions, prompted her to provide information he thought was pertinent to her care, and then talked about her treatment options. After discussing her alternatives with her physician, Mary decided to begin taking Naprosyn (naproxen) for her arthritis and to start a weight reduction program to help treat her osteoarthritis.

*With acknowledgment to Peter L. Steere and Edward Krupat.

LEARNING OBJECTIVES

Upon completion of this chapter, the student shall be able to:

- Describe factors that influence the healthcare system's focus on the treatment of diseases rather than their prevention.
- Identify and describe services and programs for individuals with limited financial resources or limited access to healthcare services.
- Explain the impact of the Internet on patients' access to health information.
- Define and explain direct-to-consumer advertising.
- Compare and contrast health practitioners' opinions of direct-to-consumer advertising to those of the pharmaceutical industry.
- Explain the following models of the practitioner–patient relationship and their application when interacting with patients:
  a. Szasz and Hollender's models of care
  b. Consumer model of care
  c. Patient-centered model of care
- Describe the role that patient autonomy plays in patient–practitioner relationships.
- Compare and contrast the biomedical and biopsychosocial models of care.
- Compare and contrast compliance and adherence.
- Explain how adherence is measured.
- Identify factors influencing patient adherence to therapeutic recommendations.
- Explain health literacy.
- Identify communication techniques that can be used regardless of patients' health literacy level.
- Explain the following health behavior models:
  a. Locus of control
  b. Health belief model
  c. Theory of reasoned action
  d. Theory of planned behavior
  e. Social cognitive theory (self-efficacy)
  f. Transtheoretical model (stages of change)
- Explain patient attitudes and behavior using the models described in the chapter when presented with a patient.
- Describe motivational interviewing (MI) and its use in behavioral change.
- Develop an approach to facilitate behavior change and indicate the rationale for the selected approach when given a patient case.

CHAPTER QUESTIONS

1. In what ways is the current crisis in healthcare financing a result of past successes of America's healthcare system?
2. How have patient expectations of and experiences in the healthcare system changed over the years?
3. How do the models of healthcare delivery address some of the classic issues of patient–practitioner relations (the balance of power, patient autonomy, and patient satisfaction)?
4. What factors influence patients' adherence to therapeutic recommendations? In which direction (more or less adherent) do you think each of these factors influence adherence?
5. How do the health behavior models help practitioners facilitate behavior change in patients?

INTRODUCTION

As reforms in health care occur, corresponding changes are also seen in patients, health professionals, and the healthcare environment. Although the healthcare system always seems to be in a state of flux, the focus remains on restoring sick patients to health. Healthcare professionals, health institutions, and insurance companies are interested in patients and their behaviors. Along with this interest is the desire to work with patients and to improve their care and satisfaction with services. This chapter explores topics related to the patient, including the shift in focus of care from acute to chronic diseases, the healthcare environment, patient expectations of care, models of care, and health behaviors.

DEFINITIONS

Being a patient perhaps at one time suggested that an individual was under the care of a physician. It suggested illnesses and a process of healing and recovery. While this definition still holds true, being a patient today may mean that a person is receiving services from a pharmacist, nurse, therapist, and/or dietician, as well as from providers of therapeutic massage, acupuncture, or a variety of other complementary services.

This multidisciplinary approach is a change in—and perhaps even in some ways a return to—the manner in which individuals seeking care find services they feel are necessary for healing. This shift comes despite the fact that medical technology is, in the United States, at its highest ever level of sophistication. While the introduction of new medical technologies has certainly changed patients' expectations and experiences, just as important are the effects that the economics of this evolving system of health care will have on the United States' financial ability to provide a reasonable standard of care for every patient.

DEMOGRAPHICS

The graying of America and its far-reaching implications are exerting serious pressure on the United States' healthcare systems. The rapid acceleration in the aging of the population and the use of medical services by the elderly, when combined, threaten to dramatically impact the healthcare system and healthcare reimbursement programs. The first of the baby boom population (those born between 1946 and 1964) turned 65 years of age in 2011. By 2040, it is estimated that 20% of Americans will be age 65 or older (National Center for Health Statistics, 2010). The number of oldest elderly—those older than 85 years—is projected to grow at a rapid rate from 5.8 million in 2010 to 19 million in 2050 (Vincent & Velkoff, 2010) (**Table 4-1**).

Because advances in technology have helped to find treatments and cures (e.g., immunizations and antibiotics) for many of the more acute forms of illness, much of the current effort in health care focuses on the management of chronic conditions. Diabetes, hypertension, cancer, human immunodeficiency virus (HIV) infections, and other long-term (lifelong), multisystem diseases have replaced scarlet fever, measles, and whooping cough as targets of the country's healthcare system. Mary, from our case scenario, is an example of this phenomenon—she has several chronic conditions to be managed.

Table 4-1 Shifts in American Population (Thousands) as of July 1 for Each Year

	2014	2010	2006
Total population	318,857	309,347	298,593
5–14 years	41,191	41,012	40,410
15–44 years	128,009	125,888	125,751
45–64 years	83,536	81,777	74,612
65–84 years	40,080	34,937	32,143
85 years and older	6,162	5,543	5,063

Source: Data from U.S. Census Bureau.

TREATMENT VERSUS PREVENTION

The U.S. system of health care, despite significant investments and experimentation with managed care and related wellness programs, remains largely a system designed to care for the sick. An emphasis on prevention has been increasing among a variety of entities in the healthcare system, as well as the federal government through its *Healthy People* initiative (http://www.healthypeople.gov/). Among these entities, one shared goal is to improve health through the development of wellness initiatives. Nevertheless, broad-based initiatives focused on wellness and prevention have met with limited success with many individuals slow to embrace some of the suggested wellness behaviors, such as dietary and exercise recommendations. Changing consumer behavior and community responsibilities to promote wellness, despite clear messages of the dangers of not doing so, is a slow and difficult task (Knowles, 1997). Cigarette smoking, for example, has long been recognized for its ability to cause cancer and emphysema but remains a frequent behavior, despite community, state, and national efforts that apply financial and cultural pressures to stop.

In addition, compliance with positive contributors to health such as consumption of a proper diet and engaging in exercise are often seen as difficult, tedious, or simply overly mundane. The relationship between such practices and actual wellness is often too unclear for many to appreciate. As a consequence, many individuals who are at risk for sedentary lifestyle diseases often experience them.

Further, while many illnesses caused by environmental factors (e.g., poor sanitation) have been minimized in the United States, many of the current preventive practices responsible for reducing chronic disease are provided by healthcare professionals, including preventive health care, such as blood pressure screening and bone density testing. Preventive health care adds costs to the healthcare system, but the reduction in future costs (money that would otherwise be spent on more acute care) can often be accomplished by making an investment in such health measures. Ideally, such an investment would come from insurers, at-risk providers, and consumers.

PATIENTS' EXPECTATIONS

Health care is different from most consumer products and services offered in the marketplace. When buying a car, a consumer can go to the car dealership and test drive a car before deciding to purchase it. Of course, a patient cannot test drive surgery. Instead, patients rely on health professionals to advise them about the most appropriate procedure or decision.

Although patients may rely on health professionals' advice on appropriate decisions, consumers are becoming increasingly more active participants in the healthcare process. In the past, healthcare professionals seemed to have all the knowledge related to health and well-being. Patients visited the physician or other health professional to obtain this information. The physician would advise, and the patient would (in theory) comply.

Today, however, a wealth of information is available. Patients can watch television and learn about medications available for various conditions. They can use the Internet to find resources and information on diseases, treatments, and medications. For example, Mary found information on arthritis through the Internet and learned of the use of Tylenol (acetaminophen) to treat this condition while watching television. Patients are becoming informed consumers. As a consequence, the dynamics of the relationship between healthcare professionals and patients is changing.

Instead of the physician telling the patient what to do, a more collaborative relationship between physician and patient is evolving. In this relationship, the patient asks questions and becomes an active participant in making healthcare decisions; in a sense, the healthcare professional and patient become partners in the care process. In some cases, the patient may actually ask the physician for a specific product or treatment for a condition based on personal research. For example, Mary went to her physician's appointment armed with specific questions about arthritis and glucosamine. (The "Models of Care" section in this chapter discusses this phenomenon in more detail.)

ACCESS TO HEALTH INFORMATION

Information Seeking

Eighty-seven percent of American adults go online and 67% of American households have broadband connections (Pew Research Center, 2014, 2015). With the increased accessibility to the Internet comes an increased volume of information. Patients can obtain data on a wide variety of topics, including information about diseases, medications, and therapies. Of Internet users surveyed in a 2012 study, 72% indicated they had used the Internet to look online for health information (Fox & Duggan, 2013). However, healthcare professionals are still relied upon during serious health episodes with 70% of adults receiving information from clinicians offline (Fox & Duggan, 2013). In addition, 60% rely on family and friends for information while 24% seek out information from others with the same condition. Health information sought by individuals online included information on: (1) a specific condition, medical problem, or procedure; (2) specific medical treatment or procedure; (3) weight control (4) alternative treatments; (5) health insurance; (6) food safety and recalls; (7) drug safety or recalls; (8) medications seen in advertisements; and (9) medical test results (Fox & Duggan, 2013).

By using the Internet, patients like Mary can easily acquire information that is written in a layperson's terms. They can go online at any time of day or night—information is immediately available around the clock. Besides finding information, patients can identify support systems through online advocacy groups, chat rooms, and message boards (Fox & Duggan, 2013; Fox & Jones, 2009; Levy & Strombeck, 2002; Sennett, 2000). Compare this ready accessibility and ease of use to the maze that must be navigated to reach many healthcare practitioners, and it is easy to see why patients might turn to the Internet for help. Health professionals are, in turn, being asked by their patients about the information they obtain from online sources. With the anticipated increase in the use of the Internet as a source for health information, patients' questions to practitioners about this information will likely become more frequent. For this reason, healthcare practitioners should be aware of how to retrieve information from the Internet, as well as how to evaluate the credibility of websites.

Self-Care

Self-care related to health is "a range of behaviors undertaken by individuals to promote or restore health" (Dean, 1989, p. 119). In other words, it consists of actions that individuals take to treat or prevent an illness. These actions can include self-medicating with nonprescription products and seeking advice from family and friends.

When individuals become ill, they go through an appraisal process of their symptoms. Is it serious? Is it getting better? Is it disruptive? Depending on the results of their assessment, patients may believe that they are sick and assume the sick role. As a part of this transformation, they begin to investigate what is occurring. They may talk to friends and family members for their advice, take medication, and consult alternative health practitioners. For example, Mary talked to her friend, Mrs. Johnson, about arthritis. In addition, patients may assume a wait-and-see attitude or they may take action. When patients perceive the illness as serious or life-threatening, they might be prompted to go to the physician (Lubkin, 1990; Suchman, 1965). In the case of Mary, she did not seek attention from the physician until she could no longer stand the pain and it became disruptive to her life.

In the last several years, pharmacies and pharmacists have played a larger role in helping patients manage their self-care. Pharmacists have implemented disease management programs for a variety of chronic diseases, including diabetes (Baran et al., 1999; Cranor & Christensen, 2003; Nau & Ponte, 2002; Simpson et al., 2011; Skinner, Poe, Hopper, Boyer, & Wilkins, 2015), hyperlipidemia (Bluml, McKenney, & Cziraky, 2000), and hypertension (Carte et al., 2015; Park, Kelly, Carter, & Burgess, 1996; Svarstad et al., 2013). In addition, preventive and screening services are being implemented in pharmacies, both chain and independent. Vaccination programs to administer the influenza vaccine are found in community pharmacies in most states. Similarly, many pharmacies offer diabetes and hypertension screening programs. Pharmacy services have grown and encompass the management of chronic diseases (e.g., diabetes, hyperlipidemia, hypertension, asthma), nutrition counseling, refill reminder programs, and medication therapy management. As pharmacists become more intimately involved in patient care, learning about models of care and health behavior theory is important to improve their interactions with patients and to facilitate health behavior change.

MODELS OF CARE

Szasz and Hollender's Three Models of Care

Two physicians, Szasz and Hollender (1956), described three models of patient care. These models, which are now recognized by many as the standard in the field, relate the nature of the patient's illness to the patient's capacity for meaningful dialogue and/or independent action. Each model of care is analogous to the relationship between parents and their children at different stages in their lives (infant, adolescent, and adult).

The activity–passivity model is characterized by an active practitioner and a passive patient; it is analogous to the relationship parents have with an infant child. This model of care is typically used in emergency situations, when the patient has been severely injured and is incapable of coherent communication and/or independent action (e.g., trauma, delirium, or coma). Szasz and Hollender described this form as the oldest type of practitioner–patient relationship; by definition, this model does not include much, if any, interpersonal communication. In this model, the patient is simply a recipient—the object of the practitioner's actions.

The guidance–cooperation model is used in situations in which the patient is capable of interpersonal communication and is actively involved in the relationship. Szasz and Hollender considered this form to be the most commonly used approach to care. Under this model, patients have more power of independent action than in the activity–passivity model of care, but still require professional attention and defer to medical expertise. This relationship is analogous to the relationship between parents and an adolescent child, and it typically applies to patients who are seeking help for some acute condition (e.g., infection or a broken bone).

The third model, mutual participation, applies most commonly when patients have some type of chronic disease (e.g., diabetes, heart disease, or arthritis). This model assumes that the patient and the practitioner are equally powerful and interdependent. Their mutual power comes from their relatively equal yet distinct knowledge bases; the practitioner possesses medical expertise, and the patient has personal experiences gained by living with the condition. In this way, both parties are interdependent; they share with and learn from each other to achieve an ongoing, successful treatment program. The patient and the practitioner relate to each other as two adults. For example, Mary and her physician exchanged information; her physician presented Mary with treatment options, and she made the decision as to which option she would try.

Szasz and Hollender described these three models of care as operating in a dynamic fashion, applied as the patient's situation dictates. That is, much as a parent's relationship with a child changes as the child gains independence, so, too, might a practitioner's relationship change with a patient. If a patient's condition evolves from traumatic to acute to chronic, as in an accident with enduring health effects, the practitioner's model of care would likewise evolve to accommodate these changes. Nonetheless, Szasz and Hollender acknowledged that (at least in the 1950s) the balance of power in physician–patient relations was significantly tipped toward physicians, with guidance–cooperation being the standard mode of practice, and mutual participation being least common.

As is suggested by the parent–child analogies of these models, the traditional imbalance of power has often been characterized as paternalistic (Beisecker & Beisecker, 1993; Emanuel & Emanuel, 1992; Parsons, 1951; President's Commission, 1982). However, as pointed out by Reeder (1972), societal changes beginning in the 1960s fostered a shift in this traditional imbalance, with patients becoming decreasingly deferential.

The Consumer Model of Care

Reeder suggested a consumer model of care that was eventually elaborated on by others (Haug & Lavin, 1981, 1983; Roter & Hall, 1992). The consumer model is characterized by greater patient autonomy in decision making, where the traditional authority of physicians has become increasingly challenged. As the word *consumer* suggests, patients are perceived as increasingly informed and skeptical buyers of medical care, whereas physicians are sellers who respond to the needs of the patient. In this conceptualization, the traditional emphasis on the physician's rights (to direct) and the patient's obligations (to follow) are essentially reversed to emphasize the patient/buyer's rights and the physician/seller's obligations. This dramatic shift in power has led some to criticize this model as going too far, by emphasizing conflict and mistrust while discrediting medical expertise.

As with most representations, the three Szasz and Hollender models and the consumer model reflect some significant proportion of reality—emphasizing the balance of power within the physician–patient relationship. This has been a popular topic, with the nature of the relationship being represented in various ways (see, e.g., Childress & Siegler, 1984; Emanuel & Emanuel, 1992; Roter & Hall, 1992; Veatch, 1972). Some observers, however, have shifted the emphasis away from issues of power and disease as the focus of the medical encounter; instead, they consider the manner in which practitioners and patients relate to each other in terms of how they define the problem at hand.

The Patient-Centered Model of Care

The patient-centered model is often contrasted with the disease-centered model of patient care (Balint, Hung, Joyce, Marinker, & Woodcock, 1970; Byrne & Long, 1976; Henbest & Stewart, 1990; Levenstein, Brown, Weston, Stewart, McCracken, & McWhinney, 1989; Mishler, 1984). In the disease-centered models, the presenting problem is understood with scientific detachment; the focus is on organic pathology and accurate diagnosis.

The patient-centered orientation shifts the focus from just the body to the person as a whole. Practitioners who adopt this model are encouraged to view the illness through the patient's eyes by considering these four key elements: (1) understanding the patient's ideas about what is wrong, (2) eliciting the patient's feelings (especially fears) about the illness, (3) assessing how the problem affects the patient's daily life, and (4) discovering what expectations the patient has regarding treatment (Weston, Brown, & Stewart, 1989). With these considerations in mind, the dialogue between practitioner and patient takes on different characteristics. Instead of the traditional closed-ended, disease-centered questions, phrased to keep the patient's responses brief and focused on pathology, a patient-centered dialogue asks open-ended questions that facilitate the patient's feedback and explore the meaning of the problem from the patient's point of view.

Consider the contrast between these two models as they are depicted in the following examples. We begin with the disease-centered interview.

Doctor: Hello, Pat. What seems to be the problem that's brought you here today?

Patient: I've been getting these stomach cramps lately, and I thought I ought to come and find out what's going on.

Doctor: I see. How long have you been having the cramps?

Patient: A couple of weeks.

Doctor: Have you been constipated?

Patient: Yes, I have.

Doctor: How about diarrhea?

Patient: That, too. It goes from one to the other.

Doctor: I see. How long does the diarrhea last?

Patient: About 3 days at a time.

Doctor: And then you get constipated?

Patient: That's right.

Doctor: What kinds of foods have you been eating?

Patient: For a while I was eating pretty much nothing except junk food, but since this has happened I've been laying off the Big Macs, and it's still no better.

Doctor: Have you tried any self-medication?

Patient: My roommate said I ought to take Pepto-Bismol, but I decided not to.

Doctor: That's good. You shouldn't take anything unless you consult first with a doctor. Are you on any medication regimen now?

Patient: No, I'm not taking anything at all.

Doctor: Yes, I see. Well, I'll have to examine you and do some tests before I can give any definite diagnosis. It's too early to tell what it could be.

[After the examination, the doctor and patient continue their discussion.]

Patient: What could it be? When will I know?

Doctor: As I said, I can't tell you anything significant without test results, but I should have something more definitive soon. The tests will rule out some possibilities and get me closer to an answer.

Patient: I guess I'll just have to wait.

Doctor: That's right. I'll have something for you soon. Is there anything else wrong that I can take care of now?

Patient: That's all for now. I'll be in touch with you soon, doc.

Now consider how a patient-centered interview with the same patient might go.

Doctor: Hi, Pat. How are you doing?

Patient: Pretty well. I'm on spring break now.

Doctor: Really? How much longer until you're done with classes?

Patient: Finals are in early May, and then I'll be back home again.

Doctor: That's good to hear. What can I do for you today?

Patient: I've been getting these stomach cramps lately, and I thought I ought to find out what's going on.

Doctor: Sounds tough. What about them have you noted?

Patient: Sometimes I get these real bad bouts of diarrhea, and sometimes I get constipated. I'm a real mess.

Doctor: It sounds as if you don't know whether you're coming or going. What do you think is the problem?

Patient: I'm not sure. For a while I was pretty much eating only junk food, but since this has happened I've been laying off the Big Macs, and it's still no better.

Doctor: So it hasn't made much of a difference? Is there anything else you've tried?

Patient: My roommate said I ought to take Pepto-Bismol, but I decided not to try it.

Doctor: I think you made a good decision. Are things going well at school? Have you been under a lot of stress?

Patient: This has been a hard semester, and I have been having a hard time keeping my grades up.

Doctor: Well, that might have something to do with it, but that's only one possibility. I'll have to examine you and do some tests before I can tell you anything for sure.

[After the examination, the discussion continues.]

Doctor: Is there anything else on your mind?

Patient: No, that's all that's on my mind for now, but I really am concerned.

Doctor: It certainly is enough to get anyone upset, but I want you to know that these kinds of symptoms are not uncommon, and, of the several possible things it could be, most are quite treatable. I hope you're not letting this ruin your life at school.

Patient: It's been tough. I run track, but this was not my idea of practicing the dash.

> **Doctor:** I'll bet not. Well, within the next week when the tests come back, I think we'll be able to come up with a number of good suggestions. Are you comfortable with the plan of attack we've set out? Is there anything else I can do for you?
>
> **Patient:** Yeah, that's all for now. I'll be in touch with you soon, doc.

If one were to assume the role of the patient while reading these brief exchanges, the first example might ring truer to most experiences with medical practitioners, whereas the second example might seem more satisfying. A review of the research strongly suggests that patients generally express greater satisfaction with their care when treated as a whole person rather than simply as a medical problem (Hall & Dornan, 1988a, 1988b).

The Biopsychosocial Model of Care

Although paternalistic disease-centered models of care may still be the norm, in recent years there has been a general movement away from these perspectives and toward the consumer- and patient-centered models. In this context, it seems appropriate to mention one more way of conceptualizing models of care that reflects this era of change. Similar to the perceived movement from disease-centered to patient-centered care, some observers have noted a broad shift in Western medicine away from the standard biomedical model and toward a more inclusive biopsychosocial model (Engel, 1978, 1979, 1980; Stroebe & Stroebe, 1995).

Thanks to its scientific roots in molecular biology, the standard biomedical model evolved to emphasize mind–body dualism; biochemical deviation became the sole basis of disease, and psychosocial matters were relegated to nonmedical status. Because the biomedical model served our purposes so well during eras in which the major killers were acute, infectious diseases (e.g., influenza, tuberculosis, and gastroenteritis), it became accepted as the standard model of patient care. As life expectancy began to increase and chronic diseases became the major killers (e.g., heart disease, cancer, and cerebrovascular disease), the scope of the biomedical model has been viewed as overly narrow and less satisfactory given our current needs. Today, psychosocial issues such as poverty, place of residence, environmental pollution, diet, exercise, and stress are recognized as increasingly significant variables in understanding what ails us. George Engel succinctly expressed the problem with the biomedical model:

> The crippling flaw of the model is that it does not include the patient and his or her attributes as a person, a human being. Yet in the everyday work of the physician the prime object of study is a person, and many of the data necessary for hypothesis development and testing are gathered within the framework of an ongoing human relationship and appear in behavioral and psychological forms, namely, how the patient behaves and what he or she reports about himself or herself and his or her life (1978, p. 536).

The biopsychosocial model takes into account health and illness as a product of a person's physical and social context as well as his or her emotional and psychological state. Thus, this model adds behavioral and other psychosocial data into the equation with biochemical processes for scientific analysis and understanding of illness. If we are to understand how individual behaviors and the meanings that people attach to their symptoms can and do affect health, we need to consider more broad-based models in treating patients.

ADHERENCE

Often health professionals refer to whether a patient is compliant to therapeutic recommendations. Compliance refers to the patient following a health professional's recommendations, or in other words, the patient complies with what a health professional tells her to do. Although the terms are often used interchangeably, adherence implies that the patient has a choice or autonomy in following a health professional's recommendations. Similar to Szasz and Hollender's models of activity–passivity and guidance–cooperation, compliance is paternal; the pharmacist represents the parent and the patient represents the child following the parent's directions. Adherence is different than a parental relationship and suggests that the patient is a participant in the decision making and adherence to a recommendation, which reflects the mutual participation model or patient-centered care.

Adherence is measured using a variety of techniques, including both direct and indirect measures. Direct measures include observation of the patient taking the medicine, as well as biochemical measurement in the urine and blood (Ho, Bryson, & Rumsfeld, 2009). Indirect measures, which are more commonly used to measure adherence, include patient questionnaires, patient self-report, patient diaries, clinical response, pill counts, electronic monitoring devices, and prescription claims data/pharmacy store data (Ho, Bryson, & Rumsfeld, 2009). There are a number of patient questionnaires available to measure adherence, such as the Morisky Medication Adherence Questionnaire (MAQ), Self-Efficacy for Appropriate Medication Use Scale (SEAMS), Brief Medication Questionnaire (BMQ), Hill-Bone Compliance Scale, and the Medication Adherence Rating Scale (MARS) (Lavsa, Holzworth, & Ansani, 2011).

When using prescription claims data, usually a medication possession ratio (MPR) or proportion of days covered (PDC) is calculated to assess medication adherence. The MPR is calculated by summing the days' supply of a specific medication for all claims during a defined period of time and dividing this sum by the number of days during the defined period of time (Fairman & Motheral, 2000). The PDC is calculated by using the days covered by prescription fills during a defined period of time (as identified by the denominator) divided by the number of days between the first fill and end of measurement period (Nau). When using these measures, patients are considered adherent when the medication is available to them (at home) 80% of the time (Ho, Bryson, & Rumsfeld, 2009).

Adherence rates vary across types of medications or medical condition. Using prescription claims data, Briesacher and colleagues compared medication adherence rates across seven different medical conditions. Rates varied widely among the conditions. Using an 80% threshold for adherence, 72.3% of patients were adherent to medications for hypertension, 54.6% for hypercholesterolemia, 65.4% for type 2 diabetes, 51.2% for osteoporosis, 68.4% for hypothyroidism, 36.8% for gout, and 60.8% for seizure disorders. The researchers did not identify all factors correlated to adherence rates, but observed that the number of comorbidities, add-on medication therapies, and previous experience with taking medications were associated with the level of adherence based on the disease state (Briesacher, Andrade, Fouayzi, & Chan, 2008).

There are two main types of nonadherence: primary and secondary. Primary nonadherence occurs when the patient does not fill or pick up the initial prescription. Secondary nonadherence occurs when the patient picks up or receives the prescription, but does not take the medication as prescribed. When a patient is nonadherent, a health professional should investigate the reasons why a patient is not following recommended advice. Often, it is assumed the patient unintentionally does not follow directions, such as in the case of forgetfulness or a change in a daily schedule. Although this does commonly occur, sometimes a patient intentionally does not take a medication or adopt a healthy behavior. Based on the National Report Card of Medication Adherence by the National Community Pharmacists Association (NCPA), approximately 75% of adults, 40 years and older, indicated at least one nonadherent behavior in the last 12 months, including missing a dose (57%), forgetting if a dose was taken (38%), not refilling a medication in time (28%), taking a lower dose (22%), not filling a new prescription (20%), and stopping a medication (14%) (National Community Pharmacists Association, 2013). In addition, 50% of respondents reported multiple types of nonadherence, with an average of two nonadherent behaviors per individual.

Factors that influenced the level of medication adherence were personal connection to pharmacist or pharmacy staff, affordability of medications, continuity of care, their feeling of importance of taking the medication as exactly as prescribed, how informed they are about their health, and extent of unpleasant side effects (National Community Pharmacists Association, 2013).

In 2003, the World Health Organization released a report reviewing adherence literature on a variety of disease states in both developed and developing countries. In the report, a framework was developed to describe the factors influencing patients' adherence to recommendations. The dimensions of the framework were: (1) health system, (2) social/economic, (3) condition-related, (4) patient-related, and (5) therapy-related. Factors, as identified by the NCPA study, are included, as well as others (**Table 4-2**). Some of these factors are discussed in this chapter.

Table 4-2 Selected Factors Influencing Patient Adherence

Dimension	Factor
Health system	Patient–provider relationship Communication Access to care and treatments
Social/economic	Living conditions Cost of therapy/treatment Literacy Financial resources Availability of social support networks
Condition-related	Severity of condition Level of disability Presence of comorbidities
Patient-related	Knowledge Illness beliefs Self-efficacy Expectations of treatment Motivation Cultural beliefs
Therapy-related	Complexity of treatment regimen Occurrence of side effects Duration of treatment Previous treatment failures Immediacy of treatment effects

Source: Reprinted with permission from Plake, K. S. Behavior Change. In: Richardson M, Chant C, Cheng JWM, et al., eds. *Pharmacotherapy Self-Assessment Program*, 6th ed. *Health Promotion and Maintenance*. Lenexa, Kansas: American College of Clinical Pharmacy, 2008:2.

CULTURAL INFLUENCE ON HEALTH

Culture is a shared system of values, beliefs, and learned patterns of behavior that specifies acceptable and nonacceptable behaviors and offers individuals guidance on dealing with aspects of life (Galanti, 2004; Halber & Halber, 2008; Loustaunau & Sobo, 1997). Culture is different in that it is dynamic and changing. It is generally passed to each succeeding generation, but it is influenced by an individual's proximity to the culture of origin, education, gender, age, and sexual preference (Loustaunau & Sobo, 1997). Aspects regarding the cultural influence on health are briefly presented in this section of the chapter. Keeping in mind that books have been written about culture and its influence on health, it is not feasible to detail every aspect of culture in this short section. The author recommends the reader seek resources to inform his or her own pharmacy practice.

It is important for a health professional to consider culture because it can influence a variety of patient behaviors and outcomes. First, cultural belief systems and health practices regarding health and illness can vary. Cultural or lay belief systems of health can range from the necessity of establishing equilibrium in the body to the supernatural, such as the belief that a disease is a punishment from a higher power (Galanti, 2004; Loustaunau & Sobo, 1997). From the point of view of the patient, treatment effectiveness will be influenced by the cultural beliefs regarding the illness. In addition, certain disease states, in particular those involving mental health, are stigmatized within some cultural groups and can influence individuals' help-seeking behaviors and treatment adherence. There also is a cultural influence on how diseases and symptoms are expressed to others, including health professionals. For example, emotional stresses may be expressed as physical symptoms or complaints (Galanti, 2004; Loustaunau & Sobo, 1997). In addition, some individuals will be very expressive about their symptoms while others will be stoic and reveal very little about their health status.

Specific health practices can be used by individuals to promote healing, such as the use of prayer, rituals, folk remedies, herbs, and alternative health practitioners (e.g., acupuncturists, massage therapists, and native healers) (Galanti, 2004; Loustaunau & Sobo, 1997). In addition, certain practices within the culture can impact health, such as dietary preferences. Although at first glance, this may not appear to be of much importance, advising a patient who has recently emigrated from Africa on dietary choices using examples from a typical Western/Anglo diet would not be very effective, nor would it promote adherence.

Communication patterns, both verbal and nonverbal, can vary among cultures as well. The use of idioms or slang, such as the use of "getting cold feet," can be misinterpreted and taken for their literal or cultural meanings (Galanti, 2004). Health professionals should avoid using such terminology. Nonverbal communication also can be interpreted differently across cultures (Galanti, 2004; Loustaunau & Sobo, 1997). Such behaviors include, but are not limited to, the appropriateness of touch, eye contact, personal space, facial expressions, silence, head movements, and hand and arm gestures. For example, in the United States, direct eye contact is expected by many as a sign that an individual is listening and interested. However, in some cultures, direct eye contact signals disrespect so a patient may avert his or her eyes to show respect and concern (Galanti, 2004).

In some cases, the use of an interpreter may be necessary when working with patients for whom English is their second language. When using an interpreter, it is recommended that he or she be fluent in both languages of interest, be trained, preferably with a medical focus, be unrelated to the patient, and never be a child, particularly the patient's child. Although it may be difficult to find an interpreter meeting these specifications, there are reasons for these guidelines. In many cultures, there are traditional gender-specific roles that each family member plays. It may be inappropriate to discuss certain topics among mixed company, such as in the case of opposite genders or with children (Galanti, 2004). As a result, the health professional's message may not be completely relayed to the patient and/or the patient may not have fully informed the interpreter and the health professional, giving an incomplete picture of the patient's health.

Health may very much be a family affair, depending on the cultural value system. At times, a large contingent of the family may attend an appointment; others may prefer a private individual appointment with a health professional. Often, there is a hierarchical approach to decision making within the healthcare context. A specific family member or head of household, such as the case of a family matriarch or patriarch, may be making the healthcare decisions for family members. As a result, these family members may play an active role in health consultations (Galanti, 2004; Loustaunau & Sobo, 1997).

HEALTH LITERACY

Navigating the healthcare system and adhering to therapeutic recommendations requires patients to be able to read and interpret prescription bottle labels, complete health insurance or informed consent forms, read and interpret nutrition information on food labels, and follow verbal or written instructions. Although literacy is an essential skill for patients in taking care of their health, it is health literacy that encompasses the skills necessary to navigate the healthcare system. Health literacy is defined "as the degree to which individuals have the capacity to obtain, process, and understand basic health information and services needed to make appropriate health decisions" (Ratzan & Parker, 2000). Health literacy is necessary for patients to accomplish health-related tasks so that their health can be maintained as well as improved.

Approximately 90 million Americans lack the necessary literacy skills to function in the current healthcare system (IOM, 2004). Based on the 2007 National Healthcare Disparities Report, 12% of adults have the necessary health literacy skills to manage all aspects of their health care (Agency for Healthcare Research and Quality, 2008). Although studies have indicated that there are individuals who are at an increased risk of having limited health literacy skills, limited health literacy can affect anyone irrespective of their cultural, educational, or socioeconomic backgrounds. Of importance to health professionals, patients with limited health literacy often find accessing healthcare resources difficult, which results in poorer outcomes as compared to those with higher health literacy (Berkman et al., 2004).

Although there are instruments available to identify individuals with low literacy skills, it is often impractical to use them in a high-paced healthcare environment. In most cases, these tools are used in research to measure patients' health literacy and its impact on outcomes, as well as to assess interventions. These tools include the Short-Form Test of Functional Health Literacy for Adults (S-TOFHLA) (Baker, Williams, Parker, Gazmararian, & Nurss, 1999), Rapid Estimate of Adult Literacy in Medicine (REALM) (Davis et al., 1993), and Newest Vital Sign (NVS) (Weiss et al., 2005). All these instruments have been used widely in the literature to assess patients' health literacy level. Screening questions also have been developed and validated against some of these health instruments in an attempt to quickly assess if a patient is at risk for having limited health literacy. These screening questions include: (1) "How often do you have someone help you read hospital materials?" using a scale all of the time, most of the time, some of the time, a little of the time, or none of the time; (2) "How confident are you filling out medical forms by yourself?" using a scale of always, often, sometimes, occasionally, or never; and (3) "How often do you have problems learning about your medical condition because of difficulty understanding written information?" using a scale of all of the time, most of the time, some of the time, a little of the time, or none of the time (Chew et al., 2007). Of these three questions, "How confident are you in filling out medical forms by yourself?" was the most predictive in identifying individuals with limited health literacy (Chew et al., 2007).

Although there are methods to identify individuals with limited health literacy, experts often advise adopting communication strategies that can be used for all patients, regardless of health literacy level (Paasche-Orlow & Wolf, 2007). This approach is suggested because individuals frequently try to hide their difficulty in understanding information. For many patients, it is embarrassing and so they often act as if they understand even when they do not. In most instances, it is recommended that health-related information be communicated at the fifth-grade level or lower in order to maximize the message for the majority of individuals. Using clear communication strategies is also suggested when working with patients. These techniques are helpful not only to those with limited health literacy skills, but also with patients who do not experience difficulty navigating the healthcare system. These strategies include to: (1) assess patient understanding through the use of open-ended questions, (2) use plain or "living room" language, (3) avoid medical jargon, including vague words and those with multiple meanings, (4) emphasize one to three key points when providing education, (5) encourage questions, (6) use the teach-back technique, (7) write down instructions in easy to understand language, and (8) provide visually appealing educational materials (Kripanlani & Weiss, 2006; Weiss, 2007; Williams et al., 2002).

There are a wide variety of techniques, guidelines, templates, and tools available to assist health professionals in ways to communicate with patients (Kripalani & Weiss, 2006; Weiss, 2007; Williams, Davis, Parker, & Weiss, 2002). For example, the U.S. Pharmacopeia website contains many health-related pictograms (http://www.usp.org/audiences/consumers/pictograms/) that can be used in educating patients. In addition, readability statistics can be calculated using Microsoft Word, allowing practitioners to estimate the grade level of their written material. Ask Me 3 is a program (http://www.npsf.org/?page=askme3) to encourage patients to become active participants in the healthcare dialogue. Additional resources include the Agency for Healthcare Research and Quality pharmacy health literacy center (http://pharmacyhealthliteracy.ahrq.gov/sites/PharmHealthLiteracy/default.aspx), Pfizer Clear Health Communication Initiative (http://www.pfizer.com/health/literacy/public_policy_researchers/overview_of_health_literacy_and_clear_health_communication), and the MedlinePlus website (https://www.nlm.nih.gov/medlineplus/).

HEALTH BEHAVIOR MODELS

Given that there appears to be a desire to move toward a more comprehensive patient care model, healthcare professionals should be aware of how to help patients change their health behaviors and comply with recommended therapies. The following models attempt to explain and predict health behaviors and behavior change based on a variety of factors. However, there is no one model that is perfect in explaining patients' behaviors. When working with patients, a therapeutic plan should not be a "one-size fits all" approach. Instead, a plan should be individualized and tailored to the patient in order to improve likelihood of adherence. The health behavior models discussed in this chapter should give the reader an overview of many of the factors that influence patients' behavior. Knowledge of these factors can help practitioners to ask appropriate questions of their patients to assist in developing a plan for change.

Locus of Control

Locus of control has its origins in Rotter's social learning theory, which states "the potential for a behavior to occur in a given situation is a function of expectancies that the behavior will lead to a particular outcome and the extent to which an outcome is valued" (AbuSabha & Achterberg, 1997,

p. 1125). Although it may sound similar to some of the models discussed later in this chapter, locus of control specifically refers to whether an individual feels that attainment of a particular outcome is within his or her control or outside of it. If an individual thinks that health outcomes are within his or her control, he or she is considered to have an internal locus of control. In other words, the individual thinks that what he or she does (or does not do) determines the outcome of personal health. If the individual believes that outcomes are outside of his or her control, the individual is said to have an external locus of control. In other words, the individual believes that forces outside of his or her control determines health outcomes.

External locus of control can be further divided into two categories: (1) powerful others and (2) chance (AbuSabha & Achterberg, 1997; Levenson, 1974; Wallston, Wallston, & Devellis, 1978). Individuals who believe that other people, such as healthcare professionals and family members, determine health outcomes are said to have a powerful others' orientation. Those with a chance orientation believe that their health outcomes and other events are attributable to fate or chance.

Health Belief Model

The health belief model is used to understand the successes and failures of health behavior change. Rosenstock and colleagues initially developed this model to explain why people practice preventive behavior, but it has since been used to explain such behaviors as compliance with drug therapy and other disease management practices (Clark & Becker, 1998; Rosenstock, 1974; Salazar, 1991).

This model focuses on the likelihood that an individual will take action or change his or her behavior. According to this model, the perceived susceptibility and severity of the disease determine the perceived threat of the disease to the individual and contribute to the likelihood of changing behavior. Susceptibility is an individual's perception of his or her risk for contracting the disease; severity is the seriousness of a disease if left untreated (Clark & Becker, 1998; Salazar, 1991).

In addition to susceptibility and severity, the perceived benefits and barriers contribute to the likelihood of taking action. Benefits are the individual's beliefs that changing the behavior will reduce the disease threat. These are weighed against the barriers to change or the negative aspects (e.g., money, effort) of such a change in behavior, which act as deterrents to behavior change. If an individual believes that he or she has a high susceptibility to a severe/serious disease, the perceived threat is high enough so he or she may see the benefits of changing behavior (Clark & Becker, 1998; Salazar, 1991). Conversely, if the susceptibility and/or severity of the disease are low, the perceived threat is low and, therefore, the behavior change may not be perceived as providing sufficient benefits. In this case, the person is unlikely to change the behavior.

Demographic (age, gender, and ethnicity), sociopsychologic (personality, social class, and peer and reference group pressure), and structural variables (knowledge about the disease and prior contact to the disease) may influence how someone perceives the susceptibility, seriousness, and threat of the disease. In addition, cues to action can influence how an individual perceives the threat of disease. These cues might include mass media campaigns, advice from others, reminder postcards from a physician, illness of a family member or friend, or a newspaper or magazine article (Clark & Becker, 1998; Salazar, 1991).

Finally, self-efficacy may play a role in the health belief model. In brief, self-efficacy or efficacy expectation pertains to a person's confidence in his or her ability to take action or change a behavior. In other words, an individual must feel competent to overcome the barriers to positive behavior change (Strecher & Rosenstock, 1997). Self-efficacy is described in more detail later in this chapter.

According to the health belief model, for an obese person to lose weight, the individual would need to believe that he or she is susceptible to the negative effects of obesity as well as the possibility of severe effects from the disease. For example, for a behavior change to occur, the person needs to believe that he or she is more susceptible to suffering a cardiovascular event because of being overweight. In addition, the individual needs to believe that the cardiovascular event is serious to perceive a threat from developing the disease. The patient may see the benefits of enrolling in a weight reduction program, but if the barriers are greater than the benefits, he or she still may not take action. In addition, modifying factors, such as social support or cues to action (e.g., an obese family member having a heart attack), may influence the likelihood that the individual will actively try to lose weight. Besides the modifying factors, the person must believe in his or her ability to overcome the barriers to losing weight (self-efficacy) before he or she will attempt the weight loss regimen.

Self Efficacy

Self efficacy is part of a broader theory of learning, social cognitive theory. Though components of social cognitive theory have applications to health behavior, the focus of this section will be on the construct, self-efficacy. Bandura identified the following two types of expectations that influence behavior: (1) outcome expectations and (2) efficacy expectations (Bandura, 1977). Outcome expectations are the individual's expectation or belief that a particular behavior will result in a particular outcome. For example, a person may believe that exercise can help her lose weight. Efficacy expectations are the individual's expectations that he or she has the ability to accomplish this behavior, such as participating in an exercise routine to lose weight.

According to the theory, the key lies in the individual's perceptions of the outcomes and efficacy in performing these behaviors—not his or her true capabilities (Clark & Becker, 1998). That is, a person might begin an exercise program to lose weight because he or she believes that exercise will result in a weight loss and that he or she can perform this activity. In addition, expectations are specific for particular behaviors (AbuSabha & Achterberg, 1997; Clark & Becker, 1998). In other words, just because a person believes that he or she can undertake an exercise program, it does not mean that he or she believes that he or she can decrease his or her caloric intake or diet. His or her outcome and efficacy expectations may be different for a diet as compared to an exercise program.

Efficacy expectations are learned through the following four mechanisms: (1) performance accomplishments, (2) vicarious experiences, (3) verbal persuasion, and (4) physiologic state (Bandura, 1977, 1986; Clark & Becker, 1998). Performance accomplishments refer to an individual's attempt at a particular behavior that is perceived to be difficult. The experience of success in accomplishing this difficult behavior increases self-efficacy. For example, if a person fears going on a diet, yet attempts to make this lifestyle change and experiences success, then his or her self-efficacy will improve.

Vicarious experiences refer to the modeling of behaviors by others and the individual observing such behaviors. To improve self-efficacy, it must be seen that the model achieved success through overcoming difficulties (as compared to being easy) and the model must be similar in characteristics (gender, age) to the observer. Perhaps a friend is successful in achieving weight loss by dieting. By observing his or her friend's weight loss and the difficulties in succeeding in this task, a person may feel more capable of attempting this same change.

Verbal persuasion encourages the individual to continue to make attempts in behavior changes, such as a pharmacist encouraging a patient to continue or advising him or her to attempt an exercise regimen or diet. The final mechanism that influences efficacy expectations pertains to the physiologic state of the individual. High physiologic arousal, such as tension and agitation, increases the likelihood of failure. For instance, a person who feels fatigued or experiences pain after exercising may believe that he or she cannot accomplish the behavior.

Theory of Reasoned Action and the Theory of Planned Behavior

According to the theory of reasoned action, a determinant of a person's behavior is one's behavioral intention or the likelihood of performing the behavior. The following two factors are hypothesized to lead to an individual's behavioral intention: (1) the attitude toward performing the behavior and (2) the subjective norm associated with the behavior.

With the first factor, the likelihood of performing a behavior is influenced by the person's beliefs about the behavior and the outcome(s) associated with it. The value associated with the outcome—whether positive or negative—is another important component of one's attitude toward the behavior (Clark & Becker, 1998; Madden, Ellen, & Ajzen, 1992; Montano, Kasprzyk, & Taplin, 1997). For example, an individual who believes that losing weight is associated with positive outcomes will have a positive attitude toward the behavior change needed to lose weight.

The second factor, subjective norm, refers to what other important individuals think about the person's behavior change or of his or her desire to perform the behavior. In other words, do others approve or disapprove of the performance of the specific behavior? As part of this evaluation of others' beliefs, the individual also is affected by his or her desire or motivation to comply with others' wishes (Clark & Becker, 1998; Madden et al., 1992; Montano et al., 1997). For example, if an individual believes that others want him or her to lose weight and is motivated by these beliefs or expectations, he or she has a positive subjective norm. Both positive attitudes and a positive subject norm will increase the likelihood of performing the behavior or carrying through on the behavioral intention.

Theory of reasoned action fails to address the issue of the person's degree of control over the behavior. Control refers to factors, both personal and external, that influence the behavior such as a workable plan, skills, knowledge, time, money, willpower, and opportunity. However, the degree of control or factors could influence both behavioral intention and the performance of a behavior. The theory of planned behavior is an extension of the theory of reasoned action in which perceived behavioral control is added to the theory of reasoned action model to address those cases in which a person does not have a high degree of control over the behavior (Clark & Becker, 1998; Madden et al., 1992; Montano et al., 1997).

Perceived behavioral control is determined by control beliefs, which refers to the presence or absence of resources for and the barriers to the performance of the behavior. In addition, the perceived power of each resource and barrier to promote or deter behavior is considered. For example, if an individual has a strong belief about the existence of resources to encourage the behavior, then he or she has a high perceived control over the behavior. By contrast, if an individual believes that factors can deter him or her from performing the behavior, such as the lack of time to exercise, the person is said to have low perceived control and is less likely to perform the behavior (Clark & Becker, 1998; Madden et al., 1992; Montano et al., 1997).

Transtheoretical Model of Change

The transtheoretical model of change was developed by Prochaska in the 1970s and 1980s to determine why the attempts to change behavior failed or succeeded. Commonly referred to as the readiness to change model, it theorizes that a patient progresses through five stages before a change in behavior, such as quitting smoking or losing weight, occurs. These stages are (1) precontemplation,

(2) contemplation, (3) preparation, (4) action, and (5) maintenance (Berger, 1997; Prochaska, Johnson, & Lee, 1998; Prochaska & Velicer, 1997).

Patients in the precontemplation stage have not thought of changing a specific behavior, and such a change is not expected to occur in the foreseeable future (the next 6 months). Patients are in the precontemplation stage for a variety of reasons, including being uninformed or underinformed about the outcomes of their behaviors and/or discouraged about their ability to change because of past failures. In addition, this category includes individuals who are unwilling to change their behaviors. Individuals in this stage of change avoid talking, reading, or thinking about the needed behavior change. Often they are perceived as unmotivated and as unprepared for action-oriented intervention programs (Berger, 1997; Prochaska, Johnson, & Lee, 1998; Prochaska & Velicer, 1997).

Unlike individuals in the precontemplation stage, patients entering the contemplation stage are beginning to consider a change in their behavior and intend to make that change within the next 6 months. These individuals recognize the benefits of changing, but also realize the costs or negative aspects of behavior change. For this reason, patients may become stuck in this stage because of their ambivalence about the benefits versus the costs of change. In other words, they have no plan for action and are not entirely ready to commit to a change (Berger, 1997; Prochaska, Johnson, & Lee, 1998; Prochaska & Velicer, 1997). Even though a 6-month timeframe is used, patients can stay in this stage for longer periods of time and become "stuck" thinking about making a change (Prochaska, Norcross, & Diclemente, 2013). Commitment to making a change will not occur until the benefits of the change outweigh the barriers to the behavior change.

In the preparation stage, patients commit to a behavior change and plan to take action, usually within the next month. In many cases, they have already taken some small steps toward action within the past year and are ready to make a change. These individuals are prepared to engage in an action-oriented intervention, such as a smoking cessation program (Berger, 1997; Prochaska, Johnson, & Lee, 1998; Prochaska & Velicer, 1997).

Patients in the action stage are in the process of changing their behavior and have taken specific steps to do so over the past 6 months (Berger, 1997; Prochaska, Johnson, & Lee, 1998; Prochaska & Velicer, 1997). In the maintenance stage, individuals do not use change processes as frequently as in the action stage. Instead, they focus on triggers (e.g., environment, friends, and family) that may make them susceptible to their old habits. The goal during this stage is to prevent relapse into the old behavior. People in this stage need help to control or become aware of these triggers for relapse. Despite the temptation, patients are more confident that they will not return to their old behaviors. The maintenance stage can last anywhere from 6 months to 5 years (Berger, 1997; Prochaska, Johnson, & Lee, 1998; Prochaska & Velicer, 1997).

Besides focusing on appropriate interventions based on the level of patient's commitment to engaging in a behavior change, the healthcare professional should facilitate movement through this model. Assessing the stage of change, or the patient's level of readiness, can be done be asking questions, such as:

"Do you think behavior X is a problem for you now?"

"When do you intend to change behavior X?"

If patient answers yes to whether it is a problem, he or she is likely in contemplation, preparation, or action stage (Prochaska, Norcross, & Diclemente, 2013). Using the previously outlined timeframes for each stage, a pharmacist can determine the patient's readiness for change. For example, if the patient says "within the next month," he or she is likely in the preparation stage, while if the patient says "now," he or she is likely in the action stage (Prochaska, Norcross, & Diclemente, 2013). Though not specially developed for the transtheoretical model, motivational interviewing (MI) (discussed later in this chapter) is a communication approach that pharmacists can use to determine the patient's commitment to change and facilitate the patient's movement through the stages of change.

One caveat to this model is that patients do not always move through the model linearly. Instead, there is often a spiral pattern (Prochaska, Norcross, & Diclemente, 2013). For example, a patient may start in contemplation move to preparation, action, and then relapse. At this point, he or she will go back to an earlier stage, such as precontemplation or contemplation. In some cases, a patient will feel like a failure and resist thinking about change. Approximately 15% of those who relapse move into the precontemplation stage while 85% move to the contemplation stage (Prochaska, Norcross, & Diclemente, 2013).

According to the transtheoretical model of change, interventions to change patient behavior should consider the patient's level of readiness to change. If someone is overweight and in the precontemplation stage, the desired intervention should be promoting awareness rather than enrolling him or her in a weight reduction plan, such as Weight Watchers. The weight reduction plan will not be successful for this individual because he or she has no intention to change at this point, or may not even know that he or she should change. Furthermore, the barriers to weight loss may seem insurmountable and enrollment in a weight reduction plan will not necessarily address those barriers. By comparison, a person in the preparation stage is ready to make a change and has already taken small steps toward weight reduction, such as reading about nutrition, talking to friends or family about diets, or searching the Internet. He or she is more likely to be successful in a weight reduction program.

INTERVENTIONS

Interventions and techniques to facilitate behavior change can be used to help patients move toward the action and maintenance stages of change. Those developed specifically in conjunction with the transtheoretical model are called processes of change (**Table 4-3**). Other interventions can be used to help patients succeed in changing behavior. These include goal setting, self-monitoring, problem solving, and skills training, (Kehoe & Katz, 1998). When goal setting with patients, both short- and long-term goals should be considered. If a long-term goal is the only focus, patients can get discouraged if they are not making the progress they desire. To provide patients with "small victories," short-term goals should be set. A key to setting short-term goals is that they are achievable. For example, instead of discussing a 30-pound weight loss with a patient, discuss losing 1 to 2 pounds per week as a short-term goal. All behavior change goals should be individualized, specific, reasonable, and measurable (Kehoe & Katz, 1998).

Self-monitoring involves patients monitoring their progress in the behavior change or the status of their disease. Examples of self-monitoring include keeping logs or diaries of blood pressure or blood glucose values, foods eaten during the day, completion of exercise, and number of cigarettes smoked. In a sense, it is documentation for the patient and a form of accountability. The use of logs and diaries also can build self-efficacy when patients observe the results of their behavior change (Kehoe & Katz, 1998).

Problem solving allows patients to visualize scenarios that may be challenging to a behavior change and identify strategies to address these challenges (Kehoe & Katz, 1998). Patients determine specific ways to cope with a barrier or difficulty prior to its actual occurrence. If the event does occur,

Table 4-3 Processes of Change

Process of Change	Definition	Example	Stage Emphasized
Consciousness raising	Increasing awareness about the causes, consequences, and cures for a problem behavior or diseases	Education, pamphlets, media campaigns	Precontemplation Contemplation
Emotional arousal (Dramatic relief)	Arousing an emotional response with a subsequent reduced effect if action can be taken	Personal testimonies, media campaigns, role-playing	Precontemplation Contemplation
Self-reevaluation	Assessing one's self-image with and without behavior	Smoker assessing what it would be like to be a nonsmoker	Contemplation
Environmental reevaluation	Assessing how a behavior impacts the social environment	Smoker assessing how his or her smoking impacts spouse, children, etc.	Precontemplation Contemplation
Self-liberation	Believing that one can change and committing to the change	New Year's resolution or telling others of changes	Preparation
Counter conditioning	Substituting healthy behaviors for unhealthy ones	Nicotine replacement, fat-free foods	Action Maintenance
Stimulus control	Removing cues for unhealthy behaviors and adding prompts for healthy behaviors for easy access	Removing high-fat foods from home, keeping exercise equipment in car	Action Maintenance
Contingency management	Using rewards to encourage behavior change	Praise, group recognition, purchase of new clothes after weight loss	Action Maintenance

(Continues)

Table 4-3 Processes of Change (continued)

Process of Change	Definition	Example	Stage Emphasized
Helping relationships	Receiving and using support from others	Buddy systems for exercise or weight loss, family involvement in change	Action Maintenance

Source: Data from Schumaker, S. A., Schron, E. B., Ockene, J. K., & McBee, W. L. (Eds.). (1998). *The Handbook of Health Behavior Change* (2nd ed.). New York, NY: Springer Publishing Company, LLC; Proschaska, Norcorss & Diclemnte, 2013.

patients are more prepared to handle it and experience a successful outcome. This technique can be used for almost any behavior change. For example, a pharmacist could ask a patient, "What will you do at a party when you are faced with unhealthy food options?" or "How would you respond when your blood sugar is 200mg/dL?" If the patient does not know how to handle a scenario, it is an opportunity for the pharmacist to provide education.

Patients also need skills to be successful in making behavior changes. Skills can range from using a blood glucose meter to reading a nutrition label to developing an exercise regimen. The pharmacist can model skills by demonstrating or showing the patient how to perform a skill and then having the patient demonstrate the skill back to the pharmacist. Guidelines for using modeling in patient education are: (1) assess patient's current level of understanding of skill or behavior, (2) specify the skill or behavior, (3) provide easy-to-follow steps when explaining complex behaviors, (4) sequence the instruction in order of steps or from the easiest to hardest step, and (5) have the patient demonstrate the skill or behavior (Kehoe & Katz, 1998).

Motivational Interviewing

Developed by Miller and Rollnick, MI is a patient-centered approach to facilitate behavior change by exploring and resolving a patient's ambivalence (Miller & Rollnick, 2002). Unlike the traditional advising or persuasive approach used by health professionals, the focus of MI is to help a patient resolve his or her ambivalence, which is often seen in the precontemplation and contemplation stages of change in the transtheoretical model. Based on reports in the literature, the use of these MI techniques is more effective in facilitating behavior change among patients as compared to the traditional advice-giving approach in patient care (Hardcastle, Taylor, Bailey, Harley, & Hagger, 2013; Lundahl et al., 2013; Rubak, Sandboek, Lauritzen, & Christensen, 2005).

In MI, a partnership is formed between the health professional and patient. Key to using this approach is preserving the patient's autonomy while eliciting a patient's motivation, or lack thereof, to adhere to healthy behaviors or therapeutic recommendations (Miller & Rollnick, 2002). Ambivalence to behavior change can result from many of the factors discussed in the health behavior change models. **Exhibit 4-1** lists factors that encourage behavior change, which can be used in the MI process. As part of the collaboration between the patient and health professional, the key

Exhibit 4-1 Selected Factors Encouraging Behavior Change

- Want to change
- Face few barriers in performing the behavior change
- Believe they have the skills necessary to change
- Believe in positive outcomes as a result of the change
- Believe important "others" support the change

principles of MI are used: expressing empathy, developing discrepancy, rolling with resistance, avoiding argumentation, and supporting self-efficacy. Descriptions of each of the principles can be found in **Table 4-4**. A detailed description of MI and its use is beyond the scope of this chapter, as books have been written about this topic alone. Readers are advised to seek some of these resources, as well as online examples, to learn more about this effective communication approach (Berger & Vallaume, 2013; Miller & Rollnick, 2002; Rollnick, Miller, & Butler, 2008).

Table 4-4 Motivational Interviewing Principles

Principle	Approach
Expressing empathy	Use of reflective listening to help the patient feel understood. Utilize statements, such as "It sounds like..." or "You seem to be saying..."
Developing discrepancy	Create cognitive dissonance by having the patient compare present behavior with his or her goals, making it difficult for the patient to ignore the discrepancy. Encourage the patient to consider the benefits of the new behavior and the negatives of the status quo.
Rolling with resistance	Develop mutually negotiated solutions with the patient. Change direction of conversation by using a different strategy or approach when experiencing resistance from the patient.
Avoiding argumentation	Resist arguing with patient about discrepancies because doing so creates defensiveness and resistance in the patient, making change unlikely. Avoid "righting reflex" or statements, such as "Yes,..., but..."
Supporting self-efficacy	Provide support and encouragement to improve the patient's confidence in changing a behavior.

Source: Adapted from Miller, W. R., Rollnick, S., & Butler C. C. (2008). *Motivational interviewing in health care: Helping patients change behavior.* New York, NY: The Guilford Press.

CONCLUSION

Patient care is currently undergoing a transition toward increased collaboration between healthcare professionals and patients. Given the increasing knowledge patients have about their health, providers will need to take a different approach to care than telling the patient what to do and expecting unquestioning compliance. Of course, not all patients are alike. They have their own unique issues and characteristics that affect their interactions with healthcare professionals as well as determine their impact on the healthcare system and the healthcare system's impact on them.

As healthcare professionals continue to try to change patient health behaviors, the models, as well as the factors affecting adherence, described in this chapter provide a basis for the development of effective interventions. By asking patients questions, healthcare practitioners can determine patients' beliefs regarding the numerous factors that influence their behaviors. In using these models, practitioners can use the information gained from patients to target specific behaviors with specific interventions.

QUESTIONS FOR FURTHER DISCUSSION

1. Would you suggest other models of care or variations on the models discussed in this chapter, based on a pharmacist–patient interaction rather than a physician–patient interaction?
2. How does your personal experiences relate to the health behavior models discussed in this chapter?
3. Do pharmacists need to make changes in the various practice settings to improve delivery of health care to patients? Why or why not?
4. How could the health behavior models and MI be implemented in pharmacy practice?
5. How will you adapt your communication when providing patient care to patients with limited health literacy?

KEY TOPICS AND TERMS

Activity–passivity model of patient care
Adherence
Compliance
Consumer model of care
Culture
Guidance–cooperation model of patient care
Health behavior models
Health belief model
Health literacy
Motivational interviewing
Mutual participation model of patient care
Patient-centered model of care
Preventive health care

REFERENCES

AbuSabha, R., & Achterberg, C. (1997). Review of self-efficacy and locus of control for nutrition and health-related behavior. *Journal of the American Dietetic Association*, *97*(10), 1122–1133.

Agency for Healthcare Research and Quality. (2008). *National healthcare disparities 2007 report*. Rockville, MD: U.S. Department of Health and Human Services.

Arias, E. (2006). United States life tables. (2003). *National Vital Statistics Reports*, *54*(14), 1–6.

Baker, D. W., Williams, M. V., Parker, R. M., Gazmararian, J. A., & Nurss J. (1999). Development of a brief test to measure functional health literacy. *Patient Education and Counseling, 38*(1), 33–42.

Balint, M., Hung, J., Joyce, D., Marinker, M., & Woodcock, J. (1970). *Treatment of diagnosis: A study of repeat prescription in general practice.* Toronto, ON: J. B. Lippincott.

Bandura, A. (1977). Self-efficacy: Toward a unifying theory of behavioral change. *Psychological Review, 84*, 191–215.

Bandura, A. (1986). *Social foundations of thought and action.* Englewood Cliffs, NJ: Prentice-Hall.

Baran, R. W., Crumlish, K., Patterson, H., Shaw, J., Erwin, W. G., Wylie, J. D., & Duong, P. (1999). Improving outcomes of community-dwelling older patients with diabetes through pharmacist counseling. *American Journal of Health-System Pharmacists, 56*, 1535–1539.

Beisecker, A. E., & Beisecker, T. D. (1993). Using metaphors to characterize doctor–patient relationships: Paternalism versus consumerism. *Health Communications, 5*, 41–58.

Berger, B. A. (1997). *Readiness for change: Improving treatment adherence.* Durham, NC: Glaxo, Inc., and Clean Data.

Berger, B. A., & Vallaume, W. S. (2013). *Motivational interviewing for health care professionals: A sensible approach.* Washington, DC: American Pharmacists Association.

Berkman, N. D., DeWalt, D. A., Pignone, M. P., Sheridan, S. L., Lohr, K. N., Lux, L., ... Bonito, A. J. (2004). *Literacy and health outcomes.* Rockville, MD: Agency for Health Care Research and Quality.

Bluml, B. M., McKenney, J. M., & Cziraky, M. J. (2000). Pharmaceutical care services and results in Project ImPACT: Hyperlipidemia. *Journal of the American Pharmaceutical Association, 40*, 157–165.

Briesacher, B. A., Andrade, S. E., Fouayzi, H., & Chan, K. A., (2008). Comparison of drug adherence rates among patients with seven different medical conditions. *Pharmacotherapy, 28*(4), 437–443.

Byrne, P. S., & Long, B. E. L. (1976). *Doctors talking to patients.* London, England: Royal College of General Practitioners.

Carter, B. L., Coffey, C. S., Ardery, G., Uribe, L., Ecklund, D., James, P., ... Vaughn, T. (2015). Cluster-randomized trial of a physician/pharmacist collaborative model to improve blood pressure control. *Circulation Cardiovascular Quality and Outcomes, 8*, 235–243.

Chan, L., Hart, L. G., & Goodman, D. C. (2006). Geographic access to health care for rural Medicare beneficiaries. *Journal of Rural Health, 22*(2), 140–146.

Chew, L. D., Griffin, J. M, Partin, M. R., Noorbaloochi, S., Grill, J. P., Snyder, A., ... VanRyn, M. (2007). Validation of screening questions for limited health literacy in a large VA outpatient population. *Journal of General Internal Medicine, 23*(5), 561–566.

Childress, J. F., & Siegler, M. (1984). Metaphors and models of doctor–patient relationships: Their implications for autonomy. *Theoretical Medicine, 5*, 17–30.

Clark, N. M., & Becker, M. H. (1998). Theoretical models and strategies for improving adherence and disease management. In S. A. Shumaker, E. B. Schron, J. K. Ockene, & W. L. McBee (Eds.), *The handbook of health behavior change* (2nd ed., pp. 5–32). New York, NY: Springer.

Cranor, C. W., & Christensen, D. B. (2003). The Asheville project: Short-term outcomes of a community diabetes care program. *Journal of the American Pharmacists Association, 43*(2), 149–159.

Davis, T. C., Long, S. W., Jackson, R. H., Mayeaux, E. J., George, R. B., Murphy, P. W., & Crouch, M. A. (1993). Rapid estimate of adult literacy in medicine: A shortened screening instrument. *Family Medicine, 25*(6), 391–395.

Dean, K. (1989). Conceptual, theoretical, and methodological issues in self-care research. *Social Science and Medicine, 29*(2), 117–123.

Emanuel, E. J., & Emanuel, L. L. (1992). Four models of the physician–patient relationship. *Journal of the American Medical Association, 267*, 2221–2226.

Engel, G. L. (1978). The biopsychosocial model and the education of health professionals. *Annals of the New York Academy of Sciences, 310*, 169–181.

Engel, G. L. (1979). The need for a new medical model: A challenge for biomedicine. *Science, 196*, 129–136.

Engel, G. L. (1980). The clinical application of the biopsychosocial model. *American Journal of Psychiatry, 137*, 535–544.

Fairman, K., & Motheral, B. (2000). Evaluating medication adherence: Which measure is right for your program? *Journal of Managed Care Pharmacy, 6*(6), 499–504.

Fox, S., & Duggan, M. (2009). The social life of health information. Pew Internet and American Life Project. Retrieved from http://pewinternet.org/~/media//Files/Reports/2009/PIP_Health_2009.pdf

Fox, S., & Duggan, M. (2013). Health online 2013. Pew Internet and American Life Project. Retrieved from http://www.pewinternet.org/files/old-media//Files/Reports/PIP_HealthOnline.pdf

Fox, S., & Jones, S. (2009). The social life of health information. Pew Internet and American Life Project. Retrieved from http://pewinternet.org/~/media//Files/Reports/2009/PIP_Health_2009.pdf

Galanti, G. (2004). *Caring for patients from different cultures.* Philadelphia, PA: University of Pennsylvania Press.

Halber, K. V., & Halber, D. A. (2008). *Essentials of cultural competence in pharmacy practice.* Washington, DC: American Pharmacists Association.

Hall, J. A., & Dornan, M. C. (1988a). Meta-analysis of satisfaction with medical care: Description of research done in and analysis of overall satisfaction. *Social Science and Medicine, 26*, 637–644.

Hall, J. A., & Dornan, M. C. (1988b). What patients like about their medical care and how often they are asked: A meta-analysis of the satisfaction literature. *Social Science and Medicine, 27*, 935–939.

Hardcastle, S. J., Taylor, A. H., Bailey, M. P., Harley, R. A., & Hagger, M. S. (2013). Effectiveness of a motivational interviewing intervention on weight loss, physical activity, and cardiovascular disease risk factors: A randomized controlled trial with a 12 month post-intervention follow-up. *International Journal of Behavioral Nutrition and Physical Activity, 10*, 40.

Haug, M. R., & Lavin, B. (1981). Practitioner or patient—Who's in charge? *Journal of Health and Social Behavior, 22*, 212–229.

Haug, M. R., & Lavin, B. (1983). *Consumerism in medicine: Challenging physician authority.* Beverly Hills, CA: Sage.

Henbest, R. J., & Stewart, M. (1990). Patient-centeredness in the consultation, 2: Does it really make a difference? *Family Practice, 7*, 28–33.

Ho, P. M., Bryson, C. L., & Rumsfeld, J. S. (2009). Mediation adherence: Its importance in cardiovascular outcomes. *Circulation, 119*, 3028–3035.

Institute of Medicine (IOM). (2004). *Health literacy: A prescription to end confusion.* Washington, DC: National Academies Press.

Kehoe, W. A., & Katz, R. C. (1998). Health behaviors and pharmacotherapy. *Annal of Pharmacotherapy, 32*, 1076–86.

Knowles, J. H. (1997). *Doing better and feeling worse: Health in the United States.* New York, NY: Norton Press.

Kripalani, S. & Weiss, B. D. (2006). Teaching about health literacy and clear communication. *Journal of General Internal Medicine, 21*, 888–890.

Lavsa, S. M., Holzworth, A., & Ansani, N. T. (2011). Selection of a validated scale for measuring adherence. *Journal of American Pharmacists Association, 51*(1), 90–94.

Leavitt, J. W., & Numbers, R. L. (1997). Sickness and health: An overview. In J. W. Leavitt & R. L. Numbers (Eds.), *Sickness and health in America: Readings in the history of medicine and public health* (3rd ed., pp. 3–10). Madison, WI: University of Wisconsin Press.

Levenson, H. (1974). Activism and powerful others: Distinctions within the concept of internal-external control. *Journal of Personality Assessment, 38*, 377–383.

Levenstein, J. H., Brown, J. B., Weston, W. W., Stewart, M., McCracken, E. C., & McWhinney, I. (1989). Patient-centered clinical interviewing. In M. Stewart & D. Roter (Eds.), *Communicating with medical patients* (pp. 107–120). Beverly Hills, CA: Sage.

Levy, J. A., & Strombeck, R. (2002). Health benefits and risks of the Internet. *Journal of Medical Systems, 26*(6), 495–510.

Loustaunau, M. O., & Sobo, E. J. (1997). *The cultural context of health, illness, and medicine.* Westport, CT: Bergin and Garvey.

Lubkin, I. M. (1990). *Chronic illness: Impact and interventions* (2nd ed.). Sudbury, MA: Jones and Bartlett.

Lundahl, B., Moleni, T., Burke, B. L., Butters, R., Tollefson, D., Butler, C., & Rollnick, S. (2013). Motivational interviewing in medical care settings: A systematic review and meta-analysis of randomized controlled trials. *Patient Education and Counseling, 93*, 157–168.

Madden, T. J., Ellen, P. S., & Ajzen, I. (1992). A comparison of the theory of planned behavior and the theory of reasoned action. *Personality and Social Psychology Bulletin, 18*(1), 3–9.

Miller, W. R., & Rollnick, S. (2002). *Motivational interviewing: Preparing people for change.* New York, NY: The Guilford Press.

Mishler, E. G. (1984). *The discourse of medicine: Dialectics of medical interviews.* Norwood, NJ: Ablex.

Montano, D. E., Kasprzyk, D., & Taplin, S. H. (1997). The theory of reasoned action and the theory of planned behavior. In K. Glanz, F. M. Lewis, & B. K. Rimer (Eds.), *Health behavior and health education* (pp. 85–112). San Francisco, CA: Jossey-Bass.

National Center for Health Statistics. (2004). *NCHS data on aging*. Hyattsville, MD: National Center for Health Statistics.

National Center for Health Statistics. (2010). *Health, United States, 2009: With special feature on medical technology*. Hyattsville, MD.

National Community Pharmacists Association. (2013). Medication adherence in American: A national report card. Retrieved from http://www.ncpa.co/adherence/AdherenceReportCard_Full.pdf

Nau, D. P. Proportion of days covered (PDC) as a preferred method of measuring medication adherence. Retrieved from http://www.pqaalliance.org/images/uploads/files/PQA%20PDC%20vs%20%20MPR.pdf

Nau, D. P., & Ponte, C. D. (2002). Effects of a community pharmacist-based diabetes patient-management program on intermediate clinical outcome measures. *Journal of Managed Care Pharmacy, 8*(1), 48–53.

Paasche-Orlow, M. K., & Wolf, M. S. (2007). Evidence does not support clinical screening of literacy. *Journal of General Internal Medicine, 23*(1), 100–102.

Park, J. J., Kelly, P., Carter, B. L., & Burgess, P. P. (1996). Comprehensive pharmaceutical care in the chain setting. *Journal of the American Pharmaceutical Association, NS36*(7), 443–451.

Parsons, T. (1951). *The social system*. Glencoe, IL: Free Press.

Pew Research Center. (2014). Internet users demographics. Retrieved from http://www.pewinternet.org/data-trend/internet-use/latest-stats/

Pew Research Center. (2015). Home broadband 2015. Retrieved from http://www.pewinternet.org/2015/12/21/home-broadband-2015/

President's Commission for the Study of Ethical Problems in Medicine and Biomedical and Behavioral Research. (1982). *Making health care decisions: The ethical and legal implications of informed consent in the patient–practitioner relationship* (Vol. 1). Washington, DC: U.S. Government Printing Office.

Prochaska, J. O., Johnson, S., & Lee, P. (1998). The transtheoretical model of change. In S. A. Schumaker, E. B. Schron, J. K. Ockene, & W. L. McBee (Eds.), *The handbook of health behavior change* (2nd ed., pp. 59–84). New York, NY: Springer.

Prochaska, J. O., Norcross J. C., & Diclemente, C. C. (2013). Applying the stages of change. *Psychotherapy in Australia, 19*(2): 10–15.

Prochaska, J. O., & Velicer, W. F. (1997). The transtheoretical model of health behavior change. *American Journal of Health Promotion, 12*(1), 38–48.

Ratzan, S. C., & Parker, R. M. (2000). Introduction. In C. R. Seldin, M. Zorn, S. C. Ratzan, R. M. Parker (Eds.), *National Library of Medicine current bibliographies in medicine: Health literacy*. NLM Pub. No. CBM 2000-1. Bethesda, MD: National Institutes of Health, United States Department of Health and Human Services.

Reeder, L. G. (1972). The patient-client as a consumer: Some observations on the changing professional –client relationship. *Journal of Health and Social Behavior, 13*, 406–412.

Rollnick, S., Miller, W. R., & Butler C. C. (2008). *Motivational interviewing in health care: Helping patients change behavior*. New York, NY: Guilford Press.

Rosenstock, I. M. (1974). Historical origins of the health belief model. *Health Education Monographs, 2*, 328–335.

Roter, D. L., & Hall, J. A. (1992). *Doctors talking with patients—Patients talking with doctors*. Westport, CT: Auburn House.

Rubak, S., Sandboek, A., Lauritzen, T., & Christensen, B. (2005). Motivational interviewing. *British Journal of General Practice, 55*, 305–312.

Salazar, M. K. (1991). Comparison of four behavioral theories: A literature review. *AAOHN Journal, 39*(3), 128–135.

Schoen, C., Osborn, R., How, S. K. H., Doty, M. M., & Peugh, J. (2008). In chronic condition: Experiences of patients with complex health care needs, in eight countries, 2008. *Health Affairs, 28*(1), w1–w16.

Sennett, C. (2000). Ambulatory care in the new millennium: The role of consumer information. *Quality Management in Health Care, 8*(2), 82–87.

Simpson, S. H., Majumdar, S. R., Tsuyuki, R. T., Lewanczuk, R. Z., Spooner, R., & Johnson, J. A. (2011). Effect of adding pharmacists to primary care teams on blood pressure control in patients with type 2 diabetes. *Diabetes Care, 34*, 20–26.

Skinner, J. S., Poe, B., Hopper, R., Boyer, A., & Wilkins, C. H. (2015). Assessing the effectiveness of pharmacist-directed medication therapy management in improving diabetes outcomes in patients with poorly control diabetes. *Diabetes Educator, 41*(4), 459–465.

Smolderen, K. G., Spertus, J. A., Nallamothu, B. K., Krumholz, H. M., Tang, F., Ross, J. S., ... Chan, P. S. (2010). *Journal of the American Medical Association, 303*(14), 1392–1400.

Strecher, V. J., & Rosenstock, I. M. (1997). The health belief model. In K. Glanz, F. M. Lewis, & B. K. Rimer (Eds.), *Health behavior and health education* (pp. 41–59). San Francisco, CA: Jossey-Bass.

Stroebe, W., & Stroebe, M. S. (1995). *Social psychology and health*. Pacific Grove, CA: Brooks/Cole.

Stuifbergen, A. (1999). Barriers and health behaviors of rural and urban persons with multiple sclerosis. *American Journal of Health Behavior, 23*(6), 415–425.

Suchman, E. A. (1965). Stages of illness and medical care. *Journal of Health and Human Behavior, 6*, 114–128.

Svarstad, B. L., Kotchen, J. M., Shireman, T.I., Brown, R. L., Crawford, S. Y., Mount, J. K., ... Wilson, D.A. (2013). Improving refill adherence and hypertension control in black patients: Wisconsin TEAM Trial. *Journal of Pharmacists Association, 53*, 520–529.

Szasz, T., & Hollender, M. (1956). A contribution to the philosophy of medicine: The basic model of the doctor–patient relationship. *Archives of Internal Medicine, 97*, 585–592.

Tebbe, J. (1998). Health care delivery in America: Historical and policy perspectives. In R. L. McCarthy (Ed.), *Introduction to health care delivery: A primer for pharmacists* (p. 18). Gaithersburg, MD: Aspen.

United States Bureau of the Census (USBOC). (2000). Retrieved from www.census.gov/population/estimates/nation/intfile2-1.txt

U.S. Census Bureau, Population Division. (2015). Annual estimates of the resident population for selected age groups by sex for the United States, states, counties, and Puerto Rico commonwealth and municipios: April 1, 2010 to July 1, 2014. Retrieved from http://factfinder.census.gov/faces/tableservices/jsf/pages/productview.xhtml?src=bkmk. Source: U.S. Census Bureau, Population Division. Release Date: June 2015.

Veatch, R. M. (1972). Models for ethical medicine in a revolutionary age. *Hastings Center Report, 2*, 5–7.

Vincent, G. K., & Velkoff, V. A. (2010). The next four decades, the older population in the United States: 2010 to 2050. *Current population reports* (pp. 25–1138). Washington, DC: U.S. Census Bureau.

Wallston, K. A., Wallston, B. S., & Devellis, R. (1978). Development of the multidimensional health locus of control (MHLC) scales. *Health Education Monographs, 6*, 160–170.

Weiss, B. D., Mays, M. Z., Martz, W., Castro, K. M., DeWalt, D. A., Pignone, M., ... Hale, F. A. (2005). Quick assessment of literacy in primary care: The newest vital sign. *Annals of Family Medicine, 3*(6), 514–522.

Weiss, B. D. (2007). *Health literacy and patient safety: Help patients understand manual for clinicians*. Chicago, IL: American Medical Foundation and the American Medical Association.

Weston, W. W., Brown, J. B., & Stewart, M. (1989). Patient-centered interviewing. Part I: Understanding patients' experiences. *Canadian Family Physician, 35*, 147–151.

Williams, M. V., Davis, T., Parker, R. M., Weiss, B. D. (2002). The role of health literacy in patient-physician communication. *Family Medicine, 24*(5), 383–389.

World Health Organization. (2003). *Adherence to long-term therapies: Evidence for action*. Geneva, Switzerland: WHO.

CHAPTER

5

Drug Use, Access, the Supply Chain, and the Role of the Pharmaceutical Industry

Kyle D. Ross, Kimberly S. Plake, and Louis P. Garrison Jr.*

Case Scenario

MPC Pharmaceuticals is a large pharmaceutical firm that does not have a presence in the erythropoietin (EPO) market. The firm has a strong desire to be selling a drug in this area, but management is divided in terms of the strategy to best achieve this. There are two main options the firm can pursue: (1) develop a new version of EPO that is superior to any drug on the market or (2) develop a copy of a current version of EPO produced by Hemocyte, Inc. called Erystim. The MPC board's last meeting on the topic was in November 2015 and a decision was reached at a meeting in July 2016.

Those on the board in favor of developing a new version of EPO like the idea of having a first-in-class drug that could command premium pricing and deliver large revenues to MPC. A new version would enjoy protection from any imitators for a number of years and could support the development of other drugs in the company. However, the drawbacks to pursuing a new EPO drug are substantial as well. One of the main disadvantages of developing a new version is that it would take many years for the drug to go from discovery to approval by the Food and Drug Administration (FDA). There is a substantial amount of clinical testing that new drugs must go through in order to gain approval by the FDA. Another drawback is that there are high costs and a high level of uncertainty when developing a new drug. Even if a drug is promising early on, there is a low probability that it will eventually be approved by the FDA for sale in the United States.

The members of the board who supported developing a copy of Erystim point to the shorter time frame and higher likelihood of success that are distinct advantages to pursuing a copy of an existing drug. They feel that there are a number of drugs in the EPO market and that by developing a copy, the firm would be able to compete by charging a lower price and thereby gaining a large market share. The downside to pursuing this strategy is that other copies can enter into the market and the market could become crowded.

(*Continues*)

*With acknowledgment to Peter L. Steere, Michael Montagne, and Dana Hammer.

In the end, MPC chose to pursue development of a copy of Erystim. The firm made this decision based in large part on relatively recent developments in the pharmaceutical sector. One of the largest changes affecting MPC's decision was the passage of the Affordable Care Act in March 2010. One of the pieces of the legislation was to lower the clinical trial burden for copies of biologics. This meant that MPC's version of EPO will be able to rely on Hemocyte's clinical trial data. By doing this, MPC would be able to save on development of their version and price it at a lower price than Hemocyte's Erystim. The board also decided that this aspect of the Affordable Care Act would make any innovative drug MPC produced less profitable, since new copies would eventually be able to rely on its clinical trial data.

Another major factor that affected MPC's decision is the emphasis on cost control they had been receiving from many major insurers in the United States. Many insurers relayed that they were not excited at the idea of covering a new, more expensive version of EPO, but they would love to have the option of adding a copy of Erystim to their formularies. MPC also felt that consumers were becoming very cost conscious, indicated in part by the rise of Internet and mail-order pharmacies. Both of these factors demonstrated to MPC that in a crowded EPO market, positioning itself to compete on price was the best decision for MPC.

Since the decision was made in July 2016 to pursue a copy of Hemocyte's drug, MPC entered into negotiations to purchase EGlobin. EGlobin is a small biotech firm that has developed a drug called Erysimilar that is a copy of Erystim. By purchasing EGlobin, MPC plans to have a copy of Erystim approved by the FDA in less than 18 months. MPC feels confident that once approved, Erysimilar will be accepted by patients and physicians as a viable substitute for Erystim. This will provide revenue for the company in a relatively short amount of time and put MPC in a desirable position in the EPO market.

LEARNING OBJECTIVES

Upon completion of this chapter, the student shall be able to:

- Discuss how consumers view drugs and their expectations of them.
- Describe the role prescribers and pharmacists play in treating patients with pharmaceuticals.
- Describe the steps a drug goes through in its development and approval.
- Describe the four stages of clinical testing of a drug.
- Explain how the intellectual property rights of drug manufacturers are protected.
- Discuss the concerns surrounding increased globalization in drug production.
- Discuss how future healthcare trends could affect both the pharmaceutical sector and pharmacists.

CHAPTER QUESTIONS

1. What are the primary ways U.S. consumers choose to approach decisions about using drugs, and what are the main factors that affect their decisions?
2. What are the FDA responsibilities for drug regulation and what can it not control?
3. What are the main differences between the regulation of intellectual property rights for small-molecule drugs and biologics?
4. In what ways are the jobs of pharmacists likely to be different 10 years from now, and what are the main factors driving those changes?

INTRODUCTION

Pharmaceuticals are some of the most visible treatments in medical care. Consumers possess a familiarity with them that is matched by little else in medicine. Many patients choose the drug they will consume (nonprescription drugs) or might advocate for the prescription of a particular drug from their physician. This familiarity is driven in part by the fact that many pharmaceuticals are advertised directly to consumers, and consumers then form their own opinions apart from healthcare providers. The simplicity of drugs is another aspect of drugs that contributes to the comfort patients have with drugs. For the most part, a patient puts a pill in his or her mouth, takes a drink of water, and swallows. For other drugs, all that is required is to inject or infuse the drug, which can often be done by the patient at home.

This simplicity and familiarity mask the true complexity of pharmaceuticals. There are multitudes of side effects and interactions to consider when selecting a drug for treatment. Not all drugs work the same in every patient. It is a costly and lengthy process to develop and produce new drugs, especially for new diseases, and many candidate drugs will never be approved. These and other complexities associated with pharmaceuticals can lead to friction and misunderstanding among the public, pharmaceutical firms, and healthcare providers. Patients may wonder why the drug they are taking costs so much when it is so simple and small, or why their physician has prescribed a certain medication when their friend takes a different one for the same condition. Managing these types of questions often falls to healthcare providers and particularly to pharmacists.

As shown in the MPC example, pharmaceutical firms must consider many factors when making a decision about developing new drugs. Even if a new or better drug can be developed, the market may dictate that it is not the best strategy to pursue development of a new drug. Concerns about length of development, its cost, regulatory approval, changes in laws, patient acceptance, and insurance reimbursement all come into play.

This chapter will explore the nature of the pharmaceutical market. It will explain and answer the questions and tensions raised previously. Included in the discussion will be the relationship between consumers and drugs, the relationship between healthcare providers and drugs, how a drug goes from an idea to a package on pharmacy shelves, the role of pharmacists in the pharmaceutical market, and how the pharmaceutical market is being changed by current trends and legislation.

DRUGS AS REMEDIES, POISONS, OR MAGICAL CHARMS

Substances that produce a change in cellular or physiologic functioning of humans are called drugs, but there is more to these chemicals than their pharmacologic activity (Montagne, 1996). Social values also affect the perception and use of drugs. Some drugs are illegal, some are highly restricted in their use, and some are readily available. The social values in the United States, for example, drive the difference in legal status of marijuana, pseudoephedrine, and naproxen sodium.

Pharmakon is the Greek term for *drug*. This term has three meanings, including remedy, poison, and magical charm. Drugs are often thought of as remedies when they alleviate symptoms or eliminate disease in patients. Drugs can be poisons at the same time. Drugs can cause unpleasant side effects while delivering therapeutic effects or cause death in an overdose. Sometimes drugs' therapeutic effects are achieved by poisoning cells in a patient, such as with chemotherapy. The fact that many patients do not know or understand how a drug works lends a sense of magic to the drug.

The term *magic bullet* is sometimes used to describe drugs and was coined by Paul Ehrlich as he searched for a treatment for syphilis that would destroy the syphilis bacterium without harming the tissue of the patient (Strebhardt & Ullrich, 2008).

Manufacturers focus on a drug's therapeutic effects. They are primarily concerned with optimizing the biochemical activity, increasing the specificity, and limiting the adverse events associated with a drug. Health professionals are similarly concerned with a drug's therapeutic effects. They want to treat their patients as quickly and efficiently as possible. They will choose drugs that maximize the treatment effects and minimize the side effects for each patient. Interestingly, in some cases, the side effects of a drug can lead to alternative therapeutic indications. For example, minoxidil was developed to treat high blood pressure, but was found to grow hair as a side effect. Now minoxidil is commonly used to promote hair growth. There are a number of attributes of a drug upon which patients and consumers focus. These can include the treatment effect, adverse events, and cost. Sometimes patients may request a particular drug from their prescriber because they believe it has a desired therapeutic effect. Unwanted side effects or high costs, however, may deter patients from taking medications as prescribed by their physicians.

As science and medicine have progressed, medical and social problems have increasingly come to be defined primarily by the biologic processes that drive them. Medicalization is the idea of defining or describing problems in medical terms or treatment through medical interventions (Davis, 2006). Medicalization has led to a reduction in the social stigma surrounding many conditions such as depression, eating disorders, anxiety disorders, and attention-deficit/hyperactivity disorder. These complex conditions include social, mental, and emotional components, however, and often require treatment with nonpharmacologic therapy as well, such as counseling, dietary changes, and environmental changes. Medicalization can sometimes minimize the importance of nonpharmacologic treatments and prevent the use of them by patients.

The difference in beliefs and values about drugs can create tension between healthcare providers and patients. The social aspects of drugs are many times of greater importance to patients than to healthcare providers and can be the main driver of the use of a drug. Healthcare providers' understanding of these differences in beliefs can improve both the treatment and satisfaction of patients.

CONSUMER PERSPECTIVE ON DRUG USE

The end use for drugs is consumption by patients. Ambulatory consumers make the final decision about whether or not they will use a drug. Consumers have a wide range of options when it comes to deciding what drug to use to treat their particular disease or symptom. For a consumer to ultimately select a drug to use, he or she must be reasonably confident that taking the drug will produce the desired treatment effect with minimal side effects. If a drug does not work in the desired way, or if adverse events are greater than expected, a consumer may lose faith in the drug or lose trust in the individual who recommended the drug. The latter can create tension between patients and healthcare providers and be problematic because future recommendations may not be trusted.

Consumer Choices in Drug Use

When faced with a non–life-threatening health problem, an individual has a number of different options from which to choose. The simplest response to the health problem is to ignore it or do nothing at all. This response occurs about one third of the time. Two-thirds of the time a consumer will choose to take an action to resolve the health issue that he or she is facing (Heller, 1992; Montagne & Basara, 1996).

When taking action, consumers most commonly choose to treat themselves, rather than see a healthcare provider. When choosing to treat themselves with a nonprescription drug or herbal remedy, consumers are influenced by a number of factors. These include personal experience, advice of friends, web-based advice, direct-to-consumer advertising, and restrictions by law. The market for nonprescription drugs is significant. U.S. consumers spent $56.9 billion in 2014 on nondurable medical products (Centers for Medicare and Medicaid Services, 2015a). Nondurable medical products are defined by the Centers for Medicare and Medicaid Services as nonprescription drugs and medical sundries (Centers for Medicare and Medicaid Services, 2015b). Complementary and alternative medicine (CAM), which are treatments that are not considered to be a part of conventional medicine, are also important options for consumers not choosing to use typical Western medicine. Consumers spent $33.9 billion on CAMs in 2007 (Nahin, Barnes, Stussman, & Bloom, 2009).

Consumers will use the medical system one-fourth of the time when they decide to take action. When they visit a doctor, two-thirds of consumers will leave with a prescription (National Association of Chain Drug Stores [NACDS], 2005). The market for prescription drugs is much larger than that for nonprescription drugs. In 2014, U.S. consumers spent $297.7 billion on prescription drugs, which accounted for 9.92% of health spending. The annual rate of expenditure increase on prescription drugs rose from 2.4% in 2013 to 12.2% in 2014. The 2014 annual rate of expenditure increase on prescription drugs was faster than that for overall health costs. Reasons for this acceleration include new medications, reduction in the impact of patent expirations, and price increases for brand-name drugs (Centers for Medicare and Medicaid Services, 2015a).

Consumer Purchases of Drugs

Where a consumer purchases a drug will depend on a number of factors. Virtually all prescriptions are filled and purchased at or through a pharmacy. Many nonprescription drug purchases also occur at pharmacies, but these purchases account for less than half of all purchases. In 2008, 35% of nonprescription drug purchases were made in pharmacies, 29% at mass merchandisers, and 21% in food stores. Online retailers, dollar stores, warehouse clubs, and other outlets accounted for 15% (Kline & Company, 2009). Convenience and price are the main factors affecting the choice of where to purchase nonprescription drugs. Pharmacies have been losing share in recent years as consumers have sought and found lower prices.

Cost is frequently an overriding factor when a consumer is choosing to purchase a drug, whether it is prescription or nonprescription. When a prescription is written, the prescription typically is covered by a patient's insurance, which usually requires a copayment (a one-time flat payment) or coinsurance (a percentage of the price) for the patient. If an individual does not have health insurance, he or she may choose not to fill a prescription due to the high cost of the drug. The market for generic drugs is driven primarily by the fact that they are cheaper than brand-name drugs. Consumers who have insurance may be required to use generics or face higher copayments when filling a prescription. Some drugs, including many new biologic drugs, are very expensive and come with coinsurance levels that make them too costly for many patients. The issue of out-of-pocket cost is a very important component of the decision of which drug to purchase. Healthcare providers may recommend a course of treatment, but if it is too costly for the patient, other treatments may need to be considered or it may result in the patient going untreated. If a patient is unable to afford a treatment, some manufacturers offer programs, commonly referred to as patient assistance programs to eliminate or reduce the cost for qualifying patients.

In the example at the beginning of the chapter, MPC weighed the purchasing and reimbursement of drugs heavily in making its decision to pursue a copy of an existing drug rather than develop a new drug. MPC decided that offering a low-cost alternative was the best strategy to pursue in the EPO market due, in part, to the belief that consumers would readily purchase a lower priced version of EPO.

HEALTH PROFESSIONALS' ROLE IN DRUG USE

Health professionals serve a guiding role for patients in treating health problems. When a person goes to a health professional, he or she expects a recommendation for a course of action to solve his or her health problem. There are many recommendations a health professional may give to an individual, including lifestyle changes, physical therapy, and surgery. One of the most common, and expected, recommendations in the United States is a prescription for drug therapy.

Prescribers

Taking a drug to remedy a health problem can be simple and satisfying for both the patient and physician. Sometimes just the act of a physician prescribing a drug can satisfy a patient. Patients will sometimes demand antibiotics for viral infections and be happy only when the prescription is written, even though the drugs will do nothing for the infection. Other times, the placebo effect is all that is needed for the patient to feel better. Most of the time, though, a physician will prescribe a drug the patient needs, and the drug will aid the patient's healing. In many of these cases, the act of prescribing a drug satisfies a patient and usually requires little follow-up by the physician.

Notable factors that affect how physicians prescribe drugs are:

- Education, especially additional training in pharmacotherapeutics and preceptors' prescribing behavior
- Promotional campaigns, such as drug advertising
- Colleagues or those health professionals who are part of the prescriber's social network
- Control and regulatory mechanisms (e.g., drug laws, formularies, triplicate prescriptions)
- Demands from patients and society (Raisch, 1990a, 1990b; Soumerai, McLaughlin, & Avorn, 1989)

Dispensers

The most common image that consumers have of pharmacists is that of the community pharmacist responsible for filling their prescriptions. In 2014, there were about 4 billion retail prescriptions filled in the United States, which is approximately a 11% increase over the 3.6 billion filled in 2009 (NACDS, 2010; Kaiser Family Foundation, 2015). While both chain and independent pharmacies earn the majority of their sales through filling prescriptions, independent pharmacies rely much more heavily on these sales than do chain pharmacies (National Community Pharmacists Association [NCPA], 2009).

As technology has developed, the need for retail pharmacists to spend their time filling prescriptions has been substantially reduced and become much more automated. This trend is also due to the rise of Internet sales and mail-order delivery of prescriptions. While the time spent physically filling prescriptions has gone down, pharmacists now must spend a greater amount of time checking and verifying more prescriptions filled by technicians and robots.

Partly in response to this dissatisfaction, the dispensing element of pharmacy practice is currently undergoing rapid change, particularly through the increase in technologies that allow pharmacists to be less involved in the manual process of counting and labeling medications. While an increase in the use and certification of pharmacy technicians has helped to remove the pharmacist from many of these technical functions, the complete drug-handling capabilities of robotics and counting equipment are also working to make pharmacies more efficient and patient centered. Similarly, while prescription writing, patient management, and billing systems were once pen and paper based, computer systems have all but replaced the paper profiles and accounting required to operate a pharmacy, and e-prescribing is commonplace. Computer and online systems also perform sophisticated screening of potential drug-related problems, adherence monitoring, and adjudication of claims during the filling process. Medication therapy management is also something pharmacists have pursued to a greater degree as they have become eligible for reimbursement for clinical activities.

Hospitals and other institutional pharmacies seeking to better manage personnel costs while maintaining quality and improving patient safety are also paying close attention to dispensing productivity. Robotics and increased technician responsibilities for filling and preparing medication orders in the central pharmacy, as well as sophisticated dispensing technologies (such as Pyxis medication-dispensing machines) on patient care units, allow pharmacists to spend more time on reviewing, recommending, and monitoring patient therapies.

PATH OF A PHARMACEUTICAL FROM IDEA TO PRESCRIPTION

When a new drug is available for consumers to purchase (sometimes only after receiving a prescription), it has undergone many years of experimentation, testing, and regulatory approval. Each new pharmaceutical approved for sale requires a large investment of resources, and developing new drugs is quite risky for pharmaceutical companies. As a result, new drugs are typically quite expensive. Given the significant value, lifesaving potential, and potential safety issues surrounding new drugs, there is a complex regulatory, development, and distribution system for them in the United States.

Regulation of Pharmaceuticals

In the United States there are two primary systems regulating the use of drugs. One of these systems is the various state laws and agencies that control the practice of pharmacy and professionals. The other is the regulation of the safety and effectiveness of the drugs, which is done by the FDA. The FDA determines which drugs are allowed to be sold and prescribed in the United States and which drugs are categorized as prescription and nonprescription drugs.

There are two main acts under which the FDA controls pharmaceuticals. The first of these is the Food, Drug and Cosmetic Act, which was first passed in 1938. For the most part, the Food, Drug, and Cosmetic Act directs the FDA in how it regulates traditional small-molecule drugs and hormones. This includes drugs such as acetaminophen, simvastatin, and insulin. The other act under which the FDA regulates drugs is the Public Health Service Act of 1944. It is under the Public Health Service Act that the FDA regulates drugs such as biologics that are made up of much larger molecules and are more complex than small-molecule drugs. Biologics include drugs such as bevacizumab, trastuzumab, and erythropoietin. The fact that small-molecule drugs and biologics are regulated by different acts has important consequences on the regulation of intellectual property rights for these two different types of drugs.

Once the FDA has determined a drug is safe and effective enough to be sold in the United States, it has little direct control over how the drug is actually used or prescribed, such as for non -FDA-approved (off-label) indications. A drug cannot, however, be sold or marketed in the United States until the FDA has approved it. To ensure the safety and effectiveness of pharmaceuticals and biological products, the FDA performs the following seven basic functions:

1. Approval of drugs on the basis of purity, safety, and effectiveness
2. Regulation of all labeling for prescription and nonprescription drugs

3. Regulation of advertising for prescription drugs (the Federal Trade Commission regulates nonprescription advertising)
4. Regulation of manufacturing processes of drugs and institution of recalls
5. Regulation of bioequivalence for generics and biosimilars
6. Monitoring of drugs postapproval to detect any problems with the use of drugs, such as unanticipated adverse reactions (e.g., postmarketing surveillance)
7. Monitoring of the safety of the nation's blood supply (U.S. FDA [n.d. e])

The FDA can only make decisions based on the information it is given. The studies used to determine the safety of a drug are generally not large enough to detect all possible adverse events. This is one of the reasons the FDA monitors drugs after they have been approved. Sometimes companies are not wholly forthright with the information they have on their candidate drugs. One recent example of this is GlaxoSmithKline's withholding and downplaying heart attack risks of Avandia (rosiglitazone). This is not common, however, and there are laws to try to prevent this from happening. Even the information the FDA has is not without uncertainty. There are times when the FDA has to develop its own interpretations of manufacturers' data. While the public would like the FDA to never make a mistake or miss a potential side effect of a drug, it is not always possible for the FDA to be completely sure about the benefit–risk balance of a new drug when it is released onto the market. The FDA acts in what it views as good faith for the public and strives to ensure drugs on the market are safe for consumers.

Development and Approval of a New Drug

The development of a new drug is a long and expensive process. The expected capitalized cost of a new drug is $2.59 billion (DiMasi, Grabowski & Hansen, 2014). Clinical testing alone can be expected to take between 6 and 7 years. The development of a drug can be broken into four main stages. The first of these is the discovery of new compounds or proteins. The second is the preclinical testing stage. The third is the clinical testing stage. The final stage is approval and postclinical testing. Very few products make it through all of these stages to become a drug that is prescribed and taken by a consumer.

The first stage of discovery is carried out primarily by scientists who identify compounds and proteins that have potential to be a viable drug. For every 250 candidates that go to preclinical testing, between 5,000 and 10,000 compounds are evaluated (Pharmaceutical Research and Manufacturers of America [PhRMA], 2010b). This corresponds to a rate of only 2.5% to 5.0% candidates moving on to preclinical testing. In preclinical testing, a company conducts tests to determine whether or not a drug is safe to test in humans. These tests are carried out through animal testing and other tests in a laboratory. Approximately 2.5% of the candidates in this stage make it through preclinical testing (PhRMA, 2010b). This results in less than 0.1% of potential drugs making it from discovery to entry into clinical testing (**Table 5-1**).

When a firm would like to start clinical testing of a product, it must first submit an Investigational New Drug (IND) application to the FDA's Center for Drug Evaluation and Research (small-molecule drugs) or the FDA's Center for Biologics Evaluation and Research (biologics). The firm must then wait 30 days before beginning any clinical testing to give the Center for Drug Evaluation and Research or the Center for Biologics Evaluation and Research time to review the application. There are four phases of clinical testing, three of which occur prior to product approval (U.S. FDA [n.d. b; n.d. c]).

The first phase of clinical testing is conducted through Phase I clinical trials. The goal of Phase I trials is to learn about how the drug works in humans. These trials determine the dosing range

Table 5-1 Drug Development to Get One Approved Drug

Stage	Length	Patients	Number in stage
Potential candidates	Varies	NA	10,000
Preclinical testing	Varies	Animals	250
Phase I clinical trial	1 year	100 healthy volunteers	10
Phase II clinical trial	2 years	300 with target disease	6
Phase III clinical trial	3–4 years	2,000–3,000 in clinical setting	2–3
FDA approval	1 year	NA	1–2
Approved drug (Some Phase IV studies)	10–14 years	Disease population	1

Data from: Pharmaceutical Research and Manufacturers of America. (PhRMA). (2010). Pharmaceutical Industry Profile 2010. Washington, DC: PhRMA.

and method, document the metabolism and excretion of the drug, and identify toxicities associated with the drug. These trials are relatively small with a group of less than 100 normal, healthy volunteers and are short term (less than 1 year). On average, 60% of drugs make it through Phase I trials to the next phase (Tufts Center for the Study of Drug Development [CSDD], 2010).

Phase II trials are the second phase of clinical testing. In this phase, the drug is studied in a few hundred patients diagnosed with the disease the drug is designed to treat. The goal is to study and determine the efficacy and safety of the drug in the actual patients who will be treated. These trials are longer than Phase I trials; they may take up to 2 years to complete. If the trial shows sufficient efficacy and safety, then the drug will proceed to Phase III trials. For drugs in Phase II testing, only 39% of drugs will be expected to move on to Phase III testing (Tufts CSDD, 2010).

The final preapproval step is completion of Phase III testing. Testing in this phase is much more extensive and is designed to provide strong evidence of safety and efficacy. Phase III trials typically involve a few thousand patients and can last up to few years. Subjects are randomized into control and experimental groups and treated with doses and in settings that are similar to what would be expected in the real world. Once Phase III testing has been completed, the firm can move on and submit their drug for approval to the FDA. The percentage of drugs coming out of Phase II trials that are submitted for approval after entering Phase III testing is 64% (Tufts CSDD, 2010).

Once clinical testing has been successfully completed, a firm will submit its drug to the FDA for approval. The firm does this by submitting a New Drug Application (NDA). The NDA specifies all of the relevant information about a drug, including how the drug is manufactured, how the drug acts in the body, how the drug will be marketed, labeling information, and toxicological information. The FDA then reviews the application and gives its decision on whether or not to approve the drug. When a new drug is submitted, 85% of the time it is approved (Tufts CSDD, 2010). When approval and all phases of preapproval clinical testing are combined, only 16% of drugs that begin the testing phase will be approved by the FDA (Tufts CSDD, 2010).

Once a drug is approved, it is often not the last time the FDA will examine the drug. Many times there are Phase IV trials that are conducted after the drug is already approved. Phase IV studies continue to evaluate the safety and effectiveness of drugs and look for any side effects that may have been missed in earlier trials. During these studies, large groups of patients are monitored over longer time periods than Phase I, II, or III trials. A firm may also want to get a drug approved as a nonprescription, or over-the-counter medication. A firm can do this through the NDA process or submit an application to switch to over-the-counter status after the drug is approved through the NDA process. If a firm would like to alter the drug's ingredients, dosage, manufacturing, or labeling, it submits a supplemental NDA to the FDA to get the changes approved. Makers of generics or biosimilars instead submit an abbreviated NDA to get their products approved with a lower clinical trial burden than the original product. The FDA will examine the bioequivalence, bioavailability, and pharmacokinetic/pharmacodynamic properties of a generic or biologic to ensure they are the same or similar to a reference product.

The high cost, long time frame, and high degree of uncertainty for drug development were all important factors in MPC deciding against developing a new version of EPO in our case scenario. The payoff in the end was simply not high enough for MPC to be willing to invest a substantial amount of time and resources into a new drug. Instead, MPC decided to go with the shorter time frame of developing a copy of an existing EPO drug.

Pricing

The pricing of drugs is not a simple process and can engender a substantial amount of ill will from patients. There are many factors that go into the pricing of a drug, including the costs of producing the drug, the drug development costs, negotiated reimbursements by a payer (e.g., a pharmacy benefit manager (PBM) agrees with a manufacturer on the price it will pay), margins for wholesalers, and margins for retailers. All of these factors combine to produce the price the consumer pays for the drug. It is important to recognize that the pricing of new, patented medicines is different from those that have gone off-patent and are therefore subject to generic entry and competition. To incentivize R&D for innovative medicines, patents provide intellectual property protection, which will be discussed in more detail later in this chapter. Sellers with patent protection are essentially empowered—during the limited patent life—to try to determine and charge what the market will bear. Their desired prices, which are typically far above short-run marginal costs, aim to recoup the costs of R&D for successful, as well as failed products. Once (small molecule) drugs go off-patent and generic competition is encouraged by regulations, then prices fall dramatically, approaching the short-run marginal cost of production and distribution. The United States has higher prices for patented medicines than other developed countries, but lower generic prices (Garrison, 2013).

In some countries with government-sponsored health systems, patients see no or very little direct, out-of-pocket cost when they are prescribed a drug. In the United States, it depends on the nature of the individual's health insurance policy. There can be substantial differences between plans. Some policies require the individual to pay a flat copayment for a prescription medication while other policies employ a percentage-based coinsurance for each prescription. If an individual has no insurance, he or she is usually responsible for the full cost of a prescription.

The largest component of the cost of drugs is the resources that were devoted to the research and development of an innovative drug. Once a drug is fully developed and tested, there is relatively little cost in actually producing and providing the drug: the short-run marginal cost of production and distribution is low. It is for this reason that many consumers and consumer advocates criticize the prices that drug companies charge for what can be lifesaving treatments. Without sufficient revenue from drug sales, however, many companies would cease to develop new drugs. There is always a trade-off between prices today and investment in new drugs. It is difficult for pharmacists to endure the ire of patients with regard to pricing, especially when they have little control over most of the costs. Educating patients about how drugs are priced can help to alleviate the tensions that may arise when patients are upset about the price of their prescriptions.

Pharmaceutical Marketing

Pharmaceutical firms use a variety of methods to market their products. One of the methods firms use is to meet with physicians and educate them on the merits of using their product. Another method is direct-to-consumer (DTC) advertising. There has been much debate over the benefits and pitfalls of allowing companies to market their products through advertising directly to patients. Those in favor of allowing DTC advertising note that pharmaceutical firms are selling a product and should be allowed to market in the same way that other products are marketed. Those against allowing DTC advertising often state that drugs are products with the potential for serious harm. The general public is generally ill equipped to evaluate the potential for serious harm and thus DTC advertising should be prohibited. This is not a settled question, but currently, firms are allowed to advertise their products to consumers in the United States as long as they meet the guidelines of the FDA.

In 1997, the Food and Drug Administration (FDA) offered new guidelines for direct-to-consumer (DTC) advertising in the form of broadcast television commercials for prescription drugs (Wilkes, Bell, & Kravitz, 2000). As a consequence of the FDA's decision, television advertisements for medications have proliferated. When watching television, a patient can learn of many different products available with or without a prescription. These commercials range from a description of a health problem/disease to an explanation of a particular brand-name product, such as Humira (adalimumab) or Lunesta (eszopiclone). In addition, print advertisements may be found in magazines and newspapers.

It appears that DTC advertising may be influencing consumer demand for a medication. Physicians are more likely to prescribe a specific drug product when patients ask (USA Today et al., 2008; Ventola, 2011; McKinlay et al., 2014). Drugs that are heavily advertised to patients are some of the best-selling medications (General Accounting Office, 2002). Many companies advertise their products in this way as part of their strategy for dealing with an increasingly competitive marketplace—that is, in an attempt to increase the demand/market share for their products (Wilkes et al., 2000). However, studies are mixed on the effect DTC advertising has on drug utilization and sales (Mukherjee & Limbu, 2013).

As with any controversial issue, both supporters and detractors of DTC advertising exist. Proponents suggest that such advertising enables consumers to become better informed by learning about new products and alternative treatment options (Kaiser Family Foundation, 2006; Ventola, 2011). Critics of DTC advertising claim that this practice promotes inappropriate prescribing, strains the patient–provider relationship, increases the costs of care, and distorts the physician's professional role (Ventola, 2011; Kaiser Family Foundation, 2006; Wilkes et al., 2000). Despite these concerns, it appears that DTC advertising will continue in the future and be a part of the healthcare dynamic.

Distribution

There are seven major players in the process of getting a medicine from the manufacturer to the patient/beneficiary. Their complex inter-relationships are shown in **Figure 5-1**.

Retail pharmacies obtain their medications from drug wholesalers or from drug manufacturers directly. They pay an amount based on wholesale acquisition cost or determined through a group purchasing organization (GPO). Drug wholesalers are firms that purchase drugs from

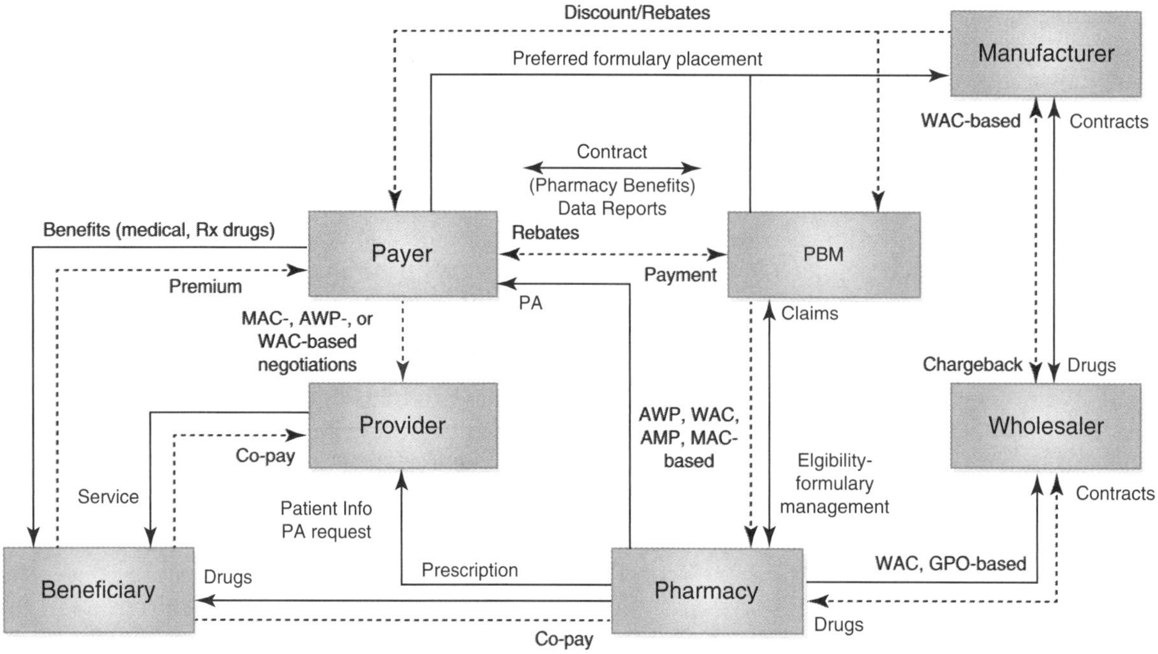

Figure 5-1 The Players in Managed Care Pharmacy.

Academy of Managed Care Pharmacy. Sept. 22, 2015 http://www.amcp.org/Newsletter.aspx?id=20076.

pharmaceutical manufacturers and then distribute them to retail pharmacies under a contractual arrangements. At one point, many large pharmacies were moving away from purchasing from wholesalers in favor of purchasing directly from manufacturers to avoid markups from wholesalers. This trend has been reversed recently as retailers have looked to avoid the cost of warehousing and maintaining inventory. The consumer/patient/beneficiary then purchases their drugs from a retailer often with a copayment that varies by "tier" based on the payer's perception of the need for cost sharing to limit spending. The retailer may be a local pharmacy, mail-order pharmacy, or Internet pharmacy.

Internet pharmacy is a growing industry though there are no reliable estimates of the volume of prescriptions obtained over the Internet (Orizio et al., 2011). However, the National Association of Boards of Pharmacy (NABP) monitors Internet pharmacies. The NABP also runs an accreditation program for Internet pharmacies, and has accredited 67 Internet pharmacy practice sites (NABP, 2016). As of December 31, 2015, 10,668 Internet drug outlets were cited for selling prescriptions that were not in compliance with state and federal laws and/or NABP patient safety and pharmacy practice standards (NABP, 2016). Internet prescribing and delivery is only one aspect of what is called "e-commerce," which more broadly involves buying and selling goods and services over the Internet. E-commerce falls into four main categories: business-to-business, business-to-customers, customer-to-business. and customer-to-customer. These business transactions among all of players in the pharmacy distribution channels are increasingly electronic.

PBMs, such as Medco Health Solutions and CVS Caremark, are companies that manage prescription drug programs for health insurers and companies that offer prescription drug coverage to their employees. As shown in Figure 5-1, PBMs interact with payers, manufacturers, and pharmacies. They design formularies and negotiate prices and rebates for the drugs dispensed to customers covered under their plan. Formularies are lists of medicines and how they will be reimbursed under a prescription drug benefit contract. For example, Medco may say that Lipitor (atorvastatin) requires a $30 copayment per prescription and may have negotiated to pay Pfizer $54 per prescription. PBMs are now responsible for the prescription drug programs of most U.S. consumers.

Global Aspects of Pharmaceuticals and Counterfeiting

As the world becomes more and more interconnected, global issues involving medication are becoming much more significant. There are many firms located outside the United States involved in the development, production, and testing of drugs. While there are many benefits to the increased globalization of the drug market, there are challenges and pitfalls difficult for regulatory agencies such as the FDA to guard against while preserving a robust international flow of drugs and ideas.

One important component of globalization for drugs is the production of drugs outside the United States. Drugs are allowed to be produced outside the United States and then sold as prescription medications in the United States. However, the FDA must approve the manufacturing process and plant where the drugs will be produced. Even as the FDA attempts to regulate and monitor the drugs in the United States, drugs that are not manufactured properly can still be a problem in the United States. The protection of patents is also a concern for U.S. companies. In many countries, enforcement of patents is not as strong as U.S. firms would like, and foreign companies sometimes copy and produce drugs in violation of patents. Developing countries must weigh the costs and benefits of recognizing international patents. The costs of recognizing the patents include raising the prices of drugs in the country. The benefits include adherence to international treaties and a more positive research environment for firms. This can help to preserve biodiversity and natural lands (Chang & Ross, 2009). Some firms have agreed to fund preservation projects in return for first access to new discoveries in these areas. In order to fully ensure patent enforcement, the U.S. government must also work with local governments to see that patents are enforced.

It is currently against the law to purchase prescription drugs in another country for use in the United States. There is an allowable exception:

> when 1) the intended use [of the drug] is unapproved and for a serious condition for which effective treatment may not be available domestically either through commercial or clinical means; 2) there is no known commercialization or promotion to persons residing in the U.S. by those involved in the distribution of the product at issue; 3) the product is considered not to represent an unreasonable risk; and 4) the individual seeking to import the product affirms in writing that it is for the patient's own use (generally not more than 3 month supply) and provides the name and address of the doctor licensed in the U.S. responsible for his or her treatment with the product or provides evidence that the product is for the continuation of a treatment begun in a foreign country/area. (U.S. FDA, 2010, Section 9–2)

Counterfeit drugs are clearly a problem in the developing world. The World Health Organization (WHO) has estimated over 30% of drugs sold in much of the developing world are counterfeit

(WHO, 2008). WHO has been directed to undertake a new study of what are called substandard/spurious/falsely-labeled/falsified/counterfeit (SSFFC) medical products (WHO, 2015). One systematic review of 44 studies found that the median prevalence of failing quality tests was 28.5%, and rates were higher in middle-income countries (Almuzaini et al., 2013). Evidence is lacking, however, on the health and economic impacts of these quality problems. Investigating these issues are the aims of the WHO study.

The problem is also large in magnitude in the United States. It is difficult to know the extent of the problem, but the Center for Medicine in the Public Interest estimated that there would be $75 billion of counterfeit drugs sales in the United States in 2010 (CMPI, 2005). The FDA is charged with stopping the sale of counterfeit drugs but has a limited budget to do so. As long as production of drugs continues outside of the United States and Internet pharmacies continue to grow, it will be difficult for the FDA to effectively halt the sale of counterfeit drugs in the United States. One example of counterfeit drugs is the sale through an Internet pharmacy of oseltamivir in the United States. The FDA warned about oseltamivir in June of 2010, and there is no approved generic version of oseltamivir, although the brand-name version, Tamiflu, has been approved.

Counterfeit drugs pose a substantial threat to consumers. At a minimum, consumers risk receiving no benefit from treatment when consuming drugs with no active ingredients. At worst, consumers stand to suffer adverse effects or even death from drugs with harmful and toxic chemicals in them. The use of counterfeit drugs can also be detrimental to patients' health if it delays their access to effective treatments. To help protect patients, pharmacists should know which drugs are most commonly counterfeited and be familiar with their colors, shapes, and symbols. Wholesalers may unintentionally distribute counterfeit drugs, so pharmacists stand as the final guard for patients. Pharmacists should also counsel patients to only buy from reputable pharmacies to minimize the risk of using counterfeit drugs. It will be difficult, if not impossible, to eliminate counterfeit drugs, but pharmacists can work to help their patients from falling victim.

An emerging trend in the globalization of drugs is conducting clinical trials in locations outside the United States. It is estimated that between 40% and 65% of clinical trials take place at sites outside the United States (Anand, Wang, & Whalen, 2008; Tufts CSDD, 2009). Additionally, the 20 largest pharmaceutical companies are conducting one third of clinical trials exclusively outside the United States (Cairns et al., 2009). In these cases, there would be no U.S. patients for trials of drugs that will be approved for use in the United States. Many foreign trials are conducted in western Europe, but a rapidly growing number of these trials are conducted in areas chosen for their low costs, such as Asia and South America.

There are a number of concerns with the growth of foreign trials. One is that the FDA is not equipped to inspect many foreign clinical trial sites. A Department of Health and Human Services Inspector General's report found that in 2008 the FDA inspected 1.9% of domestic clinical trial sites, but only 0.7% of foreign clinical trial sites. It also found that some early stage clinical trials are being conducted without IND application approval (Department of Health and Human Services, 2010). Another concern about the use of foreign clinical trials is that it is sometimes difficult to know how to attribute differences in patient outcomes from the various sites. The sites do not always follow the same standards, especially those located in emerging market countries. As a result, it can be difficult for the FDA to know whether a difference in the data is a result of chance, patient selection, ethnic differences, unblinding, method of observation, or treatment practices (Temple, 2009). There are certainly benefits to the increasing use of foreign clinical trial sites. One primary benefit is the inclusion of a wider number of populations than may be used in a U.S.-exclusive clinical trial. This can yield important results for different ethnic groups in the United States that are not usually included in U.S. clinical trials. As the use of foreign clinical trials continues to increase, the FDA works toward better oversight and inspection of these sites in the future INDs, and exploring new and innovative ways to oversee foreign clinical trials.

Intellectual Property Rights

Intellectual property rights (IPRs) are one of the most important components of the U.S. pharmaceutical system. IPRs are laws and regulations put into place to protect the ideas and products of innovators. Examples outside of drug development include copyrights on music and patents on inventions. IPRs have two main effects on the drug market. One is that they provide incentives for firms to innovate and develop new drugs that fight diseases. The other is that they provide power to firms to control the market for a drug and charge a higher price than firms would be able to without intellectual property protections. The United States has developed intellectual property regulations that attempt to balance these two effects by giving protections to innovators for a limited amount of time.

Innovations in pharmaceuticals need IPRs because innovations are a public good. A public good is considered such when it is used by a consumer, it is not used up, and it is available for others to use. It is different from a private good, such as a hamburger, that is used up once it is consumed. Knowledge is almost always considered a public good. When one gains knowledge, that knowledge is still available for others to gain and share. It takes a large amount of upfront investment to develop the knowledge of an innovative drug. If these innovations were not given intellectual property protections, others could take the knowledge and produce drugs without having to put up any kind of investment. The price for this new drug would be quite low and it would be very difficult for the innovating firm to make back their investment. Under these circumstances, few firms, if any, would be willing to develop new drugs. Having no new drugs would be an undesirable outcome from society's point of view.

To preserve incentives to innovate, IPR protection should last at least as long, on average, as it takes for a company to recoup its capitalized investment (Grabowski, 2008). However, if firms are given indefinite intellectual property protection, prices for drugs would likely remain very high. This scenario would result in fewer patients receiving drugs. This, too, is not a desirable outcome from society's point of view. Because of this, after a specified time period, other firms are allowed to copy and sell generic (or biosimilar) versions of the innovator's drug. The costs of producing the copies of the innovation are lower than developing the new drug, so prices are lower for the generic versions of the drug. This allows for lower costs of treatment and more patients being treated. The goal of IPRs is to preserve the incentive to innovate for firms, but not to subject consumers to high prices for too long.

In practice, the mechanisms for protecting IPRs are different for small-molecule drugs than for biologic drugs. This is due to differences in the complexity and nature of development of the two types of drugs. The primary driver of IPRs for small-molecule drugs is patent protection. Patents prevent other firms from copying an innovator's product while the patent is in force. The mechanism of IPR protection for biologic drugs is data exclusivity. Data exclusivity means that a firm can rely on the innovating firm's original clinical trial data to demonstrate the safety and effectiveness of its biosimilar (or generic) drug. The generic or biosimilar firm can then avoid having to conduct its own clinical trials (or at least it can conduct much smaller and less extensive trials). Using an innovator's clinical trial data allows for firms that are copying the innovator to save a substantial amount on developing their versions of biologic drugs by being able to avoid conducting clinical trials themselves.

It is important to note here that there is a substantial difference in copies of small-molecule drugs and biologic drugs; copies of small-molecule drugs are termed *generics*; copies of biologics are termed *biosimilars*. As mentioned earlier, small-molecule drugs are much less complex and are made up of smaller molecules than biologic drugs. They are also chemically synthesized rather than being produced by living cell lines. For example, atorvastatin (Lipitor), a small-molecule drug, has a molecular weight of 1209 daltons, while bevacizumab (Avastin), a biologic, has a molecular weight of 149,000 daltons. It is therefore realistic and possible to make identical copies of small-molecule drugs. It is nearly impossible to identically replicate a biologic drug. There will always be small differences in the copied drug and the original biologic. For these reasons, small-molecule drugs and biologics are not treated the same when it comes to regulating entry of copies of a drug.

IPRs for small-molecule drugs are regulated under the Drug Price Competition and Patent Term Restoration Act (commonly called the Hatch-Waxman Act) of 1984 (U.S. FDA [n.d. a]). The main provisions of the act are to give data exclusivity periods to innovators for 5 years after initial approval of the drug. They can also get additional 3-year period of data exclusivity for new indications and additional 6-month period for pediatric applications. These data exclusivity periods run concurrently with patent protection. Patents are granted for a period of 20 years and are granted at any time during a drug's development. Typically, the patent is granted many years prior to the drug being approved and launched into the market. A firm may apply to get an extension if the testing and approval process takes a long time. The patent can be extended for up to 5 years. The patent may not be in force, though, for more than 14 years after a drug is first approved. Patents are the most important form of IPR protection for small-molecule drugs, because generics are exact copies of the innovative drug and the data exclusivity period is relatively short (**Table 5-2**).

IPRs for biologic drugs are primarily regulated under the Patient Protection and Affordable Care Act of 2010. The specific provision on biologic IPRs is the Biologics Price Competition and Innovation Act of 2009 (U.S. FDA [n.d. d]). Patent regulation of biologics is almost the same as that for small-molecule drugs; patent length is 20 years with an available 5-year extension. But patents are not as important for biologics' IPRs. This is because it is easier to work around patents given the complexity of biologics and the fact that it takes longer for biologics to be developed. The most

Table 5-2 IPR Protection for Small-Molecule and Biologic Drugs

	Small-molecule drugs	Biologic drugs
Governing act	Hatch-Waxman	PPACA
Year enacted	1984	2010
Patent length	20 years from patent application with U.S. PTO	20 years from patent application with U.S. PTO
Data-exclusivity period	5 years from FDA approval	12 years from FDA approval
New clinical trials required for generics/biosimilars?	No	Yes, but limited
Interchangeability with reference drug	Yes	Yes

PPACA = Patient Protection and Affordable Care Act; U.S. PTO = United States Patent and Trademark Office.

Data from Patient Protection and Affordable Care Act; United States Patent and Trademark Office.

important form of IPRs for biologics is the data exclusivity period. The data exclusivity period is 12 years in length with little opportunity for extensions. Prior to the passage of the Patient Protection and Affordable Care Act, there was no pathway for manufacturers of biosimilars to rely on the clinical trial data of the innovators. While makers of biosimilars will still have to conduct more extensive clinical trials than those of small-molecule generics, the clinical trial burden is now much lower after enactment of the Patient Protection and Affordable Care Act.

The implementation of a limited data exclusivity period for biologic drugs was perhaps the most important factor for MPC in deciding to pursue development of a copy of Erystim. If MPC was not able to rely on the clinical trial data of Hemocyte, it would have likely decided against developing its own copy of Erystim and against purchasing EGlobin. Relying on Hemocyte's clinical trial data was a necessity for MPC to decide to pursue a biosimilar.

FUTURE TRENDS IN THE PHARMACEUTICAL SECTOR

Advances in medicine, biology, and policy reforms, along with changing demographics will influence the pharmaceutical sector over the course of the next decade. An ever-increasing understanding of the human genome will drive both the development and selection of drugs for treatment of diseases. As the U.S. population becomes older and more obese, treating diseases such as diabetes will become more and more important. The implementation of health reform, which will increase both insurance coverage and the government's role in patient care, will force a hard look at restraining spending. All of these factors will affect the drugs that patients receive to treat disease.

Personalized medicine is one of the most quickly developing areas in drug treatment. The hope of personalized medicine is that treatment selections will be optimized for each patient given his or her specific individual characteristics. This will be accomplished by testing patients for factors such as genetic markers that indicate one course of treatment over another. In its fullest realization, personalized medicine will avoid unnecessary treatments and, by extension, the costs and adverse events that go along with them. There are still a number of hurdles for personalized medicine to overcome such as the limited predictive power of genomic information, and the difficulty and costs of developing highly predictive genetic tests, as well as economic barriers, including our cost-based diagnostic test reimbursement system, among others (Garrison & Austin, 2006). Currently, there are a substantial amount of research and resources devoted to realizing the promise of personalized medicine, and that should continue in the coming years. Some areas where personalized medicine has begun to be implemented are in breast cancer treatment with trastuzumab and blood clotting with warfarin. As testing is improved and costs brought down, personalized medicine will become a larger part of the treatment of many diseases, especially in oncology, in the coming decades.

Biologic drugs are also expected to become a larger portion of new pharmaceuticals in the next few decades. As much as 71% of all new drug approvals could be biologic in nature by 2025 (BioWorld, 2009). Biologics, such as monoclonal antibodies, are a large part of new cancer treatments, and it is likely that any vaccine developed for HIV/AIDS will be a biologic. As the role of biologics increases, the number of treatments for orphan diseases is likely to increase as well. Orphan diseases are diseases that affect a very small population. In the United States, they typically affect fewer than 200,000 people. Treatments for orphan diseases are twice as likely to be classified as biologics than small-molecule drugs (Trusheim, Aitken, & Berndt, 2010). Biologics hold the promise to treat diseases that are currently untreatable and improve outcomes in those that currently are treatable. The tradeoff is that biologics often carry a high cost. As biologics assume a larger role in treatments, there will be discussion of the benefits versus the costs of using them.

Population demographics and recent government action are two other influences on the pharmaceutical sector. The U.S. population as a whole continues to become more obese and is increasingly affected by chronic diseases such as diabetes. This will make controlling these chronic diseases a high priority for physicians. As such, development of drugs to treat chronic diseases will become more important. Diabetes, for example, has 235 new medicines in development in the pharmaceutical and biotechnology sectors in the United States (PhRMA, 2010a). As for the government's role, the recently passed health reform act will lead to greater health insurance coverage across the United States. As part of this increase in coverage, there will be a greater number of individuals who are covered under government programs, such as Medicaid. For the pharmaceutical industry, this will mean that a larger number of patients may receive their drugs, but at a reduced cost.

CONCLUSION

Drugs play a large role in the delivery of health care in the United States. It is a complex and evolving role shaped by consumers, pharmaceutical firms, and healthcare providers. Pharmacists play a vital role in linking consumers to physicians and pharmaceutical firms. Understanding this role and adjusting to changes are important tasks for pharmacists as they interact with patients. Helping patients and others understand how the pharmaceutical sector works can lead to improved patient satisfaction and outcomes. Even as the role of pharmacists evolves, patients will continue to value and seek input from pharmacists.

QUESTIONS FOR FURTHER DISCUSSION

1. Which course of action would you have recommended that MPC Pharmaceuticals take? Why?
2. Do you think the way in which drugs are developed and approved in the United States should be changed? What would you suggest to improve the process?
3. How do you think intellectual property rights should be protected for innovative drug manufacturers?
4. Do you think the FDA is able to adequately oversee foreign production of drugs and foreign clinical trials? Why or why not?
5. What do you feel the role of a pharmacist should be? Do you see the changes for the role of a pharmacist outlined in this chapter as desirable?

KEY TOPICS AND TERMS

Biologics
Biosimilar
Chain pharmacy
Clinical trial
Consumer drug use
Counterfeit drugs
Data exclusivity period
Dispenser
Drug wholesaler
Generic drug
Independent pharmacy
Intellectual property rights (IPRs)
Internet pharmacy
Investigational new drug
Mail-order pharmacy
Medicalization
New drug application (NDA)
Nonprescription (over the counter)
Off-label drug use
Orphan diseases
Patent
Personalized medicine

Pharmaceutical manufacturer
Pharmaceutical marketing
Pharmaceutical research and development
Pharmakon
Postmarketing surveillance
Prescriber
Prescription
U.S. drug approval process
U.S. drug development process

REFERENCES

Almuzaini T., Choonara I., Sammons H. (2013). Substandard and counterfeit medicines: A systematic review of the literature. *BMJ Open, 3*, e002923.

Anand, G., Wang, S., & Whalen, J. (2008, December 1). Scrutiny grows for drug trials abroad. *The Wall Street Journal*. Retrieved from http://online.wsj.com/article/SB122809561842168089.html

Anon. (2014, December 14). E-commerce in pharmaceutical business: An overview. Pharmnews. Retrieved from http://www.pharmanewsonline.com/e-commerce-in-pharmaceutical-business-an-overview /BioWorld. (2009, August). *Market-leading biotechnology drugs: Blockbuster dynamics in an ailing economy.* Atlanta, GA: AHC Media, LLC.

Cairns, C., Califf, R., Glickman, S., Harrington, R., McHutchison, J., & Peterson, E. (2009). Ethical and scientific implications of the globalization of clinical research. *New England Journal of Medicine, 360*(8), 816–823.

Center for Medicine in the Public Interest (CMPI). (2005). *21st century health care terrorism: The perils of international drug counterfeiting.* Retrieved from https://www.pacificresearch.org/fileadmin /news_import/20070202_2005_Drugs_Counterfeiting_01.pdf

Centers for Medicare and Medicaid Services. (2015a). *National Health Expenditures 2014 Highlights.* Retrieved from https://www.cms.gov/Research-Statistics-Data-and-Systems/Statistics-Trends-and-Reports /NationalHealthExpendData/Downloads/highlights.pdf

Centers for Medicare and Medicaid Services. (2015b). *Quick Definitions for National Health Expenditure Accounts (NHEA) Categories.* Retrieved from https://www.cms.gov/Research-Statistics-Data-and-Systems /Statistics-Trends-and-Reports/NationalHealthExpendData/Downloads/quickref.pdf

Chang, Y. M., & Ross, K. D. (2009). Biodiversity, intellectual property rights and North-South trade. *Economics Bulletin, 29*(2), 992–1002.

Davis, J. E. (2006). How medicalization lost its way. *Society, 43*(6), 51–56.

Department of Health and Human Services, Office of Inspector General. (2010). *Challenges to FDA's ability to monitor and inspect foreign clinical trials.* Retrieved from http://oig.hhs.gov/oei/reports/oei-01-08-00510 .pdf

Dave, D., & Saffer, H. (2010). *The impact of direct-to-consumer advertising on pharmaceutical prices and demand.* Cambridge, MA: National Bureau of Economic Research.

DiMasi, J. A., Grabowski, H. G., & Hansen R. W. (2014). Cost of developing a new drug. Briefing from Tufts Center for the Study of Drug Development.

Garrison, L. P. (2013). Pharmacoeconomics and Drug Pricing. Chapter 8. In Rodney J. Y. Ho & Milo Gibaldi, *Ho and Gibaldi's Biotechnology and Biopharmaceuticals: Transforming Proteins and Genes into Drugs*, 2nd ed. New Jersy: John Wiley and Sons.

Garrison, L. P., & Austin, M. J. F. (2006). Linking pharmacogenetics-based diagnostics and pharmaceuticals for personalized medicine: Scientific and economic challenges. *Health Affairs, 25*(5), 1281–1290.

General Accounting Office. (2002, October). *FDA oversight of direct-to-consumer advertising has limitations.* Retrieved from http://www.gao.gov/new.items/d03177.pdf

Grabowski, H.G. (2008). Follow-on biologics: Data exclusivity and the balance between innovation and competition. *Nature Reviews Drug Discovery, 7*, 479–488.

Heller, H. (1992). *Health care practices and perceptions: A consumer survey of self-medication.* Washington, DC: The Proprietary Association.

Kaiser Family Foundation. (2003, June). *Impact of direct-to-consumer advertising on prescription drug spending.* Washington, DC: Kaiser Family Foundation.

Kaiser Family Foundation. (2006, November). *Prescription drugs: Advertising, out-of-pocket costs, and patient safety from the perspective of doctors and pharmacists.* Washington, DC: Kaiser Family Foundation.

Kaiser Family Foundation. (2015). *Total number of retail prescription drugs filled at pharmacies.* Retrieved from http://kff.org/other/state-indicator/total-retail-rx-drugs/

Kline & Company, Inc. (2009). *Nonprescription drugs USA 2008.* Retrieved from http://www.klinegroup.com/reports/brochures/cia6g/factsheet.pdf

McDaniel, M. R., & DeJong, D. J. (1999). Justifying pharmacy staffing by presenting pharmacists as investments through return-on-investment analysis. *American Journal of Health-Systems Pharmacists, 56*, 2230–2234.

McKinlay, J. B., Trachtenberg, F., Marceau, L. D., Katz, J. N., & Fischer, M. A. (2014). Effects of patient medication requests on physician prescribing behavior: Results of a factorial experiment. *Medical Care, 52*(4), 294–299.

Montagne, M. (1996). The pharmakon phenomenon: Cultural conceptions of drugs and drug use. In P. Davis (Ed.), *Contested ground: Public purpose and private interest in the regulation of prescription drugs* (pp. 253–294). New York, NY: Oxford University Press.

Montagne, M., & Basara, L. R. (1996). Consumer behavior regarding the choice of prescription and non-prescription medications. In M. C. Smith & A. I. Wertheimer (Eds.), *Social and behavioral aspects of pharmaceutical care.* Binghamton, NY: Pharmaceutical Products Press.

Mukherjee, M., & Limbu, Y. (2013). A review of research on direct-to-consumer advertising of prescription drugs. *International Journal of Pharmaceutical and Healthcare Marketing, 7*(3), 226–243.

Nahin, R. L., Barnes P. M., Stussman B. J., & Bloom B. (2009). Costs of complementary and alternative medicine (CAM) and frequency of visits to CAM practitioners: United States, 2007. *National health statistics reports; No. 18.* Hyattsville, MD: National Center for Health Statistics. Retrieved from https://nccih.nih.gov/research/statistics/costs

National Association of Boards of Pharmacy. (2016, January). *Internet Drug Outlet Identification Program: Progress report for state and federal regulators.* Retrieved from: http://s3.amazonaws.com/awarerx2015/app/public/ckeditor_assets/attachments/45/nabpinternetdrugoutletreport_jan_2016.pdf

National Association of Chain Drug Stores Foundation (NACDS). (2005). *The chain pharmacy industry profile 2005.* Alexandria, VA: NACDS.

National Association of Chain Drug Stores Foundation (NACDS). (2010). *2010–2011 chain pharmacy industry profile.* Alexandria, VA: NACDS.

National Community Pharmacists Association (NCPA). (2009). *2009 NCPA digest, sponsored by Cardinal Health.* Alexandria, VA: NCPA.

Orizio, G., Merla, A., Schulz, P.J., Gelatti, U. (2011, September 30). Quality of online pharmacies and websites selling prescription drugs: A systematic review. *Journal of Medical Internet Research,* Retrieved from http://www.jmir.org/2011/3/e74/

Pharmaceutical Research and Manufacturers of America (PhRMA). (2010a). *Medicines in development for diabetes 2010 report.* Washington, DC: PhRMA. Retrieved from http://www.phrma.org/sites/phrma.org/files/attachments/Diabetes_2010.pdf

Pharmaceutical Research and Manufacturers of America (PhRMA). (2010b). *Pharmaceutical Industry Profile 2010.* Washington, DC: PhRMA.

Public Health Service Act. (1944). Retrieved from http://www.fda.gov/RegulatoryInformation/Legislation/ucm148717.htm

Raisch, D. W. (1990a). A model of methods for influencing prescribing: Part I. *DICP: Annals of Pharmacotherapy, 24*, 417–421.

Raisch, D. W. (1990b). A model of methods for influencing prescribing: Part II. *DICP: Annals of Pharmacotherapy, 24*, 537–542.

Soumerai, S., McLaughlin, T. J., & Avorn, J. (1989). Improving drug prescribing in primary care: A critical analysis of the experimental literature. *Milbank Quarterly, 67*, 268–317.

Strebhardt, K., & Ullrich, A. (2008). Paul Ehrlich's magic bullet concept: 100 years of progress. *Nature Reviews Cancer, 8*, 473–480.

Temple, R. (2009). Use of non-U.S. data in NDAs. *ASCPT special session: Regulatory considerations of using non-U.S. data in NDAs: Focus on efficacy, safety, and clinical pharmacology.* Retrieved from http://www.ascpt.org/Portals/8/docs/Meetings/2009%20Annual%20Meeting/Friday/Regulatory%20Considerations.pdf

Trusheim, M. R., Aitken, M. L., & Berndt, E. R. (2010). Characterizing markets for biopharmaceutical innovations: Do biologics differ from small molecules? *Forum for Health Economics & Policy 13*(1), Article 4. Retrieved from http://www.bepress.com/fhep/13/1/4/

Tufts Center for the Study of Drug Development. (2009). *Tufts CSDD outlook 2009*. Boston, MA: Tufts CSDD.

Tufts Center for the Study of Drug Development. (2010). *Tufts CSDD outlook 2010*. Boston, MA: Tufts CSDD.

U.S. FDA. (n.d. a). *Abbreviated new drug application (ANDA): Generics*. Retrieved from http://www.fda.gov/Drugs/DevelopmentApprovalProcess/HowDrugsareDevelopedandApproved/ApprovalApplications/AbbreviatedNewDrugApplicationANDAGenerics/default.htm

U.S. FDA. (n.d. b). *Development and approval process (CBER)*. Retrieved from http://www.fda.gov/BiologicsBloodVaccines/DevelopmentApprovalProcess/default.htm

U.S. FDA. (n.d. c). *How drugs are developed and approved*. Retrieved from http://www.fda.gov/Drugs/DevelopmentApprovalProcess/HowDrugsareDevelopedandApproved/default.htm

U.S. FDA. (n.d. d). *Implementation of the Biologics Price Competition and Innovation Act of 2009*. Retrieved from http://www.fda.gov/Drugs/GuidanceComplianceRegulatoryInformation/ucm215089.htm

U.S. FDA. (n.d. e). *What we do*. Retrieved from http://www.fda.gov/AboutFDA/WhatWeDo/default.htm

U.S. FDA. (2010). Coverage of personal importations. In *Regulatory procedures manual* (Section 9–2). Silver Spring, MD: U.S. FDA. Retrieved from http://www.fda.gov/ICECI/Compliance Manuals/RegulatoryProceduresManual/ucm179266.htm

USA Today, Kaiser Family Foundation, & Harvard School of Public Health (2008, March). *The public on prescription drugs and pharmaceutical companies: Summary and chartpack*. Washington, DC: Kaiser Family Foundation.

Ventola, C. L. (2011). Direct-to-consumer advertising. *Pharmacy & Therapeutics, 36*(10), 669–684.

Wilkes, M. S., Bell, R. A., & Kravitz, R. L. (2000). Direct-to-consumer prescription drug advertising: Trends, impact, and implications. *Health Affairs, 19*(2), 110–128.

World Health Organization (WHO). (2008). *Counterfeit drugs kill*. [International Medical Products Anti-Counterfeiting Taskforce (IMPACT) brochure]. Retrieved from http://www.who.int/impact/FinalBrochureWHA2008a.pdf

World Health Organization (WHO). (2015, March 30). Document A68/33, Report by the Director General to the Sixty-Eight World Health Assembly on Substandard/spurious/falsely-labelled/ falsified/counterfeit medical products. Retrieved from http://apps.who.int/gb/ebwha/pdf_files/WHA68/A68_33-en.pdf

CHAPTER

6

Public Health

Ardis Hanson, Peter D. Hurd, and Bruce Lubotsky Levin

Case Scenario

Bob is a pharmacist in a small rural town in the Midwest. He and his group of coworkers want to take charge of the public health plans for a small group of people who will live in his community, Mars. They live in an isolated community that has become fairly adept at creating a lifestyle that is self-sustaining. While satellite TV and radio keep them up to date on world events, most of the community life is centered on neighbors and the town's pharmacy. Since Bob graduated from pharmacy school a few years ago, he has been adding various pharmacy-related services to the pharmacy (including blood pressure checks and diabetes counseling), and now he feels ready to take these services to the next level. Bob wants to promote the new pharmacy services using a public health approach. He believes that a public health approach allows him to offer additional services to improve the health of his local community. His father happens to be his boss, and although he is retired, he still watches over store details and has allocated $15,000 for a budget. What should Bob recommend?

Bob decides on a promotional program that will highlight a different pharmacy service each week. If you were in Bob's shoes, what would you do each of the next 5 weeks? What should Bob do before he implements the program? How can he identify the most important needs of his community, and how can he pick activities that will tap into the community's willingness to change and try new things? How can he identify some "sure-fire successes" that will help his community and also help his pharmacy?

Bob decides to apply the transtheoretical model (e.g., precontemplation, contemplation, preparation, action, and maintenance) in the public health programs (Prochaska, DiClemente, & Norcross, 1992) with the goal of moving people from precontemplation to maintenance on a number of health and prevention issues. This model helps him realize that one size will not always fit because some of the community members are ready for change and others have not even thought of doing anything different.

LEARNING OBJECTIVES

Upon completion of this chapter, the student will be able to:

- Define public health, prevention, and epidemiology.
- Discuss the importance of disease prevention and health promotion.
- Apply public health objectives to pharmacy practice and pharmacy education.
- Discuss the roles of pharmacists within public health systems.
- Compare and contrast specific examples of emerging public health issues pharmacists face in clinical practice.

CHAPTER QUESTIONS

1. Define the terms public health, prevention, and epidemiology.
2. What are some of the critical public health issues facing our society?
3. How has the field of public health in America changed since the 18th century?
4. How does public health differ from the practice of medicine in the United States?
5. What role can pharmacy play in public health initiatives in America?

INTRODUCTION

The purpose of this chapter is to introduce essential concepts and critical issues in public health. One of the important perspectives readers should gain from this chapter is the public health viewpoint regarding the health of people, which focuses on groups of people, communities, and at-risk populations versus individuals. Since a public health perspective centers on the health of the public or from a population perspective, interventions necessary to improve health play a central role. Interventions vary, such as the availability of community health clinics, local antismoking laws, restaurant health inspections, and clean-air messages. This chapter will also provide readers with public health strategies and concepts fundamental to help achieve society's interest in ensuring the conditions in which people can be healthy.

Public Health

Public health has been defined in a variety of ways, but definitions tend to include efforts to prevent disease as well as promote healthy lifestyles using health promotion and health education initiatives. In the early 20th century, Winslow (1920) defined public health as six essential activities: (1) preventing disease and prolonging life, (2) promoting health through environmental efforts (including sanitation measures), (3) controlling communicable diseases, (4) advocating health education through personal hygiene, (5) organizing medical and nursing services for early diagnosis and preventive treatment of disease, and (6) ensuring health as a right of every citizen. Rosen (1993, p. 1) added "Throughout human history, the major problems of health that men have faced have been concerned with community life, for instance, the control of transmissible disease, the control and improvement of the physical environment (sanitation), the provision of water and food of good quality and in sufficient supply, the provision of medical care, and the relief of disability and destitution." Thus, the focus on community and social group responses to health promotion and disease prevention are central components to the definition of public health.

In a major report on the status of public health in America, the Institute of Medicine (IOM, 2003, p. 1) recognized the concept of health for the public good and "the fundamental duty of government to promote and protect the health of the public." However, accomplishing population-level health improvement requires changes in how innovative interventions are developed, how promising tools and strategies are scaled from small test groups into community-wide interventions, and how interventions are refined and evaluated to continue to improve population health. It also requires building change into a system's infrastructure, including educational systems, community-based care, social services, and primary as well as behavioral health systems (IOM, 2015).

As an independent, nonprofit organization that works outside the government, the IOM is an arm of the National Academies of Science and works to provide advice to decision makers and the public in health-related areas. Another important component of IOM work is prevention. Health is seen as a primary good in society because it affects so many aspects of human potential and social capital. If public health is "... what we, as a society, do collectively to assure the conditions in which people can be healthy" (IOM, 1988, p. 19), then social and environmental issues become part of the public health population-based agenda.

Individual versus Population Perspectives of Health

Historically, medical care training focuses on the treatment of illnesses in individuals. Just as medical and allied medical professionals are taught to alleviate pain and suffering in individual patients, pharmacists are taught to provide appropriate medications for individual patients and to help individuals manage their illnesses. Public health, however, pursues a population-based, trans-disciplinary approach to disease prevention and health promotion in specific at-risk populations. While disease prevention, morbidity reduction, and increased longevity do benefit individuals, public health professionals examine problems, critical issues, and diseases from a broader population-based perspective. Examples might include increased wellness in a state's overweight population through nutrition, diet, and exercise programs; a smoking cessation program for a county school system; the reduction of morbidity from automobile accidents in newly licensed automobile drivers (adolescents between the ages of 16 and 21). These examples show public health initiatives are designed for targeted groups of at-risk populations and communities rather than individuals.

HISTORICAL PERSPECTIVE

Public health and healthcare delivery systems date back to 18th-century Europe and late 19th-century America. Historically, public health is an intricate combination of the sanitation, environmental, and medical sciences. As bacteriologic and immunologic advances were recognized and used to control communicable diseases, the concept of disease prevention was incorporated into public health. Eventually, public health evolved into a transdisciplinary focus on public or community health sciences that now incorporates elements from the social, political, environmental, and the behavioral health sciences.

At one time, a community-based perspective was a unique way to view disease prevention. A major typhus outbreak in New York City during the mid-1800s was such a test case. Stephen Smith, an early public health pioneer, discovered that more than 100 victims of typhus fever lived in the same tenement. The tenement was in serious disrepair, had a basement filled with sewage, and too many tenants crowded into the rooms of the building. Smith became an advocate for improved living conditions and encouraged the establishment of a citywide public health board that eventually became the New York Metropolitan Board of Health (Smith, 1973). Although Smith's efforts focused on the living conditions of an entire group of people, his efforts also addressed the health needs of individuals.

Another example is polio. Polio viruses date back to before the Common Era. However, polio viruses were not described in medical records until 1789 in Underwood's *Treatise on Diseases of Children*. In 1894, over 100 cases were recorded in Rutland County, Vermont (Caverly, 1984). By 1908, epidemic poliomyelitis had become problematic throughout the United States. Several theories of poliomyelitis were advanced. Early theories suggested that polio replicated in nervous tissue

(Flexner & Lewis, 1909). However, by 1940, Sabin and Ward had proved poliomyelitis was a viral infection (Sabin & Ward, 1941a, 1941b). By the 1950s, Salk (1953) and Sabin (1953) had developed successful vaccines to prevent poliomyelitis. In addition, numerous interventions were developed to treat persons infected with the disease and late sequelae ("post-polio") presentation (Dean, 1991; Farbu et al., 2006; Robinson, Hillel, & Waugh, 1998; Stolwijk-Swuste, Tersteeg, Beelen, Lankhorst, & Nollet, 2010). Although typhus and polio viruses are acknowledged as enteric diseases (transmitted via the fecal—oral route), other methods of transmission are also important to public health.

How diseases are spread determines the public health preparedness and response to large outbreaks of disease. Although determining the mode of contact for the spread of diseases is critical to immediacy of treatment, such determination can be very difficult. Langmuir (1964) suggested that diseases, such as diphtheria, pertussis, and influenza, might be spread both through the air and by personal contact. Proved through extensive systematic epidemiological studies and laboratory studies, airborne and personal contact have been key factors in addressing pandemics.

The experience gained during one pandemic, such as the 1918 influenza outbreak, may allow public health professionals to better detect, clarify, and understand subsequent pandemics, such as the 2009 H1N1 influenza pandemic. However, there is always a conflict between the need for data collection to guide thoughtful and appropriate implementation of an intervention and the immediate urgency to take some sort of preventive action.

EPIDEMIOLOGY

Epidemiology, a core discipline of public health, is the study of the factors that determine the frequency and distribution of disease in human populations. *Incidence* and *prevalence* are both terms commonly used to refer to measurements of disease frequency. *Incidence* is the number of new cases of a specific disease occurring in a population during a certain period of time. The *prevalence* is the total number of cases in a population who have a specific disease during a defined time period. Using data collected through surveillance systems and/or descriptive epidemiologic studies, we can examine numerous aspects of the health of a community, focusing on a specific at-risk group in a specific place over a specific period of time. The data then are used to generate hypotheses regarding cause and transmission of disease, with a focus on community intervention and prevention of disease recurrence. Social inequities, including socioeconomic status, gender, and race/ethnicity, also are key determinants of population health and are used in a variety of explanatory models (Dahlgren & Whitehead, 1991; Krieger, Williams, & Moss, 1997).

An epidemiologic approach also can be used in looking at diet and health, exposure to pollution and cancer, or radiation risk and birth defects. In each case, populations and data about groups are used to infer the possible causes of illness.

Epidemiologic approaches also provide a framework for reporting health statistics, such as the causes of death or the prevalence of health problems. For example, *Health, United States, 2014* (National Center for Health Statistics, 2015) reports the following statistics:

1. Between 2003 and 2013, life expectancy increased 1.9 years for American men and 1.5 years for American women.
2. In 2012–2013, 15.3% of women and 20.5% of men were cigarette smokers.
3. In 2013, 70% of children 19 to 35 months of age received vaccinations protecting them against seven childhood infectious diseases.
4. In 2013, 20.5% of adult Americans under 65 years of age did not have health insurance coverage.

Global and National Perspectives

Mortality and morbidity rates are two of the most important measures when examining health and disease from global and national perspectives. Mortality rates report the number of deaths in an area per year. Morbidity rates report the number of illnesses or cases of disease in a population over a given period of time. Reporting the number of people who die annually and the causes of their deaths, along with injury data, allows us to gauge the effectiveness of a state, national, or country's health system(s).

Globally, the World Health Organization (WHO) (2014) reports the overall top 10 causes of death are ischemic heart disease; stroke; chronic obstructive pulmonary disease; lower respiratory infections; trachea, bronchus, and lung cancers; HIV/AIDS; diarrheal diseases; diabetes mellitus; road injuries; and hypertensive disorders. The Global Burden of Disease study found that, for most countries, reductions in age- and/or sex-specific mortality appear to be associated with a steady shift to deaths caused by noncommunicable disease and injuries (Naghavi et al., 2015).

Meanwhile, the top five causes of death in the United States are heart disease, cancer, chronic lower respiratory diseases, unintentional injuries, and stroke. Alzheimer's disease is the sixth, followed by diabetes; influenza and pneumonia; nephritis, nephrotic syndrome, and nephrosis; and intentional self-harm (Centers for Disease Control & Prevention, 2015). Of the chronic diseases responsible for seven of the top 10 leading causes of death, heart disease and cancer alone account for nearly half of all lives lost each year. In addition, these chronic diseases are among the most costly diseases and are also the most preventable. Diabetes mellitus, for example, is a major focus of medication and disease management programs for physicians and pharmacists.

Globally, the WHO (2014) estimates that 38 million deaths are attributable to noncommunicable diseases, and of these deaths, 40% affected people 70 years of age and younger. The impact of deaths from noncommunicable disorders is felt across all nations. However, low- and middle-income countries are hit the hardest, and the majority of premature deaths occur in these countries (WHO, 2014). Cardiovascular diseases, cancer, chronic respiratory diseases, and diabetes are responsible for 82% of deaths from noncommunicable diseases. In its 2014 report on noncommunicable diseases, the WHO specifically targeted behavioral and biological risk factors. Behavioral risk factors for morbidity are alcohol use, physical inactivity, salt/sodium intake, and tobacco use. Biological risk factors are identified as elevated blood pressure, diabetes and obesity, and elevated cholesterol; low intake of fresh fruits and vegetables; and low intake of fatty acids (WHO, 2014).

Nationally, from morbidity risk perspectives in the United States, leading risk factors are diabetes, hypertension, high serum cholesterol, obesity, tobacco use, and excessive alcohol use (Johnson, Hayes, Brown, Hoo, & Ethier, 2014). The Centers for Disease Control and Prevention (CDC) argues that significant morbidity can be reduced through "improved nutrition, increased physical activity, improved vaccination rates, avoidance of tobacco use, adoption of measures to increase motor-vehicle safety, early detection and treatment of risk factors, and health care quality improvement" (Johnson et al., 2014, p. 4).

Morbidity and mortality statistics are critical to gauge how effective prevention and promotion programs are in improving population health. Periodic shifts in morbidity and mortality indicate programmatic changes in health priorities and allocation of resources. Consider there are numerous types of health risks. Each risk may be the result of a complex relationship between behavioral, social, economic, environmental factors, and/or genetic predisposition. Each of these influences may provide an opportunity for health promotion/education, prevention, and early intervention initiatives and programs. This has expanded the focus of public health to include both the prevention of acute illnesses, and minimization of the effects of chronic diseases through primary, secondary, and tertiary prevention (see the "*Prevention*" section in this chapter). Nevertheless, the effectiveness or outcomes of these programs are often measured over decades rather than in months or years.

SOCIAL DETERMINANTS OF HEALTH: PUBLIC HEALTH MODEL

For over 60 years, the WHO (1948, p. 100) has defined health as "a state of complete physical, mental, and social well-being, and not merely the absence of disease or infirmity." As this definition illustrates, health is more than simply the absence of disease, and public health issues help broaden how we conceptualize the true health of a population. Certainly, the idea of health includes the minimization of the effects of disease both on the individual and for the population as a whole. However, in today's world, the concept of health includes the notion of an ability to function in the roles that one desires, not simply the physical role, but also mental and social roles. The WHO (2001) reflects this shift in focus from disability (cause) to level of health (impact), an important construct in population health, with its latest version of the International Classification of Functioning, Disability, and Health.

In general, we think of a healthy person as one who has the ability to do things physically, mentally, emotionally, and socially. This idea of health is measured by: (1) physical tests, such as exercise; (2) mental tests, like those testing awareness of person, place, and time; (3) psychological tests for emotion including those for depression; and (4) other quality-of-life assessments. A healthy society means people are living in conditions that allow and promote physical and mental behaviors and social well-being. While safe drinking water and proper waste disposal are included in public health practice, other examples include a smoke-free eating environment, a pollution-free park, and a safe road between restaurants and homes.

While there are many reasons to emphasize the public nature of health, one of the most compelling reasons is the relationship between health and social class. Across age and cultures, lower social classes have consistently had lower levels of health (Braveman, Cubbin, Egerter, Williams, & Pamuk, 2010). While numerous factors can help explain this association (including lack of resources, less formal education, environmental risks, and dangerous occupations), there is a link between social class and individual health.

HEALTH DISPARITIES

Few people would be surprised by the fact that countries differ in the quality of health and/or the quality of health care that is provided to their citizens, but there also is a corresponding lack of equality of health within a country. Health disparity, as it was defined in the early 1990s, was to address poorer health among socially and economically disadvantaged people within any racial/ethnic group (Braveman, 2014). This is the perspective *Healthy People 2020* used in its description:

> A health disparity is a particular type of health difference that is closely linked with economic, social, or environmental disadvantage [that most often affects] groups of people who have systematically experienced greater social or economic obstacles to health based on their racial or ethnic group, religion, socioeconomic status, gender, age, or mental health; cognitive, sensory, or physical disability; sexual orientation or gender identity; geographic location; or other characteristics historically linked to discrimination or exclusion (U.S. Department of Health and Human Services, 2015).

Higher incidence of disease, shorter average length of life, and greater infant mortality are all indicators of health disparities for minorities when compared to whites in the general U.S. population. However, researchers found that people with the lowest incomes and least education, as well as groups with intermediate income and education levels, were also the least healthy compared to those with more education and higher incomes (Braveman et al., 2010). This supports the notion that health disparities are not simply issues for those at the lowest levels of socioeconomic status but for any identified cultural, social, ethnic, or racial group in any urban, suburban, or rural community located in a multitude of geographic locations in the United States.

Many factors can account for the health disparities that are found in the United States. Certainly, access to quality medical care would be one of those factors. Nevertheless, a public health approach helps us look for additional explanations, including the lack of a healthy diet, no safe place to exercise or play, pollutants in the air, lead paint in the house, insects and rodents in living areas, and lack of language skills necessary to navigate complicated healthcare systems. In addition, other factors, including the lack of transportation and the lack of sensitivity to different cultural or religious practices, further help to explain why health disparities can be so prevalent and so difficult to resolve.

Prevention and promotion are especially critical in addressing health disparities. Alvarado, Harper, Platt, Smith, and Lynch (2009) suggested that interventions to reduce the risk factors addressed by *Healthy People 2010* objectives for all populations should be targeted to low-income and less-educated populations in order to have the most impact on meeting 2010 objectives (also see the "*Healthy People 2020*" section in this chapter). This approach would not only reduce risk factors and chronic diseases across groups but would result in an overall reduction of health disparities (Alvarado et al., 2009).

Cultural competence is an integral part of addressing health disparities. Bleidt and Coleman (2008) view cultural competency as a continuum from cultural insensitivity to awareness and sensitivity to integration. They emphasize that pharmacy healthcare providers need to move from cultural insensitivity, where cultural differences simply fail to be recognized, to both an awareness and sensitivity to the cultural differences that influence personal health and the provision of health care. Ideally, healthcare providers will integrate the knowledge of other cultures into the practice of health care for the individual patient. Differences in eye contact, male/female roles, health beliefs, and healthcare practices need to be appreciated, understood, and used to optimize the provision of health care to diverse populations (Bleidt & Coleman, 2008).

CHANGING HEALTH PRIORITIES

The nature of public health problems, both in the United States and globally, has changed over the past 200 years. The variety of local public health issues (e.g., clean air, drinkable water, and waste disposal) becomes global in scope rather than specific to countries or selected populations. Historically, these changes in health priorities illustrate the growth and progress of scientific knowledge in the etiology and control of disease. Further, they illustrate the gradual acceptance of health promotion and disease intervention as a public responsibility. Finally, the development of public health practice also demonstrates that a number of public health issues and problems remain unresolved. This chapter will focus on such issues as HIV/AIDS, emergency preparedness and response to natural disasters, and the H1N1 pandemic.

HIV/AIDS

The shift in health promotion and disease prevention (and early intervention) activities, focusing on chronic rather than acute illnesses, has been complicated by new public health challenges that have developed in concert with advances in new medical technologies, such as genetic-based treatments, new drug discoveries, and online monitoring systems. As an example, infectious diseases, such as HIV/AIDS, remain a major cause of morbidity and mortality throughout the world. UNAIDS (2015) estimated that, in 2014, almost 37 million (36.9) people lived with HIV and over

1 million (1.2) people died of AIDS. Even with the new drugs and prevention initiatives, it is estimated there were 2 million new infections, or about 5,600 new infections per day (UNAIDS, 2015). In the United States, an estimated 1.2 million people live with HIV. However, the CDC estimates that one in eight individuals is unaware that he or she is infected (Hall et al., 2015; UNAIDS, 2008). Approximately 50,000 new HIV cases are reported yearly in the United States. In 2013, almost 48,000 individuals were diagnosed with HIV, and approximately 26,000 individuals were diagnosed with AIDS (Centers for Disease Control and Prevention, 2016, para. 3).

The majority of new cases of HIV infection are transmitted through sexual behavior, and approximately one half of all new cases of HIV infection are among people aged 25 years and younger. However, the death rate for HIV is higher for individuals between 35 and 54 years of age than for other ages. Children younger than 13 years accounted for less than 1% of HIV/AIDS diagnoses (Centers for Disease Control and Prevention, 2015). African Americans and Hispanic Americans have AIDS rates considerably higher than rates among Caucasian Americans. High-risk heterosexual contact also accounts for a considerable proportion of new HIV diagnoses among men of minority races/ethnicities and among women of all races/ethnicities (CDC, 2015). In addition, the percentage of individuals infected due to heterosexual activity also has increased, having surpassed the percentage infected through drug injection (CDC, 2015).

HIV/AIDS is not only an epidemic in the United States, but also is a pandemic, affecting the health of populations throughout the world. Although the number of HIV infections declined globally and HIV-related deaths also have decreased, Sub-Saharan Africa accounts for 76% of all people who have HIV/AIDS and for 75% of AIDS deaths. During 2013, 15 countries accounted for more than 75% of the 2.1 million new HIV infections that occurred (UNAIDS, 2014). Further, six countries have little or no decline in new HIV infections, low treatment coverage, and high HIV burden: (1) Indonesia, (2) Russian Federation, (3) Central African Republic, (4) Democratic Republic of the Congo, (5) Nigeria, and (6) South Sudan (UNAIDS, 2014).

From a public health practice perspective, pharmacists provide important community-based care. Hirsch et al. (2011) describe the effectiveness of a 3-year program of pharmacist-provided medication therapy management services in treating individuals with HIV/AIDS. They specifically examined patient outcomes, as well as pharmacy and medical costs. Outcomes included antiretroviral therapy medication regimens, use of contraindicated antiretroviral therapy regimens, occurrence of opportunistic infections, and patient adherence rates. They found pilot pharmacy patients received more appropriate HIV treatment and were significantly more adherent to therapy. While non-antiretroviral therapy (ART) medication costs were 30% to 40% greater in the pilot group each year, expenditures for inpatient services were found to be significantly lower for the pilot group than for the nonpilot group. Although no significant differences in mean total cost per patient per group were observed, the additional medication therapy management (MTM) services payment added less than 3% to the total cost of care for participants. Hirsch and colleagues suggest this study should not only help healthcare plans understand the value of MTM, especially for persons with HIV/AIDS, but also increase the possible implementation of more MTM services in community pharmacies. This is important in light of the Medicare Prescription Drug, Improvement, and Modernization Act of 2003 (and Medicare Part D) and the Affordable Care Act.

Emergency Preparedness and Response to Natural Disasters

Disasters often remove one's sense of well-being and security. Whether the disaster is manmade or natural, a disaster may be a cataclysmic event (such as the earthquake in Haiti in 2010) or an event with a slow onset (such as the drought in Sub-Saharan Africa during the years 1972–1993). By August 2015, there were 251 global disasters. Over 115 million people were affected, including deaths, injuries, displacements, homelessness, and trauma (Centre for Research on the Epidemiology of Disasters, 2015). By August 2015, the U.S. Federal Emergency Management Agency had issued 57 emergency and disaster declarations in the United States, of which 35 were major disaster declarations (U.S. Federal Emergency Management Agency, 2015).

In addition to natural and technological disasters, manmade disasters (genocide and war) continue to have a significant effect upon the public's health. The Global Internal Displacement Profile Project estimates that 16 million people were forced from their homes due to severe political, religious, ethnic, or social persecution during 2014 and 19.3 million were displaced due to geophysical or weather-related disasters (Internal Displacement Monitoring Centre, 2015).

Preparedness for disasters and terrorism, a critical component of protecting the health of the public, includes identifying at-risk populations, assessing community health, and mapping local and national infrastructures. The 2006 Pandemic and All Hazards Preparedness Act refocused the research priorities of the university-based Centers for Public Health Preparedness (Institute of Medicine, 2009). It recommended the Centers address the design and implementation of emergency preparedness training, how best to communicate accurate information in a timely manner to diverse audiences, create sustainable community-based preparedness systems, and develop evaluation criteria and metrics to assess the performance of public health emergency response systems (Institute of Medicine, 2009).

Most recently, an IOM workshop examined how best to improve regional disaster response coordination (Reeve et al., 2015). The three foci of this workshop were: (1) improving patient tracking and evacuation, (2) reducing surge burdens on clinical facilities, and (3) improving services within area community-based and public health programs. Major points from this workshop were the inclusion of pharmacists in planning efforts and the integration of "minute clinics" where pharmacists could provide point-of-care services during a disaster. A spokesperson for the National Association of Chain Drug Stores stated that "pharmacies could be a public health asset in mitigating surge issues in the community, also reducing the burden on hospitals" (Reeve et al., 2015). Further, regional planning responses to disasters would allow pharmacists to engage more completely in preparedness, response, and mitigation activities (Reeve et al., 2015).

With the increase in disasters nationally and globally, pharmacists have important roles in disaster and crisis response planning by providing services at disaster sites and participating in bioterrorism detection activities (Hurd & Mount, 2008). A survey of the impact of two disasters in Toronto, Canada (one health and one a major citywide blackout) emphasized the importance of pharmacies as frontline healthcare facilities (Austin, Martin, & Gregory, 2007). In lieu of official emergency preparedness guidelines and policies, pharmacists relied on their own experience and professional judgment and that of their colleagues. Austin and colleagues (2007) found that documentation systems, experience, professional judgment, and teamwork practices could be used as indicators of successful adaptation to disasters. The interview-based study highlights the importance of leadership and advanced preparation prior to actual disasters (Austin et al., 2007).

Armitstead and Burton (2006) describe a certification program designed to increase urban and rural community pharmacists' knowledge of bioterrorism. The program, located at the University of Kentucky College of Pharmacy, trained 142 licensed pharmacists during a 2-year period (Armitstead & Burton, 2006). In Birmingham, Alabama, the McWhorter School of Pharmacy at Samford University assisted the state in preparing for those who had been forced out of their homes by hurricane Katrina when it was discovered that refills for prescriptions were becoming a huge problem (Hogue, Hogue, Lander, Avent, & Fleenor, 2009). Feret and Bratberg (2012) describe their experiences as a pharmacist consulting team for statewide bioterrorism and emergency preparedness. Over 10 years of consulting have substantiated their belief of the importance of pharmacists in the development and evaluation of readiness, clinical knowledge, and capability. However, in the conclusions of the two studies by Ford (Ford, Dallas, & Harris, 2013; Ford, von Waldner, & Perri, 2013), pharmacists preferred the role of pharmaceutical supplier, with less involvement in patient management and response integration roles. This may require a paradigm shift for practicing pharmacists, as well as new emphases on pharmacy education and professional development training.

H1N1 Pandemic

Pandemics are considered widespread epidemics of infectious or contagious diseases that affect one or more countries or continents contemporaneously. The influenza pandemics of 1918–1919, 1957–1958, and 1968–1969 killed millions of people worldwide. The 1918–1919 influenza pandemic alone killed between 20 and 40 million people, and it is estimated that approximately one third of the world's population was infected (Taubenberger & Morens, 2006, para.1).

The public health implications of earlier influenza pandemics made the emergence of the H1N1 virus in 2009 particularly serious. Within 50 days of the first reported incidence of the H1N1 virus in April, 2009, the virus had spread to over 76 countries, resulting in over 160 deaths and approximately 36,000 cases (Chawla et al., 2009). By August 2009, over 2,000 deaths had occurred and over 200,000 laboratory-confirmed cases were reported (Franco-Paredes et al., 2009). Mass media coverage of hospitalizations and deaths due to the H1N1 virus, especially among younger individuals, contributed to increased awareness of disease prevention and health promotion initiatives through infectious disease control measures and mass immunization.

During the H1N1 pandemic, the CDC issued alerts on new surveillance tools to model the spread of flu and the impact of various interventions based upon disease and affected population parameters. In addition, the CDC released information for pharmacists regarding treatment guidelines, recommendations for the use of antiviral medications, emergency authorizations for medication shipment and use, situation updates, and infection control (see www.cdc.gov/h1n1flu/). Bhavsar, Kim, and Yu (2010), for example, describe their roles as pharmacists in the CDC's emergency preparedness and response activities during the H1N1 pandemic, which included emergency use requests for medications and use of the Strategic National Stockpile of medications.

An essential part of emergency preparedness and response is effective immunization strategies at the patient, provider, and system levels. Community-based promotion and prevention campaigns utilizing television, radio, and the Internet are one way to increase immunization levels at the patient level. Vlahov, Coady, Ompad, and Galea (2007) describe additional strategies for providers. At the systems level, the most important strategy is to promote broader access to influenza vaccines and reduce missed vaccination opportunities (Vlahov et al., 2007). One critical strategy is to broaden the healthcare base to include additional healthcare providers, such as nurses and pharmacists, to provide immunizations within the community setting and to provide greater access to vaccines.

MODELS FOR CHANGE

One of the methods to promote change is to design community interventions using theories or models that have proven helpful in creating changes in behavior, both at the individual and population levels. Public health has employed many change models, including the theory of planned behavior (Ajzen, 1991), the transtheoretical model (Prochaska & DiClemente, 1983), and self-efficacy theory (Bandura, 1977). Kotter and Cohen (2002) make it clear the first step for successful large-scale change is creating a sense of urgency (Kotter, 2008). Whether at the patient level or the population level, people need to feel the need to change. Without that driving force, the energy to change will be lacking. Skaff (2014) has provided an application of Kotter's work to pharmacy and provider status, which highlights the challenges in transforming the pharmacist's role.

In public health, Prochaska et al. (1992) developed a five-step model, the transtheoretical model, which classified individuals regarding their level of readiness in adopting a behavior change. Their first step is precontemplation, which is not giving any consideration for the need to change. People in this stage will resist change because there is no perceived need. The next stage is contemplation, thinking about change, and is followed by preparation. Action and then maintenance are the last two stages and include individuals actively engaging in a behavior change (Prochaska et al., 1992). In a population, individuals may be in various stages of readiness. In developing interventions, one may consider programs that address the various needs of these individuals. In the case of flu vaccination programs, one would want an information program to not only effect a change from thinking that a flu shot is unnecessary to necessary, but also to offer opportunities for people to take action and receive a vaccination.

Social marketing utilizes basic marketing techniques found in advertising and applies them to social issues (Grier & Bryant, 2005). Pharmacy students who have taken a marketing course are familiar with the four *P*s of marketing: (1) product, (2) price, (3) place, and (4) promotion. Social marketing can use these same fundamental concepts and adapt them to a public health intervention. For flu vaccinations, the product is the vaccination, the price might be free (but would need to consider transportation costs and time away from work), the place needs to be convenient, and the promotion needs to be targeted to a specific at-risk population. For example, people without access to computers will not find web pages very helpful in a campaign to increase flu awareness. The framework that models and theories provide for public health interventions is invaluable and should be a central component of health promotion and disease prevention initiatives.

PREVENTION

The traditional approach to disease prevention in public health is the primary- and secondary-tertiary models. Primary prevention (often operationalized in health promotion activities) refers to the avoidance of disease occurrence as well as actions taken prior to disease onset. Examples include immunizations, water fluoridation, and prospective medication review for potential interactions.

Secondary prevention refers to the early diagnosis (detection) and prompt treatment (early intervention) of disease and the avoidance of disability. Examples of secondary preventive efforts include hypertension and cholesterol screening, programs that encourage self-assessment for cancers, and pharmacist review of drug use in nursing homes.

Tertiary prevention refers to the limitation or reduction of disability when disease has already occurred, through rehabilitation designed to encourage recovery and prevent further problems. Examples of tertiary preventive initiatives include cardiac rehabilitation programs and occupational therapy for individuals with a variety of physical disabilities.

Institute of Medicine and the Future of Public Health

The Future of Public Health (IOM, 1988, p. 40) defined the mission of public health as "the fulfillment of society's interest in assuring the conditions in which people can be healthy." Thus, the focus on communities and their collective responses to health promotion and disease prevention are central components in the definition of public health. *The Future of Public Health* provided a guide on issues important to the health of the public, with a focus on HIV/AIDS, toxic environmental conditions, lack of health insurance, and the relationship between public and private sector care. Although these problems may have appeared as insurmountable, *The Future of Public Health* also stressed the capability of the U.S. public health infrastructure to effectively problem solve issues of quality of life and the provision of health care.

The follow-up report, entitled *The Future of the Public's Health in the 21st Century* (Institute of Medicine, 2003), depicted the United States as a nation still challenged by toxic environments (e.g., the Three Mile Island disaster), a large uninsured population, and by health disparities, as well as facing new challenges such as obesity, antimicrobial resistance, and bioterrorism. Further, it continued to frame public health as "... what we as a society do collectively to assure the conditions in which people can be healthy" (IOM, 1988, p. 1).

Another IOM report, *Informing the Future: Critical Issues in Health*, continued to emphasize improvement of the nation's healthcare systems (IOM, 2009). Nevertheless, it highlighted health as a significant component of U.S. foreign policy, with recommendations for the U.S. government to increase global health efforts over the next 4 years. In addition, *Informing the Future* emphasizes risk management and healthy communities. Priority areas for healthy communities include care for women's and children's health, U.S. military and veterans' health, improved HIV prevention and intervention, and implementation of electronic health (medical) records (Hanson & Levin, 2013).

Although the reports mentioned in this section only provide an overview of the changing public health priorities since 1980, the purpose of the IOM reports is to provide a rationale for prioritizing public health initiatives in the United States. The *Healthy People 2020* initiatives, discussed below, describe the nation's public health objectives and establish benchmarks to determine effectiveness. Tobacco use, immunizations, and obesity continue to be public health concerns, with the underlying issues for each changing and creating new health challenges. Use of electronic cigarettes continue to rise despite increasing legislation to create smoke-free environments, immunizations for sexually transmitted diseases work best if given to children that are considered too young to be sexually active (HPV prevention) raises moral questions, and obesity continues despite a national awareness of healthy eating and exercise.

Healthy People 2020

Tobacco use, poor diet, and physical inactivity are examples of behavioral risk factors that lead to chronic diseases. Seven of the 10 leading causes of death in the United States are attributable to chronic disease. An estimated 90 million individuals in the United States are affected by chronic diseases, resulting in disability and major limitations in daily living activities (Ramsey et al., 2005, p. 1).

In 1979, *Healthy People* provided national objectives for promoting health and preventing disease. Preparation of the *Healthy People* report was a cooperative effort of the federal health agencies, the National Academy of Sciences' IOM, and a federal task force on disease prevention and health promotion. The authors assessed the relative contributions of lifestyle/behavior, environment, biologic factors, and health care to health problems. They suggested that approximately 50% of U.S. mortality was due to unhealthy behavior or lifestyle choices, 20% was due to environmental factors, 20% to human biologic factors, and only 10% to issues in healthcare delivery (United States Office of the Assistant Secretary for Health and Surgeon General, 1979).

The reports set and monitor national health objectives and measure the impact of prevention activity for the nation. For example, *Healthy People 2010* provided general goals for 10 leading health indicators, such as tobacco use, immunizations, and overweight/obesity (U.S. Department of Health and Human Services, 2010). *Healthy People 2020* supports those three general goals (US DHHS, 2010), all of which have aspects that are applicable to pharmacists and to pharmacy practice.

Tobacco Use

Tobacco use and abuse is a major health risk for people across the world and is responsible for nearly 500,000 deaths in the United States annually. The *Healthy People* goal for reducing tobacco use across all ages is to increase the number of evidence-based tobacco control programs as well as the provision of insurance coverage for evidence-based treatment of nicotine dependency. Tobacco cessation programs provided by pharmacists may offer one of the most accessible ways to improve the overall health of a community (Babb & Babb, 2003, p. 58).

Historically, pharmacy has been involved in smoking cessation programs because of the interest in population health. Both pharmacy students and pharmacists have been trained to counsel in tobacco cessation programs (Dent, Harris, & Noonan, 2007; Hudmon, Prokhorov, & Corelli, 2006; Williams, 2009). Adding training in evidence-based practice requires effective teaching models to increase both the pharmacist's knowledge and self-efficacy in counseling patients on this difficult behavior change. Martin, Bruskiewitz, and Chewning (2010) described a multimedia program for community pharmacists that combined home study with live training. The combination of teaching strategies, which included problem solving, modeling, rehearsal, and feedback, significantly improved participants' knowledge. In addition, 75% of attendees implemented a tobacco cessation program after course completion. One year after completing the tobacco cessation course, more than 50% of community pharmacists were still providing tobacco cessation programs (Martin et al., 2010).

Immunizations

Healthy People also prioritizes immunizations with the objective to increase vaccination coverage levels for universally recommended vaccines for young children and for influenza and pneumococcal diseases among adults. Using the 2002–2008 National Immunization Survey, Zhao and Luman (2010) analyzed sociodemographic factors, including race, ethnicity, and number of siblings; family poverty status; urban, suburban, or rural status; mother's education level, marital status, and age; and number and type of vaccination providers (public or private). In addition, they noted if the children had participated in the Vaccines for Children program. Describing how progress has been made in meeting *Healthy People 2010* goals, the trend from 2000 to 2008 indicated a reduction in disparities among most sociodemographic groups. One noteworthy trend was a substantial decrease in disparities between children living in rural areas versus those living in suburban areas (Zhao & Luman, 2010).

However, other researchers disagree and claim disparities continue. In their study, influenza vaccination levels for adults did not meet the *Healthy People 2010* objectives (Merrill & Beard, 2009). Furthermore, Jackson and colleagues (2009) found higher levels of pneumococcal vaccination coverage only among two populations: (1) adults 65 years of age and older, and (2) younger adults with diabetes mellitus. However, Yoo and associates (2015) determined that immunization disparities among the elderly may be overrepresented based on the analytic method used (e.g., differences in the estimated coefficients and characteristics not included in the regression models). Equalizing recognized characteristics among racial/ethnic groups could provide a more accurate assessment of racial/ethnic disparities in influenza vaccination among the elderly.

Pharmacists play an important role in helping to achieve the objectives of increasing vaccination coverage levels. All states allow pharmacists to immunize patients. Some states require certification or limit the types of immunizations to flu shots and pneumococcal vaccines, while other states allow pharmacists to administer a broad range of immunizations. Studies show that in states where pharmacists are authorized to provide adult immunizations, there are a larger number of individuals who receive immunizations and an increase in immunizations in rural counties (Bearden & Holt, 2005; Crawford, Blaney, Amesty, Rivera, Turner, Ompad, & Fuller, 2011; Chun, Sautter, Patterson, & McGhan, 2016). This results in overall better individual and community health as well as reduced morbidity and mortality.

Obesity

The continuing rise in obesity among children and adults in the United States has resulted in the extension of the 2010 public health goal of reducing obesity and accompanying comorbid diseases as part of the 2020 objectives. Although overweight and obesity prevalence have increased steadily among all population groups in the United States, as of 2011–2012, approximately one third of adults, or over 72 million Americans, were obese (Ogden, Carroll, Kit, & Flegal, 2014). Furthermore, obesity in adults and more specifically in women has increased faster than obesity in children. If the current trends in obesity continue, by 2030, it is projected that over 85% of adults will be either overweight or obese, and by 2048, all American adults will be overweight or obese. Approximately 17% (or 12.7 million) of children and adolescents aged 2 to 19 years are obese (Ogden et al., 2014). Childhood obesity is more prevalent in children from lower-income families (Pan, Blanck, Sherry, Dalenius, & Grummer-Strawn, 2012, p. 2563). By 2030, it is estimated that treating diseases associated with obesity and overweight will cost between $860 and $950 billion (16–18%) of the total U.S. healthcare costs (Wang, Beydoun, Liang, Caballero, & Kumanyika, 2008). Increased obesity is associated with increased risk for premature death, increased healthcare costs, a reduced quality of life, and increased morbidity. Diseases associated with obesity include hypertension, coronary heart disease, type 2 diabetes mellitus, and certain forms of cancer.

Disease state management programs and MTM programs are essential components of managing chronic diseases. Screenings in community pharmacies for diabetes, hypertension, and dyslipidemia resulted in improved follow-up consultations with primary care providers (Snella et al., 2006). Further, as pharmacists become part of a patient's medical home, a systematic and comprehensive provision of care model, their role in advising on choice of medication, especially for obesity treatments, will become more prominent. The Healthy Habits Program, a weight management pharmaceutical care service (including educational programs, nutrition counseling, and exercise) at Auburn University's Pharmaceutical Care Center, not only helped over 150 patients decrease their risk status but also established pharmacists at the center of disease prevention and health promotion activities on campus (Lloyd et al., 2007). A number of studies have examined the role of the pharmacist in weight-loss programs with positive results (Bottorff, 2006; Harmon, Pogge, & Boomershine, 2014; Krska, Lovelady, Connolly, Parmar, & Davies, 2010; Todd et al., 2014).

PHARMACY AND PUBLIC HEALTH

Public Health Workforce

Healthy People 2020 identifies the public health workforce as a key component of the U.S. public health infrastructure. The public health workforce, often defined as individuals employed by local, state, and federal government health agencies, includes individuals working in academic settings who teach, train, or participate in public health research. In addition, the public health workforce also includes individuals who work in private sector healthcare delivery organizations and members of local communities.

The importance of the public health workforce was recognized in 1993 when a list entitled *Core Functions of Public Health* was inserted into Title III of the Health Security Act (HR 3600§3311-3312, 103rd Congress, 1993). Although the bill was defeated, it eventually resulted in the creation of a single definitive list of the 10 essential public health services (Turnock & Handler, 1997). These essential public health services include the following:

1. Monitor health status to identify community health problems.
2. Diagnose and investigate health problems and health hazards in the community.
3. Inform, educate, and empower people about health issues.
4. Mobilize community partnerships to identify and solve health problems.
5. Develop policies and plans that support individual and community health efforts.
6. Enforce laws and regulations that protect health and ensure safety.
7. Link people to needed personal health services and ensure the provision of health care when otherwise unavailable.
8. Assure a competent public health and personal healthcare workforce.
9. Evaluate effectiveness, accessibility, and quality of personal and population-based health services.
10. Research to provide new insights and innovative solutions to health problems.

As interest in competencies for the public health workforce increased, the Council on Linkages Between Academia and Practice published its first core competencies list in 2001, mapping competencies across the 10 essential public health services. In 2009, the Council (2010) published a revised list with competencies spanning eight content areas or domains: (1) Analytical/Assessment Skills, (2) Policy Development/Program Planning Skills, (3) Communication Skills, (4) Cultural Competency Skills, (5) Community Dimensions of Practice Skills, (6) Public Health Sciences Skills, (7) Financial Planning and Management Skills, and (8) Leadership and Systems Thinking Skills. In June 2014, again, the Council revised its competencies, using the eight domains and adding three career stage tiers: (1) Front Line Staff/Entry Level, (2) Program Management and/or Supervisory Level, and (3) Senior Management and/or Executive Level. These new competencies include the use of public health informatics practices at individual, programmatic, and business operations levels; development of continuous quality improvement strategies; assessment of health literacy; assessment of organizations for cultural competence; recognition of the ethical conduct of research; development of local, state, and federal agency partnerships; implementation of appropriate judicial and operational procedures; improvement of organizational performance through evaluation; and implementation of personal development opportunities for public health staff.

In addition to core competencies, public health leaders throughout the United States have created a credentialing system for public health workers as well as how best to evaluate the performance of the public health systems. Part of the discussion on public health systems performance is tied to the accreditation and credentialing of the public health workforce (Scutchfield, Bhandari, Lawhorn, Lamberth, & Ingram, 2009, p. 266).

In 2005, the National Board of Public Health Examiners was created (Gebbie et al., 2007) providing graduates of public health programs a voluntary certification examination to measure their core knowledge and skills. As the credentialing of the public health workforce continues, this examination likely will become a standard requirement to work in the public health field. Thus, issues such as whether persons without a formal professional public health education should be credentialed and how to measure the competence of workers without a formal professional public health education will need to be resolved (Gebbie, 2009). This likely will have implications for pharmacists who work within the public health workforce, especially with the continuing movement to create practice specializations within pharmacy practice.

Changing and Expanding Roles of Pharmacy and Pharmacists

One of the telling signs of the changing role of pharmacists in public health is the increasing interest in the combination of a PharmD degree with a master's degree in public health. In 2006, the American Public Health Association adopted a policy statement on the role of pharmacists in public health recognizing that the role of pharmacy in public health was still developing, expanding, and being redefined as the profession adopts more public health responsibilities. In 2008, the American Association of Colleges of Pharmacy approved a special interest group in public health (SIG), consisting of pharmacy educators with an interest in this area (American Association of Colleges of Pharmacy, 2015). By 2010, 13 colleges of pharmacy offered this dual-degree option, and the number continues to increase (American Association of Colleges of Pharmacy, n.d.).

The U.S. Public Health Service has a long history of hiring pharmacists and using them in public health roles ranging from the Indian Health Service to population disease control. As an example of the changing role of pharmacy, consider the areas of environmental and occupational health. These areas usually focus on limiting the risk for worker exposure to chemicals, regulating chemical pollutants in the environment, and the safe disposal of hazardous waste. Of specific concern is medication disposal because medications can be excreted naturally by the patient and pass through filtration plants without being removed (Stoddard & Huggett, 2015).

In the 2008–2009 annual report from the President's Cancer Panel entitled *Reducing Environmental Cancer Risk: What We Can Do Now* (Reuben, 2010), there was specific mention of the proper disposal of pharmaceuticals and the potential cancer risk to those who consume water that has been polluted by the improper disposal of pharmaceuticals by the public. Currently there are no limits in drinking water for these kinds of chemicals. The roles for pharmacists in environmental health are just beginning to be recognized and developed (Harbison et al., 2008), including the disposal of hazardous waste from the pharmacy and compliance with Occupational Safety and Health regulations in the pharmacy.

Pharmacovigilance and Risk Management

Pharmacovigilance is another example of the expanding role for pharmacy and considered part of a broader public health perspective. Pharmacovigilance is the detection, assessment, and prevention of adverse effects, particularly long- and short-term side effects, of pharmaceutical products within public health practice (Uppsala Monitoring Centre, 2015). The burden on the public's health due to adverse drug events is significant. In a review by the Agency for Healthcare Research and Quality (2010), adverse drug events were estimated to cause more than 770,000 injuries and deaths per year, with the cost to individual hospitals exceeding as much as $5 million. Furthermore, the toxicity of the medicines used in the treatment of HIV/AIDS may result in adverse consequences of a patient's dermatologic, hepatic, hematologic, metabolic, and neurologic systems.

Discovering adverse drug reactions is an important part of pharmacovigilance and can be done in patient populations rather than on a patient-by-patient basis. Being able to use large databases to detect adverse drug reactions early can play a very important role in the safe and effective use of medications. By developing a clear picture of the risks of a medication, the patient and provider can more accurately weigh the potential harm against the benefits of the medication.

To detect adverse drug reactions that are less common, countries have begun to collaborate on the creation of databases that include enough cases to find patterns in very large groups that would be missed in smaller populations (Uppsala Monitoring Centre, 2015). Counterfeit drugs and drugs used in nonapproved ways are additional examples of how international cooperation can lead to a rapid response to a problem.

Another area of pharmacovigilance is the drug resistance of antibiotics. Moreover, a large database of drug use can help pinpoint problem areas and areas of resistance. Researchers can examine the database, looking for patients who are having trouble using their medications. An example might include an asthma patient refilling a rescue inhaler too frequently while failing to refill a second inhaler that is designed for maintenance doses. Looking for these patterns can provide information to pharmacists in the identification and resolution of medication-related problems at a population level.

In one study of the VA Pharmacy Benefits Management Strategic Healthcare Group, the use of evidence-based practices and clinical and contracting processes/procedures to improve quality of care and patient outcomes was examined, as well as the safety, appropriateness of use, effectiveness, and cost-effectiveness of prescription drugs for veterans. The authors found that cooperation of the multidisciplinary teams involved in patient care, reliance on evidence-based practices, and a focus on continuous quality improvement resulted in improved practice and health outcomes (Sales, Cunningham, Glassman, Valentino, & Good, 2005).

Formularies and the management of medication therapy provide additional examples of the changing role of pharmacy. The drug benefits in some health insurance plans are managed by a pharmacy benefit management company. Its main purpose is to provide the prescription drug benefit, which would include processing the claim and providing the medication to the individual member either through a local pharmacy or through the mail. The pharmacy benefit management company can operate at a much larger scale than an individual health insurance plan, resulting in a reduction in costs of providing the drug benefit. Because the emphasis is on cost savings to the insurer, strategies are offered to the insurer to reduce costs. As one of these strategies, the pharmacy benefit manager will develop formularies (lists of drugs) that are preferred in the plan. If the drugs on the formulary are used, they will be cheaper, saving money for all involved, including the patient.

Challenges Facing Pharmacy and Public Health

There are a number of public health pharmacy areas that will offer exciting opportunities for pharmacists. Three areas of public health pharmacy that would seem to have important implications for the future include: (1) health literacy, (2) medication compliance/adherence to medication regimens, and (3) the nutrition/exercise component of drug therapy. Nevertheless, there are also many challenges facing the future of public health in the field of pharmacy. There are many examples of public health approaches that have been implemented by pharmacists, including community outreach, student services, and intervention training programs.

The broad area of healthcare reform will offer critical opportunities for pharmacy. One significant area is the development of community health teams for transitional care, which includes discharge planning with medication therapy management services under the medical home model. Healthcare reform also provides for a grant-awarding patient safety research center for medication management therapy services. A national health workforce commission will integrate healthcare training across professional schools.

Health Literacy

In *Healthy People 2010*, health literacy is defined as the degree to which an individual can obtain, process, and understand basic health information and health services and make appropriate health decisions. Zarcadoolas, Pleasant, and Greer (2005) include a number of dimensions for health literacy: fundamental literacy, scientific literacy, civic literacy, and cultural literacy. This broader definition of health literacy can be of great impact to patients and providers. Choosing a broader focus helps underscore the fact that health literacy is not simply a problem for a patient, but rather a problem for healthcare systems and the providers working within those systems (Nielsen-Bohlman, Panzer, & Kindig, 2004).

Because of the nature of public health and its work with underserved populations, it is critical that pharmacists address and detect health literacy problems that may interfere with the patient's health. Pharmacists can use a number of tools to improve their attempts to address issues related to health literacy. One of the simplest approaches is the use of plain language (Stableford & Mettger, 2007). Attempts to use nonjargon, easy-to-understand communication is one of the keys to addressing health literacy problems.

A second approach, commonly known as 'teach back', uses the technique of requesting the patient to explain to the health practitioner the message that the patient has received as if the patient was now the teacher (Dinh, Bonner, Clark, Ramsbotham, & Hines, 2016). This approach can be very helpful in detecting misunderstandings, gaps in knowledge, and potentially harmful misinterpretations.

The design of health information needs to include a consideration of the health literacy and cultural background of the target audience. The ability to use health information to make informed decisions needs to be monitored and assessed. Strengths in one area, such as fundamental literacy, may not assure strengths in scientific or mathematical areas of literacy.

Adherence to Medication Regimens

The degree to which an individual complies with a prescribed regimen (drug, diet, exercise) is often referred to as adherence. Medication adherence is one of the continuing public health issues in pharmacy. Patients may be prescribed the correct treatment, but they sometimes fail to fill the prescription, take the medication, or correctly dose the medication. Even those who initially adhere often fail to continue taking the drug. The way public health pharmacy approaches this problem can have a significant effect because multifaceted approaches to adherence have shown some success by tailoring programs to individual needs, simplifying medication regimens, and delivering programs over a longer period of time (McDonald, Chang, & Schultz, 2013).

There are many ways to measure compliance/adherence. In addition to asking a patient about his or her medication(s), pharmacists also should ask a patient what really helps him or her remember to take the medication correctly, and how they cope with the challenges of taking the medication as prescribed. One pharmacy-based measure is a pill count, basically looking at the number of pills dispensed, the frequency of dosing, and the number of pills currently in the container. A modification of this would be to predict the time when a refill should be needed and then compare the actual refill to the predicted time.

Other approaches are to measure therapeutic outcomes (lowered cholesterol) or the drug level in the body (achieved a therapeutic level). All are valuable, but some are more appropriate for particular situations. In public health pharmacy, comparing refill frequency with predicted times would enable the identification of population risks for the at-risk group that is being assessed.

Nutrition/Exercise and Drug Therapy

The health problems of the U.S. population include the management of chronic disease in an aging population. The baby boomer population (born between 1946 and 1964) will continue to develop chronic diseases as they age, diseases that parallel the current causes of death in the U.S. population (heart disease, cancer, and stroke). The management of chronic diseases (including diabetes, arthritis, and others) often requires a team-based approach that includes both proper diet and adequate exercise.

Public health approaches to encourage populations to eat healthy and to be active can be a part of public health pharmacy practice. Within this broad category, the pharmacist can also play a part in the management of obesity. As discussed earlier, obesity is a major public health problem facing the U.S. population at all ages and the pharmacist, as a part of the healthcare team, should play a vital role in helping combat this serious public health problem.

Importance of Public Health in Pharmacy

Although we may think of global public health concerns in the context of communicable diseases (such as HIV or the Ebola virus), the world population is living longer and is increasingly urbanized, challenged by poverty, and very mobile. The primary focus of future prevention and early intervention initiatives will include health, nutritional education and support, and control of infectious diseases. Adding to the disease burden of heart disease, cancer, and stroke, global public health concerns will also include depression, alcohol abuse, tobacco use, and the problems associated with the health of an aging population (Levin, Hennessy, & Petrila, 2010).

Healthy People 2020 objectives will affect pharmacy education and practice.

Objective HP2010–1-7 recommends that pharmacy education include core competencies in health promotion and disease prevention, with an emphasis on cultural diversity.

Objective HC/HIT (Health Communication and Health IT) HP2020–6 increases the number of patients involved in their own healthcare decision making. This requires the pharmacist to be more proactive and to communicate more effectively with patients regarding medication choice, use, adherence, adverse effects, and self-monitoring.

Objective DSC (Disability and Secondary Conditions) HP2020–6 increases the numbers of individuals with access to health and wellness programs, which further establishes pharmacists as a critical component in medical homes and as members of extended care and community care teams.

Objective DSC HP2020–13 increases the number of graduate courses in disability and health as part of public health programs, a move that pharmacy schools and colleges may parallel.

Objective OA (Older Adults) HP2020–6 increases the proportion of the healthcare workforce with geriatric certification, and may provide the opportunity for a new specialization in pharmacy, much like the clinical psychiatric pharmacist.

With the push toward the adoption of a national electronic health record (Levin & Hanson, 2011), two objectives for health communication and health information technology also may affect pharmacy practice. In the health communication/health information technology area, objectives HP2020–11 and HP2020–12 seek to increase the percentage of healthcare providers who use health information technology in order to improve the health of individuals and at-risk populations and to increase the percentage of healthcare providers and governmental health organizations that use advanced connectivity to maximize health information systems (U.S. Department of Health and Human Services, 2010). Increased use of health information systems also will lend itself to better surveillance of health events, disease tracking, and bioterrorism preparedness. Surveillance objectives address medical safety, especially the monitoring and analysis of adverse events associated with pharmaceutical therapies in community and specialty pharmacy practice.

CONCLUSION AND IMPLICATIONS FOR PHARMACY

This chapter has covered a variety of concepts, topics, and critical issues related to public health and pharmacy. For a pharmacist thinking about implementing a public health pharmacy program in a smaller community (as in the case scenario presented at the beginning of this chapter), there are many suggestions, topics, and approaches that might be considered. Creating a sense of urgency to change, or identifying an area where that urgency is already present, will be an important key to the success of a public health pharmacy program. Pharmacists, as members of the healthcare team, have the potential to make significant differences for their communities and for their patients in many areas and specialties within public health.

QUESTIONS FOR FURTHER DISCUSSION

1. How may health information technologies affect pharmacy practice?
2. What role does public health have in the education and training of physicians, nurses, pharmacists, and other providers of health care?
3. Is there a need in the research, academic, and practice areas for public health pharmacists?
4. What future public health issues will be most important to pharmacy?
5. What role can pharmacists play in the development of the assessment of health needs within a specific population?

KEY TOPICS AND TERMS

Epidemiology
Health
Health disparities
Incidence
Morbidity
Mortality rate
Pandemic
Prevalence
Prevention
Primary prevention
Secondary prevention
Social determinants of health
Tertiary prevention

REFERENCES

Agency for Healthcare Research and Quality. (2010). Reducing and preventing adverse drug events to decrease hospital costs. Retrieved from http://www.ahrq.gov/qual/aderia/aderia.htm

Aizen, I. (1991). The theory of planned behavior. *Organizational Behavior and Human Decision Processes, 50*(2), 179–211. doi:10.1016/0749-5978(91)90020-T

Alvarado, B. E., Harper, S., Platt, R. W., Smith, G. D., & Lynch, J. (2009). Would achieving Healthy People 2010's targets reduce both population levels and social disparities in heart disease? *Circulation: Cardiovascular Quality and Outcomes, 2*(6), 598–606. doi:10.1161/circoutcomes.109.884601

American Association of Colleges of Pharmacy. (2015). Public health SIG. Retrieved from http://www.aacp.org/GOVERNANCE/SIGS/PUBLICHEALTH/Pages/default.aspx

American Association of Colleges of Pharmacy. (n.d.). Table 4, Dual degree programs anticipated for 2015-2016. In Pharmacy school admission requirements (Ed.).

American Public Health Association. (2006, November 8). *The role of the pharmacist in public health.* Washington, DC: APHA. Retrieved from http://www.apha.org/advocacy/policy/policysearch/default.htm?id=1338

Armitstead, J. A., & Burton, D. C. (2006). Enhanced pharmacy training for counter-terrorism and disaster response. *Journal of Telemedicine & Telecare, 12*(Suppl 1), 3–5. doi:10.1258/135763306777978498

Austin, Z., Martin, J. C., & Gregory, P. A. (2007). Pharmacy practice in times of civil crisis: The experience of SARS and the blackout in Ontario, Canada. *Research in Social and Administrative Pharmacy, 3*(3), 320–335.

Babb, V. J., & Babb, J. (2003). Pharmacist involvement in Healthy People 2010. *Journal of the American Pharmacists Association, 43*(1), 56–60.

Bandura, A. (1977). Self-efficacy: Toward a unifying theory of behavioral change. *Psychological Review, 84*(2), 191–215.

Bearden, D. T., & Holt, T. (2005). Statewide impact of pharmacist-delivered adult influenza vaccinations. *American Journal of Preventive Medicine, 29*(5), 450–452.

Bhavsar, T. R., Kim, H. J., & Yu, Y. (2010). Roles and contributions of pharmacists in regulatory affairs at the Centers for Disease Control and Prevention for public health emergency preparedness and response. *Journal of the American Pharmacists Association, 50*(2), 165–168.

Bleidt, B. A., & Coleman, C. A. (2008). Understanding multicultural pharmaceutical education. In B. L. Levin, P. Hurd, & A. Hanson (Eds.), *Introduction to public health in pharmacy* (pp. 279–294). Sudbury, MA: Jones and Bartlett.

Bottorff, M. (2006). Role of the pharmacist. *Pharmacotherapy, 26*(12 pt 2), 227S–232S.

Braveman, P. (2014). What are health disparities and health equity? We need to be clear. *Public Health Reports, 129*(Suppl 2), 5–8.

Braveman, P., Cubbin, C., Egerter, S., Williams, D. R., & Pamuk, E. (2010). Socioeconomic disparities in health in the United States: What the patterns tell us. *American Journal of Public Health, 100*(Suppl 1), S186–S196.

Caverly, C. S. (1984). Preliminary report of an epidemic of paralytic disease occurring in Vermont in the summer of 1894. *Yale Medical Journal, 1*, 1–5.

Centers for Disease Control and Prevention. (2016). *HIV in the United States: At a glance.* Atlanta, GA: CDC. Retreived from http://www.cdc.gov/hiv/statistics/overview/ataglance.html

Centers for Disease Control and Prevention. (2015). Leading causes of death: Number of deaths for leading causes of death. Retrieved from http://www.cdc.gov/nchs/fastats/leading-causes-of-death.htm

Centers for Disease Control and Prevention. (2015, February). Diagnoses of HIV infection in the United States and dependent areas, 2013. *HIV Surveillance Report, 25*, 1–82.

Centre for Research on the Epidemiology of Disasters. (2015). In EM-DAT: The international disaster database. Brussels, Belgium: Author (CRED). Retrieved from http://www.emdat.be/database

Chawla, R., Sharma, R. K., Madaan, D., Dubey, N., Arora, R., Goel, R., ... Bhardwaj, J. R. (2009). Mitigation approaches to combat the flu pandemic. *Journal of Global Infectious Diseases, 1*(2), 117–130.

Chun, G. J., Sautter, J. M., Patterson, B. J., & McGhan, W. F. (2016). Diffusion of pharmacy-based influenza vaccination over time in the United States. *American Journal of Public Health*, e1-e2.

Council on Linkages Between Academia and Practice. (2010, May). *Core competencies for public health professionals* (Adopted May 10, 2010) ([revised] ed.). Washington, DC: Public Health Foundation. Retrieved from http://www.phf.org/resourcestools/documents/core_public_health_competencies_iii.pdf

Council on Linkages Between Academia and Public Health Practice. (2014, June). *Core competencies for public health professionals.* Washington, DC: Council on Linkages Between Academia and Public Health Practice. Retrieved from http://www.phf.org/resourcestools/Documents/Core_Competencies_for_Public_Health_Professionals_2014June.pdf

Crawford, N. D., Blaney, S., Amesty, S., Rivera, A. V., Turner, A. K., Ompad, D. C., & Fuller, C. M. (2011). Individual- and neighborhood-level characteristics associated with support of in-pharmacy vaccination among ESAP-registered pharmacies: pharmacists' role in reducing racial/ethnic disparities in influenza vaccinations in New York City. *Journal of Urban Health, 88*(1), 176–185.

Dahlgren, G., & Whitehead, M. (1991). *Policies and strategies to promote social equity in health: Background document to WHO—Strategy paper for Europe.* Stockholm, Sweden: Stockholm Institute for Further Studies.

Dean, E. (1991). Clinical decision making in the management of the late sequelae of poliomyelitis. *Physical Therapy, 71*(10), 752–761.

Dent, L. A., Harris, K. J., & Noonan, C. W. (2007). Tobacco interventions delivered by pharmacists: a summary and systematic review. *Pharmacotherapy, 27*(7), 1040–1051.

Dinh, H. T., Bonner, A., Clark, R., Ramsbotham, J., & Hines, S. (2016). The effectiveness of the teach-back method on adherence and self-management in health education for people with chronic disease: a systematic review. *JBI Database of Systematic Reviews and Implementation Reports, 14*(1), 210–247.

Evans, R. G., & Stoddard, G. L. (1994). Producing health, consuming health care. In R. G. Evans, M. L. Barer, & T. R. Marmor (Eds.), *Why are some people healthy and others not? The determinants of health of populations* (pp. 27–64). New York, NY: Aldine de Gruyter

Farbu, E., Gilhus, N. E., Barnes, M. P., Borg, K., de Visser, M., Driessen, A., ... Stalberg, E. (2006). EFNS guideline on diagnosis and management of post-polio syndrome. Report of an EFNS task force. *European Journal of Neurology, 13*(8), 795–801.

Feret, B., & Bratberg, J. (2012). A ten-year experience of a pharmacist consulting team for statewide bioterrorism and emergency preparedness. *Medicine and Health, Rhode Island, 95*(9), 279, 280.

Flexner, S., & Lewis, P. A. (1909). The transmission of poliomyelitis to monkeys. *Journal of the American Medical Association, 53*, 1639.

Ford, H., Dallas, C. E., & Harris, C. (2013). Examining roles pharmacists assume in disasters: A content analytic approach. *Disaster Medicine and Public Health Preparedness, 7*(6), 563–572.

Ford, H., von Waldner, T., & Perri, M., 3rd. (2013). Pharmacists' roles in post-September 11th disasters: A content analysis of pharmacy literature. *Journal of Pharmacy Practice, 27*(4), 350–357.

Franco-Paredes, C., Hernandez-Ramos, I., Del Rio, C., Alexander, K. T., Tapia-Conyer, R., & Santos-Preciado, J. I. (2009). H1N1 influenza pandemics: Comparing the events of 2009 in Mexico with those of 1976 and 1918–1919. *Archives of Medical Research, 40*(8), 669–672.

Gebbie, K. (2009). Public health certification. *Annual Review of Public Health, 30*, 203–210.

Gebbie, K., Goldstein, B. D., Gregorio, D. I., Tsou, W., Buffler, P., Petersen, D., ... Silver, G. B. (2007). The National Board of Public Health Examiners: Credentialing public health graduates. *Public Health Reports, 122*(4), 435–440.

Grier, S., & Bryant, C. A. (2005). Social marketing in public health. *Annual Review of Public Health, 26*, 319–339.

Hall, H. I., An, Q., Tang, T., Song, R., Chen, M., Green, T., & Kang, J. (2015). Prevalence of diagnosed and undiagnosed HIV infection–United States, 2008-2012. *MMWR: Morbidity and Mortality Weekly Report, 64*(24), 657–662.

Hanson, A., & Levin, B. L. (2013). *Mental health informatics*. New York, NY: Oxford University Press.

Harbison, R. D., Morris, S., III, & Harbison, C. (2008). Environmental and occupational health. In B. L. Levin, P. D. Hurd, & A. Hanson (Eds.), *Introduction to public health in pharmacy* (pp. 77-99). Sudbury, MA: Jones and Bartlett.

Harmon, M., Pogge, E., & Boomershine, V. (2014). Evaluation of a pharmacist-led, 6-month weight loss program in obese patients. *Journal of the American Pharmacists Association (2003), 54*(3), 302–307.

Hirsch, J. D., Gonzales, M., Rosenquist, A., Miller, T. A., Gilmer, T. P., & Best, B. M. (2011). Antiretroviral therapy adherence, medication use, and health care costs during 3 years of a community pharmacy medication therapy management program for Medi-Cal beneficiaries with HIV/AIDS. *Journal of Managed Care Pharmacy, 17*(3), 213–223.

Hogue, M. D., Hogue, H. B., Lander, R. D., Avent, K., & Fleenor, M. (2009). The nontraditional role of pharmacists after hurricane Katrina: Process description and lessons learned. *Public Health Reports, 124*(2), 217–223.

Hudmon, K. S., Prokhorov, A. V., & Corelli, R. L. (2006). Tobacco cessation counseling: pharmacists' opinions and practices. *Patient Education and Counseling, 61*(1), 152–160.

Hurd, P. D., & Mount, J. K. (2008). Health emergency preparedness and response. In B. L. Levin, P. Hurd, & A. Hanson (Eds.), *Introduction to public health in pharmacy* (pp. 321–336). Sudbury, MA: Jones and Bartlett.

Institute of Medicine. (1988). *The future of public health*. Washington, DC: National Academy Press.

Institute of Medicine. (2003). *The future of the public's health in the 21st century*. Washington, DC: National Academies Press.

Institute of Medicine. (2009). *Informing the future: Critical issues in health* (5th ed.). Washington, DC: National Academies Press.

Institute of Medicine. (2015). *Spread, scale, and sustainability in population health: Workshop summary*. Washington, DC: National Academies Press.

Internal Displacement Monitoring Centre. (2015). Global figures. Geneva, Switzerland: Norwegian Refugee Council. Retrieved from http://www.internal-displacement.org/global-figures

Jackson, L. A., Baxter, R., Naleway, A. L., Belongia, E. A., & Baggs, J. (2009). Patterns of pneumococcal vaccination and revaccination in elderly and non-elderly adults: A Vaccine Safety Datalink study. *BMC Infectious Diseases, 9*, 37.

Johnson, N. B., Hayes, L. D., Brown, K., Hoo, E. C., & Ethier, K. A. (2014). CDC National Health Report: Leading causes of morbidity and mortality and associated behavioral risk and protective factors–United States, 2005-2013. *MMWR Supplements, 63*(Suppl 4), 3–27.

Kotter, J. P. (2008). *A sense of urgency*. Boston, MA: Harvard Business Press.

Kotter, J. P., & Cohen, D. S. (2002). *The heart of change: Real-life stories of how people change their organizations*. Boston, MA: Harvard Business School Press.

Krieger, N., Williams, D. R., & Moss, N. E. (1997). Measuring social class in US public health research: Concepts, methodologies, and guidelines. *Annual Review of Public Health, 18*, 341–378.

Krska, J., Lovelady, C., Connolly, D., Parmar, S., & Davies, M. J. (2010). Community pharmacy contribution to weight management: identifying opportunities. *International Journal of Pharmacy Practice, 18*(1), 7–12.

Langmuir, A. D. (1964). Airborne infection: How important for public health? I. A historical review. *American Journal of Public Health and the Nation's Health, 54*, 1666–1668.

Levin, B. L., & Hanson, A. (2011). Mental health informatics. In N. A. Cummings & W. T. O'Donahue (Eds.), *Understanding the behavioral health care crisis: The promise of integrated care and diagnostic reform*. New York, NY: Routledge/Taylor & Francis.

Levin, B. L., Hennessy, K. D., & Petrila, J. (2010). *Mental health services a public health perspective*. New York, NY: Oxford University Press.

Lloyd, K. B., Thrower, M. R., Walters, N. B., Krueger, K. P., Stamm, P. L., & Evans, R. L. (2007). Implementation of a weight management pharmaceutical care service. *Annals of Pharmacotherapy, 41*(2), 185–192.

Martin, B. A., Bruskiewitz, R. H., & Chewning, B. A. (2010). Effect of a tobacco cessation continuing professional education program on pharmacists' confidence, skills, and practice-change behaviors. *Journal of the American Pharmacists Association (2003), 50*(1), 9–16.

McDonald, K. M., Chang, C., & Schultz, E. (2013). *Through the quality kaleidoscope: Reflections on the science and practice of improving health care quality: Closing the quality gap: Revisiting the state of the science*. (AHRQ Report No.: 13-EHC041-EF). Rockville, MD: Agency for Healthcare Research and Quality. Retrieved from http://www.ncbi.nlm.nih.gov/pubmedhealth/PMH0077471/

Merrill, R. M., & Beard, J. D. (2009). Influenza vaccination in the United States, 2005-2007. *Medical Science Monitor, 15*(7), PH92–PH100.

Naghavi, M., Wang, H., Lozano, R., Davis, A., Liang, X., Zhou, M., ... Abraham, B. (2015). Global, regional, and national age-sex specific all-cause and cause-specific mortality for 240 causes of death, 1990-2013: A systematic analysis for the Global Burden of Disease Study 2013. *Lancet, 385*(9963), 117–171.

National Center for Health Statistics. (2015). *Health, United States, 2014*. Rockville, MD: U.S. Dept. of Health, Education, and Welfare, Public Health Service, Health Resources Administration, National Center for Health Statistics.

Nielsen-Bohlman, L., Panzer, A. M., & Kindig, D. A. (2004). *Health literacy: A prescription to end confusion*. Washington, DC: National Academies Press.

Ogden, C. L., Carroll, M. D., Kit, B. K., & Flegal, K. M. (2014). Prevalence of childhood and adult obesity in the United States, 2011-2012. *Journal of the American Medical Association, 311*(8), 806–814.

Pan, L., Blanck, H. M., Sherry, B., Dalenius, K., & Grummer-Strawn, L. M. (2012). Trends in the prevalence of extreme obesity among US preschool-aged children living in low-income families, 1998-2010. *Journal of the American Medical Association, 308*(24), 2563–2565.

Prochaska, J., & DiClemente, C. (1983) Stages and processes of self-change in smoking: Toward an integrative model of change. *Journal of Consulting and Clinical Psychology, 51*(3), 390–395.

Prochaska, J. O., DiClemente, C. C., & Norcross, J. C. (1992). In search of how people change. Applications to addictive behaviors. *American Psychologist, 47*(9), 1102–1114.

Ramsey, F., Ussery-Hall, A., Garcia, D., McDonald, G., Easton, A., Kambon, M., ... CDC. (2005). Prevalence of selected risk behaviors and chronic diseases—Behavioral Risk Factor Surveillance System (BRFSS), 39 steps communities, United States, 2005. *Morbidity and Mortality Weekly Report (MMWR). Surveillance Summaries, 57*(11), 1–20. Retrieved from http://www.cdc.gov/mmwr/pdf/ss/ss5711.pdf

Reeve, M., Altevogt, B., Davis, M. Forum on Medical and Public Health Preparedness for Catastrophic Events, Board on Health Sciences Policy, & Institute of Medicine. (2015). *Regional disaster response coordination to support health outcomes: Summary of a workshop series*. Washington, DC: National Academies Press.

Reuben, S. H. (2010). *Reducing environmental cancer risk: What we can do now*. Washington, DC: U.S. Department of Health and Human Services, National Institutes of Health, National Cancer Institute.

Robinson, L. R., Hillel, A. D., & Waugh, P. F. (1998). New laryngeal muscle weakness in post-polio syndrome. *Laryngoscope, 108*(5), 732–734.

Rosen, G. (1993). *A history of public health*. Baltimore, MD: The Johns Hopkins University Press.

Sabin, A. B. (1953). Present status and future possibilities of a vaccine for the control of poliomyelitis. *A.M.A. American Journal of Diseases of Children, 86*(3), 301–310.

Sabin, A. B., & Ward, R. (1941a). The natural history of human poliomyelitis: I. Distribution of virus in nervous and non-nervous tissues. *Journal of Experimental Medicine, 73*(6), 771–793.

Sabin, A. B., & Ward, R. (1941b). The natural history of human poliomyelitis: II. Elimination of the virus. *Journal of Experimental Medicine, 74*(6), 519–529.

Sales, M. M., Cunningham, F. E., Glassman, P. A., Valentino, M. A., & Good, C. B. (2005). Pharmacy benefits management in the Veterans Health Administration: 1995 to 2003. *American Journal of Managed Care, 11*(2), 104–112.

Salk, J. E. (1953). Studies in human subjects on active immunization against poliomyelitis. I. A preliminary report of experiments in progress. *Journal of the American Medical Association, 151*(13), 1081–1098.

Scutchfield, F. D., Bhandari, M. W., Lawhorn, N. A., Lamberth, C. D., & Ingram, R. C. (2009). Public health performance. *American Journal of Preventive Medicine, 36*(3), 266–272.

Schillinger, D., Piette, J., Grumbach, K., Wang, F., Wilson, C., Daher, C., … Bindman, A. B. (2003). Physician communication with diabetic patients who have low health literacy. *Archives of Internal Medicine, 163*(1), 83–90.

Skaff, A. (2014, September 20). A reflection on John P. Kotter's "Leading Change: Why Transformation Efforts Fail." *ASHP Connect* [Blog]. Retrieved from http://connect.ashp.org/blogs/angela-skaff/2014/09/20/transformation-efforts-pharmacy?ssopc=1

Smith, S. (1973). *The city that was*. Metuchen, NJ: Scarecrow Reprint Corp. (Original work published 1806).

Snella, K. A., Canales, A. E., Irons, B. K., Sleeper-Irons, R. B., Villarreal, M. C., Levi-Derrick, V. E., … Nelson, A. A. (2006). Pharmacy- and community-based screenings for diabetes and cardiovascular conditions in high-risk individuals. *Journal of the American Pharmacists Association, 46*(3), 370–377.

Stableford, S., & Mettger, W. (2007). Plain language: A strategic response to the health literacy challenge. *Journal of Public Health Policy, 28*(1), 71–93.

Stoddard, K. I., & Huggett, D. B. (2015). Wastewater effluent hydrocodone concentrations as an indicator of drug disposal program success. *Bulletin of Environmental Contamination and Toxicology, 95*(2), 139–144.

Stolwijk-Swuste, J. M., Tersteeg, I., Beelen, A., Lankhorst, G. J., & Nollet, F. (2010). The impact of age and comorbidity on the progression of disability in late-onset sequelae of poliomyelitis. *Archives of Physical Medicine and Rehabilitation, 91*(4), 523–528.

Taubenberger, J. K., & Morens, D. M. (2006). 1918 influenza: The mother of all pandemics. *Emerging Infectious Diseases, 12*(1), 15–22.

Todd, A., Moore, H. J., Husband, A. K., Bambra, C., Kasim, A., Sniehotta, F. F., … Summerbell, C. D. (2014). Community pharmacy interventions for public health priorities: protocol for a systematic review of community pharmacy-delivered smoking, alcohol and weight management interventions. *Systematic Reviews, 3*, 93.

Turnock, B. J., & Handler, A. S. (1997). From measuring to improving public health practice. *Annual Review of Public Health, 18*, 261–282.

U.S. Department of Health and Human Services. (2010). *Healthy People 2020*. Washington, DC: U.S. Department of Health and Human Services.

U.S. Department of Health and Human Services. (2015). Disparities. Retrieved from http://www.healthypeople.gov/2020/about/foundation-health-measures/Disparities

U.S. Federal Emergency Management Agency (2015). *Disaster declarations for 2015*. Retrieved from https://www.fema.gov/disasters/grid/year/2015?field_disaster_type_term_tid_1=All

UNAIDS. (2008). *Report on the global HIV/AIDS epidemic*. New York, NY: United Nations.

UNAIDS. (2014). *The Gap report*. Geneva, Switzerland: UNAIDS.

UNAIDS. (2015). *How AIDS changed everything: MDG6: 15 years, 15 lessons of hope from the AIDS response*. Geneva, Switzerland: UNAIDS.

United States Office of the Assistant Secretary for Health and Surgeon General. (1979). *Healthy people: the Surgeon General's report on health promotion and disease prevention*. Washington, DC: U.S. Dept. of Health, Education, and Welfare, Public Health Service, Office of the Assistant Secretary for Health and Surgeon General.

Uppsala Monitoring Centre. (2015). Report from the WHO Collaborating Centre for International Drug Monitoring: Activities July 2013—June 2014. Uppsala, Sweden: WHO Collaborating Centre for International Drug Monitoring. Retrieved from http://www.who-umc.org/graphics/28368.pdf

Vlahov, D., Coady, M. H., Ompad, D. C., & Galea, S. (2007). Strategies for improving influenza immunization rates among hard-to-reach populations. *Journal of Urban Health, 84*(4), 615–631.

Wang, Y., Beydoun, M. A., Liang, L., Caballero, B., & Kumanyika, S. K. (2008). Will all Americans become overweight or obese? Estimating the progression and cost of the US obesity epidemic. *Obesity (Silver Spring), 16*(10), 2323–2330.

Williams, D. M. (2009). Preparing pharmacy students and pharmacists to provide tobacco cessation counselling. *Drug and Alcohol Review, 28*(5), 533–540.

Winslow, C.-E. A. (1920). The untilled field of public health. *Modern Medicine, 2*, 183–191.

World Health Organization. (1948). *Preamble to the Constitution of the World Health Organization as adopted by the International Health Conference, New York, 19-22 June, 1946; signed on 22 July 1946 by the representatives of 61 States (Official Records of the World Health Organization, no. 2, p. 100) and entered into force on 7 April 1948*. Geneva, Switzerland: World Health Organization.

World Health Organization. (2001). *International classification of functioning, disability and health (ICF)*. Geneva, Switzerland: World Health Organization.

World Health Organization. (2014). Global status report on noncommunicable diseases 2014. Geneva, Switzerland: World Health Organization. Retrieved from http://apps.who.int/iris/bitstream/10665/148114/1/9789241564854_eng.pdf?ua=1

World Health Organization. (2014, May). The top ten causes of death [fact sheet no. 310]. Geneva, Switzerland: World Health Organization.

Yoo, B. K., Hasebe, T., & Szilagyi, P. G. (2015). Decomposing racial/ethnic disparities in influenza vaccination among the elderly. *Vaccine, 33*(26), 2997–3002.

Youmans, S. L., & Schillinger, D. (2003). Functional health literacy and medication use: the pharmacist's role. *Annals of Pharmacotherapy, 37*(11), 1726–1729. doi:10.1345/aph.1D070

Zarcadoolas, C., Pleasant, A., & Greer, D. S. (2005). Understanding health literacy: an expanded model. *Health Promotion International, 20*(2), 195–203. doi:10.1093/heapro/dah609

Zhao, Z., & Luman, E. T. (2010). Progress toward eliminating disparities in vaccination coverage among U.S. children, 2000-2008. *American Journal of Preventive Medicine, 38*(2), 127–137.

CHAPTER

7

Quality Improvement and Patient Safety

Kyle E. Hultgren and John B. Hertig

Case Scenario

Community Hospital, located in Plainville, United States, is a 300-bed hospital that includes a 24-hour inpatient pharmacy. There are 12 full-time pharmacists and 12 full-time pharmacy technicians working in the central pharmacy and a satellite pharmacy in an intensive care unit. AH is a 50-year-old man who had been hospitalized for an uncomplicated spine surgery and was in recovery. As he was responsive and able to swallow, physicians decided to switch him from intravenous to oral opioids prior to discharge. The patient told the bedside nurse that he had taken liquid opioids in the past, but experienced nausea with pills (he could not recall the name of either liquid or pill opioids). The nurse informed the physician that AH was having severe pain, and noted that liquid opioids worked for him in the past per patient report. The physician searched for oral oxycodone in the computerized prescriber order entry (CPOE) and found two formulations for tablets and two for liquid (5 mg/5 mL and 20 mg/mL). The physician ordered a 5-mg dose of concentrated oxycodone liquid product (20 mg/mL) from the list.

When verifying this order, the pharmacist recognized that the higher concentration was atypical for inpatients, but assumed it was intended to limit the volume of fluid given to the patient. The pharmacist verified the order and made a comment on both the electronic medication administration record (eMAR) and the patient-specific label that the patient only required 0.25 mL (5 mg). As a safety assurance, the pharmacist delivered the medication bottle and a calibrated syringe to the bedside nurse. He also spoke to the nurse about the high-concentration formulation and the amount to be administered (0.25 mL). Soon after, the nurse went to the AH's room and administered the drug for his ongoing pain. The nurse gave the patient 2.5 mL (50 mg) of liquid oxycodone, a volume that she was more familiar with giving, and then left for the break.

When the covering nurse went to check on AH, she found him unconscious. A code blue was called. Naloxone was given to the patient and, fortunately, he responded well. He was transferred to the intensive care unit for continuous infusion of naloxone and close monitoring. By the next morning, the patient recovered to his baseline functioning with no apparent adverse effects.

What are the root causes of this adverse drug event and how would you work with this team to design a new process to prevent errors such as this from happening again?

LEARNING OBJECTIVES

Upon completion of this chapter, the student shall be able to:

- Describe the current landscape of medication errors in the United States.
- Identify the medication use process and potential associated causes of error in each step.
- Describe the theory of human error and what a culture of safety looks like.
- Identify strategies for preventing errors associated with look-alike sound-alike medications.

CHAPTER QUESTIONS

1. What are some of the most common sources of error in the medication use process?
2. How do practitioners identify the true source of an adverse drug event?
3. How do institutions systematically address patient safety and work to solve problems when they occur in the medication use process?
4. Why is it important to measure safety?

INTRODUCTION

Medication safety continues to be a priority in health care. In hospitals alone, over 700,000 emergency department visits and 120,000 hospitalizations are the result of adverse drug events (ADEs) (Cullen et al., 1995; Budnitz, et al., 2006). This results in a financial impact of up to $3.5 billion in extra medical costs annually (Institute of Medicine, 2006). This estimate may not completely account for costs associated with readmissions, malpractice and litigation, or other injuries to patients as the result of ADEs. Further, this doesn't include the impact ADEs have in the community setting where data is even harder to track.

Even though research on the cost and causes of ADEs has been reported for years in the literature, the problem was brought to the attention of a larger audience in the year 2000 in a series of reports by the Institute of Medicine (IOM). "To Err is Human," "Crossing the Quality Chasm," and "Preventing Medication Errors," sought to highlight, outline, and address the rampant problem of medication errors, the barriers preventing improvement in patient safety, and the strategies that need to be implemented to make medication use safer.

Safety is an incredible challenge in health care today. It is more complex than just making sure the right patients get the right medications. It is a journey that requires the combined efforts of interdisciplinary teams focused on preventing harm. Fortunately, there are also many tools and resources to help guide professionals on their journey toward creating a culture of safety.

In order to create a culture of safety for the medication use process, it is essential for practitioners to know and understand key terminology. These include:

Adverse Drug Event (ADE)

Any untoward medical occurrence that may present during treatment with a pharmaceutical product but which does not necessarily have a causal relationship with this treatment. It may be associated with inappropriate use of a drug or due to other confounders that occur during drug therapy that are not necessarily caused by the pharmacology of the drug itself. (World Health Organization, 1969; World Health Organization, 2005; Bates et al., 1995a; Edwards, 2000)

Adverse Drug Reaction (ADR)

An unwanted, undesirable effect of a medication that occurs during usual clinical use (World Health Organization, 1969; World Health Organization, 2005; American Society of Health-System Pharmacists, 1995; Edwards, 2000)

Medication Error

Any *preventable event* that may cause or lead to inappropriate medication use or patient harm while the medication is in the control of the healthcare professional, patient, or consumer. Events may be related to prescribing, labeling, packaging, compounding, dispensing, or administering the drug. (Bates et al., 1995a; NCC MERP, n.d.a; Nebeker, 2004)

THEORY OF HUMAN ERROR

The "Theory of Human Error" is a foundational patient safety concept. Developed in large part by the psychologist James Reason, human error theory notes that when humans work in a system there is always a risk for error and mistakes. This risk is ever-present and cannot be eliminated completely; however, by employing various strategies, many of these errors can be captured and potential harm mitigated. Reason defines human error as, "the failure of planned actions to achieve their desired ends—without the intervention of some unforeseeable event" (Reason, 1997; Reason, 1990). Human error can happen in the planning stage, during storage, or the execution of activities. Failures in the storage or execution stages are generally regarded as *slips* and *lapses*, while failures in planning are known as *mistakes*. A slip is an activity that was not completed according to the plan. Most often, slips are "attention" failures resulting from either a compromised mental state (i.e., stress, distraction) or misperception (i.e., reading a medication label incorrectly). Conversely, a lapse is forgetting to carry out an action step completely. As such, lapses tend to be failures of memory and occur frequently with interruption. An example of a lapse would be neglecting to counsel a patient on his or her new medication. Finally, mistakes result from incorrectly assessing the problem or proper next step, as well as when the right action is applied at the wrong time or in the wrong process.

As will be described later in this chapter, human errors can occur throughout the various steps in the medication use system. As demonstrated in **Figure 7-1**, these errors are most likely to occur when there is a confluence of three key factors: (1) when an individual makes a mistake, (2) the system subsequently fails, and (3) high-risk procedures are used. For instance, administering an intravenous (IV) medication to a patient is a high-risk procedure. Now, let's assume the nurse administering the medication misreads the label. Then, the nurse scans the medication, but the barcode doesn't scan correctly. As a result, the nurse in this example administers the wrong medication to the patient, potentially resulting in serious harm. This example is a simplified version of errors that occur daily in health systems throughout the world, representing the danger when individuals and systems fail in the process of high-risk procedures.

The example above can also be illustrated in Reason's famous "Swiss cheese model" of human error (Reason, 1997; Reason, 1990). As shown in **Figure 7-2**, the Swiss cheese model is based on the premise that each process step in a system is prone to some varying likelihood of error. Take, for instance, the process of packing for a vacation. One may have a very systematic packing strategy: shoes then shirts, then sunscreen. Yet, because of a system failure (maybe a distracting phone call during the packing process), the sunscreen is forgotten. Thus, this process step failed and an

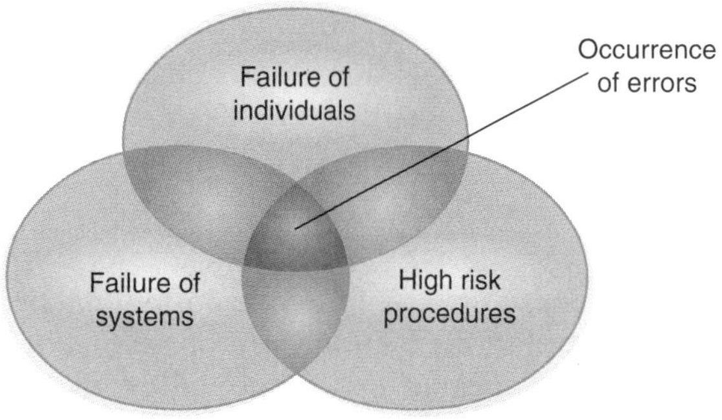

Figure 7-1 Factors Influencing Errors.

Data from Reason J. Human Error. Cambridge, UK. Cambridge University Press; 1990.

error occurred. These failures, which are inherent in each step of any process, are represented by the holes in each piece of Swiss cheese. The pieces of cheese all align perfectly for the potential error to result in an actual event.

Given this model for error, there are two broad strategies for preventing and mitigating errors. First, prevent the initial source of the error. This is not always possible given the desired outcome. Referring back to the packing example, the sunscreen is an essential component of a tropical vacation and cannot be removed from the process. However, if the vacation instead was to a destination that didn't require sun protection, this item could be removed entirely from the process; therefore, not forgotten. The second, and more commonly used, strategy is to find and fix the system problems. In this case, additional pieces of Swiss cheese are added, and the holes in each piece are made smaller. In other words, additional process steps are included, and strategies are employed to decrease the probability for failure at each step. Examples of failure reduction

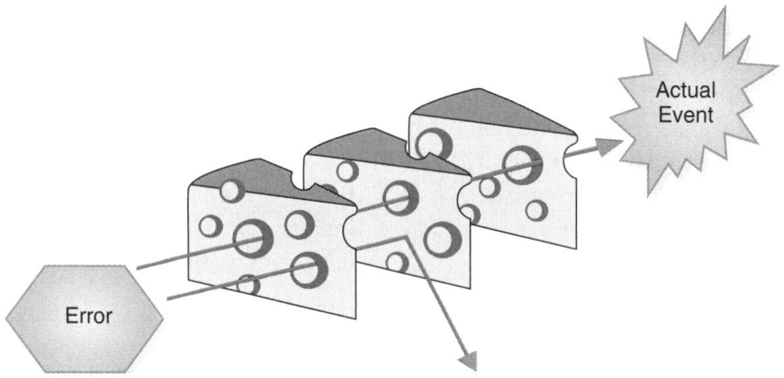

Figure 7-2 Swiss Cheese Model of Human Error.

Reason J. Managing the Risks of Organizational Accidents. Burlington, VT: Ashgate Publishing Company. 1997.

strategies may include: protocols, checklists, enhanced communication among pertinent individuals (e.g., patient, physician, nurse, pharmacist), and increased access to important information. Subsequently, these actions decrease the likelihood that all the holes will align, reducing the overall system's potential for harm (Reason, 1997; Reason, 1990).

Thinking of healthcare processes as multiple pieces of Swiss cheese with holes representing potential for harm to the system is the predominant contextual model for "systems thinking." Systems thinking requires the evaluation of the whole process rather than focusing on just one step or person. This approach forces one to consider everyone and anything that impacts the system since all process parts are interrelated. In systems thinking, adverse outcomes are comprised of both *active failures* and *latent failures*. Active failures are the human mistakes, while latent failures are at-risk situations (or holes in cheese) that have predisposed the system to having active failures becoming adverse events. When employing systems thinking, one understands that latent failures will always be present in a process. The entire system must be evaluated to ensure all identified points of failure can be reduced or eliminated altogether.

CULTURE OF SAFETY

Ensuring that an organization consistently employs systems thinking requires a positive patient safety culture. *Culture* is defined as a way of thinking, behaving, or working that exists in a place or organization (Merriam Webster, n.d.). In other words, culture is, "the way we do things." Therefore, patient safety culture in an organization is a collection of shared beliefs and attitudes regarding the reduction of patient harm. Prior to the 1990s, most organizations had a "punitive culture." This type of patient safety culture involved "punishment," and focused solely on the active failures of individuals, regardless of the potential latent, systems, and other related issues present during the error. This type of culture expected human perfection, and dissuaded the reporting and learning from adverse events. Although this model still exists today, most organizations recognize punitive culture as counterproductive when improving patient safety. By the mid-1990s, many healthcare institutions were shifting from a culture of blame and penalty to one that was blame-free and non-punitive. This type of patient safety culture became known as "non-punitive." In this model, human fallibility was recognized as an inevitable threat to patient safety. Organizations that employed this model focused on the theory of human error and used systems thinking to improve patient care processes. Unfortunately, there were still problems with addressing those individuals that behaved recklessly, endangering the patient, but now not being held accountable for dangerous actions. A model was needed to manage those few people who acted maliciously or were under the influence of substances during an adverse event. Today, "just culture," or a culture of accountability, recognizes that most errors result from systems failures, both active and latent. Hence, the focus is on improving the system rather than punishing the individual. Yet, just culture also reinforces the need for a defined line separating acceptable and unacceptable behavior. This balanced approach is considered a best practice in patient safety culture (Marx, 2001).

Creating and sustaining a positive culture of patient safety continues to be one of the biggest challenges and essential changes facing the current healthcare system (Leape et al., 2009; Nieva & Sorra, 2003). There is a growing belief that an institution's ability to avoid harm will only be accomplished through creating a culture of safety among staff (Nieva & Sorra, 2003). In 2001, the IOM published *Crossing the Quality Chasm: A New Health System for the 21st Century*. Within this report, IOM stated, "the biggest challenge to moving toward a safer health system is changing

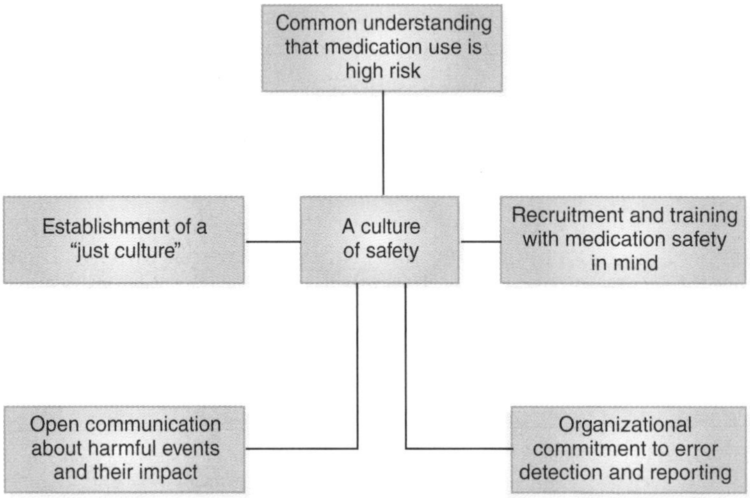

Figure 7-3 A Model of the Culture of Safety.

Data from Nieva V. F., Sorra J. Safety culture assessment: a tool for improving patient safety in healthcare organizations. *Qual Saf Health Care*, 2003;12: ii17-ii23.

the culture from one of blaming individuals for errors to one in which errors are treated not as personal failures, but as opportunities to improve the system and prevent harm," suggesting that it is imperative for institutions to create a strong safety culture that will encourage safe medication use practices among staff.

As healthcare organizations realize the importance of establishing a culture of patient safety, there is an increased demand for ways to assess the influential factors of this culture. Determining these factors is essential in first understanding a culture before attempting to improve it. Safety culture surveys can be used to identify areas for improvement in patient safety (Nieva & Sorra, 2003). In the United States, the Agency for Healthcare Research and Quality (AHRQ) created the Hospital Survey on Patient Safety Culture (HSOPSC). This survey was designed by AHRQ in 2004 to help hospitals evaluate their own culture of safety. AHRQ included multiple aspects of patient safety into their survey, as it assesses hospital staff opinions about patient safety issues, medical errors, and event reporting. Elements identified as important to establishing a safe culture are presented in **Figure 7-3**. This information is relevant to pharmacists and other health professionals seeking to improve the culture of safety at an organization.

MEDICATION USE PROCESS

The medication use process is broadly identified as the complete network of interactions spanning acquisition of the medications to be used to the monitoring and follow up after administering them. While this large view is helpful for contemplating the far reaching implications of the medication process, there are five core steps in the medication use process that are the focus of much work in patient safety and will serve as the foundation for further discussion in this chapter. Medication safety, therefore, is ensuring that all five components of this process provide the most benefit to the patient with the least risk of harm. In **Figure 7-4**, the five steps in this process are illustrated as well as the links that occur between each step. These arrows, or links, represent more than just moving from one step to another; they also represent "handoffs" between health providers and patients at any number of care settings. Additionally, the arrows in the diagram represent

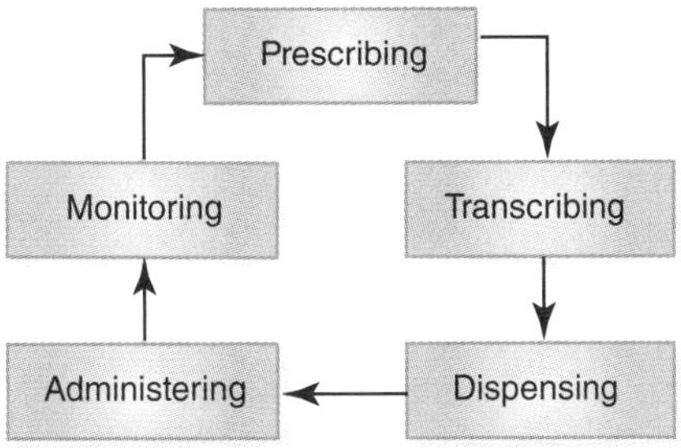

Figure 7-4 The Medication Use Process.

Data from Bates D. W. et al. Incidence of adverse drug events and potential adverse drug events. *JAMA*, 1995;274(1):29–34.

the communication that must occur with the intent to create a level of clarity. When the process is effective, patients have the opportunity to experience positive outcomes with their medication therapy with decreased risks of adverse events.

Prescribing

The first step identified in Figure 7-4 is the prescribing process. Approximately 39% of observed errors in the medication use process occur at this step (Bates et al., 1995b). It is important to note that observation of errors during this process is not an indictment of the prescriber or his or her knowledge and ability to prescribe medication therapy, but rather an evaluation of the prescribing process and how it might lead to error. Examples of the most common sources of error associated with the prescribing process are in **Figure 7-5**. If the individual prescriber is not at fault, what is the etiology of many prescribing errors? Errors generally do not occur as a result of inferior clinical knowledge, but rather how the information is communicated or translated into clinical practice. Examples include:

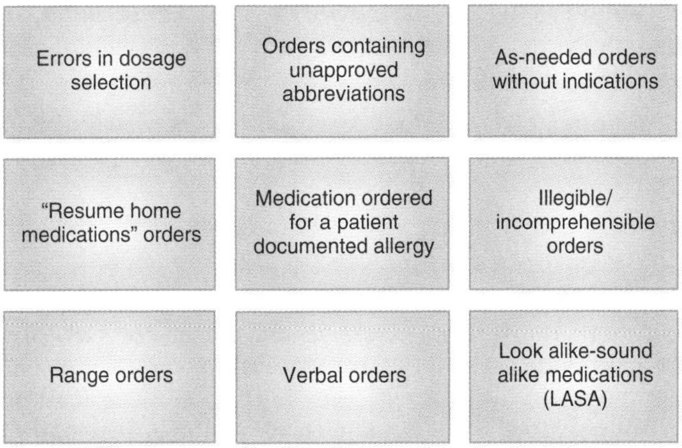

Figure 7-5 Examples of Errors Occurring in Prescribing in the Medication Use Process.

Data from Cohen M. Medication Errors. 2nd Ed.

Errors in dosage selection. This may be a result of ambiguous prescription order sets, which are a series of medication orders which create confusion due to how they are visually represented resulting in difficulty for the prescriber as to how to order them correctly or to pharmacy and nursing as to what the parameters for correct dispensing or administration are. Oftentimes, these manifest as several different formulations, concentrations, routes, and frequencies for the same medication all in close proximity to each other on a page with little or no means of differentiating which orders are to be prescribed for the patient. Additional opportunities arise in dosage selection with newly approved medications, or newly approved dosing regimens for conditions associated with preexisting medications.

Unapproved abbreviations. Whether handwritten or typed, shortened words or phrases can easily be misunderstood. A complete discussion on unapproved abbreviations occurs later in this chapter.

PRN orders without indications. An example of a PRN order is: acetaminophen 650 mg every 4 hours as needed. What does "as needed" mean? As needed for pain? What kind of pain? For fever? What is the threshold for fever? 100°F? 101°F? Ambiguity with PRN orders can lead to variation in the type of care provided to patients, as well as variation in how patients may self-medicate at home.

Resume home medications. This example is very specific to the location of the health system setting, but this type of error can easily be extrapolated to other care settings. What medications was a patient taking at home? Did changes in therapy occur that would affect home medication use? What if there are medications that represent a duplication of therapy for current medications? What if the patient is uncertain or dishonest about home medications?

Documented allergy. Imagine if the allergy information is unavailable to the prescriber. Would the prescriber be able to make sound clinical judgment during prescribing?

Illegible orders. Handwriting can be interpreted differently. For some health providers, there may be hesitation to call for clarification of an order from the prescriber. While many practitioners may take for granted the use of electronic prescribing, electronic medical records (EMRs), and many other forms of technology, utilization of these technologies is far from 100% nationally (Hsiao, 2014; Charles, 2015). Handwritten orders remain within the healthcare system and misinterpreting them remains a common source of error.

Range orders. An example of this error is acetaminophen 1 to 2 tablets every 4 to 6 hours. Is it 1 tablet every 6 hours or 2 tablets every 4 hours? Depending on the interpretation of the order, there can be variation in the amount administered and the frequency given. Orders should be clear, precise, and unambiguous. In this example, the order should be clarified and the circumstances identified for the amount administered (1 or 2 tablets) and frequency (4 or 6 hours).

Verbal orders. A verbal order may be clear, but practitioners may have difficulty processing what they were told. Interruptions are inevitable and providers are interrupted frequently throughout the day.

Transcribing

The next step in the medication use process is transcription, or translating a communicated message into a medication order. Transcribing errors account for about 12% of medication errors in the medication use process (Bates et al., 1995b). Medication orders are sent by prescribers and received by other practitioners in different ways, including verbally. While it may seem unusual to have confusion regarding a verbal order, remember for a moment the child's game of telephone. In this game, one person would whisper a statement into the ear of the person sitting next to him or her, and that person would pass it along and so forth until the final person in the chain would announce the message. It was always humorous because the message was invariably wrong, often times to a truly laughable extent. Now imagine playing this game in a patient care area where a health care provider is responsible not only for the verbal message, but a ringing telephone, patient alarms, a pager, and other medical professionals vying for attention. Not only can it be difficult to translate a verbal order to a written order, it becomes exponentially more difficult with distractions in the work environment.

Transcription errors also can be exacerbated by the number of steps in the process prior to reducing a verbal message into a medication order. For example, a prescriber calls a nurse in response to a page and prescribes medication for a patient with acute pain. The nurse writes down the prescription in shorthand because a patient call light is going off at the time. He or she hangs up the phone, answers the patient's request, deciphers his or her notes regarding the order, and calls the pharmacy to relay the order. The pharmacist writes down what he or she hears the nurse say and then enters his or her note into the computer system. From the prescriber to the pharmacy, there are multiple opportunities for the introduction of error in this process.

Why are transcription errors so prevalent? Transcription is almost an entirely human process that requires interpretation in order to synthesize a medication order. Seventy-three percent of transcription errors are associated with mental slips, or mistakes, that can be attributed to any number of workplace stressors (Cohen, 2006). Common activities that lead to transcription errors are answering telephones, answering verbal requests for information, excessive workload, multiple alerts or alarms sounding, and poorly designed work processes.

Dispensing

Once the information is transcribed into an actionable medication order, the next step is to dispense it for administration. During this step of the process, 11% of all errors in the medication use process occur (Bates et al., 1995b). Of these errors, two-thirds of them reach the patient (Institute of Medicine, 2000). Dispensing medications is a crucial step in the medication use process and represents an opportunity for pharmacist intervention. This is where words and orders and electronic transmissions become tangible drug products that get labeled for the intended consumption of patients. Although a third of medication errors associated with dispensing are caught before reaching the patient, there is room for improvement. Dispensing is also not just a pharmacy function. Nurses, physicians, and other practitioners can dispense various agents from floor stock, as well as from automated dispensing cabinets placed on patient care units. Whether it is in a pharmacy sterile compounding area or in a medication room on a nursing unit, dispensing of medications in accordance with what was ordered can be a complex and error prone process.

There are many opportunities for error when dispensing medications. Each component of the dispensing process can have a profound impact on patient care. Medications that are dispensed to the wrong patient or a patient that receives an incorrect drug can have catastrophic outcomes. A dose of chemotherapy that has the wrong time on the label for administration can cause a delay of a time sensitive chemotherapeutic agent for hours or even days, potentially impacting the effectiveness of the regimen. Similarly, an error of omission, or a dose of medication that is not given can cause a patient to experience harm. Even when the right patient gets the right dose of the right medication, it does not mean it is safe. Giving wrong information or no information to a patient on how to use his or her medication can also lead to a medication error. For example, if a patient is discharged from the hospital with accurate discharge medication directions and a 30-day supply of medications, but offered no counseling on the medications, the likelihood that a patient will misuse any one or all of the medications becomes significantly higher.

At an acute care facility, the sterile compounding at the central pharmacy is responsible for only a proportion of total doses dispensed to patients. Many medications are dispensed by nurses. Medications may come from carts that are prefilled daily by the central pharmacy or from stock bottles in supply areas, depending on the institution. One technologic approach that is commonly used in hospitals is automated dispensing cabinets or ADCs. ADCs alleviate the need for large stock bottles or the daily filling of medication carts and act as "intelligent vending machines" for patient medication storage and dispensing. In addition, profile dispensing can occur with the use of ADCs. With profile dispensing, a nurse can only withdraw medications for one patient at a time and only for patients for which she is responsible. Using this approach reduces the number of medications that a nurse can access at any given point of time. When medications are accessed, nurses obtain medications from individual pockets or locations to reduce visual distractions and avoid look-alike and sound-alike medication confusion. Other functions with this technology include the ability to sync with a pharmacy medication management system. This function provides information regarding when: a dose is dispensed for any patient in the facility, medications are dispensed on override, and a medication is accessed without a specific patient profile. The ADC interface system creates a miniature pharmacy that is only accessed for one patient and by one medication at a time—thereby decreasing the opportunity for error during medication restocking and removal.

Administration

Once the medication is dispensed, the next step is to administer it to a patient. Administration errors account for 38% of documented medication errors (Bates et al., 1995b). There are similarities between common causes of dispensing errors and administration errors (**Figure 7-6**). Once a medication is dispensed, any confusion in the dispensing step is likely carried forward to the administration step of the medication use process. For example, if a medication is dispensed for the wrong patient, it may very well likely be administered to the wrong patient as well. If a medication is dispensed and the label documents an incorrect rate of infusion, there is a chance that the medication will be infused at the incorrect rate as well.

When analyzing administration errors, one area that is a focus are workarounds (Koppel, 2008). While workarounds are prevalent in virtually all areas of the medication use process, the act

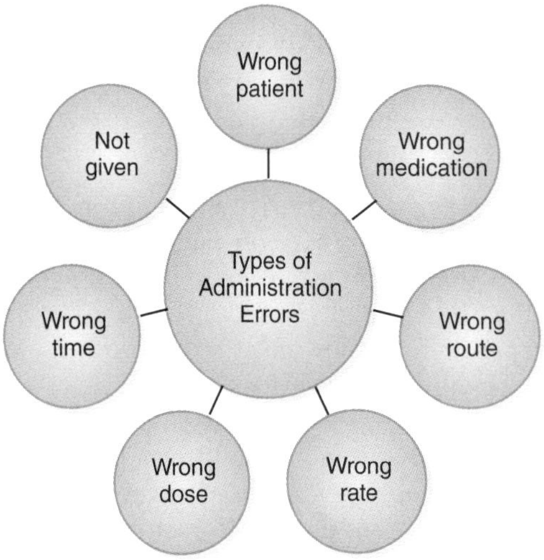

Figure 7-6 Examples of Errors Occurring in Administration in the Medication Use Process.

Data from Cohen M. Medication Errors. 2nd Ed.

of administration and the level of interaction with health information technology lend itself to additional stress and likelihood of workarounds. Workarounds are classified into three main areas: (1) omission of process steps, (2) sequencing of steps, and (3) unauthorized process steps (Koppel, 2008). Examples of each category include:

Omission of process steps: This category includes anytime that a nurse avoids completing the process of preparing medications for administration. In the case of bar code medication administration (BCMA) technology, omission includes avoiding scanning medications all together to only scanning one tablet when the prescribed dose is for two tablets.

Sequencing of steps: An example in this category is when a medication is not scanned immediately prior to administration, therefore, interrupting the sequence of events that is supposed to ensure patient safety. A situation that illustrates this kind of error is when a dose is scanned at 1300, but not given until 1400, thus avoiding the safety features offered by BCMA scanning.

Unauthorized steps: Errors in this category are ones that are contrary to policy of BCMA use and involve the intentional disabling of activated safety features built into the scanners or the scanning software itself. Examples include disabling of audible alarms or supplemental pop-up (alerts), resulting in the illusion to the practitioners of being able to scan more rapidly.

Monitoring

Finally, the act of monitoring a patient while on their medication therapy regimen is vital. Currently, there are no reliable reports in the literature on the frequency of errors in this step of the process. However, it is known that these errors occur and the impact of poor monitoring and patient follow up is seen in patient outcomes. One area that serves as an indication of the impact of patient monitoring is hospital readmission rates. Readmissions occurring within 30 days of initial discharge are a metric tracked by hospitals and used as a quality indicator. While this metric is influenced by many factors, medication use often is implicated (Budnitz et al., 2011; Ruiz et al., 2008). According to the Centers for Medicare and Medicaid Services (CMS), 20% of all discharged Medicare patients will be readmitted within 30 days, and as many as 35% will be readmitted within 90 days (Jencks et al., 2009; Beckett, Sheehan, & Redden, 2012). These events cost Medicare over $17 billion annually.

ADEs associated with a failure to monitor drug therapy can be particularly dangerous. When patients are hospitalized, they are prescribed medications that may be different from the ones they are taking at home. Upon discharge, they will be written prescriptions to continue some of these medications or to discontinue taking others. Upon discharge, patients fill their new prescriptions, often at their local community pharmacy, and may take these medications in addition to their old ones. In some instances, this may result in duplication of therapeutic effect leading to an ADE. For example, if a patient takes both the new and old medication, this results in a doubling of the dose of a medication. In the case of hypertension, the patient can experience hypotension that can lead to a fall requiring hospitalization and potential surgery. In this instance, the patient was taking medications that were prescribed for him or her at the dose they were prescribed. The sources of error are as a result of lack of patient monitoring and follow up to ensure that the patient understood the new medication therapy regimen.

ERROR PRONE DRUG PRODUCTS

Many drug names appear to look alike and/or their packaging looks similar. These similarities can create confusion and lead to errors associated with incorrect product selection in each step of the medication use process. For example, read the following sentence:

I cnat bvleiee taht I can aulaclty uesdtannrd waht I am rdnaieg.

Most likely, the message was deciphered as "I can't believe that I can actually understand what I am reading." People only require the first and last letters of the word to remain in the same position in the word and that all necessary letters are present in order to quickly identify the correct word (Shillcock, 2000). The human brain can compensate for jumbled letters in a word, which can lead to incorrect identification of medication names. Look at the following list for an example:

hydralazine, hydrocodone, hydromorphone, hydroxyzine, hydrochlorothiazide

Based on this list, one can see the potential for confusion. If a patient is prescribed hydralazine 25 mg, and it is stored on a shelf next to the hydroxyzine 25 mg, the opportunity for a dispensing and subsequent administration error is significant. In addition to the spelling of a medication, how the medication name is written on product package can also be a source of error. In **Figure 7-7**, there are two different ophthalmic medications. The packaging for these two medications is identical, as are the color of the font and the orientation of the text.

Prevention Strategies

One way to prevent errors associated with look-alike and sound-alike names is to create an emphasis on the dissimilarities in the drug names (Filik et al., 2004; Filik et al., 2006). This method is called tall man (or mixed case) lettering and it involves using capital letters to emphasize and distinguish different parts of similar looking drug names. Look once again at the example of two medications from above, but with tall man lettering applied:

hydrALAZINE, hydrOXYzine

Application of this methodology must be uniform in order to be effective. The Food and Drug Administration (FDA) and the Institute for Safe Medication Practices (ISMP) have collaborated to create an FDA approved list of medication names spelled using tall man lettering. This list is available on the FDA website on their Drug Safety page and may be downloaded, reproduced, and used within an institution (http://www.fda.gov/Drugs/DrugSafety/MedicationErrors/ucm164587.htm).

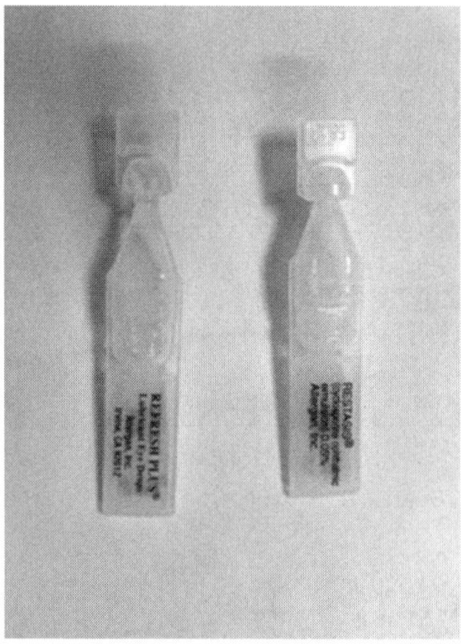

Figure 7-7 Error Prone Packaging.

Photo courtesy of Kyle E. Hultgren (author).

Another tool available to help prevent errors is an unapproved abbreviations list. When practitioners abbreviate words or medication names, they may not be used uniformly across an institution, therefore, leaving the abbreviation subject to the interpretation of another practitioner. For example, when prescribing insulin, the word "units" should not be abbreviated as "u" but instead the full word should be written. If a practitioner wrote for 10u of insulin, it could easily look like the number "100" when handwritten and a patient could accidentally receive a ten-fold overdose of a medication. There are many tables of unapproved abbreviations that have been endorsed, which are available online, with many institutions favoring the FDA and ISMP's list of unapproved abbreviations, or abbreviations that should be avoided in practice (http://www.ismp.org/tools/errorproneabbreviations.pdf).

In addition, practitioners should physically segregate similarly worded drug names in dispensing areas and ADCs. Placing these medications on different shelves or incompletely different areas or drawers will help to decrease errors associated with product selection.

ROOT CAUSE ANALYSIS AND FAILURE MODE EFFECTS ANALYSIS

Root Cause Analysis

When errors occur in the medication use process, it is imperative to understand the true nature of why they happened. It is human nature to want to assign blame for an error to a person, but this does not foster a culture of safety in an institution. Professionals need to feel safe in discussing events in an open manner in order to address and prevent events in the future. Root cause analysis (RCA) is utilized to obtain a complete understanding of why errors occur. The goal of RCA is to discover what happened, why it happened, and how to prevent it from happening again. Answering these three questions enables a team to shift the focus from punishment of individuals to prevention of patient harm (Veterans' Administration, 2015).

RCA is a retrospective tool to analyze facts about events that occurred in the past and form conclusions about why these events happened. RCA is not an individual activity that can be undertaken by a single person, rather a team of multidisciplinary professionals should be convened in order to ensure complete data collection and diversity of thought. The importance of data collection cannot be overstated. In order to make accurate assessments about the true nature of an event, a thorough understanding of the process is necessary (National Center for Patient Safety). One common pitfall that can occur when conducting a RCA is to only gather data that supports a predetermined conclusion or perception of what the root cause may be.

After the facts surrounding an event are collected, the next task is to establish causality. There are many tools that teams can use, but they all focus on understanding why an event happened. One of the most common methods is called a five "why" analysis (Veterans' Administration, 2015). It involves asking the question "why" five successive times with the goal of ultimately arriving at a root cause statement. A root cause statement is the fundamental explanation that establishes the causality of an event. Put another way, it is the true reason why something has happened. While it may be necessary to ask "why" more than five times (or possibly even fewer) in order to ascertain the true root cause, five iterations is the target for teams to pursue. An example of how this tool can be used effectively is in **Exhibit 7-1**. There are many keys to success when conducting a RCA, including:

Stick to the facts: When answering "why" to each question, do not make any assumptions. Always answer factually and with data, if it is available.

Exhibit 7-1 Example of a Five "Why" Analysis

PROBLEM: BCMA scan rates are below 90%

Why? → Nurses feel like there is not enough time to scan

Why? → They spend too much time searching for supplies

Why? → Supply room is messy, disorganized, and poorly stocked

Root Cause: Nurses spend too much time on tasks associated with organization and bookkeeping rather than nursing activities.

Solution: Create a better physical space for supplies that dramatically reduces the time wasted associated with looking for supplies.

Remember, it is "why" not "who": Questions should not blame individuals. In the example in **Exhibit 7-1**, it would be tempting to stop conducting the RCA and make the conclusion that low scan rates means nursing competency in this area is low and they must all be retrained on the technology. This false conclusion would potentially make the problem worse. Taking additional time for additional training likely would continue to strain the nurses' time that is available for scanning. Blaming individuals rather than analyzing the system can lead to an incorrect conclusion and an unsustainable solution.

Solve the right problem: Once the team has developed a root cause statement, the solution to the problem must address this statement directly. A solution that does not address a root cause will not be sustainable for the organization.

Failure Mode Effects Analysis

Another powerful tool for analyzing processes is failure mode effects analysis (FMEA). While RCA is a retrospective tool used to analyze a system after an event has already occurred, FMEA is used prospectively to predict where the greatest potential for errors may occur. Once these potential errors are identified, they are ranked to determine their significance and the likelihood of them happening. Mitigation strategies can be designed to prevent them from ever occurring (National Center for Patient Safety; National Coordinating Council for Medication Error Reporting and Prevention, n.d.b; DeRosier et al., 2002; VA NCPS, 2015). FMEA is used as a method for prospectively designing highly reliable processes in high-risk areas. The steps in conducting a FMEA are:

Step 1: Define the Problem

In order to adequately study a process, a specific focus must first be determined by the team. In this step, a project scope is identified, including what the team will and will not work on. Resources to accomplish the work are also identified.

Step 2: Describe the Process

The team develops a process flow map of the issue being studied. Process flow maps are visual tools to help people to see each step in a process, their chronology, and how each step connects to one another. This visual tool will serve as the baseline in understanding what is happening in the system.

Step 3: Conduct a Hazard Analysis

Once the process flow map is complete, the team brainstorms ways that the process may breakdown or fail at each individual step. This becomes the list of potential failure modes. Each failure mode is then given a numerical score based upon the probability that the proposed event could happen and the severity of the outcome should it come to fruition.

Step 4: Create and Act on a Plan

Each failure mode that achieves a high enough score should have a mitigation strategy created to prevent such errors from becoming a reality. The threshold for what constitutes a high enough score is a function of the scoring system the team is using and based upon a consensus decision by the team performing the analysis. One example, using the VA NCPS FMEA tool, would be a scale of possible results from 1 through 16 and anything earning greater than or equal to an 8 would merit further scrutiny (VA NCPS, 2015).

Step 5: Sustain and Evaluate the Strategy

Each mitigation strategy must be evaluated over time to ensure that it is still in place and being effective.

CONTINUOUS QUALITY IMPROVEMENT

Continuous Quality Improvement Principles

"Quality is not an act, it is a habit" –Aristotle

Improving the safety of healthcare processes requires a functional understanding of continuous quality improvement (CQI). CQI, as used in health care, can be defined as a "structured, organizational process for involving personnel in planning and executing a continuous flow of improvements to provide quality health care that meets or exceeds expectations" (McLaughlin & Kalazny, 2006). There are many CQI models and methods used today across various industries from aviation to manufacturing to health care. However, the most universally accepted and widely used model was developed by Walter Shewart, a statistician, in the 1930s. This CQI method, the *Plan-Do-Study-Act (PDSA)* (sometimes known as Plan-Do-Check Act—PDCA) cycle outlines four steps that can be continuously repeated to plan a process improvement, implement that improvement, study the results of the process change, and then modify and spread the improvement (**Figure 7-8**). W. Edwards Deming is credited with popularizing the PDSA tool, building on the concept, and introducing it to the Japanese post-World War II automotive industry (Deming, 1982). Subsequently, the PDSA cycle was adopted into health care as a standard method for the continual improvement of care and other health-related processes.

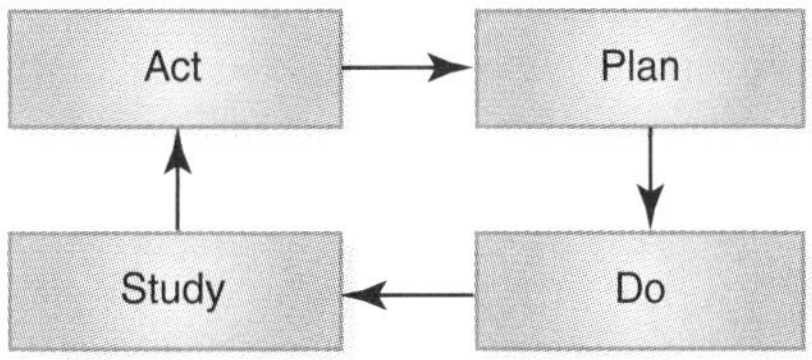

Figure 7-8 Continuous Quality Improvement Process.

Data from Institute for Healthcare Improvement. Model for Improvement. http://www.ihi.org/resources/Pages/HowtoImprove/default.aspx. Accessed July 2015.

PDSA CYCLE

Healthcare organizations commonly use PDSA as the foundation of their CQI efforts. The Institute for Healthcare Improvement (IHI) has adopted this model, integrating the step-wise approach into various patient safety educational and skills development courses. The IHI model has two phases when using PDSA. First, the project aim, measures of success, and necessary improvements are identified. Effective quality improvement requires setting clear aims; these goals should be specific, measurable, attainable, reliable, and timely (SMART). The key to effective planning is to select appropriate measures of success to determine whether effective improvement has resulted from a selected change. Importantly, teams participating in CQI should identify both qualitative and quantitative data sources, focusing on improvement trends over time rather than singular data points.

When conducting these types of projects, the focus remains on the desired improvements and not on the measures alone. Once the specific goals have been set and measures of success have been established, the next step is to identify potential changes. Ensuring that the health professionals that work within the system being evaluated are also those involved in the improvement process is essential. Changes that eliminate waste, improve process flow, increase safety, and enhance efficiency should take priority. Finally, the one change that will have greatest impact on the process is selected. For the second phase of the improvement model, the PDSA cycle should be used to test and spread the change.

Plan

As the first step in the PDSA cycle, an action plan for implementation of the change is developed. Often, a pilot study is needed to prove the change will have positive impact. This is especially important when patient care is involved in CQI efforts as small tests of change typically will be sufficient to prove success and expansion, while minimizing the potential for patient harm if a project fails. The plan should include duration, location, the measures developed previously, and an operational plan to guide implementation. Often, education assessments and tools are developed in the Plan step to ensure that all involved parties are adequately prepped, educated, and trained regarding the new change. An effective educational plan is multidisciplinary and considers the potential impact of the change on staff, patients, and their families. As the action plan is designed, a timeline should be created along with "check-steps" and a list of accountable parties. The plan will be used throughout the cycle to guide progress and clarify questions.

Do

The next step is "Do." During this phase, the action plan developed in the "Plan" step is implemented. Often, successful implementation depends heavily on having the right team members collaborating and communicating effectively. During the course of "doing," problems and unexpected observations are documented. Data should be collected according to the measure(s) selected as part of the action plan. To increase the likelihood of successful implementation, feedback should be provided regularly to all team members and staff involved in the CQI effort.

Study

Once implemented, the change needs to be analyzed during the "Study" step. Data collected should be compared to baseline measures and reconciled with what was predicted to happen. Once analyzed, the data will help the team determine whether the study impact was positive, negative, or resulted in no change. Additional quality indicator data can be added here if necessary, potentially pulled from information already collected. Barriers to change should be identified so that they can be targeted in next steps or cycles of improvement. Reflection on implementation will subsequently lead to revisions to the action plan for future change.

Act

As the final step in the PDSA Cycle, the team will use the information assessed in the previous steps. Based on the "Study" step, a change may need to be adapted, modified, and retested. If successful, the change should be adopted, and expansion of the changes into the organization should be considered. If unsuccessful, the change may need to be abandoned, and a new idea selected and tested using the PDSA Cycle. Continued monitoring and data analysis will need to be completed in order to sustain and spread the desired changes. Once the desired goals have been achieved and sustained, individuals responsible for maintaining the improvement should be assigned and held accountable using completion plans with data deadlines, reporting transparency, and feedback mechanisms.

Obviously, yet notably, the PDSA Cycle is a cyclical model for improvement. Hence, once the data has been acted on in the fourth step, the process should be repeated to develop a new "Plan." This new action plan will then be the foundation for the next round, as the team goes through the entire cycle again. Often, many PDSA cycles will be conducted at the same time with each one representing a potential positive change within an organization. With every turn of the PDSA Cycle, the process will continually improve resulting in higher quality care.

Additional Methods and Tools

There are a variety of tools that can be very useful while implementing the PDSA cycle or other CQI methods. Flowchart, Cause, and Effect Diagram (otherwise known as Fishbone or Ishikawa), Run Chart, Control Chart, Pareto Chart, RCA, and Failure Modes and Effects Analysis (as described earlier) are all tools used in performance improvement efforts. Flowcharts are constructed using various symbols (squares, diamonds, circles) and are a powerful visual tool commonly used in CQI. Otherwise known as Process Maps or Process Flow Maps, Flowcharts visually depict the flow of a process, helping those working on a particular system understand a particular sequence of events within a system. Further, Flowcharts can be effective in helping identify problem areas that can be targeted for potential change. When building a Flowchart, those individuals most familiar with the process should create it, reflecting current understanding rather than the desired or best practice process.

In addition to PDSA, the *Lean Production System* and *Six Sigma* methods are also used in CQI activities. The Lean Production System (Lean) is a method that focuses on the value of a particular process and seeks to maximize the uninterrupted flow of that value to the end customer. Unnecessary or wasteful steps that aren't of value are removed to make the resulting process more "lean" and efficient. Six Sigma is a data-driven method that focuses on customer satisfaction and defect (error) reduction. Specifically, Six Sigma refers to six standard deviations from the expected or desired process result, which in health care translates to reducing the error associated with a specific process to no more than 3.4 defects or errors per million opportunities or activities.

Measuring Safety

It was Albert Einstein who said "Not everything that can be counted counts, and not everything that counts can be counted." In health care today, measuring the relative quality and safety of patient care is essential. Data measurement, collection, reporting, and analysis are vital to an organization's continuous quality improvement efforts. As discussed earlier in this chapter, the purpose behind measurement is to learn and improve. Ultimately, measurement serves as a mechanism for feedback and accountability. Importantly, health professionals are more likely to report data on errors and events if that information is transparent and used to improve practice (Classen & Metzger, 2003). There are various sources of metrics for determining the relative safety and/or quality of a particular healthcare process. As such, it is important to pull from a variety of data sources in order to obtain a robust and complete picture of medication safety (Meyer-Massetti et al., 2011). Data may include: (1) voluntary error reports submitted through formal reporting programs; (2) automated trigger tools (i.e., using naloxone as a marker for opioid overdose for instance); (3) direct observation of errors; (4) reviewing electronic or manual patient charts; and (5) data from technology applications and hardware, including smart pumps, automated dispensing cabinets, and EMRs. There are strengths and weaknesses with each of these data sources, which is why multiple sources should be used. Multiple measures of safety are necessary to obtain a more accurate assessment of safety in an organization. Three common data collection methods are (1) voluntary error reports, (2) trigger tools, and (3) direct observations.

Voluntary Error Reports

It is important to understand the gap between errors that are reported through a voluntary incident reporting system and the actual occurrence of events in an institution. The iceberg model of accidents and errors is often used to describe this difference visually. The part of the iceberg that can be seen is far smaller than what truly exists underneath the waterline shielded from view. Voluntary error reports can also be thought of this way. The number of incidents reported is what can be seen and acted upon. Typically, these are errors that cause significant harm. The majority of events, however, may be no-harm events or those that only cause minor harm. Many of the events that do not cause harm are known as near-misses and these go largely unseen and underreported. Literature suggests that voluntary error reporting captures only 10–20% of the actual total number of events. Therefore, voluntary error reporting data should be supplemented with information from other data sources (Battles, 2001). In reviewing error reports, it can be beneficial to have first-hand knowledge of the event. However, fear of blame in a poor safety culture and misrepresentation of certain facts surrounding the event may lead to inaccurate or under-reporting. Depending on the organization, it may be mandatory to report certain events. These mandatory reporting programs will be reviewed later in the chapter.

Trigger Tools

Developed and popularized by the IHI, automated trigger tools can be an effective source of safety and quality data. Trigger tools are used to "look for clues" retrospectively as to the incidence of particular errors without examining the actual event specifically. These triggers are indicators that poor quality care has occurred. Examples of triggers used can include: prothrombin time (PTT) greater than 100 seconds, international normalized ratio (INR) greater than 6, and blood glucose less than 50 mg/dL. Each data point that meets the criteria correlates to a higher likelihood of patient harm. To use a trigger tool, roughly 10 patient charts (completed, discharged at least 30 days prior to review, and coded) should be selected every two weeks. The specific trigger data can be manually identified or automated using various technology sources. The data is tallied and then presented in three formats: adverse events per 1,000 patient days, adverse events per 100 admissions, and percent of admissions with an adverse event. The most commonly used metric is "adverse events per 1,000 patient days." Absolute numbers of potential errors should be used rather than deferring to rates and percentages. In addition, this data should only be compared internally, and not between hospitals or institutions, as too many variables exist to make accurate comparisons. Trigger tools are useful because data can be monitored over time to identify trends and patterns that can be targeted for CQI efforts. When using this tool, the benefits should be balanced against the negatives, which include labor intensive data capture, retrospective sampling, and the likelihood for false positives.

Direct Observation

As the name suggests, direct observation is a method used to watch a care process as it unfolds, recording data to help identify errors in real-time. The direct observation concept was pioneered at Auburn University, and employs independent, trained observers to watch a medication administration take place and document the process with standardized forms. Typically, an observer will watch 50 to 100 doses be dispensed or administered, while documenting any observed findings. These notes then are reconciled against the original orders to determine if there are any discrepancies between the intended therapy and the medications actually given to the patient. These discrepancies are validated, categorized, and recorded as errors. These observations can be made routinely and, as resources allow, should be conducted frequently. Considered a "best practice" in medication error detection and reporting, the direct observation method helps identify trends, creating an objective, and quantitative set of safety data. Observations can be made quite often if an organization has resources available for it. Yet, this method can be resource intensive, and prone to the "Hawthorne effect" bias, as staff may change behavior if being watched.

When measuring patient safety, it's important for health-systems to benchmark, maintaining a willingness to share best practices with other similar institutions. Benchmarking enables organizations to use measures to answer key questions, such as: (1) Where are we now in this particular patient care process? and (2) Where do we want to be or what should our goal be? There are two types of benchmarking, internal and external.

Internal Benchmarking

Internal benchmarking occurs when an organization measures performance against previously recorded internal data. Benchmarking internally allows for comparison of timely (e.g., monthly, quarterly) data elements against themselves. The measures can be validated over time, and then used to support or dispute external benchmarking data. When comparing data internally, measures should be validated, and applied consistently over time. It is important to keep context when comparing data. For instance, the frequency of use of an INR trigger tool may be substantially higher in a cardiology unit when compared to that of a pediatric unit. One must be careful not to use internal data to misrepresent error frequency or trends.

External Benchmarking

External benchmarking is how an organization measures its own performance against like institutions. Additionally, an organization may externally benchmark to meet certain quality standards or regulatory requirements. In short, these comparisons aid organizations in assessing performance relative to competitors or best practice standards. Often, once reviewed, external benchmarks are developed into internal goals. Before comparing an institution to outside benchmarks, one must realize the data may not be as accurate as the data received internally. Often, external data are filtered or "scrubbed" before being shared. It is also very important to pick an appropriate comparison group. Bed size, geographic location, affiliation, specialty, and acuity mix should be considered when checking data externally. Inappropriate external benchmarking can lead to incorrect strategic planning and frustration within institutions.

Quality Measures

To maintain compliance with various federal and state payment and accreditation programs, organizations are required to collect and report various quality metrics. Many of these are obtained through specific programs and external benchmarking. The data then are tracked internally to facilitate CQI projects. Examples of key quality measures include, but are not limited to: deep vein thrombosis prevention, readmissions within 30 days of discharge, early delivery defined as less than 39 weeks gestation, catheter-associated urinary tract infections, postoperative hemorrhage, and central line infections. Some of these quality measures have been used to determine payment penalties and rewards in pay-for-performance programs, which are covered in other chapters within this textbook.

There are many organizations in the United States that develop quality measures, and seek to incorporate them into health-systems: Agency for Healthcare Research & Quality (AHRQ), CMS, MEDMARX ADEs, The Joint Commission, Food & Drug Administration, Patient Safety Organizations (PSOs), LeapFrog Group, National Patient Safety Foundation, the National Quality Forum, Pharmacy Quality Alliance, State Departments of Health, and State Boards of Medicine, Nursing, and Pharmacy.

Patient Safety, Quality, and Regulatory Organizations

There are a multitude of professional, regulatory and quality organizations that have a role in patient safety, quality improvement, and regulatory compliance. A Patient Safety Organization (PSO) is a specific designation provided by the AHRQ. The PSO designation was enacted as a result of the Patient Safety and Quality Improvement Act of 2005, which led to the development of rules enacted by the Department of Health and Human Services (HHS) and must be followed completely. These PSOs collect error reports, and provide protection to healthcare professionals who report patient safety issues. Specifically, PSOs protect against the discovery and release of sensitive error reporting data that could be used to initiate legal recourse. There are hundreds of patient safety, quality, and regulatory organizations, which all cannot be covered in detail here. With that said, there are a few of these organizations worth reviewing; more information can be found by visiting the specific organization's website.

National Patient Safety Foundation (NPSF): The vision of NPSF is to create a world where patients and those who care for them are free from harm. This organization has a significant educational mission, includes a membership division (American Society of Professionals in Patient Safety), and manages the Certified Professional in Patient Safety (CPPS) credential.

Institute for Healthcare Improvement (IHI): Founded by Don Berwick, MD, the vision of IHI is that everyone has the best care and health possible. To accomplish this, the mission of IHI is to improve health and health care worldwide. As discussed previously, IHI is notable for their CQI best practices and various other efforts to improve patient safety (IHI Open School, Global Trigger Tool)

Agency for Healthcare Research and Quality (AHRQ): Funded through the Federal Government as part of HHS, the mission of AHRQ is to make health care safer, higher quality, more accessible, equitable, and affordable. Further, the organization works within HHS and with other partners to make sure that evidence is understood and used. This organization provides grant funding and is a well-recognized source of literature on patient safety and quality.

Institute for Safe Medication Practices (ISMP): ISMP is one of the oldest and largest organizations focused on medication safety. Founded by Michael Cohen in 1994, ISMP's mission is to be the premier independent, patient safety organization leading the effort to prevent medication errors and ADEs. The organization works to advance patient safety worldwide by empowering the healthcare community, including consumers, to prevent medication errors. A few of ISMP's activities include: reviewing medication error reports and recommendation of improvements, publishing newsletters, and consulting.

Center for Medication Safety Advancement (CMSA): Established in 2010, CMSA is an academic-based "think tank" that seeks to "make safe medication use common practice." CMSA's vision is to be the center of excellence for the creation and dissemination of best known evidence for safe medication practices. The focus at CMSA is on research/innovation, engagement with community partners and regulatory agencies, and dissemination of best practices through education.

National Coordinating Council for Medication Error Reporting and Prevention (NCCMERP): At NCCMERP, the vision is that no patient will be harmed by a medication. This vision is accomplished by maximizing the safe use of medications and increasing awareness of medication errors through open communication, increased reporting and promotion of medication error prevention strategies. NCCMERP serves as a policy group that provides standards, definitions and statements, including a standard taxonomy of classifying medication errors (A through I classification system), an algorithm for classifying errors, and peer-reviewed council recommendations.

Accreditation and The Joint Commission

Accreditation is an important concept relating directly to the quality of care provided at a healthcare institution. Specifically, "accreditation is a method for ensuring an organization achieves and maintains high-quality patient care" (Larson & Saine, 2013). Patient safety is paramount for all accrediting bodies, and typically the accreditation process is voluntary. With that said, payers, including CMS, include proper accreditation as a condition for payment for services rendered to their covered beneficiaries. Therefore, in practice, although accreditation is officially voluntary, failure to participate will significantly limit financial viability.

There are three primary accreditation bodies that have been "deemed" by CMS to provide proper and acceptable accrediting standards; these are: The American Osteopathic Association, Det Norske Veritas (DNV) Health care, and The Joint Commission (TJC). The most widely known and used accrediting agency in the United States is TJC, which has had authority for the accreditation of healthcare institutions since 1965 (Larson & Saine, 2013). In addition to accrediting hospitals, TJC develops and maintains detailed accreditation standards for a variety of healthcare institutions (i.e., hospital, long-term care). TJC also develops National Patient Safety Goals to help guide national efforts surrounding major problem areas in health care. Finally, TJC reviews sentinel events, which are defined as, "any unexpected occurrence involving death or serious physical or psychological injury or risk thereof" (Larson & Saine, 2013). Specific information on sentinel events and the resulting alert bulletins can be found on TJC's website. A working understanding of current TJC accreditation standards, related NPSGs and Sentinel Event Alerts is important as efforts are undertaken to enhance the safety and quality of care in a healthcare institution.

CONCLUSION

As the medication use experts, pharmacists play an essential role in ensuring patient safety across the continuum of care. It is vital to understand an organization's points of high risk throughout the medication use system. Special consideration should be given to getting involved in the prevention and mitigation of harm associated with medication use. Becoming increasingly acquainted with, practicing, and systematically employing the tools and concepts presented in this chapter will support pharmacists in leading medication safety and quality efforts; ultimately, resulting in substantially improved patient care.

QUESTIONS FOR FURTHER DISCUSSION

1. Much focus is given to a systems focus, but is there ever an occasion whereby it is prudent to identify human error and attribute it to a person rather than a system?
2. What are some of the implications of openly discussing medication errors as a team?
3. How could a robust CQI program help enhance reporting of medication errors?
4. What roles do patients play in the medication use process and how does this influence patient safety?
5. With many competing priorities in patient care, how do you find time to redesign systems for improved patient safety?

KEY TOPICS AND TERMS

Adverse drug events
Adverse drug reactions
Medication errors
Medication use process
Theory of human error
Continuous quality improvement
Error reporting
Measuring safety
Culture of safety
Look-alike sound-alike medications
Tall man lettering
Unapproved abbreviations
Plan-Do-Study-Act (PDSA)
Root cause analysis (RCA)
Failure modes effects analysis (FMEA)
Quality measures
Benchmarking
Lean
Six Sigma

REFERENCES

Agency for Healthcare Research and Quality. (2013, July). *Hospital survey on patient safety culture.* Rockville, MD.

American Society of Health-System Pharmacists (ASHP). (1995). ASHP guidelines on adverse drug reaction monitoring and reporting. *American Journal of Health-System Pharmacy, 52*, 417–419.

Bates, D. W., Boyle, D. L., Vander Vliet, M. B., Schneider, J., Leape, L. (1995a). Relationship between medication errors and adverse drug events. *Journal of General Internal Medicine, 10*, 199–205.

Bates, D. W., Cullen, D. J., Laird, N., Petersen, L. A., Small, S. D., Servi D.,...Hallisey, R. (1995b). Incidence of adverse drug events and potential adverse drug events. *Journal of the American Medical Association, 274*(1), 29–34.

Battles, J. B. (2001). Disaster prevention: Lessons learned from the Titanic. *Baylor University Medical Center Proceedings, 14*:150–153.

Beckett, R. D., Sheehan, A. H., & Redden, J. G. (2012). Factors associated with reported preventable adverse drug events: A retrospective, case-control study. *Annals of Pharmacotherapy, 46*(5), 634–641.

Budnitz, D. S., Lovegrove, M. C., Shehab, N., et al. (2011). Emergency hospitalizations for adverse drug events in older Americans. *The New England Journal of Medicine, 365*, 2022–2012.

Budnitz, D. S., Pollock, D. A., Weidenbach, K. N., Mendelsohn, A. B., Schroeder, T. J., & Annest, J. L. (2006). National surveillance of emergency department visits for outpatient adverse drug events. *Journal of the American Medical Association, 296*, 1858–1866.

Charles, D., Gabriel, M., & Searcy, T. (2015, April). Adoption of electronic health record systems among U. S. non-federal acute care hospitals: 2008–2014. *ONC Data Brief; No. 23.* Washington DC: Office of the National Coordinator for Health Information Technology.

Classen, D., & Metzger, J. (2003). Improving medication safety: The measurement conundrum and where to start. *International Journal for Quality in Health Care, 15*, 141–147.

Cohen, M. (2006). *Medication errors* (2nd ed.). Washington, DC: American Pharmacists Association.

Cullen, D. J., Bates, D. W., Small, S. D., et al. (1995). The incident reporting system does not detect adverse drug events: A problem for quality improvement. *Journal on Quality Improvement, 21*(10), 541–548.

Deming, E.W. (1982). *Out of crisis.* Cambridge, MA: MIT Center for Advanced Engineering Study Publishing.

DeRosier, J., Stalhandske, E., Baigian, J. P., & Nudell, T. (2002). Using health care failure mode and effects analysis. The VA National Center for Patient Safety's prospective risk analysis system. *The Joint Commission Journal on Quality Improvement, 27*(5), 248–267.

Edwards, I. R., & Aronson, J. K. (2000). Adverse drug reactions: Definitions, diagnosis, and management. *Lancet, 356*, 1255–1259.

Filik, R., Purdy, K., Gale, A., & Gerrett, D. (2004). Drug name confusion: Evaluating the effectiveness of capital ("Tall Man") letters using eye movement data. *Social Science & Medicine, 59*(12), 2597–2601.

Filik, R., Purdy, K., Gale, A., & Gerrett, D. (2006). Labeling of medicines and patient safety: Evaluating methods of reducing drug name confusion. *Human Factors, 48*(1), 39–47.

Hsiao, C J., & Hing, E. (2014). Use and characteristics of electronic health record systems among office-based physician practices: United States, 2001–2013. *NCHS data brief; No. 143.* Hyattsville, MD: National Center for Health Statistics.

Institute for Healthcare Improvement. *Model for improvement.* Retrieved from http://www.ihi.org/resources/Pages/HowtoImprove/default.aspx.

Institute of Medicine. (2000). In L.T. Kohn, J. M. Corrigan, & M. S. Donaldson (Eds.). *To err is human: Building a safer health system.* Washington, DC: National Academy Press.

Institute of Medicine. (2001). *Crossing the quality chasm: A new health system for the 21st century.* Washington, DC: National Academy Press.

Institute of Medicine. (2006). *Preventing medication errors: Quality chasm series.* Washington, DC: National Academy Press.

Jencks, S. F., et al. (2009). Rehospitalizations among patients in the Medicare fee-for-service program. *The New England Journal of Medicine*, 360, 1418–1428.

Koppel, R., et al. (2008). Workarounds to barcode medication administration systems: Their occurrences, causes, and threats to patient safety. *Journal of the American Medical Informatics Association, 15*(4), 408–423.

Larson, C. M., & Saine, D. (2013). *Medication safety officer's handbook.* Bethesda, MD: American Society of Health-System Pharmacists.

Leape, L., Berwick, D., Clancy, C., et al. (2009). Transforming healthcare: A safety imperative. *Quality & Safety in Health Care*, 18, (424–428).

Marx, D. (2001). *Patient safety and the "Just Culture:" A primer for health executives. Funded by a grant from the National Health, Lung, and Blood Institute, National Institutes for Health.* New York: Trustees of Columbia University.

Merriam Webster Dictionary. (n.d.). *Culture.* http://www.merriam-webster.com/dictionary/culture

Meyer-Massetti, C., Cheng, C. M., Schappach, D., et al. (2011). Systematic review of medication safety assessment methods. *American Journal of Health-System Pharmacists, 68*, 227–240.

McLaughlin, C. P., & Kaluzny, A. D. (2006). *Continuous quality improvement in healthcare: Theory, implementations, and applications* (pp. 3–40). Sudbury, MA: Jones and Bartlett Publishers.

National Center for Patient Safety. Available at www.patientsafety.va.gov

National Coordinating Council for Medication Error Reporting and Prevention (NCC MERP). (n.d.a). *Index for categorizing errors.* Available at http://www.nccmerp.org/medError CatIndex.html

National Coordinating Council for Medication Error Reporting and Prevention (NCC MERP). (n.d.b). *About medication errors* [homepage on the internet—undated]. Available at http://www.nccmerp.org/about-medication-errors

Nebeker, J. R., Barach, P., & Samore, M. H. (2004). Clarifying adverse drug events: A clinician's guide to terminology, documentation, and reporting. *Annals of Internal Medicine, 140*, 795–801.

Nieva, V. F., & Sorra, J. (2003). Safety culture assessment: A tool for improving patient safety in healthcare organizations. *Quality & Safety in Health Care*, 12, ii17–ii23.

Reason, J. (1997). *Managing the risks of organizational accidents.* Burlington, VT: Ashgate Publishing Company.

Reason, J. (1990). *Human error.* Cambridge, UK: Cambridge University Press.

Ruiz, B., Garcia, M., Aquirre, U., et al. (2008). Factors predicting hospital readmissions related to adverse drug reactions. *European Journal of Clinical Pharmacology, 64*(7), 715–722.

Shillcock, R., Ellison, T. M., & Monaghan, P. (2000). Eye-fixation behaviour, lexical storage and visual word recognition in a split processing model. *Psychological Review, 107*, 824–851.

U. S. Department of Veterans Affairs National Center for Patient Safety (VA NCPS). (2015a). *Root cause analysis tools.* Revision, published online. Available at http://www.patientsafety.va.gov/docs/joe/rca_tools_2_15.pdf.

U. S. Department of Veterans Affairs National Center for Patient Safety (VA NCPS). (2015b). *Healthcare failure mode and effects analysis (HFMEA).* Revision, published online. Available a http://www.patientsafety.va.gov/professionals/onthejob/hfmea.asp.

World Health Organization (WHO). (1969). International drug monitoring: The role of the hospital. *Technical Report Series No. 425.* Geneva: WHO.

World Health Organization (WHO). (2005). *WHO draft guidelines for adverse event reporting and learning systems.* Geneva: WHO.

PART

II

ORGANIZATIONAL ASPECTS OF HEALTHCARE DELIVERY

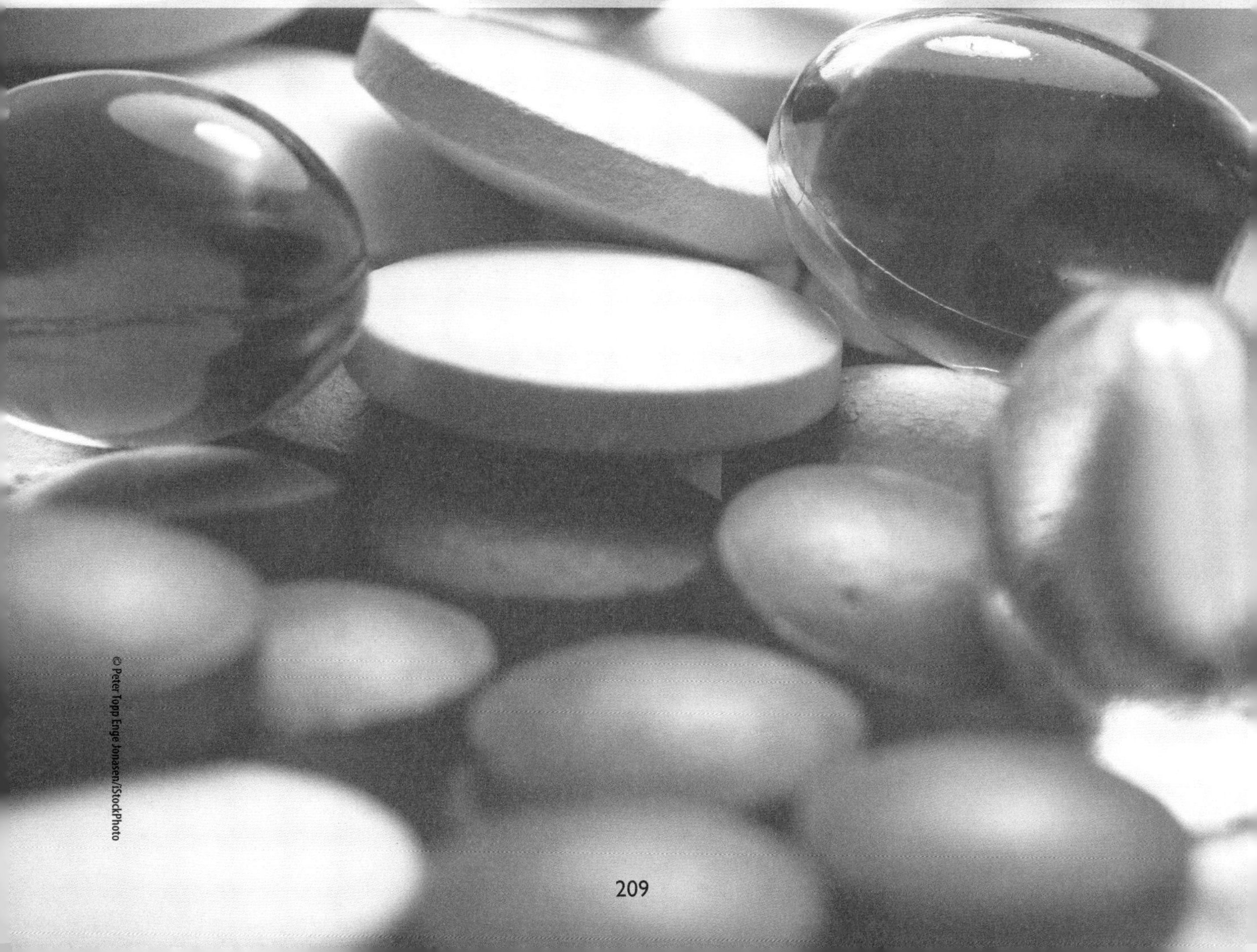

© Peter Topp Enge Jonasen/iStockPhoto

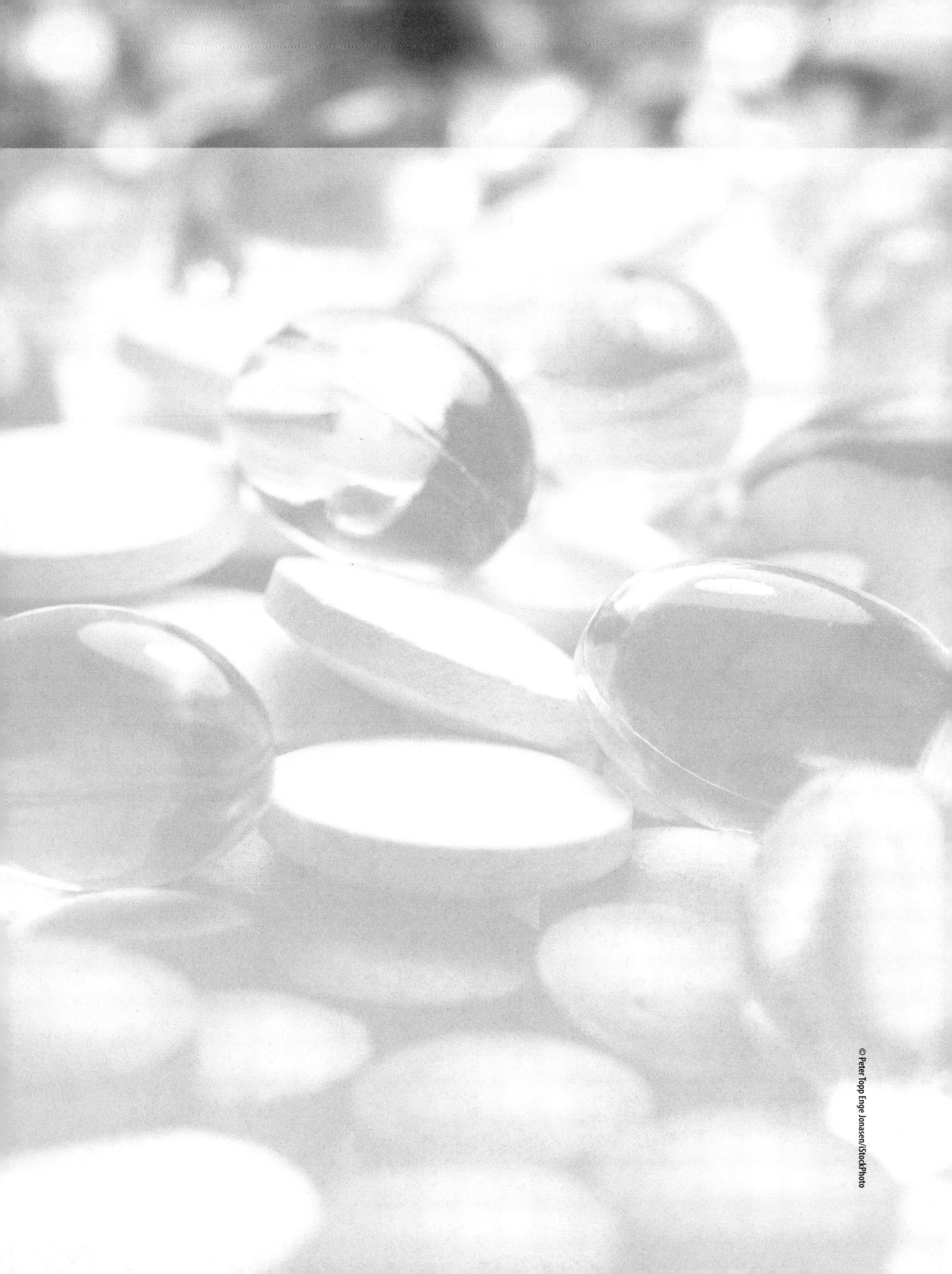

CHAPTER

8

Hospitals

Catherine N. Otto and William W. McCloskey

Case Scenario

Frank is a 60-year-old retired army officer with a history of hypertension and angina. One evening he complained of a severe tightness in his chest. His wife called 911, and Frank was rushed to the emergency department at a 250-bed community hospital affiliated with a medical school. After evaluation, Frank was admitted to the cardiac care unit for treatment of an acute myocardial infarction.

While Frank was hospitalized, a pharmacist specializing in cardiology introduced herself to him as part of the medical team. The pharmacist explained that one of the drugs for hypertension he was taking before admission was not on the hospital formulary, but that he would be given a very similar medication. Frank also noticed that his medications were prepared in tiny blister packs, not in the prescription vials with which he was familiar.

Upon Frank's discharge, an individual describing himself as a pharmacy resident reviewed with Frank those medications he would be taking at home. After discharge, Frank received follow-up care at the hospital's cardiac clinic.

LEARNING OBJECTIVES

Upon completion of this chapter, the student shall be able to:

- List and describe four factors that have influenced the role and function of the modern hospital.
- Summarize how hospitals have adapted to changes in financing of health care.
- Compare and contrast horizontal and vertical integration.
- Describe how hospitals are classified.
- Describe and give examples of general and specialty hospitals; federal and nonfederal government hospitals; nongovernment, not-for-profit, and investor-owned hospitals.
- Discuss the three sources of managerial authority in a hospital.
- Describe the purpose of hospital accreditation.

- Explain the roles and responsibilities of the following professionals: pharmacy director, staff/clinical pharmacist, pharmacy technician.
- Explain what unit-dose distribution is and describe two advantages of its use.
- Compare and contrast centralized and decentralized drug distribution systems.
- Describe how automation is utilized to support drug distribution.
- Identify four nondistributive pharmacy services provided by a hospital pharmacist.
- Define *hospital formulary.*
- Summarize the purpose of a pharmacy residency program.

CHAPTER QUESTIONS

1. What are the characteristics of hospitals?
2. How have hospitals adapted to changes in the delivery of health care?
3. What types of drug distribution systems are found in hospitals?
4. What is the role of the pharmacist in providing clinical services in the hospital?

INTRODUCTION

Since their origins as charitable institutions, hospitals have adapted to a variety of social, technologic, and political forces to become the center of the healthcare delivery system. This chapter explains how hospitals have evolved over time and discusses the challenges that they face. In addition, it introduces the role of the hospital pharmacist.

HISTORICAL PERSPECTIVE

The role and function of the modern hospital are a result of hospitals' adaptations to a number of significant developments that occurred in the first half of the 20th century. The Flexner report was one of the first factors that imposed a structural change on the hospital. In 1910, Abraham Flexner, funded by the Carnegie Foundation, conducted a survey of all medical schools in the United States and Canada. His evaluation assessed their admissions requirements, curricula, and financial basis and estimated the projected need for physicians and medical schools based on the size of the population. Flexner's recommendations included reducing the number of medical schools from 150 to 31, changing their admissions requirements to a minimum of a baccalaureate degree, and incorporating the scientific method as the foundation for medical education (Meites, 1995).

After the American Medical Association adopted the recommendations of the Flexner report, medical education in the United States was transformed into a system based on the scientific method. The scientific method bases diagnosis and treatment of disease on hypothesis formulation, experimentation, and conclusions. In response, hospitals became teaching and research centers for the practice of medicine. As medical practice increasingly came to rely on scientific principles, the use of technology became ever more important to the diagnosis and treatment of disease. It followed that the hospital became a center for technological innovations developed by researchers (see Chapter 1).

Health insurance provided financial stability for hospitals. Before the advent of such insurance, individuals paid for their hospital care with their own resources. Under that financing system, many individuals went without hospital care because it was unaffordable; others who received hospital care found it difficult or impossible to pay their bills. As a consequence, hospitals were at a significant risk for incurring large debts and possibly suffering bankruptcy. Once health insurance became widespread, hospitals no longer had to assume the financial risk and potential losses when patients could not pay their bills. Health insurance created a steady cash flow to hospitals and was critical for the funding of new technologies.

Because health insurance removed the financial barriers to hospital care for patients, the demand for health care increased. That is, health care was no longer limited by the individual's ability to pay. In addition, because health insurance initially covered only inpatient care, it provided a financial incentive to admit patients to the hospital to administer tests and procedures. Many of these admissions were unnecessary—routine diagnostic evaluation could have easily been performed on an outpatient basis. However, the availability of services in the hospital, coupled with the removal of the financial risk with health insurance, increased the demand for hospital beds, hospital services, and health care in the United States.

The Hospital Survey and Construction Act of 1946 (also known as the Hill-Burton Act) is credited with expanding the infrastructure of the healthcare delivery system by creating federal funding sources to build new hospitals, expand and renovate facilities, increase bed capacity, and add emerging technology. This legislation was particularly instrumental in supporting the building of hospitals in rural areas and small cities. Although Hill-Burton was not considered to be successful, it resulted in an increase in the number of beds in many hospitals and the incorporation of new technology, such as that currently used in emergency departments and intensive care units.

Finally, there has been a change in the types of diseases that are prevalent in the U.S. population. During the first half of the 20th century, infectious diseases were the most common types of illnesses warranting healthcare interventions. Because these disease processes were acute, hospitalizations were singular events. With the advent of preventive measures (such as immunizations and antimicrobial agents) and improvement in the water supply and general sanitation, morbidity resulting from infections has declined in recent decades. As a result, chronic diseases are now the most prevalent types of disease. Thus, hospitalizations are no longer singular events. Treatment for chronic diseases requires more than hospital care; it requires a continuum of care including ambulatory, acute, and long-term care.

Each of these factors has contributed to the development and modernization of the hospital and the U.S. healthcare delivery system. Adaptations made in the past continue to affect hospitals' reactions to the social, technological, and political forces.

FINANCING HOSPITAL CARE

Diagnosis-Related Groups

The diagnosis-related group (DRG) payment mechanism replaced the fee for service reimbursement method used for the hospitalization component (Part A) of the Medicare program when Congress instituted DRGs in 1983 as a method to control increases in Medicare spending. DRGs created incentives for hospitals to become more efficient and effective, employing utilization review and evaluating appropriateness of procedures.

As a result of the DRG payment method, now referred to as the Inpatient Prospective Payment System (IPPS), presurgical diagnostic procedures were performed on an outpatient basis instead of as a component of the hospital stay and the recovery period following surgical procedures was removed from the hospital stay by transferring the patient to a rehabilitation unit or facility. These unbundled services no longer were included in the DRG prospective payment, but were billed separately under the Medicare Part B fee schedule.

VALUE-BASED PURCHASING

Hospitals are beginning to change processes of care as a result of incentives created by the Hospital Value-Based Purchasing Program (VBP Program), a component of the Affordable Care Act (ACA) of 2010. Since October 2012, hospitals receive incentive payments for their Medicare patients based upon how well they perform or how well they improve on specified quality domains, in addition to the IPPS payments for each patient treated. The domains include measures in clinical processes of care, patient experience, outcomes and efficiency (CMS, 2013). Hospitals required to participate in the VBP Program must measure processes such as frequency of performing blood cultures in the emergency department prior to administering antibiotics, discontinuing prophylactic antibiotics within 24 hours after completion of surgery, patients' experience with pain management, and 30-day mortality rate for acute myocardial infarction (CMS, 2013). If the community hospital that Frank received treatment for his AMI participates in the VBP Program, the hospital will evaluate his health status 30 days after he is discharged.

These incentives are funded by withholding a specified percentage from the hospitals' DRG payments (CMS, 2013). One percent was withheld in 2013, the first year of the program. The amount progressively increases until 2017, when it reaches 2%, the level it is expected to remain, unless Congress makes adjustments. Hospitals receive incentive payments based upon their scores for the four domains, or on their improvement over a baseline period (CMS, 2013). Congress intended this program to be budget neutral, using 2% of total DRG payments to be allocated to high-performing hospitals. These financial rewards are used to encourage hospitals to improve their clinical processes care, in contrast to the cost containment focus of the DRG program.

Horizontal and Vertical Integration

Hospitals and other healthcare providers formed affiliations when healthcare delivery became more competitive in the 1990s. However, more integration is expected to take place as a result of the implementation of the ACA.

Horizontal integration is the term used to describe affiliations between hospitals. Sometimes the services provided by the two affiliated hospitals are similar. Often each hospital provides one or more services not provided by the other. Frequently, a partnership is formed between a smaller community hospital and a large, urban, tertiary care hospital; the urban hospital provides sophisticated technological procedures not available in the community hospital.

An organization is *vertically integrated* when it provides a continuum of services, including outpatient services, home health care, rehabilitation, and nursing home care. Vertically integrated hospitals do not have to depend solely on declining revenues from acute care. For example, in the chapter-opening case study, the hospital was able to participate in Frank's care postdischarge because it had an outpatient cardiac clinic. By integrating vertically, hospitals and the newly integrated healthcare systems are able to coordinate the entire spectrum of patient care and realize efficiencies that decrease overall costs and financial risk (American Hospital Association, 2014).

HOSPITAL CHARACTERISTICS

Hospitals are classified by length of stay, type of service provided, and ownership. Given that these classifications are not mutually exclusive, all three categories are used to classify a hospital (Health Forum, 2015). A number of other characteristics that do not fit neatly into these three categories are also used in the literature to describe hospitals—for example, community/noncommunity hospitals, teaching/nonteaching hospitals, number of beds, and multihospital chains.

Length of Stay

Classifying hospitals by the average length of stay differentiates hospitals that provide acute care from those that provide long-term care. Acute care hospitals (also referred to as short-term hospitals) have an average length of stay of fewer than 30 days. Long-term hospitals have an average length of stay of 30 or more days (Health Forum, 2015). State and local government community hospitals have a higher average length of stay—6.3 days in 2013—than investor-owned community hospitals—5.5 days reported for 2013 (Health Forum, 2015).

Type of Service

Hospitals are also classified by the type of service provided. General hospitals provide a variety of services, including general medical and surgical services. Well-known general hospitals include the Massachusetts General Hospital and the San Francisco General Hospital Medical Center. Specialty hospitals, by contrast, concentrate on one disease process (e.g., psychiatric diseases or cancer) or on one segment of the population (e.g., children's hospitals or veterans' hospitals). Noted specialty hospitals include McLean Hospital, a psychiatric hospital in Massachusetts; Memorial Sloan-Kettering Cancer Center in New York; and Shriners Hospitals for Children, located in many cities throughout the country.

Ownership

Hospitals are further characterized by their ownership and control—federal government, nonfederal government (both also referred to as public hospitals), nongovernment and not-for-profit, and nongovernment and investor owned (for-profit) (Health Forum, 2015).

The federal government operates a number of hospitals for specific populations, including veterans, military personnel, and Native Americans. Examples of hospitals under the jurisdiction of the federal government include Veterans Affairs (VA) Medical Centers throughout the nation and the Walter Reed Army Medical Center in Washington, DC.

Nonfederal government hospitals include hospitals owned and operated by city, county, or state governments. Most nonfederal government hospitals are general hospitals. State governments are primarily responsible for specialty care provided in psychiatric hospitals and caring for patients with mental disabilities.

Nongovernment-owned hospitals are divided into two groups: (1) not-for-profit (nonprofit) hospitals and (2) investor-owned (for-profit) hospitals. A number of differences exist between a nonprofit and a for-profit hospital, but the primary difference concerns what the organization does with any excess revenues at the end of the fiscal year. A nonprofit organization reinvests its excess revenues in the organization, usually in the form of capital, new equipment, remodeling, or new buildings. A for-profit organization uses its excess revenues in a similar manner; however, a portion of the excess is paid to the organization's investors in the form of a dividend. Nonprofit hospitals include those operated by the government, religious organizations, and other community hospitals.

Community Hospitals

Hospitals are described as either community or noncommunity hospitals. Community hospitals, such as the one to which Frank was admitted, include all nonfederal hospitals, short-term general, and specialty hospitals that are available to the public (Health Forum, 2015). Noncommunity hospitals are not open to the general public; they include federal hospitals for military personnel and the VA medical centers. Because Frank was a veteran of the armed services, he would have been eligible to go to a VA medical center if one was available in his area.

Teaching Hospitals

Hospitals are also classified as teaching or nonteaching hospitals. The designation of teaching hospital refers to the teaching and practice of medicine (Raffel & Raffel, 1989). Although a hospital may serve as a clinical training site for students in pharmacy, nursing, clinical laboratory, and any of the other allied health professions, it is not considered a teaching hospital unless it serves as a clinical training site for physicians. A teaching hospital may be expressly associated with a medical school, or it may have an affiliation with a medical school, serving as a site for physicians' residencies.

A teaching hospital can also be classified in another way, such as a community hospital—Frank received his medical care in this type of hospital. A teaching hospital can be a nonprofit, general, community hospital, such as Massachusetts General Hospital, or it can be a federal, general, teaching hospital, such as the many VA medical centers.

Number of Beds

American hospitals typically have fewer than 200 beds; indeed, 72.7% of U.S. hospitals fit this criterion (Health Forum, 2015). Larger hospitals are found in major urban areas, whereas smaller hospitals are found in the rural sections of the country.

Multihospital Chains

Multihospital systems emerged as a response to the changes in the healthcare environment in the 1990s, and their growth continues today. Systems of hospitals are created through mergers, acquisitions, or other legal arrangements. Multihospital systems are frequently national in scope, with hospitals being located in one or more geographic areas of the country. Not only do these national multihospital systems gain purchasing power with vendors, but they also have an advantage when competing for managed care contracts for businesses located in more than one state. Hospital Corporation of America is an example of a large multihospital system.

HOSPITAL MANAGEMENT

The following three sources of managerial authority and power exist in the hospital: the board of trustees, the hospital administration, and the medical staff.

The primary source of authority is the board of directors (in for-profit hospitals) or trustees (in nonprofit hospitals). The board is composed of members of the community who often have knowledge and skills specific to healthcare delivery. Its purpose is to determine the mission and goals of the hospital and to develop policies. It delegates more specific duties to the other two sources of managerial authority—the hospital administration and the medical staff (Raffel & Raffel, 1989).

Daily operations are the responsibility of hospital administration. The hospital administrator or chief executive officer is either a physician or an individual with an advanced degree in health administration or business. The hospital administration is responsible for implementing the policies developed by the board of trustees. The hospital management structure is usually a pyramid-like structure in which managers of departments report to assistants to the hospital administrator, who then report to the hospital administrator.

The medical staff is composed of staff physicians and community-based physicians who have staff privileges to admit and treat patients in the hospital. The medical staff is a self-governing body responsible for the quality of the medical services provided to hospitalized patients.

The organizational structure of hospitals follows the function or service provided. Direct patient care services include nursing, emergency department, urgent care, ambulatory care, surgery, and labor and delivery. Ancillary services include pharmacy, laboratory, and diagnostic imaging. Support services include housekeeping, dietary, laundry, purchasing, materials management, and security.

AMERICAN HOSPITAL ASSOCIATION

The American Hospital Association, founded in 1898, is composed of hospitals, healthcare systems and networks, and individuals. Its purpose is to provide education and resource material, collect statistics regarding its members, conduct research, and represent the point of view of hospitals in the legislative process (AHA, 2010).

HOSPITAL ACCREDITATION

The Joint Commission is a national organization founded in 1951 by the American Medical Association, American Hospital Association, American College of Physicians, and American College of Surgeons. Its purpose is to set standards and to subsequently accredit hospitals based on those standards. It accredits approximately 21,000 healthcare organizations and programs internationally and in the United States (Joint Commission, 2015a). In addition to the four founding organizations, the American Dental Association is represented as one of five corporate members. The Joint Commission accredits more than hospitals; it also accredits nursing care centers, home care organizations, ambulatory care facilities, and laboratory services (Joint Commission, 2015a). Organizations may earn certifications in areas for disease-specific care, integrated care, perinatal care, and healthcare staffing services (Joint Commission, 2015a).

Joint Commission accreditation is based on voluntary compliance with the standards. However, that accreditation has become critical for fulfilling state licensure requirements and is essential for receiving reimbursement in the Medicare and Medicaid programs.

The Joint Commission's mission is to "continuously improve health care for the public" (Joint Commission, 2015a). Its initial standards focused on the structure and the processes of healthcare delivery. However, as the environment of the healthcare delivery system changed, the Joint Commission changed the focus of its standards to include clinical processes and outcomes of care. After the Institute of Medicine published *To Err is Human,* the Joint Commission established the National Patient Safety Goals in 2002 as one method to require accredited organizations to focus upon specific activities to reduce harm to patients (Joint Commission, 2015b).

THE FUTURE OF HOSPITALS

Predicting the future of hospitals is difficult and perhaps foolish. However, considering the continuing trend of healthcare cost containment, the focus on outcomes of services delivered, and the implementation of the ACA of 2010, some directions for change can be anticipated. Hospitals will continue to try to provide state-of-the-art services and technology while operating within limited budgets. This balancing act will be coupled with greater use of healthcare services resulting from the aging of the American population and increased access for previously uninsured patients. Limited hospital budgets will likely be exacerbated by changes in the reimbursement policies of Medicare, Medicaid, health insurance companies, and managed care organizations (Institute for the Future, 2003).

As more individuals seek health care, an increasing percentage of that care will be delivered in an outpatient setting. To contend with this trend, hospitals will continue to diversify their services, to operate clinics, and to offer other diagnostic and therapeutic services on an outpatient basis.

To remain viable, hospitals will compete for health insurance and managed care contracts, physicians, and patients while focusing upon providing high quality care that improves patient outcomes.

THE PHARMACIST'S ROLE IN A HOSPITAL-BASED PRACTICE

Most hospital pharmacies have an organizational structure that consists of a director of pharmacy, an associate or assistant director, pharmacy managers or supervisors, and pharmacists with clinical and/or distributive responsibilities. Depending on the size of the department, some pharmacists may be solely dedicated to providing clinical services in a specialized area such as infectious diseases or critical care. In addition to professional personnel, the pharmacy department includes technical and support staff who may assist with product preparation, distribution, and purchasing.

Director of Pharmacy

Based on what is expected of this position, the director of pharmacy has one of the most complex jobs within the hospital (Nold & Sander, 2004). The director of pharmacy must satisfy a variety of leadership and management responsibilities, including overseeing both personnel and department budget issues. The director justifies and develops job descriptions for new pharmacy positions and generally manages the recruitment and interview process.

A major challenge facing hospital pharmacy directors today is managing the drug budget in the face of escalating medication costs. While a formulary system (as described later in the chapter) may help control costs, it is often difficult to anticipate how the cost of a new drug will affect the overall drug budget. The inability to contain drug budget costs may have a negative impact on the personnel budget and result in the loss of existing positions or failure to get approval for new ones.

In addition to leadership and fiscal responsibilities, the director often serves as the department representative on a number of interprofessional hospital committees. The director is also responsible for setting quality standards for the department, especially those concerning medication safety, evaluating policies and procedures, implementing new programs, and ensuring compliance with regulating agencies such as the Joint Commission, Department of Public Health, and Board of Registration in Pharmacy.

In hospitals with larger pharmacy departments, an associate or assistant director may assist the director with these responsibilities. In addition, managers or supervisors may be responsible for specific areas of the department such as sterile product formulation, outpatient services, or clinical services (Abramowitz & Mork, 1992). By comparison, in smaller hospitals, the pharmacy director may have to provide some staffing as well. Such directors are often referred to as working directors. In some very small institutions (fewer than 50 beds), the director may be the only full-time pharmacist and would be generally supported by part-time or per-diem personnel.

Staff and Clinical Pharmacists

The staff and clinical pharmacists provide the daily distributive and clinical services for the department of pharmacy. Since many hospital pharmacists provide a combination of both distributive and clinical services, they may not be characterized as either a staff pharmacist or a clinical pharmacist. However, some institutions may still use these terms to distinguish pharmacists whose primary responsibility may be in one area or the other. Staff pharmacists are generally more involved with routine pharmacy operations (e.g., order entry/verification, checking medication carts, sterile product preparation), and they supervise the activities of the technicians and other support staff who help with these activities. Clinical pharmacists are generally more involved with patient-care-related activities, including rounding with medical teams, obtaining medication histories, providing discharge counseling, managing adverse drug reaction programs, and responding to drug information inquiries. Job satisfaction among hospital pharmacists has been shown to be directly correlated with the number of clinical activities that one performs. Both clinical pharmacists and those with more integrated functions report being more satisfied than staff pharmacists do (Kerschen, Armstrong, & Hillman, 2006).

Because hospitals operate 24 hours a day, 7 days a week, an appropriate number of professional staff must be available to provide continuous pharmaceutical services when the pharmacy is not open. Joint Commission standards require that a qualified pharmacist be on call or available at another institution to answer questions or provide any medications that are not readily accessible to nonpharmacist personnel (Joint Commission on Accreditation of Healthcare Organizations, 2011). The Joint Commission also mandates that only pharmacists should be allowed into a pharmacy after it is closed; nurses or other nonpharmacist personnel should not be able to gain access to the pharmacy to secure medications after hours.

Joint Commission standards also require that a pharmacist review all medication orders before they are dispensed unless a licensed independent practitioner (e.g., a physician) controls the ordering, preparation, and administration of the order, or if a delay would result in patient harm. If a pharmacist is not available 24 hours a day, then a qualified healthcare professional (e.g., a nurse) must review the order and a pharmacist must conduct a retrospective review as soon as he or she is available (Joint Commission on Accreditation of Healthcare Organizations, 2011).

Technical and Support Staff

The technical personnel of a hospital pharmacy department comprise pharmacy technicians. These personnel have received special training in drug distribution, either from the hospital or from a school, such as a community college, that offers technician training programs. Pharmacy students who are fulfilling internship requirements may perform some of the tasks of a technician. Under the supervision of the pharmacist, technicians perform many of the distribution functions within the pharmacy department such as filling unit-dose cassettes, preparing intravenous admixtures, and monitoring and restocking inventory within the pharmacy and on the nursing stations.

Two national voluntary technician certification programs have been established. These include the Examination for the Certification of Pharmacy Technicians, sponsored by the Institute for the Certification of Pharmacy Technicians, and the Pharmacy Technician Certification Examination, sponsored by the Pharmacy Technician Certification Board. Certification encourages technicians to expand their knowledge and skill base, and it provides technicians with formal national recognition of their training (Murer, 1996). The expanding role of the technician allows the pharmacist to concentrate on more direct patient care or clinical activities (see Chapter 3). In the case scenario, a technician was most likely responsible for initially preparing Frank's medications, which were then checked by the pharmacist.

In addition to technicians, the support staff of the pharmacy department may include clerical personnel and individuals responsible for inventory management.

RESPONSIBILITIES OF THE HOSPITAL PHARMACY

The hospital pharmacy is responsible for the safe and effective use of drug therapy for the entire institution. Its duties include drug product selection, procurement, and distribution. The pharmacy is also responsible for ensuring that medications are prescribed appropriately and that guidelines for proper drug administration are followed (Black & Nelson, 1992).

DRUG DISTRIBUTION SYSTEMS

Floor-Stock Distribution

Floor-stock distribution was the method of drug distribution for many years. This system involved supplying the nursing staff units with a predetermined number of dosage forms, which were stored in a separate drug room in each patient care area. Nurses dispensed the medications to any number of patients from this supply, and then they reordered from the pharmacy as needed.

Two major problems have been identified with floor-stock distribution. First, the pharmacist did not have the opportunity to review the physician's order for accuracy or potential drug interactions before the medication was administered to the patient. Second, the pharmacist did not have the chance to review the patient's profile to monitor drug therapy for safety and efficacy.

Although floor-stock distribution may sometimes still be used to provide bulk supplies such as powders, some basic intravenous solutions (e.g., D5W and normal saline), and selected emergency medications, the unit-dose distribution system is now the standard distribution system in hospitals.

Unit-Dose Distribution

The unit-dose distribution system was developed in the mid-1960s to encourage the pharmacist to become more actively involved in the patient's drug therapy (Barker & Heller, 1963). The unit-dose distribution system consists of two key elements. First, a pharmacist reviews all physicians' orders for appropriateness and potential drug interactions before medications are dispensed. Second, medications are dispensed in unit doses, where each dose of medication is separately packaged and labeled with the drug name, strength, lot number, and expiration date in a ready-to-administer form (like the one that Frank received). Products may be purchased in unit-dose forms or repackaged from bulk dosage forms. While hospitals typically purchase unit-dose products when commercially available, some bulk oral and parenteral medications may be repackaged into unit dose for cost savings (Pedersen, Schneider, & Scheckelhoff, 2009).

With the unit-dose distribution system, each patient has an assigned drawer that is typically filled with a 24-hour supply of medication. For instance, if a patient is getting a medication every 8 hours, three doses of the drug would be supplied in that person's drawer. Patients' drawers are part of a medication cart for a specific patient care area; the drawers are exchanged at a predetermined time every day so they can be replenished by the pharmacy. In manual unit-dose distribution systems, the medication fill process is generally performed by a technician and verified by a pharmacist, although some hospitals use technicians to check other technicians (Woller, Stuart, Vrabel, & Senst, 1991). A recent survey of hospital pharmacy directors indicated that 37% of larger hospitals (>600 beds) employ a robotic distribution system that automates the dispensing process (Pedersen, Schneider, & Scheckelhoff, 2015). For new orders or medication changes, an alternative delivery system must be used to ensure that patients get their medication in a timely fashion. Either the pharmacy or another department is responsible for regular medication delivery to patient care areas.

A majority of hospitals (97%) surveyed reported using automated dispensing systems (Pedersen et al., 2015). Automated dispensing systems are drug storage devices that can be used to electronically dispense stat. doses of medications or doses in the absence of routine unit-dose deliveries. Those automated dispensing systems devices, such as those manufactured by Pyxis Technologies, which are available in patient care areas, interface with the pharmacy computer and dispense medications after the pharmacist reviews the order. Most of these devices require user identifiers and passwords and track usage information for billing purposes. These systems offer some potential advantages over traditional, manually processed cart exchange methods and stat. deliveries, including reduced drug delivery time and better inventory control. These devices also provide emergency doses of medications in the absence of 24-hour pharmacy services. If Frank had required an emergency medication for his heart condition, that drug would have been readily available in the cardiac care unit. Automated dispensing systems may also free up the pharmacist to engage in more patient-care-related activities.

The advantages of the unit-dose system include fewer medication errors, because the pharmacist reviews the medication order before dispensing. In addition, inventory costs are reduced by significantly cutting back on floor-stock supplies. However, labor costs are higher because more personnel are required to fill unit-dose carts. In addition, sometimes it is necessary to prepare medication in unit doses that are not commercially available. Another drawback to the unit-dose system is the potential for delays in getting the medication to patients, although the increased use of automated dispensing systems makes some drugs now more readily available. In addition, certain drugs used in emergency situations, such as cardiac arrest, are available for immediate access at the patient's bedside as part of an emergency kit or crash cart, which is located on the nursing unit. Despite minor limitations, the unit-dose system remains the preferred drug distribution system owing to its potential for enhancing patient care and controlling drug costs by reducing waste.

CENTRALIZED VERSUS DECENTRALIZED PHARMACY SERVICES

Hospital pharmacy services may be provided either from a centralized area or from two or more satellite locations. These are not mutually exclusive and some hospitals incorporate a combination of both types of services.

Centralized pharmacy services originate from a single location within the hospital. A manual (unit dose) centralized distribution system is utilized by approximately 25% of hospital pharmacies based on pharmacy directors responding to a recent survey (Pedersen et al., 2015). Because all pharmacy services are provided from a single location, fewer professional and technical resources are required than with decentralized services (John, Burkhart, & Lamy, 1976). In addition, inventory remains more consolidated, which reduces overall drug and supply costs. Survey data indicate that the use of a particular type of distribution system is dependent on the number of beds in the facility, with centralized drug distribution systems being more common in smaller hospitals than in larger ones (Pedersen et al., 2015).

Some hospital pharmacies provide pharmacy services from satellite locations in patient care areas or specialized areas, such as the operating room or emergency department. At a minimum, these decentralized services perform first-dose dispensing and pharmacist order review. Most satellites are supported by a centralized pharmacy that generally fills medication carts and performs other distributive functions. For example, Frank's first doses were provided from a satellite pharmacy in the cardiology unit to which he was admitted, but all subsequent doses were prepared in the central pharmacy. Decentralized services offer the primary advantage of having a pharmacist's presence in a patient care area, such as the pharmacist Frank encountered who specialized in cardiology. The major drawbacks of decentralization are the duplication of inventory and the additional professional and technical personnel needed to staff satellites, which increase the overall costs. Whether centralized or decentralized, some initiatives related to drug distribution systems are used to increase medication safety in hospitals. One method that has been shown to reduce adverse reactions due to medication errors is the use of computerized prescriber order entry (CPOE) (Wietholter, Sitterson, & Allison, 2009). CPOE has increased substantially over the past several years, with over 80% of hospitals reporting use of this type of system (Pedersen et al., 2015). Bar coding is another technology that can be used to scan and verify the correct patient and medication before the patient receives it in order to prevent serious administration errors. Recent survey data report that this technology is currently utilized by about 88% of hospitals to verify patient identity and check doses administered to the patient (Pedersen et al., 2015).

INTRAVENOUS ADMIXTURE SERVICES

Pharmacy personnel often prepare sterile dosage forms of medications. This requires special training in aseptic technique to ensure product integrity and to reduce infectious complications. Hospitals and other organizations that compound sterile products must be in compliance with more rigorous standards set by the *U.S. Pharmacopeia* (USP Chapter <797>). These FDA and Joint Commission—enforceable standards hold pharmacies more accountable for sterile products they compound and define how all these products should be prepared based on risk level. The risk level—low, medium, or high—is determined by factors such as how many manipulations are involved in compounding the final product and whether it is prepared from sterile or nonsterile ingredients (United States Pharmacopeial Convention, 2004).

Intravenous admixture services include the preparation of large-volume parenteral medications such as parenteral nutrition solutions and electrolyte replacement preparations (e.g., potassium chloride infusions), as well as small-volume parenteral medications such as antibiotics. Hospital pharmacies generally maintain special, environmentally controlled facilities, such as a clean room or laminar flow workbenches, in which to prepare sterile products. Such facilities are designed not only to protect the product from contamination, but also to protect the person preparing the product from potential exposure to hazardous or toxic products (e.g., chemotherapy). Some hospital pharmacies outsource bulk compounding of parenteral solutions (e.g., parenteral nutrition solutions) to an agency that specializes in sterile product preparations if this approach is more cost effective (Gates, Smolarek, & Stevenson, 1996). During his hospitalization, Frank required several large-volume intravenous solutions that were prepared by the pharmacy department in compliance with USP Chapter <797>.

NONDISTRIBUTIVE PHARMACY SERVICES

Drug Therapy Monitoring

In addition to being responsible for drug distribution, hospital pharmacists provide a wide variety of direct patient care services. The focus of most clinical pharmacy practice is drug therapy monitoring, to promote the safe and effective use of medications within the institution. Drug therapy monitoring involves verifying drug, dose, and route of administration and monitoring for medication-related problems to optimize drug therapy. By conducting admission and discharge drug histories, pharmacists also help resolve any discrepancies in what a patient may have been receiving before admission as compared to the admitting orders and any differences in the discharge orders as compared to what the patient may have been receiving while hospitalized. This is known as medication reconciliation and is now mandated by the Joint Commission. Medication reconciliation is very important during the transition of the care of patients from one healthcare setting to another (e.g., hospital to home), when they may be at increased risk of adverse events (Kirwin et al., 2012). Some pharmacists, like Frank's cardiology specialist, routinely participate in patient care rounds with the medical staff to assess the patients' status and provide point-of-care input into the patients' therapy. During these rounds, the pharmacist has the opportunity to provide input on drug therapy before an order is written. An interprofessional approach for myocardial infarction patients such as Frank has been shown to improve patient care (Coons & Fera, 2007).

Given the cost constraints so prevalent in health care, pharmacists must consider both the fiscal implications and the clinical impact of each drug order. For example, can a less expensive therapeutic alternative be prescribed, or can the patient receive the medication orally rather than intravenously? During his hospitalization, Frank's cardiology pharmacist was able to suggest a more cost-effective oral antiplatelet therapy for him.

In-Service Education

Pharmacists serve as a valuable drug therapy resource to physicians, nurses, and other healthcare personnel within the hospital. They may also counsel patients on their medications before discharge or in the ambulatory clinics of the institution. Pharmacists often provide in-service education programs on issues related to drug therapy to physicians, nurses, and other interested parties. To support these educational endeavors, hospital pharmacies may publish a newsletter to help update the hospital community on a new drug, pharmacy service, or other related topic.

Medication-Utilization Evaluation

Medication-utilization evaluation (MUE) is an interprofessional quality assurance program that was incorporated into the Joint Commission's standards in 1992. Current standards do not require a specific method be used, but rather focus on the quality improvement aspect of MUE (Joint Commission on Accreditation of Healthcare Organizations, 2011).

MUE programs objectively evaluate the use of selected drugs in the hospital by comparing them to specific criteria established for these medications, including medication-related activities such as dispensing and administration. MUE criteria typically include justification for use, monitoring parameters that should be followed, and outcome measures to determine efficacy. Results of the MUE are reviewed, opportunities for improvement are noted, and corrective actions are taken to improve drug use.

MUE programs may focus on a specific medication, a particular class of medications, or an outcome or a component of the medication use process. Drugs may be selected for MUE because of their potential risk if used inappropriately or because of their high cost compared to alternative therapies. For example, inappropriate use of an expensive antibiotic may not only increase overall drug costs to the institution but also could result in the development of drug-resistant pathogens. The pharmacy department may dictate which medications should undergo MUE (e.g., expensive medications or potentially toxic drugs) and work in collaboration with other healthcare professionals to establish the criteria for their use.

In addition to performing data collection and analysis, the pharmacy may direct the efforts to correct any deficiencies in drug use found during the MUE process. Such efforts may include in-service educational programs and pharmacy newsletters.

ADVERSE DRUG REACTION MONITORING

Adverse drug reaction monitoring is another quality assurance activity in which the pharmacy department participates. The major focus of adverse drug reaction monitoring is the reduction of preventable adverse drug reactions within the hospital. Suspected adverse drug reactions are reviewed by the pharmacy to determine the likelihood of an untoward event from a medication. In addition, the pharmacy can alert the medical staff to adverse drug reactions that may be associated with drugs that have recently been made available within the hospital.

Specialized Clinical Pharmacy Services

Pharmacists may specialize in an area of practice such as infectious diseases, nutrition support, critical care, or cardiology, such as the pharmacist on Frank's medical team. These specialists are responsible for monitoring drug therapy in a more selective patient population. For example, the infectious disease specialist may focus his or her efforts on appropriate antibiotic selection; the critical care pharmacist may be responsible for patients in the medical or surgical intensive care units of the hospital; the nutrition support specialist may monitor patients receiving parenteral nutrition; and the cardiology specialist may be responsible for monitoring anticoagulation therapy. Certification or credentialing in the area of specialization may be strongly encouraged or required for pharmacists in these positions (see Chapter 3).

Some specialized clinical pharmacy services are provided as part of a formal consultation service, and the clinical activity is performed following the written order of a physician. Pharmacokinetic consultation services are provided by many hospital pharmacies to optimize therapy using serum drug concentrations. In some cases, pharmacies may be reimbursed by third parties for such consultation services.

Although all pharmacists are responsible for providing basic drug information, some hospitals have established formal drug information services. However, the number of formal hospital and university drug information centers has decreased over the past several years. This may be due to the fact that the entry-level PharmD degree has better prepared pharmacists to answer drug information questions, and the availability of electronic databases and the Internet has made drug information easier to obtain for both healthcare professionals and the lay public (Rosenberg, Schilit, Nathan, Zerilli, & McGuire, 2009).

HOSPITAL FORMULARY SYSTEM

The purpose of a hospital formulary system is to help ensure appropriate drug therapy and control drug costs. The hospital pharmacy drug budget can be significant, with recent estimates of drug expenditures in nonfederal hospitals to be over $28 billion, which represents nearly 9% of total prescription drug costs (Schumock et al., 2014). The formulary itself is only one component of the overall system. The formulary is a "continually revised compilation of pharmaceuticals that reflects the current clinical judgment of the medical staff" (American Society of Hospital Pharmacists [ASHP], 1983). Whereas the formulary is essentially a list of medications and related products or devices routinely stocked in the pharmacy, the formulary system involves the overall process of evaluating and selecting medications to be included in the formulary. Consequently, only certain representatives of a class of drugs may be available. The decision to add or delete a drug from the formulary is based on the relative clinical benefit and cost of the medication as compared to other agents within a similar therapeutic class, or to nonpharmacotherapeutic options such as surgery.

In a hospital with a closed formulary system, physicians are directed to prescribe only those agents that are on the formulary unless the patient's medical condition dictates that a nonformulary drug is necessary. The prescriber typically has to document the reason why the alternative drug is required before the pharmacy will obtain it. As was the situation with Frank, nonformulary drugs are not routinely available within such a system and a therapeutically equivalent agent may need to be substituted for it. Therapeutic interchange is generally authorized based on previously established guidelines and allows the pharmacist to substitute an appropriate formulary equivalent without having to contact the prescriber (Tyler et al., 2008). Under an open formulary system, although physicians are encouraged to prescribe formulary drugs, nonformulary medications are generally more readily available.

The advisory group that manages the formulary system is commonly called the pharmacy and therapeutics committee. The pharmacy and therapeutics committee is an interprofessional committee made up of members of the medical, pharmacy, and nursing departments, as well as administrators and other individuals who are involved with medication use within the hospital. Pharmacy members generally include the director of pharmacy, who often is responsible for setting the committee agenda, and a drug information or other clinical pharmacist, who prepares an evidence-based, objective review of each agent requested for addition to the formulary. This review is presented to pharmacy and therapeutics committee members along with background material provided by the individual requesting the drug for formulary addition. The pharmacist's review provides an impartial perspective of the requested drug's potential benefits as compared to similar medications.

Some agents may be added to the formulary on a conditional basis; these drugs are reevaluated after a period of time to determine whether they should remain on the formulary based on clinical experience with the drug. In some cases, a drug may be added with restriction, meaning that the agent may be prescribed only by selected individuals. For example, an infectious disease specialist may have to approve an order for certain antibiotics before the pharmacy can distribute these drugs. Such restrictions usually apply to drugs that are very expensive or whose potential risks warrant that they be prescribed only by physicians who are very familiar with their appropriate use.

PURCHASING AND INVENTORY CONTROL

The pharmacy department is primarily responsible for drug management in the hospital, including purchasing and inventory control. Once the formulary status of a drug is determined, the decision regarding the brand of product acquired is ultimately made by the pharmacy; factors such as quality of manufacturer, cost, and dosage forms available all play a role in this decision.

Group Purchasing Agreements

Many hospitals participate in group purchasing agreements. Under such agreements, hospitals can collaborate with other institutions to negotiate more favorable pricing with pharmaceutical manufacturers.

Investigational Drugs

The pharmacy is also responsible for controlling the use of investigational drugs within the hospital. The pharmacist must be knowledgeable about investigational protocols being used within the hospital, including drug information, pharmaceutical data, record-keeping procedures, and proper administration techniques. In institutions that conduct a great deal of drug-related research, a specific investigational drug pharmacist is often responsible for coordinating these activities.

RESIDENCY AND FELLOWSHIP PROGRAMS

A pharmacy residency is an organized, directed, postgraduate training program designed to develop competencies in a defined area of pharmacy practice (Lazarus & Letendre, 1992). Most residency programs last 12 months and are referred to as PGY1 (postgraduate year 1) residency training. Unlike undergraduate training programs such as internships, a residency is designed to develop skills beyond those required by the state board of pharmacy for licensure. A residency is distinguished from a fellowship, another type of postgraduate program, by its preparation of the pharmacist for practice rather than independent research (see Chapter 3). Pharmacy residents typically engage in patient-care-related activities, such as counseling Frank from the chapter-opening case scenario on his discharge medications.

Some residency programs may offer training at an advanced level or specialized level (e.g., infectious diseases, cardiology) and are referred to as PGY2 programs. These programs require that the trainee complete a PGY1 program first.

In response to an increased need for qualified hospital pharmacy practitioners, the American Society of Hospital Pharmacists (ASHP) established the first accredited postgraduate training program in 1962 (Lazarus & Letendre, 1992). The ASHP (now the American Society of Health-System Pharmacists) program was the first to assess compliance with minimal standards for postgraduate training by an external review process. Programs that are ASHP accredited have been reviewed by a team of individuals from outside the hospital who determine whether the institution complies with the minimal training standards established by the ASHP.

If someone is interested in pursuing a career in hospital pharmacy, doing a residency is strongly suggested. In fact, both ASHP and the American College of Clinical Pharmacy have recommended that by 2020, all pharmacy graduates complete PGY1 residency training before they can practice in an area involving direct patient care. Whether there will be sufficient residency programs available by that date to meet this goal has yet to be determined (Knapp, Shah, Kim, & Tran, 2009).

Unlike residency programs, fellowship programs are more focused on developing one to be an independent investigator. Individuals pursing fellowships typically have the practice skills relevant to the domain the fellowship is in (e.g., infectious diseases, oncology). Those programs within a specialized area are generally sponsored by schools of pharmacy, academic medical centers, or pharmaceutical manufacturers. Fellows generally do not practice in hospital pharmacy, but pursue more academic careers where research responsibilities may be paired with patient care activities (Shord et al., 2013).

CONCLUSION

The changing healthcare environment presents significant challenges as well as opportunities for hospitals. Those institutions that adapt most quickly to these changes will position themselves more favorably to succeed in the future. Pharmacists play a significant role in the delivery of health care within the institutional setting. Individuals who wish to practice in the hospital may be advised to pursue postgraduate training experience.

QUESTIONS FOR FURTHER DISCUSSION

1. Describe the hospital of the future. Will hospitals exist as they are currently configured?
2. What role should hospitals play in the continuum of care?
3. What opportunities will be available in the future for hospital pharmacists? Will their roles expand?
4. How will automation affect drug delivery and the pharmacist's role in the hospital?

KEY TOPICS AND TERMS

- Adverse drug reaction
- American Hospital Association
- Centralized pharmacy services
- Decentralized pharmacy services
- Diagnosis-related group (DRG)
- Drug therapy monitoring
- Fellowship program
- Floor-stock distribution
- Formulary
- Horizontal integration
- Inpatient Prospective Payment System (IPPS)
- The Joint Commission
- Length of stay
- Medication-utilization evaluation (MUE)
- Residency program
- Unit-dose distribution
- Value-Based Purchasing Program (VBP Program)
- Vertical integration

REFERENCES

Abramowitz, P. W., & Mork, L. A. (1992). The hospital and the department of pharmaceutical services. In T. R. Brown (Ed.), *Handbook of institutional pharmacy practice* (3rd ed., pp. 19–29). Bethesda, MD: American Society of Hospital Pharmacists.

American Hospital Association (AHA). (2010). About the AHA. Retrieved from http://www.aha.org/aha/about/index.html

American Hospital Association (AHA). (2014, March). Trendwatch. Retrieved from http://aha.org/content/14/14mar-provintegration.pdf

American Society of Hospital Pharmacists (ASHP). (1983). American Society of Hospital Pharmacists statement on the operation of the formulary system. *American Journal of Hospital Pharmacy, 40*, 1384–1385.

Barker, K. N., & Heller, W. M. (1963). The development of a centralized unit dose dispensing system. Part one: Description of the UAMC experimental system. *American Journal of Hospital Pharmacy, 20*, 568–579.

Black, H. J., & Nelson, S. P. (1992). Medication distribution systems. In T. R. Brown (Ed.), *Handbook of institutional pharmacy practice* (3rd ed., pp. 165–174). Bethesda, MD: American Society of Hospital Pharmacists.

Centers for Medicare and Medicaid Services (CMS). (2013, March). Hospital value-based purchasing program. Department of Health and Human Services. Medicare Learning Network. Retrieved from https://www.cms.gov/Outreach-and-Education/Medicare-Learning-Network-MLN/MLNProducts/downloads/Hospital_VBPurchasing_Fact_Sheet_ICN907664.pdf

Coons, J. C., & Fera, T. (2007). Multidisciplinary team for enhancing care for patients with acute myocardial infarction or heart failure. *American Journal of Health-System Pharmacy, 64*, 1274–1278.

Gates, D. M., Smolarek, R. T., & Stevenson, J. G. (1996). Outsourcing the preparation of parenteral nutrient solutions. *American Journal of Health-System Pharmacy, 53*, 2176–2178.

Health Forum. (2015). *AHA Hospital Statistics™* (2015 ed., pp. 3–9). Chicago, IL: Health Forum (American Hospital Association).

Institute for the Future. (2003). *Health and health care 2010: The forecast, the challenge* (2nd ed.). San Francisco, CA: Jossey-Bass.

John, G. W., Burkhart, V. D., & Lamy, P. P. (1976). Pharmacy personnel activities and costs in decentralized and centralized unit dose distribution systems. *American Journal of Hospital Pharmacy, 33*, 38–43.

Joint Commission on Accreditation of Healthcare Organizations. (2011). *Comprehensive accreditation manual for hospitals*. Oakbrook Terrace, IL: Joint Commission on Accreditation of Healthcare Organizations.

Joint Commission. (2015a). Facts about the Joint Commission. Retrieved from http://www.jointcommission.org/about_us/about_the_joint_commission_main.aspx

Joint Commission. (2015b). History of Joint Commission. Retrieved from http://www.jointcommission.org/assets/1/6/TJC_history_timeline_2014.pdf

Kerschen, A. M., Armstrong, E. P., & Hillman, T. N. (2006). Job satisfaction among staff, clinical, and integrated hospital pharmacists. *Journal of Pharmacy Practice*, *9*, 306–312.

Kirwin, J., Canales, A. E., Bentley, M. L., Bungay, K., Chan, T., Dobson, E., ... Spinler, S. A. (2012). Process indicators for quality clinical pharmacy services during transitions of care. *Pharmacotherapy*, *32*, e338–e347.

Knapp, K. K., Shah, B. M., Kim, H. B., & Tran, H. (2009). Visions for required postgraduate year I residency training by 2020: A comparison of actual versus projected expansion. *Pharmacotherapy*, *29*, 1030–1038.

Lazarus, H. L., & Letendre, D. E. (1992). Residency programs in pharmacy practice. In T. R. Brown (Ed.), *Handbook of institutional pharmacy practice* (3rd ed., pp. 39–43). Bethesda, MD: American Society of Hospital Pharmacists.

Meites, S. (1995). Abraham Flexner's legacy: A magnificent beneficence to American medical education and clinical chemistry. *Clinical Chemistry*, *41*(4), 627–632.

Murer, M. M. (1996). Technician certification leads to recognition, better patient care. *Journal of the American Pharmaceutical Association*, *36*(8), 514, 519–520.

Nold E. G., & Sander, W. T. (2004). Role of the director of pharmacy: The first six months. *American Journal of Health-System Pharmacy*, *61*, 2297–2310.

Pedersen, C. A., Schneider, P. J., & Scheckelhoff, D. J. (2009). ASHP national survey of pharmacy practice in hospital settings: Dispensing and administration—2008. *American Journal of Health-System Pharmacy*, *66*, 926–946.

Pedersen, C. A., Schneider, P. J., & Scheckelhoff, D. J. (2015). ASHP national survey of pharmacy practice in hospital settings: Dispensing and administration—2014. *American Journal of Health-System Pharmacy*, *72*, 1119–1137.

Raffel, M. W., & Raffel, N. K. (1989). *The U.S. health system: Origins and functions* (3rd ed.). Albany, New York: Delmar.

Rosenberg, J. M., Schilit, S., Nathan, J. P., Zerilli T, & McGuire, H. (2009). Update on the status of 89 drug information centers in the United States. *American Journal of Health-System Pharmacy*, *66*, 1718–1722.

Schumock, G. T., Li, E. C., Suda, K. J., Matusiac, L. M., Hunkler, R. J., Vermeulen, L. C., & Hoffman, J. M. (2014). National trends in prescription drug expenditures and projections for 2014. *American Journal of Health-System Pharmacy*, *71*, 482–499.

Shord, S. S., Schwinghammer, T. L., Bradowski, M., Banderas, J., Burton, M. E., Chapleau, C. A., ... Yunker, N. (2013). Desired professional development pathways for clinical pharmacists. *Pharmacotherapy*, *33*, e34–e42.

Tyler, L. S., Cole, S. W., May, J. R., Millares, M., Valentino, M. A., Lee, C., ... Wison, A. L. (2008). ASHP guidelines on the pharmacy and therapeutics committee and the formulary system. *American Journal of Health-System Pharmacy*, *65*, 1272–1283.

United States Pharmacopeial Convention. (2004). Pharmaceutical considerations—sterile preparations (general information chapter 797). In *The United States pharmacopeia* (26th rev.)/*National formulary* (22nd ed., pp. 2350–2370). Rockville, MD: United States Pharmacopeial Convention, Inc.

Wietholter, J., Sitterson, S., & Allison, S. (2009). Effects of computerized prescriber order entry on pharmacy order-processing time. *American Journal of Health-System Pharmacy*, *66*, 1394–1398.

Woller, T. W., Stuart, J. S., Vrabel, R., & Senst, B. (1991). Checking of unit dose cassettes by pharmacy technicians at three Minnesota hospitals. *American Journal of Hospital Pharmacy*, *48*, 1952–1956.

CHAPTER

9

Ambulatory Care

David M. Scott

Case Scenario

As a consultant to Susan, a 35-year-old pharmacist, you have been asked to provide her with some advice about whether she should integrate pharmacists' patient-centered care with particular emphasis on medication therapy management (MTM) into her community pharmacy practice. For the past 5 years, Susan has developed a successful independent community pharmacy practice in a rural community of 2,500 persons in a Midwestern state. Prescriptions for seniors have increased considerably over the past decade, and this trend is expected to continue in the next 10 years. Susan is considering developing a pharmacists' patient-centered care practice. If she decides to pursue this route, Susan plans to market the program to local insurance providers for the Medicare-insured population. Common chronic disease states that are most prevalent in this rural community are cancer, diabetes, heart failure, and hypertension. Susan has maintained an adequate level of prescription care; however, Susan realizes that a high-level pharmacist's patient-centered care practice does require a major shift in her practice.

What should you advise her to do? When formulating your answer, consider the trends in ambulatory care, the impact that pharmacists' patient-centered care has made on community pharmacy practice, and the training and workforce changes that Susan must incorporate to implement this change in her practice.

LEARNING OBJECTIVES

Upon completion of this chapter, the student shall be able to:

- Explain what is meant by the term ambulatory care.
- Describe the impact of common disease states on medication use.
- Explain the types of medical practices.
- Describe the pharmacist's role in patient-centered medical homes.
- Describe what settings provide ambulatory care (e.g., hospital-related, freestanding, government).

- Explain how managed care and the Affordable Care Act are affecting ambulatory care.
- Describe the pharmacist's role in patient-centered medical homes.
- Describe the contributions the Indian Health Service has made in pharmacists' patient-centered care.
- Depict the pharmacist's role in ambulatory care.

CHAPTER QUESTIONS

1. What settings provide ambulatory care services?
2. How is managed care altering ambulatory care?
3. What contributions did the Indian Health Service make in pharmacists' patient-centered care?
4. How is pharmacists' patient-centered care affecting ambulatory care?

INTRODUCTION

Ambulatory care services have rapidly evolved and expanded since 1980. Managed care has spirited the change away from the inpatient side of hospitals to less costly forms of services provided in the outpatient settings. As costs of health care continue to rise, employers, insurance companies, and policy makers are continually searching for new ways to provide care that maintain quality, yet are accessible and cost effective. This chapter will examine the settings that provide ambulatory care, depict how managed care and the Affordable Care Act are affecting ambulatory care, and describe the pharmacist's role in ambulatory care.

GROWTH OF AMBULATORY CARE

Ambulatory care comprises healthcare services that can be delivered on an outpatient basis and do not require overnight hospitalization. Ambulatory care services have greatly expanded in recent years because of the rapid growth of managed care and the greater emphasis placed on outpatient hospital care. One significant event underlying this change in focus was the 1983 introduction of the Medicare Prospective Payment System for inpatient hospitalizations. The prospective payment system stimulated hospitals to change from rendering more services to providing shorter lengths of stay and getting patients out of the hospital faster and sicker. A second significant event was the implementation of the 2010 Patient Protection and Affordable Care Act (ACA or ObamaCare) that includes incentives to encourage ambulatory care. The ACA also requires health insurance policies to cover "10 essential benefits" that include: ambulatory patient services, emergency services, maternity and newborn care, mental health and substance use services (behavioral health), prescription drugs, preventive and wellness services and chronic disease management, and pediatric services, including oral and vision care, rehabilitative services and devices, laboratory services, and hospitalization. Prior to the ACA, most health insurance policies covered hospitalization and physician visits. Most of the benefits have been significantly improved and some services like prevention and wellness are new. Emphasis has been placed on providing lower cost options to hospitalization such as ambulatory care services.

These changes (e.g., managed care, prospective payment, ACA) encouraged the development of ambulatory care programs and are referred to in the case scenario.

Common Problems

What types of problems are seen in ambulatory care settings? The National Hospital Ambulatory Care Survey is an ongoing survey of ambulatory care. **Table 9-1** lists the distribution of outpatient

Table 9-1 Distribution of Selected Chronic Conditions by Age Categories in Outpatient Department Visits in the United States, 2011

	Total visits	% age			
Chronic condition*	*N* or %	< 45	45–64	65–74	>75
All visits (*N*) %	125,721 (100.0)	65,208	37,980	12,529	10,005
None	44.8	66.9	24.4	17.0	12.4
One or more	53.4	31.2	73.4	81.2	86.3
One	23.2	21.5	27.4	21.4	20.5
Two	13.9	6.4	21.2	24.0	23.3
Three or more	16.3	3.4	25.2	35.8	42.5
Hypertension	26.4	7.3	40.7	53.9	62.1
Hyperlipidemia	14.0	2.9	22.4	31.2	33.1
Diabetes	13.6	4.7	21.5	25.8	25.8
Depression	12.0	9.1	17.2	12.5	10.1
Arthritis	10.6	3.4	16.4	19.8	24.1
Obesity	8.7	6.9	12.9	9.1	4.7
Asthma	7.6	7.7	7.6	7.5	7.5
Cancer	7.2	2.1	10.3	16.8	17.3
Chronic obstructive pulmonary disease (COPD)	3.4	0.7	4.8	8.4	9.5

*Presence was based on response to the items on the checklist of chronic conditions and reported diagnoses. Combined total visits with chronic conditions and patients of visits exceeds 100% because more than one chronic condition may be reported per visit.

Note: Numbers may not add to totals because more than one chronic condition may be reported per visit.

Source: Data from CDC/NCHS, National Hospital Ambulatory Care Survey (2011). Table 14, p. 18. Hyattsville, Maryland: National Center for Health Statistics.

department visits in the United States by the top chronic conditions. As age increases the number of patients with chronic conditions increases and the number of visits also increases. Three of the top chronic conditions are hypertension, hyperlipidemia, and diabetes.

Table 9-2 lists the distribution of outpatient department visits for the top 20 most frequently mentioned drugs by therapeutic drug categories. The top ranked therapeutic drug category was analgesics, followed by antidiabetic agents, antihyperlipidemic agents, and antidepressants.

Table 9-2 Top 20 Most Frequently Mentioned Drugs by Therapeutic Drug Categories by Outpatient Department Visits in the United States, 2011

Therapeutic drug category*	Drug Mentions *N* (1,000)	% of Total†
Analgesics‡	41,130	12.5
Antidiabetic agents	15,610	4.7
Antihyperlipidemic agents	14,547	4.4
Antidepressants	14,286	4.3
Immunostimulants	12,923	3.9
Anxiolytics, sedatives, and hypnotics	12,337	3.7
Bronchodilators	10,937	3.3
Anticonvulsants	10,412	3.2
Dermatological agents	10,287	3.1
Antiplatelet agents	10,128	3.1
Beta-adrenergic blocking agents	10,124	3.1
Vitamins	9,206	2.8
Diuretics	9,161	2.8
Angiotensin converting enzyme inhibitors	9,140	2.8
Proton pump inhibitors	8,247	2.5

(Continues)

Table 9-2 Top 20 Most Frequently Mentioned Drugs by Therapeutic Drug Categories by Outpatient Department Visits in the United States, 2011 (continued)

Therapeutic drug category*	Drug Mentions *N* (1,000)	% of Total†
Antiemetic or antivertigo agents	8,063	2.4
Antihistamines	7,898	2.4
Calcium channel blocking agents	6,251	1.9
Vitamin and mineral combinations	5,996	1.8
Minerals and electrolytes	5,564	1.7

*Based on Multum Lexicon therapeutic drug category (http://www.multum.com/lexicon.html).

†Based on an estimated 329 million drug mentions at outpatient department visits in 2011.

‡Includes narcotic and non-narcotic analgesics and nonsteroidal anti-inflammatory drugs.

Note: Numbers may not add to totals because of rounding.

Source: Data from CDC/NCHS, National Hospital Ambulatory Care Survey (2011). Table 20, p. 25. Hyattsville, Maryland: National Center for Health Statistics.

Table 9-3 lists outpatient department drug mentions by physician specialty type. Given that primary care includes all but surgery, about 80% of all visits are in primary care. Substance abuse is an increasing trend in outpatient department visits.

Table 9-4 lists the outpatient department drug visits by expected source of payment in the United States for 2011. Most of the visits were covered by private insurance (39.3%), followed by Medicaid (35.0%) and Medicare (19.7%).

Upon review of the tables, one can see that most of the diagnoses and prescribed drugs in ambulatory care settings come from a few common chronic disease states. For this reason, primary care providers and pharmacists should receive extensive training in the management of these common diseases.

Primary Care Providers

Primary care providers include physicians, midwives, nurse practitioners, and physician assistants. Although training programs and practice responsibilities vary among states, the primary care capabilities are similar. Scheffler and colleagues have estimated that nurse practitioners and physician assistants can perform about three fourths of services that physicians perform in adult practices and about 90% of services in pediatric practices (Scheffler, Waitzman, & Hillman, 1998). At both the federal and state levels, there is interest in increasing the number of these practitioners, especially in underserved areas (Mezey, 1999).

Table 9-3 Outpatient Department Drug Visits and Drug Mentions in the United States by Type of Physician, 2011

Clinic type	Drug Visits* N (1,000)	% of Drug Visits	% of Drug Mentions†
All visits*	91,208	100.0	100.0
General and family practice†	57,219	62.7	68.9
Pediatrics	9,704	10.6	7.7
Obstetrics and gynecology	6,074	6.7	4.7
Surgery	12,274	13.5	12.7
Substance abuse and other‡	5,937	6.5	6.0

*Visits at which one or more drugs were provided, prescribed, or continued by the clinic type.

†Drug mention is documented in a patient's record of a drug provided, prescribed, or continued at a visit (up to eight per visit).

‡Substance abuse and other (includes psychiatric and mental health clinics).

Source: Data from CDC/NCHS, National Hospital Ambulatory Care Survey (2011). Accessed April 24, 2015, Table 19, p. 24. Hyattsville, Maryland: National Center for Health Statistics.

Table 9-4 Outpatient Department Drug Visits by Expected Source of Payment in the United States, 2011

Expected source(s) of payment	Total Visits* N (1,000)	% of Total
All visits*	125,721	100.0
Private insurance	49,395	39.3
Medicaid or CHIP†	44,005	35.0
Medicare	24,808	19.7
Medicare and Medicaid‡	5,482	4.4
No insurance§	8,544	6.8
Self-pay	6,510	5.2
No charge or charity	2,342	1.9

(*Continues*)

Table 9-4 Outpatient Department Drug Visits by Expected Source of Payment in the United States, 2011 (continued)

Expected source(s) of payment	Total Visits* *N* (1,000)	% of Total
Worker's compensation	759	0.6
Other	8,092	6.4
Unknown or blank	8,081	6.4

*Combined total of expected sources of payment exceeds "all visits" and "percent of visits" exceeds 100% because more than one source of payment may be reported per visit.

†CHIP is Children's Health Insurance Program.

‡Visits are included in both the Medicare and Medicaid or CHIP categories.

§No insurance is defined as having self-pay, no charge, or charity as payment source. Note: categories are not mutually exclusive.

Note: Numbers may not add to totals because of rounding. More than one category could be indicated.

Source: Data from CDC/NCHS, National Hospital Ambulatory Care Survey (2011). Accessed April 24, 2015, Table 4, p. 6. Hyattsville, Maryland: National Center for Health Statistics.

TYPES OF MEDICAL PRACTICES

Two major types of medical practices exist. The predominant form is care provided by private-practice physicians in solo, partnership, and private group practice settings on a fee-for-service basis. The second form, which has experienced dramatic growth in recent decades, is ambulatory care provided in organized settings that have an identity independent of that of the physicians practicing in it. This second category includes managed care programs such as health maintenance organizations and preferred provider organizations.

Solo Practice

Traditionally, solo medical practice has attracted the largest number of physicians. In recent years, however, the number of solo practitioners has been rapidly decreasing, largely because of managed care pressures. From a physician's perspective, solo practice offers an opportunity to avoid organizational dependence and to be self-employed. Primary care services provided by solo practitioners include family practice, internal medicine, pediatrics, and obstetrics and gynecology. These solo practitioners care for patients in office space owned or leased by the physician or in the physician's home. When patients are hospitalized, the physician sees them and provides care for them in the hospital.

Group Practice

Besides solo practice, office-based practice includes group practice. Group practice is an affiliation of three or more providers, usually physicians who share income, expenses, facilities, equipment, medical records, and support personnel, and who provide services through a formal organization (Roemer, 1981). Although other definitions exist, the essential elements are formal sharing of resources and distribution of income. The first successful nonindustrial group practice was the Mayo Clinic in Rochester, Minnesota. The Mayo Clinic was organized as a single-specialty group practice in 1887; later it was broadened into a multiple-specialty group that showed that group practice was feasible in the private sector.

Advantages of group practice from a physician's perspective include shared operation, joint ownership, centralized administrative functions, and availability of a professional business manager. From a financial viewpoint, the group practice relieves the provider of having to provide the large initial investment often required to establish a practice. Disadvantages of group practice from a provider's perspective include less individual freedom, less income, weak provider–patient relationships, and greater restrictions on referral practices (Williams, 1993).

MANAGED CARE

Managed care is the use of a planned and coordinated approach to providing health care, with the goal being delivery of quality care at the lowest cost, including emphasis on preventive care. The defining feature of managed care is the use of provider networks through a contractual arrangement specifying the types of services to be provided and the reimbursement to be received in return. With health maintenance organizations, the provider usually receives prepayment for services on a per-member, per-month basis. Thus a provider is paid the same amount of money every month for a member regardless of whether that member receives services and how much those services cost (a service contract). A health maintenance organization is a prepaid (capitation) health plan in which enrollees pay a fixed fee (often with a copayment) for designated health services.

A preferred provider organization is an insurance plan in which the managed care organization contracts with health providers to provide health services under a discounted-fee schedule. Such a healthcare plan is prepaid, and the member or family is enrolled usually for 1 year and is entitled to certain agreed-upon services. Healthcare services usually include physician visits, hospital services, prescription drugs, mental health services, and home healthcare services.

Typically, a primary care physician (gatekeeper) is chosen or assigned to coordinate an individual or family's healthcare services. When a specialist referral or hospital service is required, the gatekeeper physician must approve these services. If an individual or family goes outside the plan for these services, these services are usually not fully reimbursed or may not be reimbursable at all. Strong incentives are built in to encourage members to stay within the system.

MEDICAL HOMES

Role of the Primary Care Provider

The medical home also known as a patient-centered medical home (PCMH) is a team-based delivery model led by a primary care provider (i.e., family practice, internal medicine, pediatrician, Ob-Gyn) who is the leader of the PCMH team that provides comprehensive primary medical care to patients with the goal of obtaining optimal health outcomes. Principles that define a PCMH have been established through the joint efforts of the American Academy of Pediatrics, American Academy of Family Physicians, American College of Physicians, and the American Osteopathic Association. The PCMH is a model of primary care that aims to reinvigorate primary care and achieve the goals of better quality and lower costs of care. The Affordable Care Act has several provisions that support the PCMH. One provision is expanded Medicaid eligibility providing increased access to care for low-income Americans. The second provision is both the Medicare and Medicaid payment increases for primary care and designated preventive services.

The PCMH coordinates care across elements of the healthcare system, including specialty care, hospitals, home health care, and community services. Such coordination among patients and families and members of the care team is particularly critical during transitions between sites of care, such as when patients are being discharged from the hospital (http://www.pcmh.ahrq.gov/page/defining-pcmh). Examples of successful programs include: Blue Cross Blue Shield Plans of various states, Veteran Health Administration Patient Aligned Care Team (PACT), and Group Health Cooperative PCMH program of Seattle and Idaho (www.pcpcc.org/about/medical-home).

Role of the Pharmacist

Given the team-based nature of the PCMH, the role of the pharmacist is well established in some settings, yet is still evolving in other settings. Examples of integrated pharmacist's roles that have been developed includes academic health centers, the Veterans Administration, Indian Health Services, and community health centers. Medication management in PCMH is a major challenge since medications are involved in the majority of treatments. While pharmaceutical research has produced effective treatments for many disorders, unfortunately, low adherence can undermine the effectiveness of care at many steps of the process. Adherence has been defined as the extent to which a patient's behavior including medication use, diet, exercise, and other lifestyle factors coincides with medical or health-related advice. Medication adherence is a major public health problem in the United States with only an estimated 50% of patients with chronic conditions that are adherent to their medication regimens (WHO, 2003; Osterberg, 2005).

Since most PCMH patients reside in community settings, the communication between the primary care physician and the community pharmacist is an important issue. Unfortunately, the pharmacist in most settings does not have ready access to important medical home information. One of the significant issues in medical homes is that primary care providers often do not share this important information (electronic health records [EHRs]) with some health professionals, particularly the community pharmacist. Similarly, a community pharmacist has access to their own prescription dispensing programs, yet this information is typically not shared with the prescriber. Without this vital information, the prescriber and the pharmacist rely on suboptimal information that can result in suboptimal patient health outcomes.

One attempt to remedy this issue, is where the pharmacist has access to medical information provided to them by either the pharmacy benefit manager (such as Prime Therapeutics) and/or medication therapy management (MTM) systems designed to improve chronic disease management (Outcomes MTM). Although access to this information is a positive opportunity for the community pharmacist, the chronic disease information provided is often dated information (based on medical and pharmacy claims data and not real-time EHR information).

A second attempt to remedy this issue is that the federal government has spent billions of dollars for health information exchanges with the aim to share information between providers and patients. While technology companies, hospitals, and providers have received federal payments to implement EHRs, they have also intentionally blocked the electronic exchange of health information. They fear that they will lose business if they share information with competing providers (New York Times 5/29/15). Consequently, the crucial issue of sharing information between providers and pharmacists must be resolved before the pharmacist is fully integrated into the PCMH.

Evidence of Success

Recent literature examines the effectiveness of medical homes. Researchers concluded that continuous primary care in a medical home was associated with higher rates of vaccinations for the respondents' children (Allred, Wooten, & Kong, 2007). Reid showed within the Group Health system in Seattle that a medical home was associated with 29% fewer emergency visits, 6% fewer hospitalizations, and total savings of $10.30 per patient per month over a 21-month period (Reid, 2010). Some of the approaches being used to evaluate PCMH are summarized in the link (http://www.pcmh.ahrq.gov/page/evidence-and-evaluation).

An advocacy organization [Patient-Centered Primary Care Collaborative, (PCPCC)] also reports on the health outcomes (cost and quality) impact of PCMHs throughout the United States (https://www.pcpcc.org/initiatives). Overall, the PCMH studies demonstrate improvements across a broad range of categories including cost, utilization, population health, prevention, access to care, and patient satisfaction (https://www.pcpcc.org/initiatives).

HOSPITAL-RELATED AMBULATORY SERVICES

Hospital Clinics

Hospital clinics developed as American dispensaries in the 1700s and were intended to serve the urban poor and individuals who did not require inpatient care. Dispensaries were often freestanding buildings, so indigent patients did not mix with the paid hospital patients. The first U.S. dispensary was established in Philadelphia in 1786, followed by facilities in New York City, Boston, and Baltimore. A physician and/or apothecary who provided minor surgery, extracted teeth, and prescribed medications generally staffed the dispensary. By the mid-1850s, larger dispensaries had both a physician and a pharmacist. Financial support was meager and reliant on private donations. Most physicians volunteered their services without compensation. Freestanding dispensaries grew to about 100 by 1900 (Roemer, 1981).

By 1916, public health dispensaries' clinics experienced rapid expansion and numbered 1,300 sites, including about 500 for tuberculosis, 400 for baby hygiene, 250 for school children, and 150 for other purposes. Clinics maintained their preventive orientation, and clientele were usually limited to low-income groups. Private medical practitioners increasingly saw dispensaries as competitive and spoke of the abuse of the dispensary by patients who could properly afford private medical care. Since the end of World War I, private medical practice and hospitals have continued to flourish, causing the steady decline and closure of charitable dispensaries (Roemer, 1981). Hospital clinics have continued to provide health care for poor persons, although very little free care remains. Those patients not covered by Medicare, Medicaid, or commercial insurance usually pay according to a means-tested sliding fee scale. In some states, a free-care pool exists to offset the costs of providing unreimbursed care.

Teaching Hospital Clinics

In response to the managed care movement, teaching hospitals have reorganized their clinics to function as group practices. Many teaching hospitals now have three groups of clinics—(1) medical, (2) surgical, and (3) other. General medical clinics approximate a family practice or general internal medicine clinic but may also include other medicine areas, such as dermatology and cardiology. Surgical clinics generally include general surgery, urology, orthopedics, and plastic surgery, and they provide follow-up care for these patients. The other category of clinics includes pediatrics, obstetrics and gynecology, and other specialties, such as rehabilitation medicine (Mezey & Lawrence, 1995).

As the managed care movement casts its net even further, hospitals will become more responsive to community needs and move toward organizing medical care in a model that Madison (1983) has described as community-oriented primary care. Within this model, greater attention will be paid to common disease states, and the primary care practitioner will play an even more important role (Mezey & Lawrence, 1995). Academic health centers, for example, have been aggressively developing primary care networks to maintain their missions of clinical research, resident and student training, and patient care. Academic health centers have constructed new facilities, bought existing practices, or created partnerships with other hospitals to increase their primary care clinic base. For instance, the University of Nebraska Medical Center (a public, state-owned teaching hospital) merged with Clarkson Hospital (private, nonprofit) in Omaha, Nebraska, to expand its network of primary care clinics.

Veterans Affairs medical centers have been among the leaders in the expansion of pharmacists' roles in ambulatory care. Pharmacists have participated in Veterans Affairs primary care clinics' initiatives to improve blood pressure and increase medication compliance. Pharmacists have also become involved in pharmacist-managed anticoagulation clinics, where they have provided benefits over usual care in the form of desired therapeutic control with fewer adverse effects (Alsuwaidan, Malone, Billups, & Carter, 1998). Foss reported that two-thirds of clinic patients were within the therapeutic range following such interventions, and the percentage of thromboembolic complications was one third that of usual-care patients (Foss, Shoch, & Sintek, 1999).

The Impact of Managed Pharmaceutical Care on Resource Utilization and Outcomes in Veterans Affairs Medical Centers study has been one of the largest studies to date to examine the outcomes with pharmacists' patient-centered care. Nine Veterans Affairs medical centers participated in this study, in which patients were randomized to either an intervention group (n = 523) or a control group (n = 531). After identifying patients at high risk for developing drug-related problems, pharmacists implemented 3,048 therapy-specific interventions. Following these interventions, both hemoglobin A1C and low-density-lipoprotein cholesterol levels measurements were more improved in the intervention group compared with the control group. Total healthcare costs increased in both groups over the 12-month period; however, this increase was lower in the intervention group ($1,020) compared to the control group ($1,313) (Carter et al., 2001).

With the growth of pharmacist roles in ambulatory care, guidelines have been developed outlining the minimum requirements for the operation and management of pharmaceutical services for patients in the ambulatory care setting. Clinical practice guidelines are being developed and increasingly incorporated into health information systems. Murray and colleagues, for example, reported on a study to measure the effects of the electronic display of guideline-based, patient-specific treatment suggestions on pharmacist work patterns (Murray, Loos, Eckert, Zhou, & Tierney, 1999). The results showed that a dramatic change in work patterns occurred when pharmacists were provided with an electronic display of guidelines. In comparison with the control group, pharmacists with access to treatment suggestions spent less of their time preparing and filling prescriptions and more of their time functioning in an advisory role with patients, physicians, and nurses. Pharmacists in the intervention group also spent more of their time solving problems (Murray et al., 1999).

Ambulatory Surgery Centers

Response to the prospective payment system and managed care pressures on hospitals has led to the establishment of ambulatory surgery centers. Ambulatory surgery centers can be housed in hospital-based settings or in a freestanding ambulatory surgical center. Numerous surgeries that in the past required lengthy hospital stays can now be done in outpatient surgery centers in less time and at a lower cost. Patients having surgeries such as hernia repair are often admitted by 7:00 a.m. and discharged before noon. In fact, many third-party payers require surgical procedures to be done on an ambulatory basis unless evidence suggests that the procedure would be unsafe for the patient. As a consequence, the majority of surgical procedures are now done on an outpatient basis. Generally, surgery centers report a high level of patient satisfaction, and patients think that the quality of care is good.

Other Outpatient Services

Other outpatient services include freestanding diagnostic imaging centers, home intravenous services, home care services, and women's health centers. Additional ambulatory services will undoubtedly emerge as government and managed care organizations continue to seek delivery of care at a reduced cost.

EMERGENCY SERVICES

Hospital Emergency Services

Approximately 90% of community hospitals in the United States have emergency departments. Misuse of the emergency department has drawn intense scrutiny because it leads to routine care being delivered in expensive facilities at high costs. Emergency departments are seen as "safety nets" for uninsured and Medicaid patients, as well as off-hours care sites for other patients.

According to the 2009 National Ambulatory Care Survey, the reasons for visits ranged from life-threatening (immediate or emergent) visits to routine care (nonurgent). Immediate care is intended for patients' life-threatening conditions such as major trauma and heart attacks where an emergency department is staffed and ready to see patients that require to be seen immediately in the emergency department. About 50% of emergency department visits comprise nonurgent categories (e.g., common colds). Consequently, most of the nonurgent conditions presenting at emergency departments involve delivery of costly services that could be provided at a less expensive venue, such as a clinic, urgent care center, or physician's office. For this reason, some managed care systems require enrollees to get prior approval before authorizing emergency services. Medicaid patients often seek care from an emergency department because it is the only option available when they believe they need immediate attention. After some states implemented Medicaid managed care programs, they showed substantial declines in emergency department use (American College of Healthcare Executives, 1993).

Emergency Medical Services

Federal legislation has stipulated the creation of greatly improved emergency medical services throughout the United States. The National Highway Safety Act of 1966, for example, established performance criteria that required states to submit their emergency medical services plans for federal approval. The Emergency Medical Services System Act of 1973 authorized funding over 3 years to states, counties, and nonprofit agencies in an effort to expand and modernize their emergency medical services. Components of these services were expected to include a uniform emergency telephone number (911) and modernization of ambulance design from a hearse-type vehicle to a light van with equipment to provide cardiopulmonary resuscitation. Ambulance attendants were given emergency medical training so they could provide life-support services and trauma treatment on route to the hospital. Thanks to the improved training and equipment, emergency medical services have increased survival rates for victims of both traumatic injuries and myocardial infarction (Hoffer, 1979; Roth, Stewart, Rogers, & Cannon, 1984; Sherman, 1979).

The same legislative acts that set the emergency medical services standards also established community trauma centers and developed trauma teams to handle emergencies. Level I trauma centers offer around-the-clock care, including medical and surgical specialists, diagnostic imaging, and operating rooms staffed by well-trained personnel in well-equipped, intensive care units (Mezey, 1999).

FREESTANDING SERVICES

Urgent Care Centers

Urgent Care Centers (sometimes called emergency centers or emergi-centers) are designed to provide medical care from 12 to 24 hours a day, 7 days a week. The centers are designed to provide care for urgent and nonurgent problems. Urgent Care Centers are popular for: school physicals, patients with no family physician, and urgent problems (asthma), nonurgent problems (colds) and minor trauma. However, most do not receive ambulance cases or serve emergent cases.

In comparison to services provided at the emergency department, costs are generally lower at urgent care centers. Advantages of these centers include the convenience of and access to services without appointments and long delays, and that health insurance carriers generally prefer them to emergency department treatment (Mezey, 1999).

GOVERNMENT PROGRAMS

Health Department Services

In large European cities, boards of health were established in the 1800s and 1900s to halt the spread of communicable diseases such as plague, cholera, and typhus. Generally, these bodies were temporary boards—once the disease was eradicated, they were dissolved.

In the United States, Massachusetts set up the first state department of health in 1869. In the early days, U.S. health departments dealt largely with the prevention of tuberculosis. Another health department initiative dealt with the reduction of infant mortality by establishing milk stations where mothers who could not breastfeed could obtain clean cow's milk to feed their babies. Later, this initiative was expanded to provide advice to low-income mothers on the care of infants; it also established child health clinics and the Visiting Nurse Association.

As an outgrowth of two federal acts passed in the 1920s, maternal and child health grants were provided to states for the development of well-baby clinics. In the late 1920s, however, a conservative antigovernment wave swept over the country, led by the American Medical Association, which attacked these maternal and child health grants as socialistic programs. As a result, the U.S. Congress ended this program in 1929. It was reactivated during the Great Depression as part of Title V of the 1935 Social Security Act (Roemer, 1981).

Most public health agencies in the early 1900s were devoted to environmental problems, sanitation, and collection of statistics on communicable diseases. The 1929 stock market crash and the massive poverty during the 1930s led to a resurgent American public health movement. Currently, the following four major categories of public health services exist: (1) communicable disease control, (2) maternal and child health services, (3) chronic diseases, and (4) general ambulatory care.

Communicable disease control, the first major category, involves the control of contagious diseases and sexually transmitted diseases such as AIDS. Immunizations against diseases such as diphtheria, pertussis (whooping cough), tetanus, polio, and measles are given to infants as part of well-baby clinics and other health department–sponsored activities.

The second major category encompasses the maternal and child health clinics that have risen and fallen based on funding provided at federal, state, and local levels. Federal funding for maternal and child health services has generally come from Title V of the Social Security Act and supports local health department services for babies and pregnant women. Maternal and child health services are provided to low-income families, while families with moderate to high income are referred to private physicians. As part of President Lyndon Johnson's Great Society program, comprehensive health care (treatment and prevention) was also established under Social Security Act amendments that authorized grants for maternal and infant care clinics and children and youth clinics.

In 1976, the author of this chapter established clinical and distributive pharmaceutical services in an ambulatory children and youth clinic serving low-income families in south Minneapolis (Scott & Nordin, 1980). Instead of filling prescriptions from a prescription blank, the prescriptions were filled from the patient's chart. The pharmacy was located inside the primary patient care area, so the pharmacist could consult with the appropriate health professional or refer the patient for more extensive evaluation. As part of the patient counseling program, the pharmacy staff also administered the first dose of medication prescribed for pediatric patients, including liquid preparations (e.g., antibiotics), ophthalmic drops and ointments, and otic preparations. As part of the clinic's interdisciplinary team, pharmacists provided therapeutic and pharmacokinetic consultations, drug monitoring, drug information, educational programs for the community, and poison prevention services. The pharmacy closed in 1984 because of federal and state funding cutbacks. However, such pharmacists' patient-centered care services are possible in clinic settings, community health centers, staff model health maintenance organizations, and other ambulatory care settings.

The third major category of public health services focuses on chronic (noncommunicable) diseases—for example, the cancer detection clinic. Other efforts have targeted smoking reduction, Pap smears for cervical cancer detection, breast examinations, and hypertension screening.

The fourth major category of public health services consists of generalized ambulatory care clinics. In the mid-1960s, health departments influenced by the War on Poverty movement expanded the scope of these clinics from preventive functions to the provision of general ambulatory care. These clinics were predominantly found in low-income neighborhoods, but the prevailing policy was to turn no one away on grounds of inability to pay. Patients with complex problems were typically referred to a contracted hospital outpatient department. Today, public health clinics are vulnerable to governmental funding priorities and organized medicine pressures to eliminate or reduce the services offered there. Accordingly, health departments generally provide services in areas where most physicians are not interested in working (Roemer, 1981).

Local health departments often provide services that private practice medicine have little interest (i.e., immunizations, infectious disease case finding and control) and that fill service gaps for needy and Medicaid patients (i.e., family planning, well-baby care). The three fundamental purposes that are essential for public health are assessment, policy development, and assurance. While these fundamental purposes and essential services are basic, local and state health departments often have difficulty meeting all of them, since they are chronically under-funded and understaffed and consequently, they focus their efforts on meeting monitoring and reporting requirements.

Community Health Centers

In 1965, Congress funded the Neighborhood Health Center Act to provide comprehensive health care to low-income populations (about 2/3 of patients are uninsured or on Medicaid) in urban and rural areas of the United States in an attempt to stimulate societal growth and decrease poverty (Mezey & Lawrence, 1995). The first Neighborhood Health Center, established in 1965, was the Gouverneur Health Center, which served poor persons from New York's lower east side. Other early health center projects were developed in Boston, Chicago, and south-central Los Angeles. Evaluations of these initiatives concluded that Neighborhood Health Center program performance was generally equal, and sometimes superior, to that of other established providers of health care (Morehead, Donaldson, & Servavelli, 1971; Sparer & Anderson, 1975). In 1973, the entire

Neighborhood Health Center program under the Office of Economic Opportunity was ended, and the Neighborhood Health Center facilities were transferred to the U.S. Public Health Service (PHS) and were designated as community health centers (CHCs) (Roemer, 1981).

In 1974, Congress passed the Community Health Centers Act, which defined the scope of CHC services that must be offered to warrant receipt of federal grants. The criteria defining underserved areas were quantified and included poverty level as defined by local per-capita income, an excessive infant mortality rate, and a shortage of primary care physicians. Administering organizations include health department, community organization and a not-for profit agency. Mandated services in these federally supported CHCs were diagnostic treatment, consultation, and other services by a physician or physician extender; laboratory and X-ray services; dental services; social services; and pharmaceutical services (Roemer, 1981). Approximately 1,250 CHCs in the United States serve more than 20 million with limited financial resources. Recognized as a safety net, the Affordable Care Act of 2010 has funded expansion of community health centers. The 1978 amendments to Sections 329 and 330 of the Public Health Services Act changed the supplemental services designation and made pharmacy a primary service in CHCs. All CHCs are required to provide prescription drugs for their patients either through on-site licensed pharmacies or through a contracted arrangement with an off-site pharmacy.

The Siouxland Community Health Center (SCHC) is an example of a CHC that provides in-house pharmacy services. SCHC is located in Sioux City, Iowa. The city has become more racially mixed and culturally diverse over the past 20 years, in part because of the changing demographics of the meat packing industry workforce. Hispanics account for more than one half of the minority population, followed by a significant number of Asian Americans, African Americans, and Native Americans. SCHC manages more than 50,000 patient visits per year, and the majority of clients are at or below 100% of the federal poverty level. SCHC facilities include 18 examination rooms, 2 minor procedure rooms, 8 dental operatories (dental chairs), a basic laboratory, and a pharmacy. The major health concerns encountered by the center's practitioners are diabetes and hypertension. The on-site pharmacy fills more than 300 prescriptions per day.

A number of colleges/schools of pharmacy are developing partnerships with CHCs to integrate clinical pharmacy services in CHCs and to provide training sites for pharmacy students. SCHC, in conjunction with the University of Nebraska's College of Pharmacy, was one of the first seven CHCs to receive funding from the U.S. Health Resources and Services Administration's clinical pharmacy demonstration project to develop and deliver clinical pharmacy services. The project objective was to determine whether provision of education services by the clinical pharmacist working with the SCHC team would improve glycosylated hemoglobin (A1C) levels and quality of life for patients with diabetes in an intervention group more than improvement shown by members of the control group (who received standard care) (Scott, Boyd, Stephans, Augustine, & Reardon, 2006). Based on a national evaluation, the SCHC project was deemed a successful clinical pharmacy demonstration project; it was one of only two clinical pharmacy demonstration projects in which the regression analysis showed significantly better health outcomes than the average project. It reached and retained patients in its diabetes disease management program better than most, and it has been sustained since the end of the grant period in August 2003. The Siouxland project used an intensive program of mostly individual diabetes counseling, along with incentives, as a means to encourage patient retention (Mathematic Policy Research, 2004).

In another study, Leal and colleagues assessed the improvement that a clinical pharmacist at a CHC can make as a provider for patients with diabetes and comorbid conditions (hypertension and hyperlipidemia) by using a medical staff–approved collaborative practice agreement. Although this study did not include a comparison group, the intervention at the El Rio Health Center in Tucson, Arizona, produced a statistically significant 2% drop in mean A1C in 199 patients compared to baseline. Regarding attainment of treatment goals, the pharmacist-managed service showed an almost sevenfold increase in the number of patients at target A1C levels (Leal, Glover, Herrier, & Felix, 2004).

Indian Health Service

Treaties signed between Native American tribes and the U.S. government stipulated that American Indians would be provided certain medical and hospital services, and this obligation continues to the present day. Management of the Indian Health Service (IHS) is provided by the U.S. Department of Health and Human Services' PHS. Currently, the majority of IHS pharmacists are members of the PHS Commissioned Corps. Healthcare and pharmacy services are provided to 1.5 million American Indians and Alaska Natives living on or near reservations in 35 states. IHS programs are carried out through 49 hospitals (7–150 beds) and 180 ambulatory clinics. Although they are distributed throughout the country, most of these facilities are concentrated in the western half of the continental United States and Alaska (Flowers et al., 2009; Paavola, Kermanoski, & Pittman, 1997).

Pharmacists were first assigned as PHS officers to hospitals in 1953 to establish dispensing policies and practices. During the 1960s, several IHS innovations set the stage for a more active clinical role for pharmacists. The first innovation was that the patient's medical record replaced the traditional prescription blank as the primary document used to fill all prescriptions. By accessing the patient's chart, the pharmacist could provide a concurrent review of prescribed drug therapy for appropriateness before dispensing. The second innovation was that IHS pharmacists were the first to use private consultation rooms and provide patient counseling to every patient receiving a prescription.

The third major innovation was the provision of primary care to ambulatory patients with both acute and chronic health problems. This program began as pharmacists independently initiated and extended drug therapy. The primary care program has now progressed to pharmacists taking histories, doing physical assessments, and prescribing treatment including prescription medication. These programs were developed under the leadership of Dr. Allen J. Brands, an IHS pharmacist from 1955 through 1981, and they remain an important part of pharmacy practice today.

Since 1972, IHS pharmacists have obtained didactic and clinical training that enables them to become certified as pharmacist practitioners (Copeland & Apgar, 1980). These trained pharmacists perform physical assessments and manage both acute and chronic disease states using protocols. The protocols provide guidelines for pharmacists, including the requirement that complex and severe cases be referred to physicians. The notion of the pharmacist as a primary care provider similar to a physician assistant or nurse practitioner is more comprehensive in the IHS than the roles found in most ambulatory care settings. This unique conception of the pharmacist's primary care role was originally evolved to counteract a physician undersupply and the unmet needs of the underserved American Indian population, but it is also well suited for many other rural areas.

IHS encourages pharmacists to broaden their scope of practice. Advantages include full access to patient records, collegial relationships with health professionals, opportunities to participate in pharmacy specialized clinics, and direct patient care and emergency life support. IHS pharmacists also have opportunities to become disease state experts, often managing and participating in chronic care specialty clinics (e.g., anticoagulation, asthma, congestive heart failure, diabetes, dyslipidemia, HIV/AIDS, hypertension, immunization, pain management, and smoking cessation) (Flowers et al., 2009). Although the pharmacists' patient-centered care role has recently been advocated in the ambulatory setting, most of these innovations were first developed in the IHS.

MISCELLANEOUS PROGRAMS

School Health Clinics

The vast majority of children older than age 5 attend school in the United States; when first aid is needed or acute illness occurs, schools must provide at least limited services for these children. School health services in the United States can be traced back to 1840, when William Alcott, a distinguished educator, called for periodic visits to schools by physicians who would see children referred by teachers (Roemer, 1981). The first permanent school medical officer was appointed in New York City in 1892, followed by one in Boston, to ensure that school children with contagious diseases were identified, removed from school, and treated. School nursing services were brought into schools in New York City in 1902 and later adopted in other U.S. cities.

A wide disparity of nursing services exists in U.S. schools because communities have different socioeconomic levels, and local property taxes are usually the schools' major financial support. Ambulatory services vary between education levels because health needs change from childhood to young adult years (Roemer, 1981).

At the elementary school level, the following three components are ideally addressed: (1) health education of the child, (2) maintenance of a safe and healthy school environment, and (3) personal health services. To control communicable diseases, immunizations are required for entrance into school. Personal health services include health status appraisals (examinations), first aid to trauma cases, referral for needed medical care, psychologic services, and dental care. School nurses are the most commonly employed school health personnel, although the number working in full-time and part-time positions is unavailable.

Secondary schools require a different pattern of health services than in elementary schools to serve adolescent needs. Passage through puberty requires programs for sexuality, sexually transmitted diseases, premarital pregnancy, substance abuse prevention and treatment, violence prevention, and sports medicine. The pharmacist as a health educator is well trained to provide accurate and appropriate information on alcohol, tobacco, and other drug usage. Some colleges of pharmacy have speakers' bureaus that give presentations on a variety of substance abuse topics (e.g., smoking prevention and cessation, alcohol use, anabolic steroid use, amphetamines, marijuana, opioids, and diet pills). Health education programs on sexually transmitted diseases and birth control can be given at the school and then augmented at the community pharmacy level.

The first school health clinic was developed at a high school in St. Paul, Minnesota. Since then, clinics have been established in other schools throughout the country. Students can receive personal health services at school health clinics, which are especially important in underserved population areas.

Prison Health Services

The U.S. Department of Justice operates a system of federal prisons or penitentiaries through its Federal Bureau of Prisons. Federal prisons' capacities range from 200 to more than 2,200 inmates, and prisons are linked to more than 28 hospitals, each with a clinic for ambulatory care. Larger prisons are staffed by the PHS with full-time salaried physicians, and smaller prisons are staffed by part-time private physicians working under contract (Roemer, 1981). As part of the PHS, more than 150 pharmacists work in the Bureau of Prisons. Practice settings range from ambulatory care sites to 500-bed hospitals. Responsibilities of the pharmacist include distributing drugs from a national drug formulary, counseling patients, providing drug use reviews, monitoring labs, working in chronic care clinics, immunizing patients, administering medications, and assisting in the daily duties of the correctional facility (Flowers et al., 2009).

Since 2004, selected PHS pharmacists were trained in HIV disease and pharmacotherapy, and they manage care for Bureau of Prisons patients with HIV/AIDS under collaborative practice agreements. Here they initiate treatment, order laboratory tests to stage the severity of the infection, and modify existing antiretroviral therapy (Flowers et al., 2009).

Voluntary Agencies and Free Health Clinics

Many voluntary health agencies exist in the United States, including those run by the American Red Cross, the Salvation Army, and some overseas church missions that provide ambulatory care services in developing countries.

Another voluntary health service was the free clinic movement, a dramatic innovation in ambulatory care. Its first facility was the Haight-Ashbury Free Medical Clinic, which opened in a bohemian section of San Francisco, California, in the summer of 1967. These clinics opened without substantial grants from the federal government and were planned and supported by consumers, who were usually groups of young adults. Other free clinics opened in Cincinnati, Ohio; Detroit, Michigan; Seattle, Washington; and Minneapolis, Minnesota. By 1971, about 175 free clinics had been established throughout the country, with the greatest concentration in California. Roemer (1981) suggested that the rationale for these clinics was the feeling of distrust by socially alienated youths (such as hippies) of the establishment in the American healthcare system.

These alienated youths generally did not want to go to hospital outpatient departments and public health clinics. Free clinics were often located in vacant stores, old houses, and church basements, and they were open to everyone who came—at no charge—although donations were welcomed.

Jerome Schwartz (1971) defined free clinics as having the following seven characteristics: (1) a physical facility; (2) trained health personnel; (3) other health staff or volunteers; (4) direct provision of medical, dental, or psychologic service, including treatment of drug abuse; (5) availability to everyone without eligibility tests; (6) specified hours of service; and (7) no set payment required, although small fees might be charged for specified services and donations might be requested (Schwartz, 1971). Services are provided predominantly by volunteer physicians, nurses, pharmacists, and paraprofessionals.

Free clinics provide professional and community service opportunities to pharmacy, medical, dental, and nursing students. The author of this chapter participated as a pharmacy student at the Union Gospel Mission Free Clinic in St. Paul, Minnesota, from 1970 through 1973. Services provided at this free clinic included medical care, dental care, nursing care, and pharmacists' patient-centered care. Clientele included homeless men, women, and children, and runaway youth. Many homeless men had a variety of medical problems, including alcoholism. A pharmacist oversaw distribution of medications when possible, although a volunteer pharmacist was not always at the site. Consequently, a pharmacy student dispensed medication and provided counseling under the supervision of a volunteer physician. Medical students diagnosed and prescribed following consultation with the pharmacist and physician. Medications were generally donated to this free clinic by community hospitals and by some drug companies. Opportunities to provide pharmacists' patient-centered care increased as pharmacists and pharmacy students gained further insight and skills.

Free clinics' major obstacles are continual financial crises and staffing by voluntary health professionals. Since the 1971 Schwartz study, no general survey has been conducted of the free clinic movement (Roemer, 1981). Many free clinics remain, under the name of free health clinic, free medical clinic, or the local health department. The National Association of Free and Charitable Clinics is the nonprofit organization whose mission is focused on the issues and needs of the more than 1,200 free clinics and the people they serve in the United States (http://www.nafcclinics.org/content/clinics). Many of the free clinics have changed their names to community clinics, and some have evolved into community health centers or migrant health centers as described earlier.

AMBULATORY PHARMACY SERVICES

Hospital Outpatient Clinics

Since 1983, community hospitals in the United States have experienced a significant reduction on the inpatient side and a significant increase in outpatient visits. To compensate for the loss of inpatient revenue, most community hospitals have moved toward expansion and modernization of ambulatory care clinics (Iglehart, 1993).

Clinical pharmacy is evolving from primarily an inpatient hospital focus to a greater concentration on ambulatory care. To meet the mandatory counseling requirements of OBRA 1990 (covering Medicaid) and state-passed legislation (extension to non-Medicaid patients), outpatient hospital pharmacies are undergoing layout redesign by incorporating semiprivate consultation areas and patient consultation rooms. Pharmacist participation in the management of specific disease states (e.g., anticoagulant therapy, hypertension, asthma, and diabetes) has already been described. Pharmacists and physicians working together have developed practice guidelines for pharmacists' management of patients with these chronic disease states (Reinders, 1986). Thanks to the pharmacist's contribution in these clinics, patient compliance with both medication therapy and future clinic appointments has improved.

Primary Care and Family Practice Clinics

Carter & Helling (1992) have described pharmacy services in primary care clinics and family practice clinics, and some of the following review is based on their description. Pharmacists' patient-centered care services have been reported in clinics associated with Appalachian Regional Hospitals, especially clinics for patients with specific diseases. As members of an interdisciplinary team, pharmacists lend their expertise to physicians and other healthcare professionals who are caring for their patients. Typically, the pharmacist performs physical assessments, orders laboratory tests, and changes medication regimens (Carter & Helling, 1992). Clinical pharmacists' participation in physician group practices in area health education centers and in North Carolina and South Carolina has also been documented (Eichelberger, 1980; Johnston & Heffron, 1981; Robertson & Groh, 1982).

Pharmacists' interventions have been shown to improve care. Morse and colleagues showed that blood pressure control could be improved and its cost reduced by pharmacy interventions (Morse, Douglas, Upton, Rodgers, & Gal, 1986). In a clinic for diabetic patients, intensive monitoring and follow-up by the pharmacist resulted in improved compliance, improved control, and reduced hospitalizations (Sczupak & Conrad, 1977).

Chrischilles and colleagues' cost-effectiveness analysis of pharmacy services' effects on family practice identified pharmacy services as improving physician efficacy, reducing adverse reactions, improving compliance, and improving the quality of care (Chrischilles, Helling, & Rowland, 1984a, 1984b). Given their expanding role in ambulatory care settings, pharmacists should aggressively pursue these practice opportunities, document their effectiveness, and publish these findings after developing good research designs (Carter & Helling, 1992).

Another study compared newly anticoagulated patients who were treated with usual medical care with those treated at an anticoagulation clinic. The anticoagulation clinic group had lower rates of significant bleeding (8.1% vs. 35.0%) and thromboembolic events (3.3% vs. 11.8%), significantly lower annual rates of warfarin-related hospitalizations (5% vs. 19%) and emergency department visits (6% vs. 22%), and reduced annual healthcare costs by $132,086 per 100 patients. Hence, a pharmacist-run anticoagulation clinic improved anticoagulation control, reduced bleeding and thromboembolic event rates, and was cost effective (Chiquette, Amato, & Bussey, 1998).

Community Pharmacy

Pharmacists are in a unique position in the healthcare system: They are the most accessible of healthcare professionals, and they are highly regarded by their patients. Pharmacists know that their everyday activities benefit patients. They are responsible for saving money for patients and third-party payers, improving therapeutic regimens, and averting therapeutic failures. Recent Gallup Public Opinion polls shows that pharmacists are listed among the most trusted professionals in society. This trust, along with the fact that most people visit their pharmacist several times for every visit they make to their physician, means that the pharmacist plays a crucial role in providing pharmacists' patient-centered care and improving patient outcomes.

Many independent pharmacies have survived by diversifying their revenue bases, including consulting with skilled nursing facilities, selling durable medical equipment, and building home healthcare businesses. Chain pharmacies have also been faced with declining revenues as they compete with mail-order pharmacies, web-based pharmacies, supermarket pharmacies, and super drugstores (big box stores, mass merchants). Part of chain pharmacies' acceptance of lower margins on prescriptions reflects the thought that pharmacy departments generate more foot traffic through their stores; thus, the lower margins on prescriptions are thought to be more than offset by increases in nonprescription and sundry sales and/or increased prescription volume (Tootelian & Gaddeke, 1993).

Retail Clinics

One way that community pharmacies have diversified is through the development of retail clinics (also called "mini-clinics," "minute clinics," "convenient care clinics," or "walk-in-clinics"). The retail clinic is located in retail stores, such as grocery stores and drugstores (e.g., CVS, Walgreens), and offers relatively inexpensive healthcare services, including camp and school/sport physicals, care for minor ailments (e.g., colds, ear infections, asthma, flu, strep throat, rashes, urinary tract infections, and minor wounds) and common vaccinations.

Retail clinics are usually staffed by nurse practitioners, who (in most states) can write prescriptions and conduct basic medical examinations and procedures. Not surprisingly, such clinics have met with some resistance from competing health providers (family practitioners and urgent care centers) and are seen as providing limited service competition. Critics suggest that they present problems in areas of continuity of care, quality of care, referral, and insurance issues. Nevertheless, the cost of a retail clinic visit is typically about one half the cost of a physician visit, so retail clinics are drawing interest from both health insurance companies and employers, which are constantly seeking innovative ways to reduce healthcare costs (Kher, 2006).

Pharmacists' Patient-Centered Care

Another way that community pharmacists have diversified is through the provision of pharmacists' patient-centered care. Hepler and Strand (1990) define pharmaceutical care as "the responsible provision of drug therapy for the purpose of achieving definite outcomes that improves a patient's quality of life" (p. 539). The four possible outcomes include (1) cure of a disease, (2) elimination and reduction of a patient's symptomatology, (3) arresting or slowing of the disease process, and (4) preventing a disease or symptomatology. Traditionally, pharmacists have been primarily concerned with the process of care—that is, what they do when the patient receives care (determining whether the correct drug and the right dose at the right time are provided). With the focus on outcomes, the pharmacist also takes responsibility for what happens to the patient when the drug is given (the outcome of care). Examples of outcome criteria include increased patient knowledge of the specific disease, improved medication adherence, improved medication therapy, decreased adverse reactions, decreased misuse and abuse, and higher patient satisfaction levels.

Given that more independent community pharmacies are facing the threat of closure because of steadily declining gross margins and increasing competition by high-volume pharmacies and mail-order centers, an increasing impetus exists for pharmacists to adopt the pharmaceutical care role. As insurance programs continue to lower prescription drug reimbursements, pharmacists should investigate other revenue sources, such as providing cognitive services.

To assume this role, community pharmacists must be trained to provide pharmacists' patient-centered care. The emphasis in such training programs is to encourage the community pharmacist to assume the role of the drug therapy expert and to be responsible for the reduction of drug-related problems. This training should include documenting clinical and financial successes rather than assuming savings. These programs also strive to get the pharmacist more involved in patient care in the hope that it will result in improved treatment outcomes and reduce utilization of more expensive services, such as hospitalization and unnecessary physician visits, thereby reducing the overall cost of health care.

Although the pharmacist's role in pharmacists' patient-centered care is promoted by pharmacy academia and organizational leaders, the concept of pharmacists' patient-centered care is not yet widely accepted by consumers, physicians, and health insurance carriers. Some of the research supporting their effectiveness is presented next. Pharmacist responsibilities have evolved from the traditional dispensing of medications to an expanded patient-oriented profession known as pharmacists' patient-centered care. Studies conducted in the 1990s and early in the 2000s have confirmed the effectiveness of pharmacists' clinical services in helping to assure the safe, effective, and cost-conscious use of medications (Schumock, Meek, Ploetz, & Vermeulen, 2008; Giberson, 2011. (http://www.accp.com/docs/positions/misc/improving_patient_and_health_system_outcomes.pdf).

Evidence for Pharmacists' Patient-Centered Care

Pharmacists in the Asheville project in North Carolina have been providing services to patients with diabetes since 1997. Pharmacists received reimbursement from local employers for providing cognitive services (e.g., education, assessment, monitoring, follow-up, and referral). The pharmacists' patient-centered care group's A1C concentrations and satisfaction with services improved more significantly than a comparison group. The Asheville project showed that face-to-face meetings between diabetic patients and trained pharmacists resulted in significant improvements in clinical, humanistic, and economic outcomes (Cranor & Christensen, 2003; Cranor, Bunting, & Christensen, 2003a, 2003b).

In the Diabetes Ten City Challenge, 30 employers in 10 U.S. cities established a voluntary health benefit for employees, dependents, and retirees with diabetes. Employers used incentives, such as waiving co-payments for diabetes medications and supplies, to encourage people to manage their diabetes. Local pharmacists were trained as coaches, who helped patients track their blood sugar levels and cholesterol and to control their disease through exercise, nutrition, and lifestyle changes. Data on 573 diabetic patients enrolled in the program for at least 1 year reported that average total healthcare costs per patient were reduced by 7.2%, compared to projected costs.

Significant improvements were observed for clinical measures including a decreased mean glycosylated hemoglobin level, and a decreased mean low-density lipoprotein cholesterol level, and a decreased mean systolic blood pressure (Fera, Blumi, & Ellis, 2009). Both the Asheville study and the Diabetes Ten City Challenge study demonstrate the value of pharmacists' patient-centered care provided by the community pharmacist.

During a 3-year cholesterol management program, Project ImPACT (Improve Persistence and Compliance with Therapy) included 26 ambulatory care pharmacists who managed patients with lipid disorders. The rate for adherence with lipid-lowering drug therapy improved to about 90%, and nearly two-thirds of participants maintained accepted treatment goals (Blumi, McKenney, & Cziraky, 2000).

In another project, an asthma project was incorporated into the Asheville project and the objective was to assess the health outcomes of a community-based MTM program for adult patients with asthma over 5 years. The intervention was done by 18 certificate-trained community and hospital pharmacists who were trained by a certified asthma educator; follow-up was conducted using scheduled consultations, monitoring, and recommendations to physicians. The results reported significantly improved measures of asthma control (forced expiratory volume in 1 second and severity classification) that were sustained for as long as 5 years. The percentage of patients with asthma action plans increased from 63% to 99%, emergency department visits decreased from 9.9% to 1.3%, and hospitalizations from 4.0% to 1.9%. While spending on asthma medications increased, the total asthma-related costs were significantly lower than the projections, based on the study population's historical trends. The authors concluded that patients with asthma who received MTM services had maintained both significant improvements and decreased overall asthma-related costs (Bunting & Cranor, 2006).

In 2006, the Centers for Medicare and Medicaid Services implemented the Medicare Prescription Drug Benefit (Part D) for seniors. As part of this program, some Medicare beneficiaries will receive MTM services. The intention of this program is to ensure that seniors who have multiple chronic disease states, and are taking multiple chronic prescription medications receive management assistance with their medication regimens, thereby ensuring that their drugs are used safely, effectively, and within a reasonable cost range. While pharmacists continue to be the leading provider of MTM services, it is also performed by other providers (e.g., nurse or physician). Sponsors can use internal and/or outside personnel (e.g., pharmacy benefit manager, MTM vendor, disease management vendor, community pharmacists, long-term care pharmacists, etc.) to provide the MTM services. Some of the research supporting the pharmacist's role in providing MTM is presented next.

In the first study, pharmacist-based MTM service for the North Carolina State Health Plan enrollees was assessed. Pharmacists identified 3.6 potential drug therapy problems per resident at the initial visit and recommended a drug therapy change in about 50% of residents and contacted the prescriber about 85% of the time, and about 50% of residents with a potential drug therapy problem had a change in drug therapy (Christensen, Roth, Trystad, & Byrd, 2007).

In a second study, MTM services were assessed for hypertension and dyslipidemia provided by pharmacists for six Minnesota ambulatory clinics. Since total health expenditures decreased significantly, they reported that every $1 invested in MTM services saved $12 in other healthcare expenses (Isetts et al., 2008). In a systematic review (meta-analysis) of MTM interventions in outpatient settings, MTM was found to reduce the frequency of some medication-related problems including nonadherence and lower health care use and costs. However, this report concluded that further evidence needs to be collected to demonstrate an improvement in health outcomes (Viswanathan, 2015; http://www.pharmacist.com/CEOBlog/ahrq-report-companion-jama-article-focus-evidence-mtm).

Multiple studies have been done to assess the clinical, humanistic, and economic impact of pharmacists' patient-centered care. Despite the evidence presented and the valuable inroads that community pharmacists have made into patient care, pharmacists' patient-centered care to the average patient remains an enigma, primarily because it is not provided on a broad scale and in an identifiable manner in the community pharmacies, where most people encounter pharmacists. National and state pharmaceutical organizations, community pharmacists, and researchers need to work together to demonstrate the impact of pharmacists' patient-centered care programs before the concept will be broadly accepted. For example, in the case study, Susan is considering whether she should integrate pharmacists' patient-centered care into his community pharmacy practice.

CONCLUSION

Ambulatory care services have undergone rapid development and expansion over the last three decades. Given the need for healthcare reform, there will be continued emphasis on developing innovative and cost-effective services.

QUESTIONS FOR FURTHER DISCUSSION

1. What pharmacists' patient-centered care innovations from the Indian Health Service can be adapted for use in community pharmacy practice?
2. Several ambulatory care services have developed in the past decade. What new services do you envision in the next decade?
3. Contrast ambulatory medical practice in rural and urban areas in your state.
4. Contrast ambulatory pharmacy practice in rural and urban areas in your state.

KEY TOPICS AND TERMS

Community health centers
Community pharmacy
Emergency services
Health department
Hospital clinics
Indian Health Service (IHS)
Managed care
Patient-centered medical homes
Pharmacists' patient-centered care
Primary care
Public health

REFERENCES

Allred, N. J., Wooten, K. G., & Kong, Y. (2007). The association of health insurance and continuous primary care in the medical home on vaccination coverage for 19- to 35-month-old children. *Pediatrics, 119* (Suppl 1), S4–S11. doi:10.1542/peds.2006-2089C. PMID 17272584

Alsuwaidan, S., Malone, D. C., Billups, S. J., & Carter, B. L. (1998). Characteristics of ambulatory care clinics and pharmacists in Veterans Affairs medical centers. *American Journal of Health-Systems Pharmacy, 55,* 68–72.

American College of Healthcare Executives. (1993). *Managed care in Medicaid: Lessons for policy and program design.* Melrose Park, IL: Health Administration Press.

Blumi, B. M., McKenney, J. M., & Cziraky, M. J. (2000). Pharmaceutical care services and results in Project ImPACT: Hyperlipidemia. *Journal of the American Pharmacists Association, 40*, 157–165.

Bunting, B. A., & Cranor, C.W. (2006). The Asheville project: Long-term clinical, humanistic, and economic outcomes of a community-based medication therapy management program for asthma. *Journal of the American Pharmacists Association, 46*, 133–147.

Carter, B. L., & Helling, D. K. (1992). Ambulatory care pharmacy services: The incomplete agenda. *Annals of Pharmacotherapy, 26*, 701–708.

Carter, B. L., Malone, D. C., Billups, S. J., Valuck R. J., Barnette, D.J., Sintek, C.D., ... Amato, M. (2001). Interpreting the findings of the IMPROVE study. *American Journal of Health-Systems Pharmacy, 58*, 1330–1337.

Chiquette, E., Amato, M. G., & Bussey, H. I. (1998). Comparison of an anticoagulation clinic with usual medical care. *Archives of Internal Medicine, 158*, 1641–1647.

Chrischilles, E. A., Helling, D. K., & Rowland, C. R. (1984a). Clinical pharmacy services in family practice: Cost-benefit analysis. I: Physician time and quality of care. *Drug Intelligence in Clinical Pharmacy, 18*, 333–341.

Chrischilles, E. A., Helling, D. K., & Rowland, C. R. (1984b). Clinical pharmacy services in family practice: Cost-benefit analysis. II: Referrals, appointment, compliance and cost. *Drug Intelligence in Clinical Pharmacy, 18*, 436–441.

Christensen, D. B., Roth, M., Trystad T., & Byrd, J. (2007). Evaluation of a pilot medication therapy management project within the North Carolina state health plan. *Journal of the American Pharmacists Association, 47*, 471–483.

Copeland, G. P., & Apgar, D. A. (1980). The pharmacist–practitioner training program. *Drug Intelligence in Clinical Pharmacy, 14*, 114–119.

Cranor, C. W., & Christensen, D. B. (2003). The Asheville project: Short-term outcomes of a community pharmacy diabetes care program. *Journal of the American Pharmacists Association, 43*, 149–159.

Cranor, C. W., Bunting, B. A., & Christensen, D. B. (2003a). The Asheville project: Factors associated with outcomes of a community pharmacy diabetes care program. *Journal of the American Pharmacists Association, 43*, 160–172.

Cranor, C. W., Bunting, B. A., & Christensen, D. B. (2003b). The Asheville project: Long-term outcomes of a community pharmacy diabetes care program. *Journal of the American Pharmacists Association, 43*, 173–184.

Eichelberger, B. N. (1980). Family practice clinical pharmacy opportunities in the community setting. *American Journal of Hospital Pharmacy, 37*, 740–742.

Fera, T., Blumi, B. M., & Ellis, W. M. (2009). Diabetes Ten City Challenge: Final economic and clinical results. *Journal of American Pharmacists Association, 49*, e52–e60.

Flowers, L., Wick, J., Figg, W. D., McClelland, R. H., Shiber, M., Britton, J. E., ... Huntzinger, P. (2009). U.S. public health service commissioned corps pharmacists: Making a difference in advancing the nation's health. *Journal of the American Pharmacists Association, 49*, 446–452.

Foss, M. T., Shock, P. H., & Sintek, C. D. (1999). Efficient operation of a high-volume anticoagulation clinic. *American Journal of Health-Systems Pharmacy, 56*, 43–48.

Giberson, S., Yoder, S., Lee, M. P. (2011). Improving patient and health system outcomes through advanced pharmacy practice. A report to the U.S. Surgeon General. (http://www.accp.com/docs/positions/misc/improving_patient_and_health_system_outcomes.pdf).

Hepler, C. D., & Strand, L. M. (1990). Opportunities and responsibilities in pharmaceutical care. *American Journal of Hospital Pharmacy, 47*, 533–542.

Hoffer, E. (1979). Emergency medical services. *New England Journal of Medicine, 301*, 1118.

Iglehart, J. K. (1993). The American health care system: Community hospitals. *New England Journal of Medicine, 329*, 372–376.

Isetts, B. J., Schondelmeyer, S. W., Artz, M. B., Lenartz, L. A., Heaton, A. H., Wadd, W. B, Brown, L. M., & Cipolle, R. J. (2008). Clinical and economic outcomes of medication therapy management services: The Minnesota experience. *Journal of the American Pharmacists Association, 48*, 203–211.

Johnston, T. S., & Heffron, W. A. (1981). Clinical pharmacy in family practice residency programs. *Journal of Family Practice, 13*, 91–94.

Kher, U. (2006, March 20). Get a check-up in Aisle 3. *Time,* pp. 52–53.

Leal, S., Glover, J. J., Herrier, R. N., & Felix, A. (2004). Improving quality of care in diabetes through a comprehensive pharmacist-based disease management program. *Diabetes Care, 27,* 2983–2984.

Madison, D. L. (1983). The case for community oriented primary care. *Journal of the American Medical Association, 249,* 1279–1282.

Mathematic Policy Research, Inc. (2004, November 30). Evaluation of HRSA's clinical pharmacy demonstration projects. Final report, volume II: Case studies, chapter II. *Siouxland Community Health Center Network,* pp. 11–20.

Mezey, A. P. (1999). Ambulatory care. In S. Jonas & A. R. Kovner (Eds.), *Health care delivery in the United States* (pp. 183–205). New York, NY: Springer.

Mezey, A. P., & Lawrence, R. S. (1995). Ambulatory care. In A. R. Kovner (Ed.), *Jonas's health care delivery in the United States* (pp. 122–161). New York, NY: Springer.

Morehead, M. A., Donaldson, R. S., & Servavelli, M. R. (1971). Comparisons between OEO neighborhood health centers and other health care providers of ratings of the quality of health care. *American Journal of Public Health, 61,* 1294–1306.

Morse, G. D., Douglas, J. V., Upton, J. H., Rodgers, S., & Gal, P. (1986). Effect of pharmacist intervention and control of resistant hypertension. *American Journal of Hospital Pharmacy, 43,* 905–909.

Murray, M. D., Loos, B., Eckert, G. J., Zhou, X., & Tierney, W. M. (1999). Work patterns of ambulatory care pharmacists with access to electronic guideline-based treatment suggestions. *American Journal of Health-Systems Pharmacy, 56,* 225–232.

New York Times. (2015, May 29, Pear, Subscription Publication). Officials say companies are intentionally blocking health data exchange.

Osterberg L., & Blaschke T. (2005). Adherence to medication. *New England Journal of Medicine, 353,* 487–497.

Paavola, F. G., Kermanoski, K. R., & Pittman, R. E. (1997). Pharmaceutical services in the United States Public Health Service. *American Journal of Health-Systems Pharmacy, 54,* 766–772.

Reid, R. J., Coleman, K., Johnson, E. A., Fishman, P. A., Hsu, C., Soman, M. P...., Larson, E. B. (2010). The group health medical home at year two: cost savings, higher patient satisfaction, and less burnout for providers. *Health Affairs, 29,* 835–843.

Reinders, T. P. (1986). Clinical services and ambulatory care. In T. R. Brown, & M. C. Smith (Eds.), *Handbook of institutional pharmacy practice* (pp. 509–515). Baltimore, MD: Williams and Wilkins.

Robertson, D. L., & Groh, M. (1982). Activities of the clinical pharmacist in a private family practice. *Journal of Family Practice Research, 1,* 188–194.

Roemer, M. (1981). *Ambulatory health services in America.* Rockville, MD: Aspen Systems.

Roth, R., Stewart, R. D., Rogers, K., & Cannon, G. M. (1984). Out of hospital cardiac arrest: Factors associated with survival. *Annals of Emergency Medicine, 13,* 237–243.

Scheffler, R. M., Waitzman, N. J., & Hillman, J. M. (1998). The productivity of physician assistants and nurse practitioners and health force policy in the era of managed care. *Journal of Allied Health, 25,* 207–217.

Schumock, G. T., Meek, P. D., Ploetz, P. A., & Vermeulen, L. C. (1996). Economic evaluations of clinical pharmacy services—1988–1995. *Pharmacotherapy, 16,* 1188–2008.

Schwartz, J. L. (1971). Preliminary observations of free clinics. In D. E. Smith, D. J. Bentel, & J. L. Schwartz (Eds.), *The free clinic: A community approach to health care and drug abuse* (pp. 144–206). Beloit, WI: Stash Press.

Scott, D. M., Boyd, S. T., Stephans, M., Augustine, S. C., & Reardon, T. P. (2006). Outcomes of pharmacist-managed diabetes care services in a community health center. *American Journal of Health-Systems Pharmacy, 63*(21), 116–122.

Scott, D. M., & Nordin, J. D. (1980). Pharmacist role in projects for children and youth. *American Journal of Hospital Pharmacy, 37,* 1339–1342.

Sczupak, C. A., & Conrad, W. F. (1977). Relationship between patient-oriented pharmaceutical services and therapeutic outcomes of ambulatory patients with diabetes mellitus. *American Journal of Hospital Pharmacy, 34,* 1238–1242.

Sherman, M. A. (1979). Mobile intensive care units: An evaluation of effectiveness. *Journal of the American Medical Association, 241,* 1899–1901.

Sparer, G., & Anderson, A. (1975). *Cost of services at neighborhood health centers: A comparative analysis.* Washington, DC: Office of Economic Opportunity.

Tootelian, D. H., & Gaddeke, R. M. (1993). *Essentials of pharmacy management.* St. Louis, MO: Mosby-Yearbook.

Viswanathan, M., Kahwati, L. C., Golin, C. E., Blalock, S. J., Coker-Schwimmer, E., Posey, R., Lohr, K. N. (2015). Medication therapy management interventions in outpatient settings: A systematic review and meta-analysis. *Journal of the American Medical Association Internal Medicine, 175*(1), 75–87. (http://www.ncbi.nlm.nih.gov/pubmed/22964778).

Williams, S. J. (1993). Ambulatory health care services. In S. J. Williams & P. R. Torrens (Eds.), *Introduction to health services* (4th ed., vol. 1, pp. 108–113). Albany, NY: Delmar.

World Health Organization. (2003). Adherence to long-term therapies: Evidence for action. (http://www.who.int/chp/knowledge/publications/adherence_introduction.pdf). Geneva: World Health Organization. ISBN 92-4-154599-2.

CHAPTER

10

Long-Term Care

Aleda M. H. Chen and Emily M. Laswell*

Case Scenario

Anna was a vibrant and active woman all her life. She was a star athlete in college, taught English and physical education at high schools, and volunteered extensively in her local community. In her 70s, her family began to notice some changes; Anna was forgetting little things. Over the years, the forgetfulness became more apparent, and by the time Anna was in her 80s, it was clear she had Alzheimer's disease. At first, her husband cared for her as much as he could, but with arthritis, many of the tasks he simply could not perform.

Her daughter, Marie, lived down the street with her husband and daughter. She started regularly providing care for her aging mother and father, postponing a return to the teaching career she put on hold while her own daughter was young. For years, Marie would go grocery shopping for her parents, help with the housework, and take them to medical appointments. Then, she would go home and care for her family. The years of caring started to take a toll on Marie as she entered her 50s, and her health began to deteriorate as she had little time for a proper diet or exercise. Eventually, Anna needed round-the-clock care for her activities of daily living, particularly toileting and bathing. Her husband's arthritis left him wheelchair-bound and unable to provide care, and the tasks became harder and harder for Marie to complete. One day, Anna fell and went to the hospital. The healthcare providers recommended that the family either hire home care or go to a long-term care (LTC) facility due to the advanced nature of her Alzheimer's and the level of care required. Medicare would pay for the first 90 days of the stay in a LTC facility, and since Anna's husband had purchased long-term care insurance years ago, they chose to go with long-term care. However, the long-term care insurance did not cover all the costs, and each month, Anna's husband spent more and more of their dwindling savings on her care.

*With acknowledgment to Kimberly S. Plake, Kristin B. Meyer and Ernest J. Dole.

LEARNING OBJECTIVES

Upon completion of this chapter, the student shall be able to:

- Define *long-term care (LTC)*.
- Compare and contrast Medicare and Medicaid regarding their coverage of LTC.
- Explain the reasons patients face financial difficulties in paying for LTC services.
- Identify and explain the types of institutional and community-based LTC services available to patients and their families.
- Describe the types of patients who use LTC services.
- Explain why there is a need for extended-care services.
- Distinguish between the philosophies of institutional and community-based LTC.
- Define *aging in place*.
- Compare and contrast medication regimen review (MRR), drug utilization evaluation (DUE), and drug utilization review (DUR).
- List the opportunities for pharmacist involvement in the care of residents in LTC facilities.
- Describe the benefits of pharmacist involvement in the care of residents in LTC facilities.
- Identify resources available to consultant pharmacists who wish to further develop their patient care skills.

CHAPTER QUESTIONS

1. What factors have led to the increasing need for long-term care (LTC) facilities?
2. What opportunities are available for pharmacists in the LTC setting?
3. What are the financing mechanisms available to persons who use LTC services?
4. What types of patients use LTC services?

INTRODUCTION

In the United States, many types of healthcare services are available. One type of care for which use is increasing is called extended-care or long-term care (LTC). LTC is defined as a "set of health, personal care, and social services delivered over a sustained period of time to persons who have lost or never acquired some degree of functional capacity" (Kane & Kane, 1987, p. 4). In addition, it is defined as "health, social, and residential services provided to chronically disabled persons with functional or cognitive impairments" (Liu, 1994, p. 476). Primarily, LTC assists people who have disabilities due to limitations in performing activities of daily living (ADLs) such as bathing, dressing, and toileting, or instrumental activities of daily living (IADLs) such as shopping and food preparation (Katz, Ford, Moskowitz, Jackson, & Jaffe, 1963; Lawton & Brody, 1969). For example, Anna, in our case scenario, had problems with the ADLs of bathing and toileting and needed additional care beyond the capabilities of her family. It was at this time that she entered the nursing home, which could provide assistance with those activities.

Many people assume that LTC refers only to nursing home care, but LTC can occur in both community and institutional settings. Estimates indicate that nearly 8.4 million individuals received LTC in 2013 (Harris-Kojetin, Sengupta, Park-Lee, & Valverde, 2013). The determination of the type of care received is based on the individual patient's needs and circumstances. The factors determining the type of LTC needed include the level of disability, availability of informal caregivers, financial circumstances, availability of public programs, and other personal circumstances (Andel, Hyer, & Slack, 2007; Liu, 1994). The main risk factors for institutionalization include advanced age, number and types of chronic conditions, difficulties with ADLs, and living alone (Andel et al., 2007; Gaugler, Duval, Anderson, & Kane, 2007; Nihtila et al., 2008). Other risk factors include cognitive impairment, ethnicity (minorities are generally at a lower risk), low social support, poverty, difficulties with IADLs, outpatient admission, and hospital admission (Andel et al., 2007; Banaszak-Holl et al., 2004; Bharucha, Pandav, Shen, Dodge, & Ganguli, 2004; Gaugler et al., 2007).

This chapter addresses many of the LTC options available to individuals in the United States, including institutional services (such as nursing homes, continuing care retirement communities, and psychiatric institutions), community-based services (such as home health care and hospice), and community facility services (such as adult day care). In addition, it examines the changing role of pharmacy and pharmacists in these healthcare environments.

PATIENTS WHO MAY REQUIRE LONG-TERM CARE SERVICES

Older Adults

Although the majority of older adults are not seriously impaired and do not need LTC services, the primary users of these services are individuals older than age 65 (Harris-Kojetin et al., 2013). In general, the need for LTC services increases with age (Andel et al., 2007). As people age, they are more likely to develop chronic diseases, incur disabilities, or develop dementia, similar to Anna's. Indeed, chronic disease is on the rise for older adults, with 92.2% having at least one chronic disease (Hung, Ross, Boockvar, & Siu, 2011). Approximately 68.4% of Medicare patients have at least two chronic diseases, and 36.4% have four or more such conditions (Lochner & Cox, 2013). In addition, 61.1% of noninstitutionalized adults over the age of 65 experience disability or physical limitations, which leads to difficulty in performing IADLs or ADLs (Centers for Disease Control, 2015).

For people with a disability, LTC services may be provided by family and friends—often called informal caregiving—as was the case initially with Anna (Wolff & Kasper, 2006). In 2013, approximately 37 billion hours of adult care were provided by around 40 million family caregivers in the U.S. (Reinhard, Feinberg, Chuoula, & Houser, 2015). Although friends may contribute to care, the primary providers of informal caregiving are spouses and adult children, with children providing 72% of care (Mendes, 2011).

In the case of informal caregiving, the typical caregiver is a woman who is 49 years old, has some college education, lives within 20 or 30 minutes of the care recipient, and provides care for her mother approximately 24 hours per week (National Alliance for Caregiving & American Association of Retired Persons, 2015; Wolff & Kasper, 2006). Males are increasingly providing care, as 40% of caregivers were men in 2014 (National Alliance for Caregiving & American Association of Retired Persons, 2015; Wolff & Kasper, 2006).

Approximately 70% of older adults will require LTC at some point during their lifetime and at least 35% will spend time in a nursing home (Family Caregiver Alliance: National Center on Caregiving, 2015; U.S. Department of Health and Human Services, 2015; Werner, 2011). In 2012, nearly 85.1% of the 1.3 million U.S. nursing home residents were older than age 65, and 42.3% were 85 years or older. The majority of these residents were female (67.7%) and white (78.7%) (Harris-Kojetin et al., 2013). The majority of the residents needed some assistance with bathing (96.1%), dressing (90.9%), and toileting (86.6%). In addition, 56% needed help with eating (Harris-Kojetin et al., 2013). Conditions that are commonly found in older adults who reside in nursing homes include diseases of the circulatory system (e.g., hypertension, diabetes, atherosclerosis, congestive heart failure, cerebrovascular disease, anemia), mental disorders (e.g., dementia, depression), skeletomuscular diseases (e.g., arthritis), diseases of the nervous system and sensory organs (e.g., Parkinson's disease), gastrointestinal disorders (e.g., gastroesophageal reflux disease), and bowel and bladder incontinence (Moore, Boscardin, Steinman, & Schwartz, 2012).

The use of LTC services is expected to increase in coming years, primarily because of the aging of the baby boomer population (born from 1946 to 1964). In 2011, the first of the baby boomers began reaching age 65. Although the current population of older adults have decreasing rates of disability due to advances in health care (Manton, 2008), the baby boomer generation is expected to have greater rates of disability, which may be attributed to rising rates of obesity (Martin, Schoeni, Freedman, & Andreski, 2007; Seeman, Merkin, Crimmins, & Karlamangla, 2010). According to current predictions, disabilities among older adults will increase, which will increase healthcare utilization (Seeman et al., 2010). Currently, 53.7% of older adults have some physical or mental impairment, with an estimated 25.4% having a disability that impacts IADLs or ADLs (Hung et al., 2011). Given that LTC use is more predominant in persons 65 years of age and older, demand for LTC is expected to grow even more from 2011 to 2050, as 27 million older adults are expected to need LTC services in 2050 (Harris-Kojetin et al., 2013).

Patients with Chronic Diseases

Although the elderly are the primary users of LTC, other individuals also use these services. Some patients younger than age 65 who live with chronic diseases and terminal illnesses require assistance beyond the informal caregiving provided by family and friends (Jones, Dwyer, Bercovitz, & Strahan, 2009; Kaye, Harrington, & LaPlante, 2010). For example, a younger adult with end-stage renal failure may need nursing home care as the disease progresses. Besides nursing home care, these patients often receive services from hospice, home health care, and other community-based care providers. Because of the progressive nature of chronic disease, these patients may require assistance in performing daily activities and complying with their healthcare regimens. Diagnoses commonly associated with LTC services include dementia, Parkinson's disease, stroke, depression, hip fractures, and diabetes (Nihtila et al., 2008).

Alzheimer's disease is an example of a chronic disease that often requires LTC services. Approximately 48.5% of older adults in nursing homes have Alzheimer's disease or other dementias (Harris-Kojetin et al., 2013). Individuals with Alzheimer's begin to experience memory impairment and have difficulty remembering new things. Over time, these individuals lose the ability to manage their finances, perform IADLs or ADLs, and may forget family and friends. These patients typically require assistance with ADLs and with maintaining health (such as taking medications), regardless of whether they reside in the home or in an institution. In addition, individuals with Alzheimer's disease have a tendency to wander from their homes or rooms and may not be able to return. They become disoriented and often cannot provide information, such as their name or the address where they live (National Institute on Aging, 2015).

While Alzheimer's disease generally strikes individuals 60 years or older, other illnesses requiring LTC services can occur in individuals much younger. Any disease that can limit physical functioning to a significant extent can increase the likelihood that the affected individual will need some type of LTC services, regardless of his or her age. For example, individuals who have severe head or spinal injuries as the result of an accident often require LTC as they often cannot perform ADLs.

Patients with Rehabilitative Needs

Some patients may need LTC services for a short time. These patients generally require additional time to recover before returning home after discharge from a hospital or some type of rehabilitative services. Because of the emphasis on cost containment, patients frequently are released from the hospital earlier—and sicker—than in past years. If they are not ready to return to their homes, they may be discharged for additional care in a nursing home setting or to a rehabilitation center.

Other patients may be ready to return home but need assistance there (such as patients recovering from a broken hip, other broken bones, or major surgery). In such cases, home health care may be provided. As stated earlier, the type of service used depends on the level of care required, the availability of informal caregivers (such as family and friends), and the patient's insurance coverage and other financial resources (Andel et al., 2007; Liu, 1994). The patient's physical and mental health also play a role in the decision-making process (Marengoni, Aguero-Torres, Timpini, Cossi, & Fratiglioni, 2008).

Patients with Terminal Illness

Patients who are terminally ill include individuals whose prognosis is poor and are thought to be close to death (typically within 6 months). For these patients, hospice care is often used to help with physical, social, and spiritual aspects of their illnesses. Although there are increasing numbers of institutional hospice facilities available, hospice services do not necessarily require institutionalization of the patient. Instead, they may allow patients to remain at home with family and friends while receiving palliative (comfort) care (Grant, Elk, Ferrell, Morrison, & von Gunten, 2009). Hospice or palliative care services can also provide informal caregivers with relief and support systems (Stevens, Lynm, & Glass, 2006).

FINANCING LONG-TERM CARE

This section provides a brief description of the types of financing available to individuals to pay for LTC services. Extended care services are financed in four major ways: (1) Medicare, (2) Medicaid, (3) private insurance, and (4) out-of-pocket resources.

Medicare is a federally operated insurance program primarily intended for individuals older than age 65. In addition, younger persons with disabilities or with end-stage renal disease may have coverage through Medicare. Eligibility for these individuals depends on the length of the person's disability, the type of disability, and the severity of the kidney damage. For instance, renal dialysis patients automatically qualify for Medicare coverage (Centers for Medicare and Medicaid Services, 2015e).

Medicare has several components. Medicare Part A provides limited benefits for LTC institutional services such as skilled nursing care in residential homes. It also covers in-home or institutional-based hospice services for individuals who are expected to live 6 months or fewer (Centers for Medicare and Medicaid Services, 2015e). In 2007, approximately 25% of nursing home care was paid for by Medicare (Ng, Harrington, & Kitchener, 2010). For Medicare to reimburse these services, the patient must be hospitalized at least three consecutive days and admitted to a skilled nursing facility within 30 days of discharge, and a doctor must certify that the patient requires rehabilitation or skilled nursing care on a daily basis for a hospital-treated condition (Centers for Medicare and Medicaid Services, 2015e, 2015l). Medicare will pay for covered services for the first 20 days of care. For days 21 through 100, the patient must pay a copayment for each day the service is used. For example, patients paid $157.50 per day in 2015. After 100 days, patients are expected to pay the full costs associated with their care in a skilled nursing facility. In addition, Medicare reimburses home healthcare services through Part A. Home healthcare services also are reimbursed by Part B (Centers for Medicare and Medicaid Services, 2015e). Although Medicare pays for skilled nursing care, it usually does not pay for those who need only custodial care (e.g., help with bathing, dressing, using the bathroom, or eating) or other residential care services that older adults like Anna need. These services are primarily financed by Medicaid, private insurance, or out-of-pocket resources (Centers for Medicare and Medicaid Services, 2015e).

With the advent of Medicare Part D in 2006 (i.e., the prescription drug benefit for Medicare beneficiaries), there is now an added level of payment complexity for those receiving LTC services. For Medicare beneficiaries receiving LTC services, the type of service or the setting in which the services are delivered determines who pays for the prescription medications. For example, if a patient receives skilled nursing care in a nursing home within his or her benefit period, then Medicare Part A pays for the patient's prescription medications. Once the benefit period offered through Medicare Part A ends, the patient's prescriptions are paid for by Medicare Part D (if the patient is enrolled in the program) (Centers for Medicare and Medicaid Services, 2015e). Since Anna, in our example, had Medicare Part D, her medications in the nursing home would be paid for by Medicare Part D. For hospice patients, symptom management and pain medications are covered by Part A, and Part D covers nonhospice medications (such as cardiac medications) (Centers for Medicare and Medicaid Services, 2015e). Chapter 18 describes the Medicare program in detail.

Medicaid is a federally regulated, public welfare program for the poor. Although the program is regulated by the federal government, it is financed by both the federal and state governments and administered by the state. As a consequence, Medicaid programs vary from state to state with different qualifications for eligibility (usually based on income and assets) and services. In the example, Anna would become eligible for Medicaid once she and her husband used up the majority of their personal financial resources (excluding their home). Because custodial care is not reimbursed by Medicare, Medicaid often is the primary payer for nursing home care in many, if not all, states. In 2009, 43% of nursing home care was paid by Medicaid and less than 25% was paid by Medicare (Zigmond, 2013).

In the past, much of the LTC paid for by Medicaid was institutional care or nursing home care. Today, however, there is increasing interest in community-based healthcare services, such as assistance with ADLs in the home setting. In fact, Medicaid expenditures for LTC services and supports have been growing over the last several years, with $123 billion going to this type of care in 2013 (Reaves & Musumeci, 2015). These care services often provide help with ADLs, such as bathing, toileting, and dressing. Community-based health care is likely to become even more popular in the future, given the desire of individuals to remain in the community and the lower costs associated with this type of care as compared to nursing home care (Ng et al., 2010).

Patients also use private insurance to finance their care. Many older individuals have policies that pay for those charges not covered by traditional Medicare. These health insurance policies are called Medigap insurance policies because they fill in the gaps in Medicare reimbursement. Depending on the policy, benefits may include payment of Medicare deductibles, Medicare copayments, and extended home healthcare services. For example, many Medigap policies pay for the $157.50 copayment during days 21 to 100 of eligible nursing home stays. Like Medicare itself, these policies do not include custodial or residential care benefits. Older adults who choose to participate in Medigap plans must pay monthly insurance premiums in addition to copayments (Centers for Medicare and Medicaid Services, 2015e).

Like Anna, many older adults purchase LTC insurance for the following two primary reasons: (1) Medicare and Medigap do not cover custodial care and skilled care beyond 100 days and (2) to avoid the spend-down of their assets before meeting financial eligibility requirements for Medicaid. This private insurance provides financial assistance in the event that a person needs to enter an assisted living or LTC facility. Some policies also assist individuals in paying for home healthcare services, hospice care, and adult day centers. Other popular benefits include case management services, homemaker services, transportation to medical appointments, and some medical equipment. Limits to these LTC policies are based on the expense, scope, duration of benefits, and exclusion of high-risk applicants. Individuals who already receive LTC services are not eligible for LTC insurance. These policies also can be expensive, with the average yearly premium cost in 2015 being $2,170 for a 60-year-old couple, which provides $328,000 of coverage. Costs for LTC insurance policies rose 8.6% from 2014 to 2015 (American Association for Long-Term Care Insurance, 2015).

In addition, some policies do not provide inflation protection, which would allow the benefit paid to increase as inflation increases. If a policy does not have such a clause, the benefit paid is the one stated at the time of purchase (Schleich-Williams, 2015). At first, this may not seem like a problem; however, if a person buys a policy at age 50 and does not need to use the policy until he or she is 70, there will be a significant difference in the benefit paid and the actual cost of care. Of course, inflation protection can greatly increase the premium, rendering some policies unaffordable. For example, the same couple above who pays $2,170 for $328,000 in coverage can pay an additional $1,760 per month to adjust for inflation and increase their coverage to $730,000 at age 80 (American Association for Long-Term Care Insurance, 2015). In addition, it is not certain that everyone will need LTC services, which makes it difficult for consumers to decide whether to purchase a policy. Also, policies are generally less expensive when purchased at a younger age. This purchase decision is more difficult for younger consumers; however, because they do not know whether they will need LTC or LTC insurance benefits.

LTC insurance policies have been improving over the past several years, and some now include lifetime benefits, coverage for home health care, short deductible periods, and inflation protection. Nevertheless, this type of insurance is not as tightly regulated as Medigap policies are, and it may be confusing to some consumers. Consumers should compare policies and identify the benefits of these policies before purchasing. Buying policies at a younger age is cheaper, and individuals considering buying a policy should consult a professional if they have questions.

If a patient does not have private insurance that covers LTC or if he does not qualify for Medicaid, the costs of care must be paid from the patient's financial resources. Family resources may be quickly depleted, depending on the location and type of nursing home selected. Nursing home care for a sustained period of time can prove catastrophic to a patient's financial stability. In such cases, patients may have to spend down their assets to qualify for Medicaid. Anna's husband was expected to pay for her nursing home bills until their assets were exhausted.

Since paying for LTC services often can exhaust some families' financial resources, some older adults are seeking the advice of estate planners to set up trusts, LTC annuities, and other financing options. An example of a financing option for older adults needing additional healthcare services is the reverse mortgage. Many older adults are homeowners, and a reverse mortgage allows them to receive a lump-sum payment, monthly payments, or a line of credit, thereby enabling them to remain in their own home despite a cash flow crunch. The borrower never owes more than the value of the home, and the loan comes due when the borrower moves, sells the home, or dies (Federal Trade Commission, 2015).

INCREASING NEED FOR FACILITIES

In 1935, when the Social Security Act was adopted, the United States used the age of 65 or older as one of the criteria for eligibility (Social Security Administration, 2010). Thus, the older adult population was defined as 65 years or older from then forward. Today's older adults can be divided into three categories: (1) the young old—aged 65–74; (2) the middle old—aged 75–84; and (3) the old old—85 years old and older (Rosenwaike, 1985). In 2014, 13% of the U.S. population was 65 years of age and older (U.S. Census Bureau, 2015). A rapid increase in the number of older adults is expected between 2010 and 2030, when the baby boomers will reach age 65. By 2030, approximately one in five Americans will be 65 years of age or older (Colby & Ortman, 2015). The fastest growing segment of the elderly population consists of those 85 years and older. By 2050, the number of people of age 85 years and older will more than triple to 18 million (Ortman, Velkoff, & Hogan, 2014). In addition, life expectancy has been increasing, such that the average life expectancy was 81.2 years for women and 76.4 years for men in 2013 (Kochanek, Murphy, Xu, & Arias, 2014).

Not only is America aging, but the demographics of the population also are changing. In 2014, 77.5% of the population was recognized as non-Hispanic white, 17.4% as Hispanic, 13.2% as African American, 5.4% as Asian American, and 1.2% as American Indian (some people identified themselves as belonging to more than one ethnic group). By 2060, non-Hispanic white Americans will account for approximately 44% of the country's population, becoming minorities (Colby & Ortman, 2015; U.S. Census Bureau, 2015). Similarly, older adults will become more diverse as non-Hispanic whites will comprise 58% of the elderly population in 2050 (Centers for Disease Control and Prevention, 2013). The changing demographics of the older population, along with the cultural expectations within various minority groups, will undoubtedly influence the provision of LTC services.

In addition, the roles of women are changing. This trend is of prime importance to the delivery of LTC services because wives, daughters, daughters-in-law, and even granddaughters provide two-thirds of all informal caregiving services. One of a woman's primary societal roles is as a mother. The nature of the life cycle does provide some insulation against a woman's shouldering the responsibilities for aging parents and child care responsibilities at the same time. In recent decades, however, some women have postponed childbearing until their late 20s, 30s, or even 40s. Because of this delay in starting their own families, they may have to balance the dual responsibilities of caring for parents and children as Marie did in the case scenario. Some women also have assumed responsibility for raising their grandchildren. The average age of an informal caregiver was 49 in 2014, so these women could be assuming several family roles (National Alliance for Caregiving & American Association of Retired Persons, 2015). In addition to their familial responsibilities, many women work outside the home; which can make it difficult to care for an elderly parent. Approximately 67% of informal caregivers with children continue to work outside the home while caregiving (National Alliance for Caregiving & American Association of Retired Persons, 2015). The average family caregiver spends 24.4 hours per week in care-related activities, and women who must bear the double burden of performing paid work and caregiving for a parent deal with the situation in a variety of ways, such as transitioning to working part-time, taking a less demanding job, leaving the workforce, or utilizing LTC services (National Alliance for Caregiving & American Association of Retired Persons, 2015).

The growth and increased interest in extended care have been primarily driven by the changing economics of health care. In 2013, U.S. national health expenditures were 17.4% of the country's gross domestic product, amounting to more than $2.9 trillion (Centers for Disease Control and Prevention, 2015). Spending by the government for Medicare and Medicaid totaled over $1 trillion (Centers for Medicare and Medicaid Services, 2015g). With baby boomers continuing to turn 65, health expenditures are expected to increase by 5.8% per year to 19.6% of the gross domestic product in 2024 (Centers for Medicare and Medicaid Services, 2015g). In 2014, the median rate for a semiprivate room in a nursing home was $212 a day and $3,500 per month for a one-bedroom assisted living unit (Genworth Financial, 2015).

Although extended care facilities are less costly than hospitals, their cost is still a major concern. National health expenditures for nursing home care totaled $155.8 billion in 2013, with Medicare spending $34.6 billion and Medicaid $46.9 billion (Centers for Medicare and Medicaid Services, 2015g). LTC expenditures are predicted to increase by over 5% a year between 2015 and 2024, costing $274.4 billion in 2024 (Centers for Medicare and Medicaid Services, 2015j). The aging of America coupled with a stressful economic climate makes it necessary to construct creative solutions to funding extended care.

INSTITUTIONAL SERVICES

As defined earlier, LTC or extended care is care that is delivered over extended time. LTC is not environment specific; it encompasses a spectrum of care levels ranging from acute hospitalization to ambulatory, home-based health care. LTC facilities offer continuity of care and services to optimize a patient's recovery. In addition, LTC facilities are based on an interdisciplinary philosophy of care (Voisine, Walke, & Jeffery, 2009).

Nursing Facilities

Nursing facilities (NFs) encompass a wide spectrum of care, with nursing homes being the most recognizable form. Since the passage of the Omnibus Budget Reconciliation Act of 1987 (OBRA, 1987), it is preferable to refer to nursing homes as nursing facilities.

Although the average length of stay in a nursing facility is 13.7 months, the length of stay in an NF can vary greatly (Kelly et al., 2011). Approximately 19.4% of the admissions into NFs are short stayers who remain in the facility fewer than 3 months (Jones et al., 2009). Short stayers can be further classified as residents who enter the NF extremely ill and with a short life expectancy or as residents who enter the NF for short-term rehabilitation. Approximately 24.2% of residents will stay more than 3 months, with 56.4% staying longer than 1 year (Jones et al., 2009). These long-stayers can be further classified as residents with impairments primarily of cognitive function (such as ambulatory patients with dementia) or impairments of physical function (such as residents with severe degenerative joint disease or end-stage heart failure) or as residents with both impairments.

The most medically and therapeutically intensive of the NFs are the skilled nursing facilities, which must comply with Medicare and Medicaid regulations in order to receive reimbursement. Skilled nursing facilities provide medical and nursing care in addition to restorative therapy, physical therapy, and occupational therapy (Centers for Medicare and Medicaid Services, 2015f). Pharmacists' roles in these facilities are typically related to dispensing or consultant activities, which are discussed in greater detail later. Skilled nursing facilities that are associated with a hospital are referred to as long-term acute care hospitals or long-term acute care facilities (Munoz-Price, 2009).

Long-term acute care hospitals are designed for patients who need clinical and rehabilitative services and for patients who need continuous care that may not be available in all NFs. They were originally started to decrease the costs associated with hospitalization for patients who were not ready to be discharged to a nursing facility. Patients with clinical conditions, such as postcerebrovascular accident or chronic obstructive pulmonary disease, and those who require parenteral nutrition, intravenous antibiotics, postsurgical wound care, and mechanical ventilator weaning may use long-term acute care hospitals. The average stay in these facilities is 35.3 days (Eskildsen, 2007; Kahn et al., 2013; Munoz-Price, 2009). Pharmacists have a variety of roles in a long-term acute care hospital, as these facilities must have an inpatient pharmacy. Besides dispensing activities, pharmacists can participate in interdisciplinary team rounds and educational services. In these settings, pharmacists often have clinical backgrounds, specializing in acute care (Chander & Kirkwood, 2006).

Psychiatric Facilities

Psychiatric facilities provide a distinctive environment for a pharmacist's practice. Although little of the literature has focused on this practice site, pharmacists in these settings can provide treatment recommendations, patient education, medication reviews, and group patient medication clinics. Pharmacists also can participate in interdisciplinary team conferences regarding the therapy of patients and contribute to pharmacy and therapeutics committees, quality assurance activities, and activities to ensure that the facility meets the standards set by the Joint Commission.

Studies have demonstrated that pharmacists in mental health facilities improve patient outcomes (Finley, Crismon, & Rush, 2003) and contribute by providing many different kinds of services (Richardson, O'Reilly, & Chen, 2014).

Correctional Facilities

Correctional facilities often provide long-term health care to their residents. As the general population ages, so does the inmate population. Approximately 2.3% of inmates are age 65 and older (Federal Bureau of Prisons, 2015), and older adults are the fastest growing segment of the prison population, with the number of older prisoners increasing by 79% during the 2000s (Williams, Stern, Mellow, Safer, & Greifiner, 2012). Older adult inmates have chronic diseases and medical problems, just like the general population, and they typically experience them sooner than their cohort due to lifestyle differences and lack of routine medical care. However, many prisons were built decades ago and are not currently equipped to care for prisoners with ADL impairments. The need for pharmaceutical care in this population offers a unique practice opportunity for pharmacists, such as providing medication information, monitoring HIV therapy, monitoring adverse drug events, helping with the newly evolving geriatric wards in prisons, and providing palliative care services (Wick & Zanni, 2009b; Williams et al., 2012).

Specialized Institutional Care

Patients with cognitive deficits are a distinct population that is often overlooked in the LTC setting. However, there are a growing number of LTC facilities that specialize in care of patients with cognitive decline, such as Alzheimer's disease or other forms of dementia. Depending on their specialized needs, these patients may reside in intermediate care facilities (which provide 24-hour care on a temporary basis) for patients with cognitive deficits, foster homes, group homes, assisted living facilities, and state homes. Adult day centers also have services for patients with cognitive decline (Alzheimer's Association, 2015). Pharmacists working with these patients can offer many of the same services found in psychiatric hospitals and in LTC facilities, such as dispensing and consultant work.

Hospice and Palliative Care

The word *hospice* comes from the Latin root for hospitality and hospitable (Storey, 1996). The focus of hospice, or palliative care, is the humane and compassionate management of patients with terminal diseases. The goal of therapy is to maintain the quality of the patient's life rather than to cure the patient's disease. Growth in hospice care has been spurred on by its transformation from an alternative healthcare choice to a Medicare-reimbursable benefit with the 1982 enactment of the Medicare Hospice Benefit program (National Hospice and Palliative Care Organization, 2014). For a patient to be eligible for hospice under Medicare, a physician must certify that death is imminent (expected within 6 months). Medicare will reimburse services related to palliative care, or comfort care (Center for Medicare and Medicaid Services, 2015e). Although services provided to patients may vary from organization to organization, services include physician services, regular home visits by registered and licensed practical nurses, home health aide and homemaker services to help patients with ADLs, social work and counseling services, medical equipment (e.g., hospital beds), medical supplies, medications for symptom control and pain relief, volunteer support for the patient and family, physical therapy, speech therapy, occupational therapy, and dietary counseling (Centers for Medicare and Medicaid Services, 2015e; National Hospice and Palliative Care Organization, 2014).

In 2013, The National Hospice and Palliative Care Organization (NHPCO) estimated that there were approximately 5,800 hospice programs in the United States serving 1.5 to 1.6 million patients. Although the majority of hospice patients are 65 years and older, approximately 16.1% are younger than 65. Approximately 36.5% of patients are admitted with a cancer diagnosis. The rest are admitted with noncancer diagnoses such as end-stage heart disease, dementia, disability, lung disease, stroke, and end-stage renal disease. In 2013, the average length of stay in hospice care was 72.6 days, with a median of 18.5 days (National Hospice and Palliative Care Organization, 2014).

In 2013, 58.3% of hospices were independent, freestanding agencies; 19.8% were hospital based; 16.7% were home-health agency based; and 5.1% were based in LTC facilities. Hospice patients are primarily covered by Medicare (87.2%), with 6.2% of care covered by private insurance and 3.8% covered by Medicaid. Approximately 94.1% of hospice care days are provided in patients' homes, thereby avoiding more expensive hospitalizations (National Hospice and Palliative Care Organization, 2014). It is estimated that hospice care reduces Medicare costs by at least $2,561 per patient (Kelley, Deb, Du, Carlson, & Morrison, 2013).

Hospice care teams are highly interdisciplinary, as doctors, nurses, pharmacists, social workers, counselors, and many other healthcare professionals work together to provide palliative care (Martin, 2006). Furthermore, these teams include over 355,000 hospice volunteers who provide patient care through spending time with patients and families, providing support services for hospice staff, and assisting with fund-raising efforts (National Hospice and Palliative Care Organization, 2014). Within the hospice interdisciplinary care team, there is a broadening role for pharmacists. Medicare is the primary payer for hospice services, and in order to continue to receive funding, hospice facilities must comply with Medicare's conditions of participation. New rules went into effect in 2008 that require that the hospice team work with an individual who is educated and trained in drug management. Comprehensive medication therapy assessments must be done within a few days of entering hospice care and updated every 15 days. Patients and family members must also be educated in medication disposal (Martin, 2009).

While the rule does not specifically require a pharmacist to provide these services, pharmacists are uniquely qualified through their training and experience to provide drug management services. Working with hospice programs offers the pharmacist the opportunity to show their drug expertise, especially in the management of patients' pain and other palliative care. Pharmacists also can participate in patient and family education about medications, review and manage patients' medication therapy, and ensure compliance with state, local, and federal regulations (Martin, 2009).

HOME AND COMMUNITY-BASED SERVICES

Home and community-based services is care that falls between institutional LTC and care for the ambulatory patient. In other words, the patient does not need nursing home care, yet he or she cannot live completely independently. To help these individuals, home and community-based services often include a combination of housing, health care, and social support. In addition, home and community-based services can provide help to patients with their ADLs, such as eating, dressing, bathing, and transferring (Voisine et al., 2009).

Adult Day Care Services

Adult day care services are community-based group programs for adults with functional or cognitive impairments, giving families relief from care for several hours. Adult day care services are typically available during normal business hours, Monday through Friday, but some adult day care centers now offer evening hours and weekend care. However, none offer 24-hour care. A wide variety of services are offered, including therapy (physical and mental), health monitoring, personal care, caregiver support, social activities, transportation, and provision of meals/snacks (National Adult Day Services Association, 2015; Voisine et al., 2009).

Often patients enrolled in adult day care are functionally impaired and need to be cared for in a supervised environment. The care focuses primarily on maintenance and rehabilitation. Patients reside in their own or their families' homes and travel to a central location for services. The individual's family can continue their daily activities, such as work, because their loved one can be cared for in a supervised setting. There are three different models for adult day care services, which include the medical model, the social model, and the specialized model. In the medical model, the most intensive health-related services, such as therapy and nursing care, are provided in addition to social activities. The social model provides social activities, meals, and recreation. Some health services are provided in the social model, such as medication administration. The specialized model focuses on specific groups of patients, such as those with cognitive impairment or developmental disabilities (e.g., dementia, Alzheimer's disease, or mental retardation) (National Adult Day Services Association, 2015; Voisine et al., 2009).

In 2012, there were an estimated 4,800 adult day care centers in the United States, serving 273,200 patients on any given day (Harris-Kojetin et al., 2013). Adult day care centers can be stand alone or can be affiliated with or part of larger organizations, such as home healthcare agencies, skilled nursing facilities, medical centers, or senior citizen centers. No federal regulations exist yet for these centers, but the National Adult Day Services Association has developed standards of care (National Adult Day Services Association, 2015). Medicare does not cover adult day services, and the average cost per day for adult day care services is $69, with a range of $10 to $242 (Genworth Financial, 2015). The cost depends on the type of services offered. Medicaid in some states will cover adult day care services, and private medical or LTC insurance companies also may include coverage in their plans (Voisine et al., 2009). There are many potential opportunities for pharmacist involvement, as consultant pharmacists providing staff, patient, and family education; advice on medication use and storage; maintenance of medication profiles; and drug-utilization review (DUR).

Assisted Living Facilities

Group residential settings are available in the community. Assisted living communities provide supportive, individualized, and personal services in a residential setting. The amount of care needed typically depends on the individual's ability to perform ADLs. In general, the level of care is not as extensive or as skilled as that found in a nursing home setting, even though assisted living facilities may house people who are disabled enough to qualify for nursing home care. Individuals in assisted living facilities have their own room or apartment and receive support services, such as meals, personal care assistance, nursing assistance (e.g., help with medications), and housekeeping. The services offered can vary, however, depending on the assisted living facility and the needs of the residents (Centers for Medicare and Medicaid Services, 2015k; Voisine et al., 2009). Assisted living facilities promote independence, privacy, and choices, along with providing care services (Cameron & Pinkowitz, 2009).

As of 2013, there were over 31,000 licensed assisted living residencies with over 1 million residents (Assisted Living Federation of America, 2013a). The average cost per month in 2015 was $3,600, but these costs varied by services offered (Genworth Financial, 2015). Costs associated with assisted living facilities are not covered by Medicare or Medigap insurance policies. Some state-run Medicaid programs pay for components of assisted living facility care, but do not pay for room and board. Private health insurance or LTC insurance may cover assisted living facility costs (Assisted Living Federation of America, 2013b).

There are opportunities for pharmacists within assisted living facilities, since approximately 85% of the residents need help with their medications. Residents are free to obtain medications from their pharmacy of choice, but some assisted living facilities now contract with LTC pharmacies and consultant pharmacists to provide medication management services. These services can include medication reviews, special packaging of medications, and medication education for patients, families, and assisted living staff (Cameron & Pinkowitz, 2009; Voisine et al., 2009).

FUTURE OF LONG-TERM CARE

Because the accessibility and affordability of LTC are major concerns, the federal government and state governments are exploring alternative financing and care options. In 2010, President Barack Obama signed the Patient Protection and Affordable Care Act (ACA) into law, which provides several opportunities for the care of the aging population. The ACA seeks to improve healthcare for the aging population in several ways, including lowering costs by providing higher quality services, promoting health through disease prevention and education, as well as providing improved care by coordinating medical care with a patient-centered medical home (PCMH) and community-based services (U.S. Department of Health and Human Services: Administration for Community Living, 2015). Other alternatives include expanding home and community-based services, encouraging the purchase of LTC insurance, waiving Medicaid requirements for certain groups, and implementing personal care service programs (Centers for Medicare and Medicaid Services, 2015k; Doty, Mahoney, & Sciegaj, 2010; Ng et al., 2010).

In looking for alternatives, the idea of aging in place has gained momentum. Aging in place refers to staying in the same home and community as care needs change. The definition has broadened to include moving to a new community and staying there as care needs change. This approach seeks to support independent living, social activity, and community ties. Many older adults prefer to age in place, and court rulings have upheld this idea (Wick & Zanni, 2009a). In 1999, the Supreme Court ruled in the *Olmstead* case that older adults have the right to remain in their homes if able (as determined by a healthcare professional) and willing, as moving older adults to facilities before necessary would isolate and limit them from community-based interactions. This and subsequent rulings prompted states to increase the number of home and community-based services available. For example, home and community-based waivers through Medicaid allow states greater flexibility in providing extended care services to older adults (Ng et al., 2010).

One of the fastest-growing types of senior housing is the continuing care retirement community (CCRC). CCRCs are based on the aging-in-place philosophy and provide a continuum of independent living, assisted living, and skilled nursing care on a single campus. As an older adult's health status changes, he or she can move among the different levels of care without having to relocate from the campus (United States Government Accountability Office, 2010). In 2014, there were over 2000 CCRCs with at least 600,000 residents (Powell, 2014). Most CCRCs require an entry fee. The average entry fee was $280,618 in 2012 but can be as high as $1,000,000. In addition, residents pay a monthly fee, depending on the level of care, that typically ranges between $3000 and $5000 (Powell, 2014). None of these fees are covered by Medicare, Medicaid, or insurance. Depending on the CCRC, a variety of services and amenities may be offered to residents, such as golf courses, swimming pools, specialized facilities, concierge services, and restaurants (Voisine et al., 2009; Wick & Zanni, 2009a). Some CCRCs are even affiliated with universities and offer college classes (Larkin, 2007). Individuals in CCRCs typically have Medicare Part D insurance, so pharmacists can implement medication therapy management (MTM) services in these settings and help provide continuity of care (Voisine et al., 2009).

Another example of an aging-in-place approach is the Medicare Program of All-Inclusive Care for the Elderly (PACE). This program integrates all aspects of care covered by Medicare and Medicaid, including medical, social, and LTC services, in addition to services not traditionally covered, such as meals, transportation, and adult day care. Interprofessional teams provide these services for eligible patients. Older adults who are frail and individuals who are disabled are eligible for the program, but they must meet the following criteria to qualify: (1) age 55 or older, (2) live in an area with a PACE, (3) certified eligible for care, and (4) can live safely in the community with program services. If they do not qualify for Medicaid, individuals enrolled in the PACE pay only small fees (Center for Medicare and Medicaid Services, 2015h). In 2015, there were 114 PACE programs in 32 states (National PACE Association, 2015).

PHARMACY SERVICES IN LONG-TERM CARE

Pharmacy services in LTC can be divided into two categories—distribution and consulting. Medications can be provided to residents in a facility from a pharmacy in a variety of unit-dose packaging systems, according to the needs of the facility. Distribution-related services also can address problems on an individual level. Many older adults have problems with packaging of medications, dosage forms, and picking up prescription medications. Pharmacies that service LTC facilities can help provide specialized packaging, discuss dosage form alternatives with the healthcare team, and provide delivery services and on-site counseling services (Mort, 2009). For example, pharmacies can provide patients with individual packets of medications with presorted packets containing the date and time to be taken. In addition to medications, the pharmacy may provide other distribution-related services, forms, and reports and be involved in the development of policies and procedures (see **Exhibit 10-1**).

In the case of consultant services, a consultant pharmacist may be employed by the distribution pharmacy, employed by a network of LTC facilities, or self-employed as an independent consultant who contracts individually with a facility. Pharmacy consulting offers the practitioner a number of special opportunities (**Exhibit 10-2**), and many pharmacists have found a rewarding practice niche in this area. In this setting, pharmacists are hampered only by their imagination. Pharmacists provide special pharmaceutical care services such as medication regimen review (MRR) as well as monitoring for patient outcomes, identifying and resolving drug interactions, selecting cost-effective medications, using pharmacokinetic dosing principles to ensure proper dosing, following good formulary management practice, conducting drug utilization reviews (DURs), educating healthcare providers, and providing case management to coordinate medication use

Exhibit 10-1 Distribution Pharmacy Functions

Drug Distribution
Initial screening of medication orders
Drug packaging and labeling
Drug delivery (routine and emergency)
Medication reordering
Audit system for controlled medications
Emergency medication supply
Monitoring of proper storage of medication

Provision of Forms and Reports
Computer-generated patient medication profile
Medication administration record
Treatment records
Patient cardex
Physician order forms
Automatic stop orders
Treatment records
Patient care plans
Drug utilization reports
Billing statements

Other
Policy and procedure development
Drug information
Durable medical equipment
Medical/surgical supplies
Enteral products
Intravenous services

Source: Reprinted with permission from W. Simonson, *Consultant Pharmacy Practice,* (2nd ed.), 1996, p. 71.

Exhibit 10-2 Selected Pharmacist Activities in the Long-Term Care Environment

Drug regimen review (DRR)
Nutrition assessment and support services
Enteral feeding products
Durable medical equipment (DME)
Home diagnostic services
Laboratory test ordering and interpretation
Pain management counseling
Patient counseling
Medical and surgical supplies
Quality assurance programs
Computer-generated forms and reports
Committee participation
Resident assessment and care planning
Specialized clinical activities
Drug utilization or use review (DUR)
Drug information
In-service education programs
Outpatient compliance packaging
Surgical appliance fitting
Clinical research programs
Pharmacokinetic dosing services
Specialized medication delivery systems
Intravenous therapy services
Therapeutic drug monitoring
Formulary development
Medication pass observation
Infection control
Participation in state survey process
Drug use evaluation (DUE)

as a patient moves through various case settings (Levenson & Saffel, 2007; Voisine et al., 2009). Additional opportunities may exist in some settings for creating collaborative practice agreements with physicians for disease state management services in areas such as anticoagulation, asthma, diabetes, hypertension, lipid management, pain management, and smoking cessation.

Both skilled nursing facilities and intermediate care facilities are governed at the federal level by the Centers for Medicare and Medicaid Services. The Centers for Medicare and Medicaid Services develops and periodically updates guidelines to help nursing facility staff and consultant pharmacists provide the best care possible to the residents of the facilities they serve. These regulations and interpretive guidelines can be found in the *State Operations Manual* (see https://www.cms.gov/Regulations-and-Guidance/Guidance/Manuals/Downloads/som107c07.pdf). Historically, as part of OBRA 87, federal legislation was enacted to address quality and care issues of nursing home residents. An important concept in the OBRA 87 requirements was that outcome indicators should be measurable and objective. In particular, this law mandated the use of a resident assessment instrument, which is a standardized review instrument to provide comprehensive, accurate, standardized, and reproducible assessments of each resident's functional capacity. It is also required to be completed in order for a LTC facility to be Medicare and Medicaid certified.

Assessment of the resident is the essential first step in the care planning process. This process includes the utilization of the resident assessment instrument upon patient admission to collect information regarding the patient's functional capabilities and health problems. The resident assessment instrument is used to promote an outcome-oriented resident care plan so as to ensure the quality of care and the resident's quality of life through the early identification of problems and risk factors that can be avoided, managed, or reversed (American Society of Consultant Pharmacists, 2015; Centers for Medicare and Medicaid Services, 2015d). This instrument includes three sections: (1) the minimum data set, a tool used to collect the information needed to evaluate a resident; (2) the care area assessment process, which address and assess the issues identified from the information on the resident's minimum data set using evidence-based clinical resources; and (3) the utilization guidelines (Centers for Medicare and Medicaid Services, 2015d).

The minimum data set helps to identify issues that place a resident at risk for an adverse outcome. These issues or triggers are addressed by using the resident assessment protocol, a protocol that helps to mitigate the trigger. The resident assessment protocols are structured, problem-oriented frameworks developed by clinical experts to address the areas that represent the most common problem areas or risks for nursing home residents. Through this process, the resident assessment protocols provide a systematic linkage to the resident's care plan (American Society of Consultant Pharmacists, 2015; Centers for Medicare and Medicaid Services, 2015d; Rahman & Applebaum, 2009). As part of these requirements, the medication regimen for each resident must be reviewed monthly by a pharmacist (American Society of Consultant Pharmacists, 2015; Centers for Medicare and Medicaid Services, 2015d; Levenson & Saffel, 2007).

Another part of OBRA 87 dealt with the use of unnecessary drugs. Under this section of the legislation (F329), patients' medication regimens must be free from unneeded medications—defined as any medications used in excessive doses (including duplicate therapy), for excessive durations, without adequate monitoring, without indications for use, in the presence of adverse drug reactions that indicate that the dose should be reduced or discontinued, or any combination of these reasons (Centers for Medicare and Medicaid Services, 2015i). The Centers for Medicare and Medicaid Services *State Operations Manual* guidelines promote appropriate drug and dosage selection and monitoring of medication therapeutic efficacy. They also emphasize monitoring of adverse drug events. This can directly affect the consultant pharmacist's practice in LTC (Levenson & Saffel, 2007). For additional information, please consult *State Operations Manual* Appendix PP (Centers for Medicare and Medicaid Services, 2015i).

Pharmacy services (F425) and MRR (F428) encourage interdisciplinary collaboration between pharmacists and other LTC providers and place emphasis on identifying and solving medication-related issues. MRR continues to be, at minimum, a monthly requirement, and includes a comprehensive review (Centers for Medicare and Medicaid Services, 2015i). Included in Appendix PP of the *State Operations Manual* are general guidelines for the MRR process performed by the consultant pharmacist and guidance for the use of medications in the elderly (Centers for Medicare and Medicaid Services, 2015i). Identification of use of inappropriate medication in this population is primarily based on the Beers criteria, which specifically outlines inappropriate medications for older adults. Many of the medications are included in the Beers criteria because of age-associated changes in physiology leading to increased prevalence of adverse effects. Examples of medications included in the Beers criteria are amitriptyline, lorazepam, diazepam, and cyclobenzaprine (Campanelli, 2013).

Medication Regimen Review

The role of pharmacists has evolved since MRR first emerged in 1974 as part of a quality assurance program for the care of Medicare recipients in skilled nursing facilities and was expanded due to the Omnibus Budget Reconciliation Act of 1987 (OBRA '87) that imposed stricter minimum standards for LTC facilities (Clark, Gruber, & Sey, 2010b). The Centers for Medicare and Medicaid Services (CMS), in Appendix PP, began to issue standards regarding the use and monitoring of antipsychotic and other related medications for nursing homes. Thus, pharmacists were increasingly included in LTC to provide medication-related services, such as MRR (Clark et al., 2010b). The term MRR was previously known as drug regimen review, and these abbreviations can be used interchangeably in LTC and the literature. However, according to the Medicare *State Operations Manual*, MRR is a thorough evaluation of the medication regimen of a resident, with the goal of promoting positive outcomes and minimizing adverse consequences associated with medication. The review includes preventing, identifying, reporting, and resolving medication-related problems, medication errors, or other irregularities, and collaborating with other members of the interdisciplinary team (Center for Medicare and Medicaid Services, 2015i; Clark, Gruber, & Sey, 2010a; Clark et al., 2010b; Clark, Gruber, & Sey, 2011). Pharmacists should not only evaluate the appropriateness of each medication and the management of diseases and conditions, but they also should evaluate patient preferences (Clark et al., 2010b).

As directed by federal mandate, the guidelines for MRR can be divided into several categories—for example, unnecessary medications/excessive doses, excessive duration of drug therapy, inadequate drug monitoring, and absence of documented diagnosis or clinical symptoms (Center for Medicare and Medicaid Services, 2015i). To be efficient in the process of MRR, a pharmacist must develop a systematic approach of identifying actual and potential drug therapy problems (Clark et al., 2010a, 2010b). **Exhibit 10-3** provides an organized framework for the pharmacist to utilize when conducting MRR, along with examples for each category.

MRR can be prospective (at the point of admission into a LTC facility or with the initiation of a new medication), concurrent (while the medication is being used), or retrospective (after discharge or completion of medication therapy) (Clark et al., 2010b). Prospective MRR has been shown to be an effective mechanism to reduce medication use and costs. The North Carolina Polypharmacy initiative (for more information see the "Examples of Consultant Pharmacy Services" section) had

Exhibit 10-3 Drug Regimen Review Framework

1. Drug use without indication. The resident is taking a medication for no medically valid indication.
2. Untreated indication. The resident has a medical problem that requires drug therapy but is not receiving a drug for that indication.
3. Improper drug selection. The resident has a drug indication but is taking the wrong drug or is taking a drug that is not the most appropriate for the special needs of the resident.
4. Subtherapeutic dosage. The resident has a medical problem that is being treated with too little of the correct medication.
5. Overdosage. The resident has a medical problem that is being treated with too much of the correct medication.
6. Adverse drug reaction. The resident has a medical problem that is the result of an adverse drug reaction or adverse effect.
7. Drug interaction. The resident has a medical problem that is the result of a drug-drug, drug-food, or drug-laboratory test interaction.
8. Medication errors. A deficiency or weakness of the medication use process of the facility has resulted in an actual or potential medication error.
9. Medication monitoring. Evaluation of medications for effectiveness and toxicity or adverse effects.
10. Medication costs. Intervention is needed to assist the resident with obtaining access to a lower-cost medication or overcoming a barrier to medication access, such as formulary restriction or prior authorization.

Source: From "Introduction to medication regimen review – Part 2," *The Consultant Pharmacist,* 25(12), pp. 788–802, 2010. Reprinted with permission of The American Society of Consultant Pharmacists, Alexandria, VA.

pharmacists perform MRRs for nursing home Medicaid patients. Researchers found that MRRs and subsequent therapy recommendations decreased polypharmacy and cut medication costs by $30.33 per patient each month. The savings in 1 month compensated for pharmacist services (Christensen, Trygstad, Sullivan, Garmise, & Wegner, 2004). Other studies have shown MRRs to reduce unnecessary medication use (Suhrie et al., 2009) and to reduce anti-psychotic drug prescribing (Nishtala, McLachlan, Bell, & Chen, 2008).

Drug Utilization Evaluation

Drug utilization evaluation (DUE) entails a sophisticated analysis of medications, their uses, and their contributions to various patient outcomes. Institutions accredited by the Joint Commission regularly perform DUEs. A DUE may focus on a particular medication, evaluate the use of an entire class of medications, or monitor the therapy of a medical condition (The Joint Commission, 2010).

DUE is a criteria-based, ongoing, planned, and systematic review of medication. It is often prospective, in that the criteria to be applied are determined first, and then the medication for review is evaluated. Patient data and laboratory data are often included and available for review. DUEs are frequently population based in a specific institution and often part of an institution's quality assessment program. The Joint Commission recommends that a medication's inclusion be based on the following criteria: frequently prescribed, known or suspected to present significant risk, known or suspected to be problem prone, or a critical component of the care provided for a specific diagnosis, condition, or procedure.

As of 1995, the Joint Commission encouraged the use of an interdisciplinary approach to DUEs and development of collaborative medication use review. Standards continue to support an interdisciplinary approach and focus on how patient care can be improved in LTC facilities as a result of problems identified through the review process (Kubacka, 1996).

Drug Utilization Review

Drug utilization reviews (DURs) were established by the 1990 Omnibus Budget Reconciliation Act (OBRA, 1990). Pharmacists performing DURs are required to review past patterns of medication misuse, monitor current medication therapy, and offer patient counseling. By some practitioners' definition, DUR is a subset of DUE. Whereas DUE is prospective, DUR is frequently retrospective. DURs may use large databases and become part of a system's quality assurance program. In the past, use of such reviews has decreased medication costs and the use of inappropriate medications in LTC facilities (Kubacka, 1996).

MRR, DUE, and DUR have comparable functions, and the outcomes they measure can be classified into the following four categories: (1) therapeutic, (2) functional, (3) quality of life, and (4) economic (Gore, 1994; Kubacka, 1996). Documenting the patient outcomes of pharmacists' recommendations allows the practitioner to chronicle internal quality assurance. Documentation of patient outcomes also provides evidence that the pharmacists themselves are delivering quality patient care (Gore, 1994).

Medication Reconciliation

LTC facilities accredited by the Joint Commission have also performed medication reconciliation since 2005. Medication reconciliation is a process by which medications are accurately and completely accounted for throughout the care process. At admission, a complete list of medications is obtained, including dosage, route of administration, and dosing frequency. The indication for each medication also is obtained. As medications are added during the care process, they are compared to the list generated at admission and any discrepancies are reconciled. Upon discharge to another facility or home, the new facility or the patient and his family are informed about the current medication list. The goal of medication reconciliation is to avoid adverse drug events due to inadequate communication between and among healthcare providers, especially during the transfer process. Pharmacists can play a critical role in this process by designing and managing the medication reconciliation process (Steeb & Webster, 2012).

Examples of Consultant Pharmacy Services

Fleetwood Project

In an effort to demonstrate how consultant pharmacists can influence patient care in the nursing home environment, the American Society of Consultant Pharmacists initiated the Fleetwood Project. This project includes the following three phases: (1) assessment of the baseline costs of medication-related problems in the nursing home setting and the impact pharmacist MRR has on patient outcomes and costs; (2) assessment of prospective interventions utilizing a formal pharmaceutical care planning model for nursing home patients at high risk for medication-related problems (the Fleetwood model); and (3) assessment of the effectiveness of the Fleetwood model in assisted living facilities and nursing homes (Lombardi & Kennicutt, 2002).

In the first phase of the model, researchers conducted a cost-of-illness study to assess medication therapy in nursing homes. This study estimated that consultant pharmacists reduce medication-related morbidity and mortality costs by $3.6 billion annually in the United States (Bootman, Harrison, & Cox, 1997).

The second phase of the project focused on the feasibility of implementing formal pharmaceutical care planning in the nursing home setting. A 6-month pilot program was implemented in six nursing homes in Wisconsin. From the pilot study, it appeared that this approach to care was feasible (Moskowitz, 2003).

The third phase of the Fleetwood Project tested the effectiveness of the Fleetwood model and was conducted in 26 nursing facilities in North Carolina (Cameron, Feinberg, & Lapane, 2002). The investigators developed screening tools to help pharmacists identify patients at high risk for adverse events and treatment algorithms for alternatives to potentially inappropriate medications (Christian, vanHaaren, Cameron, & Lapane, 2004; Lapane & Hughes, 2004a). In addition, Fleetwood phase III reported high job satisfaction among pharmacists participating in the project (Lapane & Hughes, 2004b).

North Carolina Nursing Home Polypharmacy Initiative

After determining that many nursing home patients covered by Medicaid were taking six or more prescription medications daily, the state of North Carolina initiated a pharmacy case management program. Thirteen nursing homes were selected to participate in this program. The goal was to reduce the total number of prescription medications taken by addressing problems such as therapeutic duplication, inappropriate drug utilization, multiple prescriber issues, and higher-than-normal drug use. In addition, there was an effort to switch brand prescription medications to generics or other therapeutic alternatives. After analysis by pharmacist–physician teams, 37% of patients were identified as needing medication changes. Results from the analysis indicated that the economic benefits outweighed the costs of implementing the program by a ratio of 13 to 1 (Henry, Mendelson, & Fallieras, 2003).

Medication Therapy Management (MTM)

With the advent of Medicare Part D and the ability to be compensated for managing medications, many pharmacies and pharmacists are providing MTM services to the community. These services can improve patient outcomes and reduce healthcare costs in older adults. A pharmacy practice resident (postgraduate year 1) evaluated the medication therapies of older adults in an assisted living facility and provided drug-therapy recommendations to their primary care physicians. The goal of the project was to examine the economic impact of the intervention. The analysis identified problems such as missed drug therapy, inappropriate dosing, adverse drug reactions, and high costs; these problems were then addressed with the primary care physician. A total of 125 recommendations were made, and 72 were acted upon. The recommendations that were accepted resulted in a cost savings greater than the cost of the pharmacy services provided (Maack, Miller, Johnson, & Dewey, 2008).

Opportunities for Pharmacists in Long-Term Care

Participation in other quality assurance activities and on the pharmacy and therapeutics committees of LTC institutions offers the pharmacist more chances to expand beyond the traditional dispensing role (Levenson & Saffel, 2007). The areas of palliative care, prison inmate care, and managing patients with substance abuse problems also offer distinctive practice opportunities (Martin, 2006, 2009; Wick & Zanni, 2009b). While pharmacist presence in palliative care is increasing, other areas have little pharmacist involvement. In addition, pharmacists are teaming up with primary care providers in providing disease state management. Collaborative efforts include patient-specific medication recommendations, identification of inappropriate medication prescribing, and working with the interdisciplinary team to gather information to provide optimum care (Levenson & Saffel, 2007). There has been increasing national focus on the costs of healthcare. With the federal and state governments seeking to reduce healthcare costs, pharmacists can provide expertise in optimizing medications in terms of efficacy, safety, and cost (Stefanacci, 2012).

Pharmacists also can provide important services in assisted living facilities and PACE programs by evaluating participants for medication-related problems. At least 30 states also require that MRR be performed in assisted living facilities, which provides substantial opportunities for pharmacists (Simonson, Novak, & Jennewine, 2013). Participants in the PACE program should receive a medication review twice a year by a medical provider, and in many states, a pharmacist may fulfill that role. Additionally, pharmacists can provide other services, such as patient education, medication adherence promotion, adverse drug event monitoring, clinical services (e.g., anticoagulation, diabetes), and formulary creation (Bouwmeester, 2012).

The Medicare Prescription Drug, Improvement, and Modernization Act of 2003 also provided an opportunity for pharmacists to offer MTM services to Medicare beneficiaries since 2006. The eligible providers, covered services, and reimbursement structures vary among the prescription drug plans, but pharmacists can offer services related to medication therapy review, personal medication records, and medication-related action plans, as well as provide interventions and/or referrals, medication documentation, and follow-up (Truong, Layson-Wolf, Rodriguez de Bittner, Owen, & Haupt, 2009). Community and consultant pharmacists can provide MTM services in adult day care centers, CCRCs, and assisted living facilities, in addition to offering them in community pharmacies (Cameron & Pinkowitz, 2009; Voisine et al., 2009).

Additionally, the ACA (2010) has provided several opportunities for the expansion of pharmacist services in the LTC setting, particularly related to the PCMH, Accountable Care Organizations, and home-based care (Kaldy, 2010). In the PCMH model mentioned earlier, healthcare providers perform comprehensive care of the whole patient, from preventative care to chronic care, including patient values and preferences. Care also is led by at least one independent clinician, such as a physician or nurse practitioner, and coordinated to avoid issues with transitions of care (Agency for Healthcare Research and Quality, 2015; Stack and Kier, 2014a). The National Committee for Quality Assurance (NCQA) evaluates the quality of care provided by PCMHs, including: (1) access to care, (2) identifying and managing patient populations, (3) preappointment planning by the clinician, (4) provision of self-care support and community resources, (5) tracking and coordination of care, and (6) measuring and improving performance (Stack and Kier, 2014b, 2014c). Because of the comprehensive nature of the care as well as the focus on quality and safety, pharmacists can perform services similar to MTM and engaging in evidence-based, decision-making (Kaldy, 2010).

Accountable Care Organizations, or ACOs, consist of a group of providers and facilities that work together to ensure the consistent, quality, and cost-efficient care of Medicare beneficiaries (Centers for Medicare and Medicaid Services, 2015a). As of 2014, there were 626 ACOs serving 20.5 million patients (Gardner, 2014). While pharmacists are not mandated to be part of the team, they can provide a crucial role by assisting in medication management activities to improve outcomes and reduce costs (Kaldy 2012).

Another provision in the ACA is for an "Independence at Home Pilot Program" to test the effectiveness of providing primary care in the home setting. Teams of healthcare professionals will provide care for Medicare beneficiaries with multiple chronic conditions. These teams, led by physicians or nurse practitioners, may include pharmacists. The pilot test of the program began in 2012, with the first year of the program saving at least $25 million ($3,070 per beneficiary). Given the early success of this model and the provision to include pharmacists as part of the team, this is an excellent opportunity for pharmacists to expand their role as part of the healthcare team (Batshon, 2010; Centers for Medicare and Medicaid Services, 2015b, 2015c).

Many training programs are offered for pharmacists who are interested in working with the elderly population. The American Society of Consultant Pharmacists (ASCP) Research and Education Foundation is just one organization that has partnered with industry sponsors to offer advanced training in this area.[1] Programs available from the American Society of Consultant Pharmacists Foundation and its partners include those that focus on Alzheimer's disease/dementia, geriatric psychiatric/behavioral disorders, pain management, and Parkinson's disease. In addition, there are specific disease-related education and materials, such as prescription labeling for those dealing with vision loss.

Some pharmacists may choose to enhance their practices by obtaining certification in geriatric pharmacy. This is an optional process beyond required pharmacy licensure. A certified geriatric pharmacist has met certain educational and experiential requirements and passed an examination designed to test his or her knowledge and skills in geriatric pharmaceutical care. Continuing education guidelines must be met to maintain this certification.[2]

Rotations, residencies, and fellowships also are available for those interested in working with older adults. Many pharmacy schools offer introductory and advanced pharmacy practice experiences in geriatrics, which can introduce pharmacy students to pharmaceutical care of older adults (Odegard, Breslow, Koronkowski, Williams, & Hudgins, 2007). There are several American Society of Health-System Pharmacists–accredited postgraduate year 2 residencies available in geriatric pharmacy.[3] Typical postgraduate year 2 residencies in geriatric pharmacy give experience in ambulatory, acute, intermediate, and LTC, as well as in therapeutic monitoring of chronic diseases such as anticoagulation and diabetes. Fellowships can offer opportunities for research regarding older adults in addition to providing clinical training.

---

[1] For more information on these training programs, contact the foundation at: 1321 Duke Street, Alexandria, VA 22314-3563; phone: (703) 739-1300, fax: (703) 739-1500, email: info@ascpfoundation.org, website: http://www.ascpfoundation.org/index.cfm.

[2] For more information on becoming a certified geriatric pharmacist, contact the Commission for the Certification of Geriatric Pharmacy, 1321 Duke Street, Suite 400, Alexandria, VA 22314-3563; phone: (703) 535-3036, fax: (703) 739-1500, website: http://www.ccgp.org/.

[3] For more information, see: http://accred.ashp.org/aps/pages/directory/residencyProgramSearch.aspx.

CONCLUSION

LTC encompasses a variety of services that are provided to individuals who have lost some aspect of functioning. Like Anna in the case scenario, many individuals need help with normal daily activities, such as bathing, toileting, or dressing, which family or friends may be unable to provide. As the number of older adults continues to rise, there will be increasing demands for LTC services. Costs associated with LTC services also continue to rise with the demand for services. Many individuals purchase LTC health insurance to defray some of the costs. However, the majority of LTC costs are covered by Medicare and Medicaid, and creative solutions are needed to address the high costs of LTC for the future.

The roles for pharmacists in LTC are expanding and evolving to meet patient needs. Pharmacists provide many different services, including dispensing medications, consulting with LTC facilities and healthcare providers, and managing complex medication regimens. Training for pharmacists interested in working in LTC is available through numerous outlets, including advanced pharmacy practice experiences, residencies, fellowships, and geriatric pharmacy certification programs. Through efforts such as the Fleetwood Project and MTM services, pharmacists have demonstrated that they are well-prepared to provide LTC services and address patient care needs.

QUESTIONS FOR FURTHER DISCUSSION

1. Given that the population of older adults is growing and that healthcare dollars are finite, how would you guarantee access to LTC facilities for all patients who need that access?
2. The role of the pharmacist in the LTC setting is evolving. How would you ensure this role's continued progress? (Suggest curricular, research, and legislative solutions.)
3. Given the current financing mechanisms of LTC, how would you recommend that your parents or grandparents prepare for their potential future LTC needs?
4. Because the baby boomer population will significantly affect the need for health services, how should the healthcare community and country prepare for 2030?

KEY TOPICS AND TERMS

Activities of daily living
Adverse drug reaction
Aging-in-place
Community-based health care
Consultant pharmacist
Continuing care retirement community
Drug utilization evaluation (DUE)
Drug utilization review (DUR)
Health insurance
Hospice
Informal care or caregiving
Instrumental activities of daily living
Interdisciplinary
Long-term care services
Medication regimen review (MRR)
Older adults
Skilled nursing facility

REFERENCES

Agency for Healthcare Research and Quality. (2015). *Defining the PCMH*. Retrieved from https://pcmh.ahrq.gov/page/defining-pcmh

Alzheimer's Association. (2015). *Adult day centers*. Retrieved from https://www.alz.org/care/alzheimers-dementia-adult-day-centers.asp

American Association for Long-Term Care Insurance. (2015). Average costs for long term care insurance rise 8.6 percent. Retrieved from http://www.aaltci.org/news/long-term-care-insurance-association-news/average-costs-for-long-term-care-insurance-rise-8-6-percent

American Society of Consultant Pharmacists. (2015). Nursing facility survey and regulations. Retrieved from https://www.ascp.com/articles/nursing-facility-survey-regulations

Andel, R., Hyer, K., & Slack, A. (2007). Risk factors for nursing home placement in older adults with and without dementia. *Journal of Aging and Health, 19*(2), 213–228.

Assisted Living Federation of America. (2013a). *Assisted living*. Retrieved from http://www.alfa.org/alfa/Assisted_Living_Information.asp

Banaszak-Holl, J., Fendrick, A. M., Foster, N. L., Herzog, A. R., Kabeta, M. U., Kent, D. M., … Langa, K. M. (2004). Predicting nursing home admission: Estimates from a 7-year follow-up of a nationally representative sample of older Americans. *Alzheimer's Disease and Associated Disorders, 18*(2), 83–89.

Batshon, L. (2010). Health care reform law offers opportunities for pharmacists. *The Consultant Pharmacist, 25*(6), 388.

Bharucha, A. J., Pandav, R., Shen, C., Dodge, H. H., & Ganguli, M. (2004). Predictors of nursing facility admission: A 12-year epidemiological study in the United States. *Journal of the American Geriatrics Society, 52*(3), 434–439.

Bootman, J. L., Harrison, D. L., & Cox, E. (1997). The health care cost of drug-related morbidity and mortality in nursing facilities. *Archives of Internal Medicine, 157*(18), 2089–2096.

Bouwmeester, C. (2012). The PACE program: Home-based long-term care. *The Consultant Pharmacist, 27*(1), 24–30.

Cameron, K., Feinberg, J. L., & Lapane, K. (2002). Fleetwood Project phase III moves forward. *The Consultant Pharmacist, 17*(3), 181–198.

Cameron, K., & Pinkowitz, J. (2009). Connecting with assisted living consumers. *The Consultant Pharmacist, 24*(1), 16–28.

Campanelli, C. M. (2013). American Geriatrics Society updated Beers Criteria for potentially inappropriate medication use in older adults. *Journal of the American Geriatrics Society, 60*(4), 616–631.

Centers for Disease Control. (2015, April 29, 2015). Fast facts: Disability and functioning (adults). Retrieved from http://www.cdc.gov/nchs/fastats/disability.htm.

Centers for Disease Control and Prevention. (2013). The state of aging and health in America 2013. Atlanta, GA: Centers for Disease Control and Prevention, US Dept of Health and Human Service.

Centers for Disease Control and Prevention. (2015). FastStats-health expenditures. Retrieved from http://www.cdc.gov/nchs/fastats/health-expenditures.htm

Centers for Medicare and Medicaid Services. (2015a). Accountable Care Organizations (ACO). Retrieved from https://www.cms.gov/Medicare/Medicare-Fee-for-Service-Payment/ACO/index.html?redirect=/aco

Centers for Medicare and Medicaid Services. (2015b). Affordable Care Act payment model saves more than $25 million in first performance year. Retrieved from https://www.cms.gov/Newsroom/MediaReleaseDatabase/Press-releases/2015-Press-releases-items/2015-06-18.html

Centers for Medicare and Medicaid Services. (2015c). Independence at home demonstration. Retrieved from http://innovation.cms.gov/initiatives/Independence-at-Home/

Centers for Medicare and Medicaid Services. (2015d). MDS 3.0 RAI Manual. Retrieved from https://www.cms.gov/Medicare/Quality-Initiatives-Patient-Assessment-Instruments/NursingHomeQualityInits/MDS-30RAIManual.html

Centers for Medicare and Medicaid Services. (2015e). Medicare & you. Retrieved from https://www.medicare.gov/pubs/pdf/10050.pdf

Centers for Medicare and Medicaid Services. (2015f). Medicare coverage of skilled nursing facility care. Retrieved from www.medicare.gov/Publications/Pubs/pdf/10153.pdf

Centers for Medicare and Medicaid Services. (2015g). NHE fact sheet. Retrieved from https://www.cms.gov/Research-Statistics-Data-and-Systems/Statistics-Trends-and-Reports/NationalHealthExpendData/NHE-Fact-Sheet.html

Centers for Medicare and Medicaid Services. (2015h). PACE. Retrieved from https://www.medicare.gov/your-medicare-costs/help-paying-costs/pace/pace.html

Centers for Medicare and Medicaid Services. (2015i). *State Operations Manual Appendix PP: Guidance to surveyors for long term care facilities (Rev. 133, 02-06-15).* Retrieved from https://www.cms.gov/Regulations-and-Guidance/Guidance/Manuals/downloads/som107ap_pp_guidelines_ltcf.pdf

Centers for Medicare and Medicaid Services. (2015j). Table 02: National health expenditures amounts and annual percent change by type of expenditure. Retrieved from https://www.cms.gov/Research-Statistics-Data-and-Systems/Statistics-Trends-and-Reports/NationalHealthExpendData/NationalHealthAccountsProjected.html

Centers for Medicare and Medicaid Services. (2015k). What are my other long-term care choices? Retrieved from https://www.medicare.gov/what-medicare-covers/part-a/other-long-term-care-choices.html#collapse-4921

Centers for Medicare and Medicaid Services. (2015l). Your Medicare coverage: Skilled nursing facility (SNF) care. Retrieved from https://www.medicare.gov/coverage/skilled-nursing-facility-care.html

Chander, M., & Kirkwood, K. L. (2006). Pharmacist's role in long-term acute care hospitals. *Drug Topics, 150*(4), 56.

Christensen, D., Trygstad, T., Sullivan, R., Garmise, J., & Wegner, S. E. (2004). A pharmacy management intervention for optimizing drug therapy for nursing home patients. *The American Journal of Geriatric Pharmacotherapy, 2*(4), 248–256.

Christian, J. B., vanHaaren, A., Cameron, K. A., & Lapane, K. L. (2004). Alternatives for potentially inappropriate medications in the elderly population: Treatment algorithms for use in the Fleetwood phase III study. *The Consultant Pharmacist, 19*(11), 1011–1028.

Clark, T. R., Gruber, J., & Sey, M. (2010a). Introduction to the medication regimen review: Part 2. *The Consultant Pharmacist, 25*(12), 788–802.

Clark, T. R., Gruber, J., & Sey, M. (2010b). Introduction to the medication regimen review: Part 1. *The Consultant Pharmacist, 25*(11), 710–720.

Clark, T. R., Gruber, J., & Sey, M. (2011). Introduction to the medication regimen review: Part 3. *Consult Pharm, 26*(1), 16–27.

Colby, S. L., & Ortman, J. M. (2015). Projections of the size and composition of the U.S. population: 2014 to 2060, *Current population reports* (pp. 25–1143). Washington, DC: U.S. Census Bureau.

Doty, P., Mahoney, K. J., & Sciegaj, M. (2010). New state strategies to meet long-term care needs. *Health Affairs, 29*(1), 49–56.

Eskildsen, M. A. (2007). Long-term acute care: A review of the literature. *Journal of the American Geriatrics Society, 55*(5), 775–779.

Family Caregiver Alliance: National Center on Caregiving. (2015). Selected long-term care statistics. Retrieved from https://caregiver.org/selected-long-term-care-statistics

Federal Bureau of Prisons. (2015). Inmate statistics: Inmate age. Retrieved from http://www.bop.gov/about/statistics/statistics_inmate_age.jsp

Federal Trade Commission. (2015). Consumer information: Reverse mortgages. Retrieved from http://www.consumer.ftc.gov/articles/0192-reverse-mortgages

Schleich-Williams, C. (2016). Inflation protection for long-term care. Retrieved from http://www.advisortoday.com/archives/article.cfm?articleID=229

Finley, P. R., Crismon, M. L., & Rush, A. J. (2003). Evaluating the impact of pharmacists in mental health: A systematic review. *Pharmacotherapy, 23*(12), 1634–1644.

Gardner, P. (2014). How many patients are in ACOs? Retrieved from http://www.beckershospitalreview.com/accountable-care-organizations/how-many-patients-are-in-acos.html

Gaugler, J., Duval, S., Anderson, K., & Kane, R. (2007). Predicting nursing home admission in the U.S: A meta-analysis. *BMC Geriatrics, 7*(1), 13.

Genworth Financial. (2015). Genworth 2015 cost of care survey: Home care providers, adult day health care facilities, assisted living facilities and nursing homes. Retrieved from https://www.genworth.com/dam/Americas/US/PDFs/Consumer/corporate/130568_040115_gnw.pdf

Gore, M. J. (1994). Embracing pharmaceutical care: Consultant pharmacists lead the way. *The Consultant Pharmacist, 9*(2), 143–156.

Grant, M., Elk, R., Ferrell, B., Morrison, R. S., & von Gunten, C. F. (2009). Current status of palliative care: Clinical implementation, education, and research. *CA: A Cancer Journal for Clinicians, 59*(5), 327–335.

Harris-Kojetin, L., Sengupta, M., Park-Lee, E., & Valverde, R. (2013). Long-term care services in the United States: 2013 overview. *Vital Health Statistics, 3*(37), 1–94.

Henry, D., Mendelson, D., & Fallieras, A. (2003). *Clinical pharmacy management initiative: Integrating quality into Medicaid cost containment.* Lawrenceville, NJ: Center for Health Care Strategies.

Hung, W. W., Ross, J. S., Boockvar, K. S., & Siu, A. L. (2011). Recent trends in chronic disease, impairment and disability among older adults in the United States. *BMC Geriatrics, 11*, 47.

The Joint Commission. (2010). *The Joint Commission requirements for hospitals.* Retrieved from http://www.jointcommission.org/standards_information/tjc_requirements.aspx

Jones, A. L., Dwyer, L. L., Bercovitz, A. R., & Strahan, G. W. (2009). The National Nursing Home survey: 2009 overview. *Vital Health Statistics, 13*(167), 1–164.

Kahn, J. M., Werner, R. M., David, G., Ten Have, T. R., Benson, N. M., & Asch, D. A. (2013). Effectiveness of long-term acute care hospitalization in elderly patients with chronic critical illness. *Medical Care, 51*(1), 4–10.

Kaldy, J. (2010). Medical home 101: The pharmacist's role in this growing patient-centered care model. *The Consultant Pharmacist, 25*(8), 468–474.

Kaldy, J. (2012). Carving out the pharmacist's role in the elusive ACO. *The Consultant Pharmacist, 27*(3), 165–170.

Kane, R. A., & Kane, R. L. (1987). *Long-term care: Principles, programs, and policies.* New York: Springer.

Katz, S., Ford, A. B., Moskowitz, R. W., Jackson, B. A., & Jaffe, M. W. (1963). Studies of illness in the aged: The index of ADL: A standardized measure of biological and psychosocial function. *Journal of the American Medical Association, 185*(12), 914–919.

Kaye, H. S., Harrington, C., & LaPlante, M. P. (2010). Long-term care: Who gets it, who provides it, who pays, and how much? *Health Affairs, 29*(1), 11–21.

Kelley, A. S., Deb, P., Du, Q., Carlson, M. D. A., & Morrison, R. S. (2013). Hospice enrollment saves money for Medicare and improves care quality across a number of different lengths-of-stay. *Health Affairs, 32*(3), 552–561.

Kelly, A., Conell-Price, J., Covinsky, K. E., Cenzer, I. S., Chang, A., Boscardin, W. J., & Smith, A. K. (2011). Lengths of stay for older adults residing in nursing homes at the end of life. *Journal of American Geriatrics Society, 58*(9), 1701–1706.

Kochanek, K.D., Murphy, S.L., Xu J., & Arias, E. (2014). Mortality in the United States, 2013. *NCHA Data Brief, no 178.* Hyattsville, MD: National Center for Health Statistics.

Kubacka, R. T. (1996). A primer on drug utilization review. *Journal of American Pharmacy Association, 36*(4), 257–262, 279.

Lapane, K. L., & Hughes, C. M. (2004a). Identifying nursing home residents at high-risk for preventable adverse drug events: Modifying a tool for use in the Fleetwood phase III study. *The Consultant Pharmacist, 19*(6), 533–537.

Lapane, K. L., & Hughes, C. M. (2004b). Job satisfaction and stress among workers providing long-term care pharmacy services. *The Consultant Pharmacist, 19*(11), 1029–1037.

Larkin, M. (2007). University-based retirement communities on the rise. *The Journal of Active Aging, 6*(2), 52–59.

Lawton, M. P., & Brody, E. M. (1969). Assessment of older people: Self-maintaining and instrumental activities of daily living. *Gerontologist, 9*(3 Part 1), 179–186.

Levenson, S. A., & Saffel, D. A. (2007). The consultant pharmacist and the physician in the nursing home: Roles, relationships, and a recipe for success. *The Consultant Pharmacist, 22*(1), 71–82.

Liu, K. (1994). A data perspective on long-term care. *Gerontologist, 34*(4), 476–480.

Lochner K. A., & Cox, C. S. (2013). Prevalence of multiple chronic conditions among Medicare beneficiaries, United States, 2010. *Preventing Chronic Disease, 10*, E61.

Lombardi, T. P., & Kennicutt, J. D. (2002). Promotion of a safe medication environment: Focus on the elderly and residents of long-term care facilities. *Medscape Pharmacists, 2*(1). Retrieved from http://www.medscape.com/viewarticle/421217

Maack, B., Miller, D. R., Johnson, T., & Dewey, M. (2008). Economic impact of a pharmacy resident in an assisted living facility-based medication therapy management program. *The Annals of Pharmacotherapy, 42*(11), 1613–1620.

Manton, K. G. (2008). Recent declines in chronic disability in the elderly U.S. population: Risk factors and future dynamics. *Annual Review of Public Health, 29*(1), 91–113.

Marengoni, A., Aguero-Torres, H., Timpini, A., Cossi, S., & Fratiglioni, L. (2008). Rehabilitation and nursing home admission after hospitalization in acute geriatric patients. *Journal of the American Medical Directors Association, 9*(4), 265–270.

Martin, C. M. (2006). Understanding palliative care. *The Consultant Pharmacist, 21*(9), 698–713.

Martin, C. M. (2009). Exploring new opportunities in hospice pharmacy. *The Consultant Pharmacist, 24*(2), 114–119.

Martin, L. G., Schoeni, R. F., Freedman, V. A., & Andreski, P. (2007). Feeling better? Trends in general health status. *The Journals of Gerontology. Series B, Psychological Sciences and Social Sciences, 62B*(1), S11–S21.

Mendes, E. (2011). Most caregivers look after elderly parent; Invest a lot of time. Retrieved from http://www.gallup.com/poll/148682/caregivers-look-elderly-parent-invest-lot-time.aspx

Moore, K. L., Boscardin, W. J., Steinman, M. A., & Schwartz, J. B. (2012). Age and sex variation in prevalence of chronic medical conditions in older residents of U.S. nursing homes. *Journal of American Geriatrics Society, 60*(4), 756–764.

Mort, J. (2009). Implications and management of decline for the elderly patient. *The Consultant Pharmacist, 24*(8), 611–625.

Moskowitz, D. B. (2003). The pharmacist as care provider: Three projects support role. *Drug Benefit Trends, 15*(7), 43–46.

Munoz-Price, L. S. (2009). Healthcare epidemiology: Long-term acute care hospitals. *Clinical Infectious Diseases, 49*(3), 438–443.

National Adult Day Services Association. (2015). *About adult day services.* Retrieved from http://www.nadsa.org/ learn-more/about-adult-day-services/

National Alliance for Caregiving & American Association of Retired Persons. (2015). *Caregiving in the U.S. 2015: A focused look at those caring for the 50 +.* Retrieved from http://www.caregiving.org/caregiving2015/

National Hospice and Palliative Care Organization. (2014). NHPCO's facts and figures: Hospice care in America. Retrieved from http://www.nhpco.org/sites/default/files/public/Statistics_Research/2014_Facts_Figures.pdf

National Institute on Aging. (2015). About Alzheimer's disease: Alzheimer's basics. Retrieved from https://www.nia.nih.gov/alzheimers/topics/alzheimers-basics

National PACE Association. (2015). What is PACE? Retrieved from http://www.npaonline.org/website/article.asp?id=12

Ng, T., Harrington, C., & Kitchener, M. (2010). Medicare and Medicaid in long-term care. *Health Affairs, 29*(1), 22–28.

Nihtila, E. K., Martikainen, P. T., Koskinen, S. V. P., Reunanen, A. R., Noro, A. M., & Hakkinen, U. T. (2008). Chronic conditions and the risk of long-term institutionalization among older people. *European Journal of Public Health, 18*(1), 77–84.

Nishtala, P. S., McLachlan, A. J., Bell, J. S., & Chen, T. F. (2008). Psychotropic prescribing in long-term care facilities: Impact of medication reviews and educational interventions. *The American Journal of Geriatric Psychiatry, 16*(8), 621–632.

OBRA. (1987). *Omnibus Reconciliation Act (1987). Public Law 100–203.*

OBRA. (1990). *Omnibus Reconciliation Act (1990). Public Law 101–108.*

Odegard, P. S., Breslow, R. M., Koronkowski, M. J., Williams, B. R., & Hudgins, G. A. (2007). Geriatric pharmacy education: A strategic plan for the future. *American Journal of Pharmaceutical Education, 71*(3), article 47.

Ortman, J. M., Velkoff, V. A., & Hogan, H. (2014). An aging nation: The older population in the United States, *Current population reports* (pp. 25–1140). Washington, DC: U.S. Census Bureau.

Powell, R. (2014). Pros, cons: Continuing care retirement community. *USA Today.*

Rahman, A. N., & Applebaum, R. A. (2009). The nursing home minimum data set assessment instrument: Manifest functions and unintended consequences—past, present, and future. *Gerontologist, 49*(6), 727–735.

Reaves, E. L., & Musumeci, M. (2015). Medicaid and long-term services and supports: A primer. Retrieved from http://kff.org/medicaid/report/medicaid-and-long-term-services-and-supports-a-primer/

Reinhard, S.C., Feinberg, L.F., Choula, R., & Houser, A. (2015). Valuing the invaluable: 2015 update. *AARP Public Policy Institute, 104*, 1–25.

Richardson, T. E., O'Reilly, C. L., & Chen, T. F. (2014). A comprehensive review of the impact of clinical pharmacy services on patient outcomes in mental health. *International Journal of Clinical Pharmacy, 36*, 222–232.

Rosenwaike, I. (1985). A demographic portrait of the oldest old. *The Milbank Memorial Fund Quarterly. Health and Society, 63*(2), 187–205.

Seeman, T. E., Merkin, S. S., Crimmins, E. M., & Karlamangla, A. S. (2010). Disability trends among older Americans: National Health and Nutrition Examination surveys, 1988–1994 and 1999–2004. *American Journal of Public Health, 100*(1), 100–107.

Simonson, W., Novak, R., & Jennewine, T. (2013). Requirements for medication monitoring in assisted living facilities. *The Consultant Pharmacist, 28*(9), 569–578.

Social Security Administration. (2010). *Historical background and development of Social Security*. Retrieved from http://www.socialsecurity.gov/history/briefhistory3.html

Stack, E., & Kier, K. (2014a). Key aspects and health care benefits of patient-centered medical homes. *The Consultant Pharmacist, 29*(3), 196–199.

Stack, E., & Kier, K. (2014b). Patient-centered medical homes: Recognition and reimbursement-part 3. *The Consultant Pharmacist, 29*(5), 347–350.

Stack, E., & Kier, K. (2014c). Patient-centered medical homes: Standards for approval-part 2. *The Consultant Pharmacist, 29*(4), 275–278.

Steeb, D., & Webster, L. (2012). Improving care transitions: Optimizing medication reconciliation. Retrieved from http://www.pharmacist.com/medication-management-care-transitions-best-practices

Stefanacci, R. G. (2012). Financial oversight of medication use: An expanded role for consultant pharmacists. *The Consultant Pharmacist, 27*(4), 290–295.

Stevens, L. M., Lynm, C., & Glass, R. M. (2006). Palliative care. *Journal of the American Medical Association, 296*(11), 1428.

Storey, P. (1996). *Primer on palliative care.* Gainesville, FL: American Academy of Hospice and Palliative Care.

Suhrie, E. M., Hanlon, J. T., Jaffe, E. J., Sevick, M. A., Ruby, C. M., & Aspinall, S. L. (2009). Impact of a geriatric nursing home palliative care service on unnecessary medication prescribing. *American Journal of Geriatric Pharmacotherapy, 7*(1), 20–25.

Truong, H.-A., Layson-Wolf, C., Rodriguez de Bittner, M., Owen, J. A., & Haupt, S. (2009). Perceptions of patients on Medicare Part D medication therapy management services. *Journal of the American Pharmacists Association, 49*(3), 392–398.

U.S. Census Bureau. (2015). Annual estimates of the resident population by sex, age, race, and Hispanic origin for the United States: April 1, 2010 to July 1, 2014. Retrieved from http://www.census.gov/popest/data/national/asrh/2014/index.html

U.S. Department of Health and Human Services: Administration for Community Living. (2015). Administration on Aging (AoA): Affordable Care Act: Opportunities for the aging network. Retrieved from http://www.aoa.gov/Aging_Statistics/Health_care_reform.aspx

United States Government Accountability Office. (2010). *Older Americans: Continuing care retirement communities can provide benefits, but not without some risk*, Report to the Chairman, Special Committee on Aging, U.S. Senate, GAO-10-611. Retrieved from http://www.gao.gov/new.items/d10611.pdf

Voisine, J., Walke, L., & Jeffery, S. (2009). Home is where the heart is: Living arrangements for older adults. *The Consultant Pharmacist, 24*(2), 134–145.

Werner CA. (2011). The older population: 2010, *2010 Census Briefs*, C2010BR-09,

Washington, DC: U.S. Census Bureau.

Wick, J., & Zanni, G. (2009a). Aging in place: Multiple options, multiple choices. *The Consultant Pharmacist, 24*(11), 804–812.

Wick, J., & Zanni, G. (2009b). Challenges in caring for aging inmates. *The Consultant Pharmacist, 24*(6), 424–436.

Williams, B. A., Stern, M. F., Mellow, J., Safer, M., & Greifiner, R. B. (2012). Aging in correctional custody: Setting a policy agenda for older prisoner health care. *American Journal of Public Health, 102*(8), 1475–1481.

Wolff, J. L., & Kasper, J. D. (2006). Caregivers of frail elders: Updating a national profile. *Gerontologist, 46*(3), 344–356.

Zigmond J. (2013). As D.C. waits for a new panel to explore how to pay for long-term care, Medicaid is bearing the brunt. *Modern Healthcare, 43*(10), 6–7.

CHAPTER

11

Behavioral Health Services

Ardis Hanson, Carol A. Ott, and Bruce Lubotsky Levin

Case Scenario

You have newly graduated from pharmacy school and have taken a position in a community pharmacy setting that is near a community mental health center. Many of the clients of the center come to your pharmacy to have their prescriptions filled. In pharmacy school, you learned about the treatment of individuals with behavioral health problems (including alcohol, drug abuse, and mental disorders), but were never taught how to interact with people having serious behavioral health problems. You understand that empathy is a part of your professional demeanor, but you find you have beliefs about people with behavioral health and their ability to understand your patient counseling efforts. Occasionally, pharmacy technicians interact with these patients and you feel uncomfortable with the jokes and laughter that sometimes follows these patient visits.

On one occasion, DL, a 42-year-old man with chronic paranoid schizophrenia, comes to the pharmacy to pick up his antipsychotic prescription. It is apparent that he hasn't been taking care of himself and is becoming more ill. On previous visits, the pharmacy staff has simply handed him his prescription without offering to discuss it with him. When DL approaches the counter, you move to the window to dispense his prescription to him. You ask him how his medicine is working for him, if he has any problems, and if he recognizes the pills as ones he has taken previously. He doesn't look at you and seems surprised that you would take the time to speak with him. Upon further questioning, you realize that DL has tremors in his hands and has difficulty finding the words to express himself, although he tries. You review his medications with him, including the fact that his tremors may be due to his medicine and that he should talk to his physician about this, as there are treatments available. He thanks you and leaves the store. Several days later, DL returns to the pharmacy to pick up a prescription for a medication to treat his tremors and again thanks you for the time you took to explain this problem to him. You realize that taking the step of engaging DL and providing him encouragement has caused him to make an effort to take care of himself. You have also provided your technicians and coworkers with a model for your expectations in working with people with serious behavioral health problems.

LEARNING OBJECTIVES

Upon completion of this chapter, the student shall be able to:

- Provide a brief overview of current behavioral health services in the United States.
- Understand the role of epidemiology, service delivery systems, and healthcare professionals, such as clinical psychiatric pharmacists, in caring for individuals with behavioral health problems.
- Understand evidence-based practice/treatment guidelines for the clinical and community psychiatric pharmacist.
- Better assess the potential role for pharmacists as members of behavioral health services teams.
- Identify emerging issues, including medical homes, the Employee Retirement Income Security Act (ERISA), and rural behavioral health services.

CHAPTER QUESTIONS

1. Which two national laws had the most significant impact on the organization, financing, and delivery of behavioral health services in the United States?
2. Explain the importance of measuring the burden of disease.
3. What are some of the implications of disparities in access and utilization of behavioral health services?
4. Discuss the difference between evidence-based practice and expert consensus.
5. Describe the use of preferred drugs lists (PDLs) as a means to control drug costs. Give an example of a statewide implementation.

INTRODUCTION

This chapter presents a brief overview of behavioral health (defined as alcohol, drug abuse, and mental health) services in the United States, including epidemiologic evidence from national studies on the prevalence of mental disorders in noninstitutionalized populations. It reviews the critical issues involved in behavioral health services delivery, disease prevention and health promotion, the treatment of individuals with behavioral health problems, and ethical and legal issues in behavioral health services. In addition, the chapter identifies emerging issues critical to pharmacists who must understand the increasingly complex nature of health and behavioral healthcare delivery in the United States. The chapter is designed to help pharmacy students develop a better understanding of the needs of individuals with serious behavioral health problems, illustrated in the chapter scenario.

Global Burden of Disease

Behavioral health problems are a significant global public health issue. The World Health Organization (WHO) (2005) estimates that 14% of the global disease burden is due to mental disorders. The global disease burden uses three measures: (1) disability-adjusted life years (DALYs); (2) years of life lost to premature mortality (YLLs); and (3) years lived with disability (YLDs). Behavioral health problems accounted for 183.9 million DALYs (7.4%) of all DALYs worldwide; 8.6 million YLLs (0.5%); and 175.3 million YLDs (22.9%) of all YLDs (Whiteford et al., 2013).

What do these numbers mean? We know that the global disease burden has continued to shift away from communicable to noncommunicable diseases and from premature death to years lived with a disability (Murray et al., 2012). Behavioral health problems are considered chronic diseases, require long-term management, affect work productivity, and cause individuals to leave the workforce prematurely due to disability. Therefore, when we look at global DALYS, YLLs, and

YLDs, we recognize that mental, neurologic, and behavioral disorders cause considerable suffering and are common to individuals living in countries throughout the world. Individuals with behavioral health problems also endure social isolation, poor quality of life, and increased mortality. Individuals with behavioral health problems also suffer from poor access to care, if care even exists. Less than 70% of all WHO countries have mental health programs, much less substance abuse programs, and the majority of low- and middle-income countries devote less than 1% of their health budget to mental health care. The WHO also estimates that 25% of all patients using a health service suffer from at least one mental, neurological, or behavioral disorder; however, these disorders are often undiagnosed or untreated (WHO, 2005).

Costs of Treatment for Behavioral Health Problems Globally and in the United States

It is difficult to estimate the costs associated with behavioral health problems, since cost estimates are not available globally for all behavioral health problems. Nevertheless, a World Economic Forum report (Bloom et al., 2011) estimated that the costs of behavioral health problems will be more than double by 2030, from $2.49 billion in 2010 to $6.01 billion in 2030 (in U.S. dollars) as populations increase and age over the next 20 years.

Both the United Nations and the WHO stress the importance of treating behavioral health problems to improve population health by focusing on vulnerable and at-risk populations (Miranda & Patel, 2005). Behavioral health problems also increase the risk for developing many physical illnesses and are major risk factors for communicable and noncommunicable diseases and unintentional and intentional injury. At the same time, many health conditions increase the risk for behavioral health problems and complicate diagnosis and treatment (WHO, 2011). The aggregate social costs of these adverse consequences are enormous.

In 2013, health care spending in the United States increased 3.6% to reach $2.9 trillion, or $9,255 per person (Centers for Medicare and Medicaid Services, 2014). In 2009, spending on behavioral health services accounted for $172 billion (7.4%) of all health expenditures, with prescription drugs accounting for 28% of the costs (Substance Abuse and Mental Health Services Administration, 2013). However, this does not reflect the total (direct and indirect) costs of behavioral health care. Although it is possible to note the direct costs of medications, treatment visits, and hospitalizations, these costs likely would exclude the indirect costs of incarceration, homelessness, public benefits, supported programs and services, reduced labor supply, reduced educational attainment, and the medical complications associated with behavioral health problems (Insel, 2008). From 2008 to 2014, there was a 6.6% annual increase in spending for the utilization of behavioral health services in the United States (Levit et al., 2008).

Complexity Exacerbated by Co-Occurring Disorders

Providing high-quality health care for persons with co-occurring disorders is difficult. A number of factors, such as lifestyle issues, at-risk behaviors, service utilization, and barriers to care affect service provision. Persons with co-occurring disorders often have more instances of premature death and higher rates of disability than those who do not have co-occurring disorders. Gender also plays a role in the incidence and treatment of co-occurring disorders. In the United States, depression is the second leading cause of disability-adjusted life years in women but the tenth leading cause in men (Michaud, Murray, & Bloom, 2001). Globally, the burden of depressive disorders also is higher in women than in men (Ferrari et al., 2013). Although the interaction between co-occurring disorders with regard to prevalence, disease severity, and causative factors (Welch, Czerwinski, Ghimire, & Bertsimas, 2009) is not completely understood, it is estimated that for every dollar invested in drug treatment, $7 are saved in health and social costs (WHO, 2003).

Criminal Justice Settings as de Facto Behavioral Health Treatment Facilities

In the United States, an estimated 6,899,000 persons were in adult correctional systems in 2013, which includes offenders supervised in the community on probation or parole and those incarcerated in prisons or local jails (Glaze & Kaeble, 2014). U.S. state and federal prisons held an estimated 1,574,700 inmates (Carson, 2014), local jails held 731,200 individuals, and an estimated 4,751,400 persons were on probation or parole (Glaze & Kaeble, 2014). To place these numbers in more understandable terms, 1 in 35 adults in the United States was under some type of correctional supervision during 2013 and approximately 1 in 51 adults was on probation or parole (Glaze & Kaeble, 2014).

More than half of all prison and jail inmates have a behavioral health problem. Seventy-five percent of women in jail exhibit symptoms of mental disorders compared to 63% of men. In state prisons, 73% of females and 55% of males have a mental disorder. In federal prisons, 61% of females and 44% of males have a mental disorder (James & Glaze, 2006). Steadman and colleagues (2009) estimated that 14.5% of men and 31% of women in jails met the criteria for a serious mental illness, which is three times higher than prevalence rates for the general population. Sixty-eight percent of jail inmates report having an alcohol or drug use disorder prior to entering jail (Osher, D'Amora, Plotkin, Jarrett, & Eggleston, 2012). Persons with mental illnesses also are over-represented in probation and parole populations, with estimates ranging from two to four times the general population (Prins & Draper, 2009).

In the community, law enforcement officials are increasingly concerned with calls to apprehend individuals with behavioral health problems. At the same time, there have been reports of "mercy arrests," in essence, taking an individual with a behavioral health problem into custody because he or she was involved in a minor scuffle (or similar incident) on the street (Torrey, National Alliance for the Mentally Ill, & Public Citizen Health Research Group, 1992). Law enforcement officials report this is often their only solution to ensuring a person receives food, shelter, and medical care, since psychiatric beds in community hospitals are often unavailable and many state residential treatment facilities have been closed.

Prisons and jails, much like nursing homes, have become the nation's de facto behavioral healthcare provider (Torrey et al., 1992; Torrey et al., 2014). With the closing of state hospitals and residential treatment facilities, the transinstitutionalization of persons with serious behavioral health problems has shifted to alternative public settings. James and Glaze (2006) concluded that only one in three state prisoners, one in four federal prisoners, and one in six jail inmates who have behavioral health problems received treatment while incarcerated. Further, while a patient leaving a behavioral healthcare facility may have a discharge plan, a drug regimen, and a referral for medical assistance or an aftercare program, jails and prisons have no obligation to help the released person re-entering society cope with his or her behavioral health problems. The burden falls upon local community-based behavioral healthcare facilities.

EPIDEMIOLOGY OF MENTAL DISORDERS

A Global Epidemiologic Perspective

Fundamental to a discussion of behavioral health services is an understanding of the epidemiology of mental disorders: the study of the factors that determine the frequency and distribution of mental disorders in populations. Global estimates by the WHO (2014) indicate that 400 million people suffer from depression, 21 million people suffer from schizophrenia, and 60 million people suffer from bipolar disorders. In addition, the WHO (2002) estimates that 91 million people are affected by alcohol use disorders, and 15 million people are affected by drug use disorders. If one adds traumatic brain injuries, dementia, and other neuropsychiatric disorders, the estimated population suffering from behavioral health problems is far above the approximately 450 million people the WHO estimated in 2002.

DALYS is a measure developed by the WHO that represents the loss of 1 year of full health. Using DALYS, one is able to compare the burden of diseases that cause premature mortality (but little or no disability) to diseases that do not cause death (but do cause disability). The following behavioral health problems are among the top 20 leading causes of disability (Mathers, Boerma, & Fat, 2008): Depression is the third leading cause of disease burden in the world; alcohol use disorders (7th); bipolar disorders (12th); schizophrenia (14th); and substance use disorders (20th).

National Epidemiologic Studies

The most comprehensive mental health epidemiologic study conducted in the United States was the Epidemiologic Catchment Area study in 1978 (Robins & Regier, 1991). The Epidemiologic Catchment Area study included more than 20,000 respondents from five catchment areas (New Haven, Connecticut; Durham, North Carolina; Baltimore, Maryland; Los Angeles, California; and St. Louis, Missouri).

The major objective of the Epidemiologic Catchment Area study was to obtain prevalence rates of specific mental disorders rather than overall prevalence rates of all mental disorders. In summary, 20% of the people interviewed had a diagnosable mental disorder during a given year, with a lifetime prevalence of 32% for a behavioral health problem. Annually, more than 5% of adults in the United States had a severe mental disorder, for example, schizophrenia, major depression, panic disorder, or manic-depressive disorder (Kessler et al., 1996). In addition, nearly 6% of adults in the United States had an addictive disorder (alcohol and drug problems). Approximately 75% of individuals who were in need of services for alcohol and drug abuse did not receive treatment, which potentially has an enormous impact upon the health and stability of individuals, families, and communities.

Another important national study on serious mental illness and co-occurring disorders was the National Comorbidity Survey (NCS) (Kessler et al., 1994). The NCS incorporated revised nomenclature from the *Diagnostic and Statistical Manual of Mental Disorders* (DSM), *Third Edition* (American Psychiatric Association, 1987), examined risk factors that affect particular mental disorders, and estimated the comorbidity of mental disorders (Blazer, Kessler, McGonagle, & Swartz, 1994). The NCS study found that 21% of patients had a single mental disorder. Seventy-nine percent of the respondents had a comorbid disorder, that is, a combination of one or more mental, physical, or alcohol/substance use disorders occurring simultaneously. In addition, more than half of all lifetime mental disorders occurred in 14% of the population.

In 2003, in the National Comorbidity Survey Replication Study (NCS-R), Kessler and associates (2003) found that the prevalence of mental disorders did not change significantly from the earlier NCS. However, what did change was an increase in the rate of treating individuals with mental disorders, from approximately 20% in the NCS to nearly 33% in the NCS-R. Nevertheless, despite an increase in treating individuals with mental disorders from the NCS to the NCS replication, the majority of individuals with mental disorders did not receive treatment. While space does not permit a more extensive review of the results of epidemiologic studies of behavioral health problems in the United States, Levin, Hennessey, and Petrila (2010) present additional information about the epidemiology of behavioral health problems in selected at-risk populations.

Other Vulnerable Populations

Disparities in behavioral health care result in at-risk populations, such as cultural and linguistic minorities, rural populations, and women and children who have a lower socioeconomic status, often delaying or receiving inadequate care and terminating care early (Alang, 2015; Cook, Liu, Lessios, Loder, & McGuire, 2015; Heflinger, Shaw, Higa-McMillan, Lunn, & Brannan, 2015; Miranda, McGuire, Williams, & Wang, 2008). For example, although rates for most behavioral health problems are lower in Hispanics and African Americans than in whites, Hispanics and African Americans have poorer prognoses and more chronic disorders (Cook et al., 2014; Lo, Cheng, & Howell, 2014; Saloner & Le Cook, 2013).

On a given night in the United States, it is estimated that 578,424 people are homeless (Henry, Cortes, Shivji, & Buck, 2015). This translates to approximately 18 individuals out of every 10,000 people in the United States who are homeless. Sixty percent of these are individuals who are homeless live in shelters; 37% of all homeless people are individuals in homeless families (216,261 people were homeless in 67,613 families). Nearly one-quarter of all homeless individuals were children under the age of 18 (135,701 individuals).

Chronic homelessness is defined as homelessness among people who have a disability (e.g., serious mental illness, chronic substance use disorders, or chronic medical issues) and who are homeless repeatedly or for long periods of time (National Alliance to End Homelessness, 2014). Of almost 600,000 people, 99,434 persons are chronically homeless (84,291 individuals and 15,143 [7%] people in families) (Henry et al., 2015). Almost two-thirds of persons who are chronically homeless (53,088) lived unsheltered, under bridges, in cars, or in abandoned buildings.

More than one in ten homeless adults was a veteran (49,933). Thirty-six percent of homeless veterans live unsheltered. Four percent of homeless veterans were members of families with children. Just fewer than 10% (4,722) of homeless veterans were female (Henry et al., 2015).

Approximately 30% of individuals who are homeless have a serious mental disorder, and 17% have a physical disability (City Policy Associates, 2013). In addition, 38% of individuals who are homeless report an alcohol dependency problem, 26% report other drug use/abuse problems, and an estimated 37% of individuals who are homeless have chronic substance abuse issues (U.S. Department of Housing and Urban Development, 2009).

Finally, persons who are the most vulnerable are the elderly who receive both Medicaid and Medicare. These persons (dually eligible) are among the oldest, poorest, sickest, and most disabled individuals in the United States. Their services utilization makes them the most expensive population served by publicly funded healthcare programs. They account for a disproportionate share of Medicaid utilization and payments. The Medicare Payment Advisory Commission (2015) provides the following demographics. Approximately 9.6 million individuals in the United States were dually eligible during FY 2010. Fifty-nine percent of dual-eligible beneficiaries were 65 years of age or older. Seventy-five percent of dual-eligible beneficiaries were eligible for full Medicaid benefits. Although dual-eligible beneficiaries under age 65 were more likely to be male (48%), more than half (55%) of individuals dually eligible for Medicare and Medicaid benefits had at least one activity of daily living (ADL) limitation. Dual-eligible beneficiaries aged 65 years and older had more ADL limitations than those under age 65 (38% had 3–6 ADL limitations vs. 25% with 3–6 ADL limitations). More of the dual-eligible beneficiaries who were under age 65 reported being in poor health (19%). Behavioral health problems and intellectual disabilities and related conditions were more common among the dual-eligible population under age 65.

Fourteen percent of individuals dually enrolled in Medicaid and Medicare accounted for 36% of all Medicaid expenditures, and dual-eligible beneficiaries accounted for 33% of Medicare spending (Young, Garfield, Musumeci, Clemans-Cope, & Lawton, 2013). In addition, approximately 75% of persons who live in nursing homes are dually eligible (Liu, Wissoker, & Swett, 2007) (see **Table 11-1**).

Table 11-1 Behavioral Health Conditions in Persons who are Dually Eligible

Behavioral health conditions	Under age 65	Ages 65 and older
Anxiety disorders	19%	11%
Bipolar disorder	13%	3%
Depression	30%	20%
Schizophrenia and other psychotic disorders	14%	6%
Intellectual disabilities and related conditions	8%	1%

LANDMARK REPORTS AND LEGISLATION IN MENTAL HEALTH

Historically, the organization, financing, and provision of behavioral health services in the United States have been complicated by a confusing assortment of uncoordinated public and private delivery systems and multiple funding mechanisms that have been parallel to, rather than integrated with, general (somatic) health services (Levin, Hennessy, & Petrila, 2010).

The post–World War II era fostered optimism that behavioral health problems were treatable as well as preventable. Based upon the findings of the Joint Commission on Mental Health and Illness in 1961, the U.S. Congress initiated the largest commitment to prevention and treatment of behavioral health problems in the history of the United States with passage of the Community Mental Health Centers Act of 1963. At the height of the Community Mental Health Center (CMHC) movement in 1981, 52% of the U.S. population was living in areas served by a community mental health center (U.S. Department of Health and Human Services, 1999). For a more comprehensive review of the history of behavioral health services in America, see Deutsch (1949).

Other than the CMHC legislation in 1963, no other federal legislation has affected the financing and delivery of behavioral health services more than the 1965 passage of Titles XVIII and XIX of the Social Security Act, which established the Medicare and Medicaid programs (Social Security Act Amendments, 1965). These programs pay for health services provided to the elderly and the poor, two populations who historically have not been covered by private health insurance. While care for the elderly and medically disabled (Medicare) is administered by the Federal government, Medicaid is a jointly administered federal/state program that finances long-term and acute care.

Two seminal federal reports on behavioral health include *Mental Health: A Report of the Surgeon General* (U.S. Department of Health and Human Services, 1999) and *Achieving the Promise* (President's New Freedom Commission on Mental Health, 2003). Both reports examined the multiple, disjointed, and dysfunctional behavioral healthcare delivery systems in America, the insurance and financial limitations placed upon individuals with behavioral health problems, and the long-term consequences of the stigma of behavioral health problems.

The goals of the two reports were remarkably similar. Both reports framed behavioral health as an essential component of overall (somatic) health and well-being and focused on consumer and family-focused outcomes of care. Both reports also addressed disparities of services, urged implementation of early screening, assessment, and referral to behavioral health services, and prioritized behavioral health services delivery and services research initiatives. Finally, both reports urged increased utilization of science and technology in behavioral health.

The Paul Wellstone and Pete Domenici Mental Health Parity and Addiction Equity Act

The Paul Wellstone and Pete Domenici Mental Health Parity and Addiction Equity Act was part of the Emergency Economic Stabilization Act of 2008. The Act requires a group health plan of 50 persons or more (that provides both medical/surgical and behavioral health benefits) to ensure that mental health or substance use disorder benefits are equal in benefits and treatment offered for medical/surgical services. Therefore, there are no separate cost sharing requirements or treatment limitations placed upon behavioral health benefits that are different than the requirements or limitations placed upon medical/surgical benefits.

The Patient Protection and Affordable Care Act

With the implementation of the Patient Protection and Affordable Care Act (ACA) in 2010, a number of comprehensive health insurance reforms were established. These included: a new Patient's Bill of Rights (consumer protections); preventive services for Medicare populations (wellness visits and personalized prevention plans) and discounts on covered prescription drugs in the Medicare Part D formulary; and expanded Medicaid services to cover more low-income Americans, including prevention services. Building upon the parity provisions, the ACA requires providers to deliver rehabilitative and habilitative services to help support individuals with behavioral health problems. While states determine which of these services to cover for adults, Medicaid and CHIP requires that children enrolled in Medicaid receive a wide range of medically necessary services, including behavioral health services.

BEHAVIORAL HEALTH SERVICES DELIVERY AND THE COMMUNITY PHARMACIST

Medication adherence is a significant difficulty for many people who suffer from chronic behavioral health problems. While it is often assumed that people with behavioral health problems have greater medication nonadherence than those with long-term medical or physical illnesses, in reality, studies evaluating adherence maintain that those with chronic conditions do not take approximately one half of the doses they are prescribed, regardless of the condition (Haynes, Ackloo, Sahota, McDonald, & Yao, 2008). The reasons for nonadherence in persons with behavioral health problems are similar to those for chronic medical conditions, with a few additions. Lack of insight into the severity, or even the presence, of a serious behavioral health problem is a common factor in medication adherence in behavioral health. Other factors include difficulty paying for medications, unstable housing and support systems, and the lack of access to care. It has been documented that improving medication adherence may decrease rates of hospitalization and utilization of acute medical care services in persons with schizophrenia (Ascher-Svanum, Zhu, Faries, Furiak, & Montgomery, 2009).

The role of the pharmacist in medication adherence is expanding. Several studies have assessed the roles of both clinical and community pharmacists in interventions to improve the use of medications in individuals with behavioral health problems. Crockett, Taylor, Grabham, and Stanford (2006) studied patient outcomes related to the involvement of rural community pharmacists who provided greater patient counseling and support upon dispensing antidepressant medications. The patients who received extra support had improvement in their symptoms sooner than those patients who received care as usual (Crockett et al., 2006). Since the majority of studies of pharmacist intervention have focused on depression, there is a lack of published evidence of pharmacist impact on other serious behavioral health problems. However, clinical pharmacists working in psychiatry commonly provide extended counseling to and interventions for individuals with behavioral health problems.

To assess adherence problems, practitioners must recognize both behaviors and attitudes associated with medication use (Velligan et al., 2010). Providers commonly assume that patients take all of their doses. However, in the face of seemingly noneffective treatment, providers increase medication doses. This decision results in adverse consequences to the patient, including receiving an excessive dose, increased nonadherence, and/or development of side effects. It is important to question patients closely about their medication use, in a nonjudgmental way, to ascertain adherence.

There are numerous reasons for nonadherence, such as patient beliefs about taking medication, an unwillingness to take medications, finances, living conditions, or forgetfulness. Hence, it is critical for the pharmacist to build an alliance in which the individual feels in control of his or her treatment options as well as to provide complete patient counseling related to medications. Both of these strategies will promote adherence to the treatment plan.

EVIDENCE-BASED PRACTICE/TREATMENT GUIDELINES

Evidence-based practice, which evolved from evidence-based medicine, is defined as "the conscientious, explicit, and judicious use of current best evidence in making decisions about the care of the individual patient. It means integrating individual clinical expertise with the best available external clinical evidence from systematic research" (Sackett, Rosenberg, Gray, Haynes, & Richardson, 1996). Evidence-based practice is the foundation of health and allied health curricula now offered by schools and colleges. Treatment guidelines developed for medical conditions can be evidence-based or be expert consensus guidelines. There is an important difference between evidence-based guidelines and expert consensus guidelines. Expert consensus guidelines often consist of surveys that are completed by experts in a particular area, based upon their current practice, which may or may not be informed by the clinical literature (Kane, Leucht, Carpenter, & Docherty, 2003; Yager et al., 2014). After collating the surveys, the most preferred treatment is listed first. It is essential to understand that expert consensus guidelines are prone to individual provider bias (preference), whereas evidence-based treatment guidelines provide treatment recommendations established by the clinical literature. Many guidelines in psychiatry are a combination of clinical consensus and published research studies.

Two examples of these guidelines are the American Psychiatric Association practice guidelines and the Texas Medication Algorithm Project (TMAP). The American Psychiatric Association guidelines are more extensive in scope and cover a wider range of psychiatric disease states, including assessment of the person with mental illness. The American Psychiatric Association revises its guidelines routinely to provide consistent, informed clinical treatment of psychiatric disorders. The Schizophrenia Patient Outcomes Research Team recently published evidence-based guidelines for the treatment of schizophrenia (Kreyenbuhl, Buchanan, Dickerson, & Dixon, 2010).

Created by the Texas Department of Health Services in 1996, the TMAP uses a combination of clinical expertise and evidence-based practice to form algorithms for treatment, with a goal of improving quality of care and patient outcomes (Gilbert et al., 1998; Moore et al., 2007). The TMAP has developed algorithms for the treatment of major depressive disorder, schizophrenia, and bipolar disorder in adults. The Children's Medication Algorithm Project, part of the TMAP, focuses on attention deficit/hyperactivity disorder and major depressive disorder treatment in children. These guidelines routinely are revised and updated on the TMAP website.

The authors recommend pharmacologic and nonpharmacologic treatment of schizophrenia based upon literature reviews and rate the strength of their recommendations. While algorithms used to treat psychiatric disorders may name specific drugs, most often the clinician using the guidelines finds a class of drugs or several drugs listed. Broad interpretation of treatment guidelines often requires a further knowledge of the clinical literature to provide individualized patient treatment.

While there is increasing interest among psychiatric providers in treatment guidelines, there is also concern that the use of treatment guidelines will decrease the control that the clinician has over individual practice or may be affected by financial motivations for guideline implementation (Forsner, Hansson, Brommels, Wistedt, & Forsell, 2010).

It is clear that the practice of psychiatry is becoming ever more complex. Every year, new drug therapies are marketed, requiring pharmacists to regularly refresh their knowledge of drug mechanisms of action, pharmacology, drug interactions, and adverse events. FDA medications approved for a particular use in psychiatry are regularly used off-label for other psychiatric indications. The role of the pharmacist in managing the drug therapy regimens of persons with behavioral health problems is expanding beyond simply dispensing and counseling. The community pharmacist is in a unique position to offer specialized medication therapy management (MTM) services to this vulnerable population to improve adherence and patient understanding.

Open Access to Behavioral Health Drugs: The Indiana Example

Medicaid programs in the United States frequently utilize preferred drugs lists (PDLs) as a means to control drug costs. The PDL process requires that the physician prescribes and the patient takes certain medications in a therapeutic class prior to employing other options. Concern exists related to the overall cost-effectiveness of PDLs, the criteria that is used to develop PDLs, and the impact of the use of PDLs on quality of care (West et al., 2009). Medication access problems related to PDLs can result in a delay in treatment, increased adverse events, diminished continuity of care, and increased rate of acute medical care services (Lieberman et al., 2005). The argument for preferred drug lists and limiting access to medications often centers on the increasing costs of behavioral health drug therapy, as well as recent clinical trial publications that show similar effectiveness of older, generic drug therapies relative to newer, more expensive treatments (Caballero, Souffrant, & Heffernan, 2008).

In 2005, the State of Indiana enacted legislation known as House Bill 1325 that prohibited prior authorization for mental health drugs except under very specific circumstances and created the Mental Health Quality Advisory Committee (IC 12, 2004; HB 1325, 2005). The Mental Health Quality Advisory Committee is comprised of seven members who represent managed care, psychiatry, community pharmacy, and Indiana Medicaid and is a subcommittee of the Indiana Drug Utilization review board. The Mental Health Quality Advisory Committee applies HB 1325 to maintain open access to behavioral health drugs without PDLs, while utilizing efforts directed at cost-effective care of those with a mental illness. In Indiana Medicaid, there are what is termed *quality of use* edits, which require that drug therapy be adherent to principles of quality of care. These edits reduce polytherapy and inappropriate medication use. Currently, data are in development to determine the impact of these edits on patient outcomes, including rate of hospitalization, refill utilization, and rate of prior authorization.

MENTAL HEALTH TEAMS AND THE ROLE OF THE PHARMACIST

The mental health treatment team consists of a psychiatrist, clinical nurse specialist, psychiatric nurse, social worker, vocational/occupational therapist, psychologist, and care manager. In many treatment settings, including Veterans Administration hospitals and clinics and university teaching hospitals and clinics, a clinical psychiatric pharmacist plays a pivotal role. The clinical psychiatric pharmacist may function as a part of the team or see patients on an individual basis under a scope of practice in collaboration with a psychiatrist. Potential responsibilities of the clinical pharmacist include medication management, including initiation and adjustment of therapy, laboratory monitoring, authorization/monitoring of prescription refills, and interaction with the treatment team. In some states, clinical pharmacists are able to bill insurance plans for their services.

The role of the clinical psychiatric pharmacist expanded from 2000 to 2010. In 1996, the Board of Pharmaceutical Specialties authorized and began to administer a board certification examination in psychiatric pharmacy. To be eligible to sit for this examination, the pharmacist needs to graduate from an accredited school or college of pharmacy and have at least four years of primary practice (at least 40% of that time) in psychiatric pharmacy. The pharmacist may also complete a postgraduate year two residency specializing in psychiatric pharmacy, which reduces the number of years required to sit for the examination to 1-year postresidency. Completion of a postgraduate year, two psychiatric pharmacy residency and the board-certified psychiatric pharmacist designation provides the pharmacist with the training and certification necessary to be an active and productive provider of psychiatric pharmacy services. To date, more than 500 clinical pharmacists have received the board-certified psychiatric pharmacist designation.

Because of the lack of psychiatric providers in many settings, the role of the clinical psychiatric pharmacist is expanding into underserved areas of the population. In rural areas, clinical psychiatric pharmacists are working with primary care physicians as physician extenders to improve behavioral health services, often functioning as the psychiatric provider for an outpatient clinic (Knight, Draeger, Heaton, & Patel, 2008).

Pharmacists also provide depression screening in primary care settings (Finley, Crismon, & Rush, 2003). Simple screening tools are available that are easy for the patient to complete while in the waiting room prior to an appointment. The pharmacist evaluates the screening responses and provides feedback to the physician to improve patient care. If a screen is positive, the pharmacist can utilize the patient medical record to make appropriate treatment recommendations prior to the patient leaving the clinic. Psychiatric pharmacists also work in state hospitals, prison and jail systems, and nonteaching hospital settings.

The community pharmacist is in a unique position to provide behavioral health services. As the professional who sees the patient on a routine basis for medication refills, the pharmacist is often the first person to understand if a patient is missing refills, suffering from side effects, or beginning to have symptoms of their behavioral health problem. It is very important in behavioral health treatment that new symptoms are identified early in order to prevent a relapse or decrease the severity of a mood or psychotic episode.

The community pharmacist can form alliances with both the patient and area behavioral health providers to build a network of support for the individual suffering from a behavioral health problem. Because he or she is an integral part of the behavioral health treatment and support team, the community pharmacist should work to improve his or her understanding of behavioral health problems and increase his or her comfort level in working with these patients.

Community pharmacists should take advantage of additional professional development opportunities to first become familiar with basic psychiatric screening tools and then become certified to administer and interpret them. This is especially important if the pharmacist is part of a medical home or other treatment team.

PREVENTION AND PROMOTION

The field of public health has long utilized the triad concept of prevention. Primary prevention prevents disease occurrence of major public health problems. Secondary prevention prevents recurrences or exacerbations of diseases already diagnosed. Tertiary prevention reduces the amount of disability caused by diseases in order for at-risk populations to reach the highest possible level of functioning.

Health promotion enables people to increase control over and to improve their health. Behavioral health promotion activities enhance an individual's competence, self-esteem, and sense of well-being rather than intervene in the prevention of behavioral health problems. Behavioral health promotion initiatives are found in a variety of organizations, including schools, health organizations, industry, government organizations, and in religious institutions. In addition, societies and their multiple cultures vary in their ability to provide behavioral health promotion activities.

Starting in 1979, *Healthy People* provided 10-year national objectives for promoting health and preventing disease. It sets and monitors national health objectives and measures impacts of prevention activity. *Healthy People 2010* established 14 mental health objectives for the United States, grouped under the following three categories: (1) mental health status improvement; (2) treatment expansion; and (3) state activities (USDHHS, 2000).

Healthy People 2020 continues to refine national objectives for promoting health and preventing disease. However, a new focal area emphasizes the reduction of depression through screening and treatment (USDHHS, 2010). Objectives retained from *Healthy People 2010* include those relating to eating disorders, children with mental disorders, and specialized services for the elderly. A modified objective focuses on increasing treatment for persons with co-occurring mental and substance use disorders.

In *Informing the Future: Critical Issues in Health*, now in its sixth edition, the Institute of Medicine (2011) has consistently recommended a framework that integrates health, behavioral health, and public health, with a focus on improving the mental, emotional, and behavioral health among young people. Additional recommendations to ensure healthy communities addressed improving vaccines, educating the public regarding immunizations, and helping to improve medication safety and chronic diseases, such as cardiovascular disease, HIV/AIDS, Hepatitis B and C, and hypertension. While many of the issues addressed here are well-known to pharmacists and other health professionals, a persistent question remains how do we address prevention and promotion services in addition to general pharmacy practice in rural America?

THE ROLE OF PHARMACISTS IN RURAL AMERICA

The need for pharmacists and changing pharmacy practice to address the needs of persons with behavioral health problems in rural areas continues. The term "frontier health professional shortage area" means an area with a population density less than six persons per square mile within the service area and the time and/or distance to primary care is considered excessive (Wilger & Alfero, 2015). Since 90% of the United States is defined as rural and 20% of Americans live in rural areas, medically underserved areas occur in almost every state in the country (Thrasher, O'Connor, & Joyner, 2012). In addition to the approximately 6,100 designated primary care and 4,000 mental health HPSAs (Health Professional Shortage Areas), only 12% of pharmacists practice in rural locations (National Rural Health Association, 2005). To meet the needs of rural populations will require continuous professional development and increased competencies (Scott, 2010) and significant changes to how pharmacy practice is legislated, regulated, and delivered.

Health promotion is a growing service area for rural pharmacy practice. Although studies report that 65% of patients never discuss health issues with their pharmacists (Black, Murphy, & Gardner, 2009) or that traditional pharmacy services are more important than more clinically oriented services (Laubscher, Evans, Blackburn, Taylor, & McKay, 2009), rural pharmacists reported increased provision of disease state management programs and MTM services (Gadkari, Mott, Kreling, & Bonnarens, 2009). Concerns about privacy and pharmacists' time did not outweigh patients' perceptions that MTM services can improve medication use. A Texas study indicated that pharmacists want to expand their roles as patient care providers (Moczygemba, Barner, & Roberson, 2008).

Pharmacists working in the U.S. Public Health Service Commissioned Corps have expanded their practice outside of the traditional role of the pharmacist (Flowers et al., 2009). The Indian Health Service employs pharmacists to work in multidisciplinary teams in isolated areas in the Western part of the United States and Alaska to reach approximately 1.5 million Native Americans and Alaska Natives. These pharmacists not only dispense prescriptions, but also monitor laboratories, conduct physical assessments, and provide MTM under physician-approved treatment guidelines.

The National Rural Health Association (2009, May) made a number of recommendations to assist in rural pharmacy practice. One recommendation was a transition from a product-based reimbursement payment system to a more realistic reimbursement system that accounts for the differences in rural pharmacy services, including an exemption to antitrust law to provide rural pharmacies more leverage when negotiating Medicare Part D and third-party contracts. One policy recommendation specifically addresses the expansion of the Medicare definition of the term "nonphysician practitioners" in rural health centers and federally qualified health centers to include clinical pharmacists.

Another recommendation was the development of alternative models for pharmacy service, including the creation of national models for the provision of cognitive pharmacist services across state lines without multiple state licensures. Although the ACA has increased access to services and medications through Medicare D, it has increased the financial and administrative challenges for many rural pharmacies. One significant challenge is the use of a pharmacy benefit manager (PBM), particularly when we are looking at coverage for behavioral health.

ERISA AND PHARMACY BENEFITS MANAGERS

The Employee Retirement Income Security Act of 1974 (ERISA), originally designed to regulate employee pension plans, also covers employee welfare plans and employee welfare benefits plans. Benefits may include coverage for physical and behavioral health conditions, accidents, unemployment, and disability. Companies and employers may operate their pension and healthcare benefit plans across and within state and municipal borders under the protection of ERISA. This type of self-funding has grown increasingly popular as a means to control costs, promote wellness initiatives, and provide improved access to claims utilization data. Approximately 55% of employees in firms with 200 to 999 workers are self-funded (Kaiser Family Foundation, 2014).

ERISA defines a person (or organization) who provides services to an employee health plan as a party-in-interest. Any party-in-interest exercises any discretionary authority or control with regard to managing an employee benefit plan or its assets is considered a fiduciary. A *fiduciary* is any individual or entity that enters into a legal or ethical relationship of confidence or trust between two or more parties, with the intent of acting on the behalf of another individual, group, or system. For example, a fiduciary may administer or manage a health plan package (or a part of a package) for state employees.

A PBM may fall under ERISA as a fiduciary. PBMs administer outpatient prescription drug benefits for most Americans, who have employer-based healthcare coverage. Contracted by health plans, PBMs provide drugs at set prices to plan participants, negotiate volume discounts and rebates with pharmaceutical manufacturers, and provide drug utilization reviews. Therefore, as a fiduciary, a PBM must operate in a manner that ensures full transparency and full disclosure and acts in the best interest of its health plan beneficiaries (Slade, 2009).

In recent state and federal court cases, PBMs have been accused of alleged breaches of their fiduciary duties to self-funded employee benefit plans. Alleging violations of ERISA's fiduciary duty requirements and breach of contract, class action and civil lawsuits have launched federal fraud investigations into price manipulations and financial rebates surrounding pharmaceutical care and formularies. This has led to organizations, such as the National Community Pharmacists Association (1998), to create guides for company benefit managers on questions they should ask their PBMs.

Because ERISA originally regulated employee pension plans, it contains few codes pertaining to health care, and even fewer specific codes for behavioral health. Further, ERISA, as a Federal law, preempts state laws that attempt to regulate private-sector health plans, but it allows states to regulate the business of insurance. Since ERISA does not allow states to consider self-funding employee plans to be insurers, state insurance commissioners cannot regulate self-funding employee plans. In addition, ERISA does not establish standard employee health plan protections. Therefore, the federal government created a regulatory gap. This gap has frustrated states' efforts to bring successful individual or class action lawsuits against companies protected under the ERISA law, especially since negligence or breach of contract cannot be litigated if it relates to employee benefits plans. However, recent legal cases may change ERISA's oversight role regarding the provision of healthcare benefits.

LEGAL AND ETHICAL ISSUES

There remain a number of legal and ethical issues in behavioral health services delivery systems. These range from the capacity of individuals with behavioral health problems to decline health care and mental health care (the right to refuse treatment and informed consent) to coercion and the sexual or financial exploitation of patients by clinicians (i.e., regulation of the patient–therapist relationship). Additional issues include confidentiality, professional licensing laws (particularly in this era of continuous emerging technology), and the protection of patients from decisions made by clinical self-interest. For a more complete discussion on these issues, see Levin & Petrila, 2010.

Two issues pertinent to pharmacists are: (1) resource limitations or rationing of health and behavioral health services; and (2) denial of service. Both, of course, have practice implications for pharmacists. Not only will pharmacists require more time- and labor-intensive interactions with their patients, but they will also need to spend more time with other members of the patient or healthcare team's medical home.

The second issue, denial of service, was at the very heart of the debates in Congress during 2009–2010. The idea of health provider "refusal clauses" (also known as "conscience clauses") is contentious. Griswold v. Connecticut, 381 U.S. 479 (1965) recognized that pharmacist conscience laws conflict with the constitutional right to privacy (a woman was denied her right to use a contraceptive when a pharmacist refused to fill a prescription). Conscience clauses also may address constitutional Equal Protection issues, since not filling contraceptive prescriptions "legalizes" the unequal treatment of men and women.

The denial of coverage issue becomes more complicated under the mental health parity laws. Rosenbach and colleagues (2009) found mental health providers may select a "parity diagnosis" for patients in order to ensure insurance coverage for diagnosis and treatment. A parity diagnosis is a diagnosis selected from a subset of mental conditions eligible for coverage under the parity law, instead of covering all mental disorders in the *DSM*. States, for example, may provide parity for a limited number of mental disorders but not include any substance use disorders. If a provider changes the patient's diagnosis to a nonparity diagnosis, there would be no insurance coverage.

The fact that a provider chooses a parity diagnosis for a patient in order to ensure insurance coverage for the patient and reimbursement for the provider is a potentially problematic outcome of having lists of approved versus unapproved and nonreimbursable diagnoses. This remains a potential ethical problem despite parity law implementation in 2012.

All patients with behavioral health problems have a right to know about their therapists' credentials, procedures, services, and policies regarding access to patient records. There is an expectation of confidentiality and privacy regarding records. In the context of the Health Insurance Portability and Accountability Act (HIPAA), privacy determines who should have access, what constitutes the patient's rights to confidentiality, and what constitutes inappropriate access to health records.

Confidentiality establishes how the records, or the systems that hold the records, are protected from unauthorized or inappropriate access. Privacy and confidentiality become issues when a patient is expected to share health information, if he or she brings charges against the mental health therapist, or if the mental health professional believes the patient posed a clear danger to self or others.

A behavioral health professional may expect that the patient automatically opts-in (agrees) to share health information with all members of the practice or with other providers that the patient sees by becoming a patient. However, patients need to be informed explicitly of opt-out options to retain control over his or her information.

HIPAA provides protection for psychotherapy notes, which must be kept separate from medical profiles and may not be transferred without consent (DeLettre & Sobell, 2010). However, other behavioral information outside of psychotherapy notes may need to be protected, such as multi-axis DSM-IV diagnoses, prescribed medications, suicidal impulses or attempts, or past history (Clemens, 2012). A patient also waives his or her right to confidentiality and/or privacy when he or she enters into litigation, such as malpractice or breach of confidentiality.

The Tarasoff rule, varies extensively across state "duty to warn or protect" statutes. California, for example, recently revised its Tarasoff legislation unambiguously solely as a duty to protect potential victims (Weinstock, Bonnici, Seroussi, & Leong, 2014). Questions also are being raised about whether patient privacy is violated when mental health providers conduct an Internet search for information on their own patients (Clinton, Silverman, & Brendel, 2010).

IMPLICATIONS FOR PHARMACISTS AND PHARMACY PRACTICE

Growing collaboration among healthcare providers, with the passage of the health reform bill, creates a more integral role in the public and the private health and behavioral health sectors for the community pharmacist and the psychiatric clinical pharmacist. MTM and the medical home become increasingly important with the move toward the integration between primary care services and behavioral healthcare services. The increased collaboration also will affect pharmacy education.

Skills needed for working on an integrated team are not generally part of the academic preparation for healthcare professionals. For pharmacy education, this may require a retooling of curriculum and internships to provide more in-depth knowledge and practice for pharmacy students as well as returning professionals, especially for community pharmacists. It also may require added emphasis on community-centered approaches to pharmacy practice. These include increased awareness of current epidemiologic and disease surveillance information as well as an increased emphasis on health information technologies, such as electronic health record systems and use of additional public health information systems.

Federal and state policies are not structured to promote collaborative practice. State regulations for collaborative practice, including the definition of collaborative practice, differ significantly across states. For example, in one Midwest state, a clinical psychiatric pharmacist provides medication management services, including drug initiation and discontinuation, dose changes, refill authorizations, laboratory monitoring, and assessment for an outpatient mental health practice that includes more than 50 patients with early psychosis. The pharmacist practices under a scope of practice that is approved by the institution and signed by the clinic psychiatrists, which allows patients to be scheduled for individual clinic appointments with the pharmacist for medication management.

Pharmacists should take advantage of opportunities to engage in policy work groups. This allows them to keep abreast of critical public health issues and to bring their concerns regarding quality of care, care coordination, and patient-centered outcomes to policy makers and legislators.

Education of physicians about the training and ability of pharmacists to manage and monitor complex drug therapy regimens is paramount in gaining strong advocates for the expanded role of pharmacists in patient care. These are important considerations as community pharmacists and psychiatric clinical pharmacists continue to become a more integral part of behavioral health services and treatment teams.

QUESTIONS FOR FURTHER DISCUSSION

1. Should mental health services be integrated into healthcare delivery systems?
2. What are some of the ethical issues in behavioral health services delivery?
3. What can be done to address the needs of homeless individuals with behavioral health problems?
4. How involved should pharmacists become in caring for individuals with behavioral health problems?

KEY TOPICS AND TERMS

Behavioral health
Disability-adjusted life years
Disease state management
Medication adherence
Medication therapy management (MTM)
Mental health
Pharmacy benefit manager (PBM)
Psychiatric clinical pharmacist
Substance abuse disorders

REFERENCES

Alang, S. M. (2015). Sociodemographic disparities associated with perceived causes of unmet need for mental health care. *Psychiatric Rehabilitation Journal*, Advance online publication. doi:10.1037/prj0000113

American Psychiatric Association. (1987). *Diagnostic and statistical manual of mental disorders: DSM-III-R.* Washington, DC: American Psychiatric Association.

Ascher-Svanum, H., Zhu, B., Faries, D. E., Furiak, N. M., & Montgomery, W. (2009). Medication adherence levels and differential use of mental-health services in the treatment of schizophrenia. *BMC Research Notes, 2*, 6. doi:10.1186/1756-0500-2-6

Black, E., Murphy, A. L., & Gardner, D. M. (2009). Community pharmacist services for people with mental illnesses: Preferences, satisfaction, and stigma. *Psychiatric Services, 60*(8), 1123–1127. doi:10.1176/appi.ps.60.8.1123

Blazer, D. G., Kessler, R. C., McGonagle, K. A., & Swartz, M. S. (1994). The prevalence and distribution of major depression in a national community sample: The National Comorbidity Survey. *American Journal of Psychiatry, 151*(7), 979–986.

Bloom, D. E., Cafiero, E. T., Jané-Llopis, E., Abrahams-Gessel, S., Bloom, L. R., Fathima, S., Weinstein, C. (2011). *The global economic burden of non-communicable diseases: A report.* Geneva, Switzerland: World Economic Forum. Retrieved from http://www3.weforum.org/docs/WEF_Harvard_HE_GlobalEconomicBurdenNonCommunicableDiseases_2011.pdf

Caballero, J., Souffrant, G., & Heffernan, E. (2008). Development and outcomes of a psychiatric pharmacy clinic for indigent patients. *American Journal of Health-System Pharmacy, 65*(3), 229–233. doi:10.2146/ajhp070266

Carson, E. A. (2014). *Prisoners in 2013* (NCJ 247282). Washington, DC: U.S. Department of Justice, Office of Justice Programs, Bureau of Justice Statistics. Retrieved from http://www.bjs.gov/content/pub/pdf/p13.pdf

Centers for Medicare and Medicaid Services. (2014). *National health expenditures 2013 highlights.* Baltimore, MD: CMS. Retrieved from http://www.cms.gov/Research-Statistics-Data-and-Systems/Statistics-Trends-and-Reports/NationalHealthExpendData/downloads/highlights.pdf

City Policy Associates. (2013, December). *Hunger and homelessness survey: A status report on hunger and homelessness in America's cities: A 25-city survey.* Washington, DC: United States Conference of Mayors. Retrieved from http://www.usmayors.org/pressreleases/uploads/2013/1210-report-HH.pdf

Clemens, N. A. (2012). Privacy, consent, and the electronic mental health record: The Person vs. the System. *Journal of Psychiatric Practice, 18*(1), 46–50. doi:10.1097/01.pra.0000410987.38723.47

Clinton, B. K., Silverman, B. C., & Brendel, D. H. (2010). Patient-targeted googling: The ethics of searching online for patient information. *Harvard Review of Psychiatry, 18*(2), 103–112. doi:10.3109/10673221003683861

Cook, B. L., Liu, Z., Lessios, A. S., Loder, S., & McGuire, T. (2015). The costs and benefits of reducing racial-ethnic disparities in mental health care. *Psychiatric Services, 66*(4), 389–396. doi:10.1176/appi.ps.201400070

Cook, B. L., Zuvekas, S. H., Carson, N., Wayne, G. F., Vesper, A., & McGuire, T. G. (2014). Assessing racial/ethnic disparities in treatment across episodes of mental health care. *Health Services Research, 49*(1), 206–229. doi:10.1111/1475-6773.12095

Crockett, J., Taylor, S., Grabham, A., & Stanford, P. (2006). Patient outcomes following an intervention involving community pharmacists in the management of depression. *Australian Journal of Rural Health, 14*(6), 263–269. doi:10.1111/j.1440-1584.2006.00827.x

DeLettre, J. L., & Sobell, L. C. (2010). Keeping psychotherapy notes separate from the patient record. *Clinical Psychology & Psychotherapy, 17*(2), 160–163. doi:10.1002/cpp.654

Ferrari, A. J., Charlson, F. J., Norman, R. E., Patten, S. B., Freedman, G., Murray, C. J., & Whiteford, H. A. (2013). Burden of depressive disorders by country, sex, age, and year: Findings from the Global Burden of Disease Study 2010. *PLoS Medicine, 10*(11), e1001547 doi:10.1371/journal.pmed.1001547

Finley, P. R., Crismon, M. L., & Rush, A. J. (2003). Evaluating the impact of pharmacists in mental health: A systematic review. *Pharmacotherapy, 23*(12), 1634–1644.

Flowers, L., Wick, J., Figg, W. D., Sr., McClelland, R. H., Shiber, M., Britton, J. E., & Huntzinger, P. (2009). U.S. Public Health Service Commissioned Corps pharmacists: Making a difference in advancing the nation's health. *Journal of the American Pharmacists Association, 49*(3), 446–452. doi:10.1331/JAPhA.2009.08036

Forsner, T., Hansson, J., Brommels, M., Wistedt, A. A., & Forsell, Y. (2010). Implementing clinical guidelines in psychiatry: A qualitative study of perceived facilitators and barriers. *BMC Psychiatry, 10*, 8. doi:10.1186/1471-244x-10-8

Gadkari, A. S., Mott, D. A., Kreling, D. H., & Bonnarens, J. K. (2009). Pharmacy characteristics associated with the provision of drug therapy services in nonmetropolitan community pharmacies. *Journal of Rural Health, 25*(3), 290–295. doi:10.1111/j.1748-0361.2009.00232.x

Gilbert, D. A., Altshuler, K. Z., Rago, W. V., Shon, S. P., Crismon, M. L., Toprac, M. G., & Rush, A. J. (1998). Texas Medication Algorithm Project: Definitions, rationale, and methods to develop medication algorithms. *Journal of Clinical Psychiatry, 59*(7), 345–351.

Glaze, L., & Kaeble, D. (2014). *Correctional populations in the United States, 2013*. U.S. Department of Justice, Office of Justice Programs, Bureau of Justice Statistics. Retrieved from http://www.bjs.gov/index.cfm?ty=pbdetail&iid=5177

Haynes, R. B., Ackloo, E., Sahota, N., McDonald, H. P., & Yao, X. (2008). Interventions for enhancing medication adherence. *Cochrane Database of Systematic Reviews*(2), CD000011. doi:10.1002/14651858.CD000011.pub3

Heflinger, C. A., Shaw, V., Higa-McMillan, C., Lunn, L., & Brannan, A. M. (2015). Patterns of child mental health service delivery in a public system: Rural children and the role of rural residence. *Journal of Behavioral Health Services and Research*. doi:10.1007/s11414-015-9464-9

Henry, M., Cortes, A., Shivji, A., & Buck, K. (2015). *The 2014 Annual Homeless Assessment Report (AHAR) to Congress: Part 1: Point-in-time estimates of homelessness*. Washington, DC: U.S. Department of Housing and Urban Development, Office of Community Planning and Development. Retrieved from https://www.hudexchange.info/resources/documents/2014-AHAR-Part1.pdf

Insel, T. R. (2008). Assessing the economic costs of serious mental illness. *American Journal of Psychiatry, 165*(6), 663–665. doi:10.1176/appi.ajp.2008.08030366

Institute of Medicine. (2011). *Informing the future: Critical issues in health* (6th ed.). Washington, DC: National Academies Press. Retrieved from http://www.nap.edu/openbook.php?record_id=13180

James, D. J., & Glaze, L. E. (2006). *Mental health problems of prison and jail inmates*. Washington, DC: U.S. Dept. of Justice, Office of Justice Programs, Bureau of Justice Statistics. Retrieved from http://www.bjs.gov/content/pub/pdf/mhppji.pdf

Kaiser Family Foundation, & Health Research & Educational Trust. (2014). *Employer health benefits survey: 2014 annual survey*. Menlo Park, CA; Chicago, IL: Kaiser Family Foundation; Health Research & Educational Trust. Retrieved from http://files.kff.org/attachment/2014-employer-health-benefits-survey-full-report

Kane, J. M., Leucht, S., Carpenter, D., & Docherty, J. P. (2003). The expert consensus guideline series. Optimizing pharmacologic treatment of psychotic disorders. Introduction: Methods, commentary, and summary. *Journal of Clinical Psychiatry, 64 Suppl 12*, 5–19.

Kessler, R. C., Berglund, P., Demler, O., Jin, R., Koretz, D., Merikangas, K. R., & Wang, P. S. (2003). The epidemiology of major depressive disorder: Results from the National Comorbidity Survey Replication (NCS-R). *Journal of the American Medical Association, 289*(23), 3095–3105. doi:10.1001/jama.289.23.3095

Kessler, R. C., Berglund, P. A., Zhao, S., Leaf, P. J., Kouzis, A. C., & Bruce, M. L. (1996). The 12-month prevalence and correlates of serious mental illness (SMI). In R. W. Manderscheid & M. A. Sonnenschein (Eds.), *Mental health, United States 1996* (pp. 59–70). Washington, DC: Government Printing Office.

Kessler, R. C., McGonagle, K. A., Zhao, S., Nelson, C. B., Hughes, M., Eshleman, S., & Kendler, K. S. (1994). Lifetime and 12-month prevalence of DSM-III-R psychiatric disorders in the United States. Results from the National Comorbidity Survey. *Archives of General Psychiatry, 51*(1), 8–19.

Knight, D. E., Draeger, R. W., Heaton, P. C., & Patel, N. C. (2008). Pharmacist screening for depression among patients with diabetes in an urban primary care setting. *Journal of the American Pharmacists Association, 48*(4), 518–521. doi:10.1331/JAPhA.2008.07048

Kreyenbuhl, J., Buchanan, R. W., Dickerson, F. B., & Dixon, L. B. (2010). The Schizophrenia Patient Outcomes Research Team (PORT): Updated treatment recommendations 2009. *Schizophrenia Bulletin, 36*(1), 94–103. doi:10.1093/schbul/sbp130

Laubscher, T., Evans, C., Blackburn, D., Taylor, J., & McKay, S. (2009). Collaboration between family physicians and community pharmacists to enhance adherence to chronic medications: Opinions of Saskatchewan family physicians. *Canadian Family Physician, 55*(12), e69–e75.

Levin, B. L., Hennessy, K. D., & Petrila, J. (2010). *Mental health services: A public health perspective*. New York, NY: Oxford University Press. Retrieved from http://site.ebrary.com/id/10400775

Levin, B. L., & Petrila, J. (2010). Law, services delivery, & policy. In B. L. Levin, K. D. Hennessy & J. Petrila (Eds.), *Mental health services a public health perspective* (3rd ed., pp. 43–66). New York, NY: Oxford University Press.

Levit, K. R., Kassed, C. A., Coffey, R. M., Mark, T. L., Stranges, E. M., Buck, J. A., & Vandivort-Warren, R. (2008). Future funding for mental health and substance abuse: Increasing burdens for the public sector. *Health Affairs, 27*(6), w513–w522. doi:10.1377/hlthaff.27.6.w513

Lieberman, J. A., Stroup, T. S., McEvoy, J. P., Swartz, M. S., Rosenheck, R. A., Perkins, D. O., Hsiao, J. K. (2005). Effectiveness of antipsychotic drugs in patients with chronic schizophrenia. *New England Journal of Medicine, 353*(12), 1209–1223. doi:10.1056/NEJMoa051688

Liu, K., Wissoker, D., & Swett, A. (2007). Nursing home use by dual-eligible beneficiaries in the last year of life. *Inquiry, 44*(1), 88–103.

Lo, C. C., Cheng, T. C., & Howell, R. J. (2014). Access to and utilization of health services as pathway to racial disparities in serious mental illness. *Community Mental Health Journal, 50*(3), 251–257. doi:10.1007/s10597-013-9593-7

Mathers, C., Boerma, T., & Fat, D. M. (2008). *The global burden of disease: 2004 update.* Geneva, Switzerland: World Health Organization. Retrieved from http://www.who.int/healthinfo/global_burden_disease/GBD_report_2004update_full.pdf

Medicare Payment Advisory Commission. (2015). *Beneficiaries dually eligible for Medicare and Medicaid: Data book.* Washington, DC: Medicare Payment Advisory Commission (MEDPAC); Medicaid and CHIP Payment and Access Commission. Retrieved from http://medpac.gov/documents/data-book/january-2015-medpac-and-macpac-data-book-beneficiaries-dually-eligible-for-medicare-and-medicaid.pdf?sfvrsn=2

Michaud, C. M., Murray, C. J., & Bloom, B. R. (2001). Burden of disease–implications for future research. *Journal of the American Medical Association, 285*(5), 535–539.

Miranda, J. J., McGuire, T. G., Williams, D. R., & Wang, P. (2008). Mental health in the context of health disparities. *American Journal of Psychiatry, 165*(9), 1102–1108. doi:10.1176/appi.ajp.2008.08030333

Miranda, J. J., & Patel, V. (2005). Achieving the Millennium Development Goals: Does mental health play a role? *PLoS Medicine, 2*(10), e291 doi:10.1371/journal.pmed.0020291

Moczygemba, L. R., Barner, J. C., & Roberson, K. (2008). Texas pharmacists' opinions about and plans for provision of medication therapy management services. *Journal of the American Pharmacists Association, 48*(1), 38–45. doi:10.1331/JAPhA.2008.07015

Moore, T. A., Buchanan, R. W., Buckley, P. F., Chiles, J. A., Conley, R. R., Crismon, M. L., & Miller, A. L. (2007). The Texas Medication Algorithm Project antipsychotic algorithm for schizophrenia: 2006 update. *Journal of Clinical Psychiatry, 68*(11), 1751–1762.

Murray, C. J., Vos, T., Lozano, R., Naghavi, M., Flaxman, A. D., Michaud, C., & Memish, Z. A. (2012). Disability-adjusted life years (DALYs) for 291 diseases and injuries in 21 regions, 1990-2010: A systematic analysis for the Global Burden of Disease Study 2010. *Lancet, 380*(9859), 2197–2223. doi:10.1016/s0140-6736(12)61689-4

National Alliance to End Homelessness. (2014). *The state of homelessness in America 2014: A research report on homelessness.* Washington, DC: National Alliance to End Homelessness. Retrieved from http://b.3cdn.net/naeh/d1b106237807ab260f_qam6ydz02.pdf

National Community Pharmacist Association. (1998). *Ten questions company benefits managers must ask their PBMs.* Alexandria, VA: National Community Pharmacist Association. Retrieved from https://www.ncpanet.org/pdf/leg/leg_pbm_ten_questions.pdf

National Rural Health Association. (2005, May). *Recruitment and retention of a quality health workforce in rural areas.* Alexandria, VA: Author. Retrieved from http://www.ruralhealthweb.org/index.cfm?objectid=4075DEAB-1185-6B66-88E95A371EF681D6

National Rural Health Association. (2009, May). *Pharmacy.* Washington, DC: Author. Retrieved from http://www.ruralhealthweb.org/index.cfm?objectid=297140D6-3048-651A-FE20F640AF515516

Osher, F. C., D'Amora, D. A., Plotkin, M., Jarrett, N., & Eggleston, A. (2012). *Adults with behavioral health needs under correctional supervision a shared framework for reducing recidivism and promoting recovery.* New York, NY: Council of State Governments Justice Center Criminal Justice/Mental Health Consensus Project. Retrieved from http://csgjusticecenter.org/wp-content/uploads/2013/05/9-24-12_Behavioral-Health-Framework-final.pdf

Paul Wellstone and Pete Domenici Mental Health Parity and Addiction Equity Act of 2008, Pub. L. 110–343, 42 USC 201 §511 et seq. (2008).

President's New Freedom Commission on Mental Health. (2003). *Achieving the promise: Transforming mental health care in America: Final report.* Rockville, MD: President's New Freedom Commission on Mental Health. Retrieved from http://govinfo.library.unt.edu/mentalhealthcommission/reports/FinalReport/downloads/downloads.html

Prins, S. J., & Draper, L. (2009). *Improving outcomes for people with mental illnesses under community corrections supervision a guide to research-informed policy and practice.* New York, NY: Council of State Governments Justice Center. Retrieved from https://csgjusticecenter.org/wp-content/uploads/2012/12/Community-Corrections-Research-Guide.pdf

Robins, L. N., & Regier, D. A. (1991). *Psychiatric disorders in America: The epidemiologic catchment area study.* New York, NY: Free Press.

Rosenbach, M. L., Lake, T. K., Williams, S. R., & Buck, J. A. (2009). Implementation of mental health parity: Lessons from California. *Psychiatric Services, 60*(12), 1589–1594. doi:10.1176/appi.ps.60.12.1589

Sackett, D. L., Rosenberg, W. M., Gray, J. A., Haynes, R. B., & Richardson, W. S. (1996). Evidence based medicine: What it is and what it isn't. *British Medical Journal, 312*(7023), 71–72.

Saloner, B., & Le Cook, B. (2013). Blacks and Hispanics are less likely than whites to complete addiction treatment, largely due to socioeconomic factors. *Health Affairs, 32*(1), 135–145. doi:10.1377/hlthaff.2011.0983

Scott, D. M. (2010). Assessment of pharmacists' perception of patient care competence and need for training in rural and urban areas in North Dakota. *Journal of Rural Health, 26*(1), 90–96. doi:10.1111/j.1748-0361.2009.00270.x

Slade, D. H. (2009). ERISA preemption and the question of pharmacy benefit managers' fiduciary duty. *Journal of Legal Medicine, 30*(3), 409–425. doi:10.1080/01947640903146659

Social Security Act Amendments of 1965, Pub. L. 89–97, 42 USC Title 42 §§1395 to 1395lll (1965).

Steadman, H. J., Osher, F. C., Robbins, P. C., Case, B., & Samuels, S. (2009). Prevalence of serious mental illness among jail inmates. *Psychiatric Services, 60*(6), 761–765. doi:10.1176/appi.ps.60.6.761

Substance Abuse and Mental Health Services Administration. (2013). *National expenditures for mental health services and substance abuse treatment, 1986–2009* (HHS Publication No. SMA-13-4740). Rockville, MD: Substance Abuse and Mental Health Services Administration. Retrieved from https://store.samhsa.gov/shin/content/SMA13-4740/SMA13-4740.pdf

Thrasher, K., O'Connor, S. K., & Joyner, P. U. (2012). Rural health in pharmacy curricula. *American Journal of Pharmaceutical Education, 76*(9), 180. doi:10.5688/ajpe769180

Torrey, E. F. National Alliance for the Mentally Ill, & Public Citizen Health Research Group. (1992). *Criminalizing the seriously mentally ill: The abuse of jails as mental hospitals, a joint report of the National Alliance for the Mentally Ill and Public Citizen's Health Research Group.* Washington, DC; Arlington, VA: Public Citizen's Health Research Group; National Alliance for the Mentally Ill.

Torrey, E. F., Zdanowicz, M. T., Kennard, A. D., Lamb, H. R., Eslinger, D. F., Blasotti, M. C., & Fuller, D. A. (2014, April 8). *The treatment of persons with mental illness in prisons and jails: A state survey.* Arlington, VA: Treatment Advocacy Center. Retrieved from http://www.tacreports.org/storage/documents/treatment-behind-bars/treatment-behind-bars.pdf

U.S. Department of Health and Human Services. (1999). *Mental health: A report of the Surgeon General.* Rockville, MD: Dept. of Health and Human Services, U.S. Public Health Service. Retrieved from http://purl.access.gpo.gov/GPO/LPS3863

U. S. Department of Health and Human Services. (2000). *Healthy people 2010.* WorldCat database. Retrieved from http://purl.access.gpo.gov/GPO/LPS8595

U. S. Department of Health and Human Services. (2010). *Healthy People 2020.* Washington, DC: U. S. Department of Health and Human Services. Retrieved from http://www.healthypeople.gov/2020/

U.S. Department of Housing and Urban Development. (2009). *The 2008 annual homeless assessment report to Congress.* Washington, DC: U.S. Department of Housing and Urban Development. Retrieved from http://www.huduser.org/portal/publications/pdf/4thHOmelessAssessmentReport.pdf

Velligan, D. I., Weiden, P. J., Sajatovic, M., Scott, J., Carpenter, D., Ross, R., & Docherty, J. P. (2010). Strategies for addressing adherence problems in patients with serious and persistent mental illness: Recommendations from the expert consensus guidelines. *Journal of Psychiatric Practice, 16*(5), 306–324. doi:10.1097/01.pra.0000388626.98662.a0

Weinstock, R., Bonnici, D., Seroussi, A., & Leong, G. B. (2014). No duty to warn in California: Now unambiguously solely a duty to protect. *Journal of the American Academy of Psychiatry & Law, 42*(1), 101–108.

Welch, C. A., Czerwinski, D., Ghimire, B., & Bertsimas, D. (2009). Depression and costs of health care. *Psychosomatics, 50*(4), 392–401. doi:10.1176/appi.psy.50.4.392

West, J. C., Wilk, J. E., Rae, D. S., Muszynski, I. S., Stipec, M. R., Alter, C. L., ... Regier, D. A. (2009). Medicaid prescription drug policies and medication access and continuity: Findings from ten states. *Psychiatric Services, 60*(5), 601–610. doi:10.1176/appi.ps.60.5.601

Whiteford, H. A., Degenhardt, L., Rehm, J., Baxter, A. J., Ferrari, A. J., Erskine, H. E., ... Vos, T. (2013). Global burden of disease attributable to mental and substance use disorders: Findings from the Global Burden of Disease Study 2010. *The Lancet, 382*(9904), 15751586. doi:10.1016/S0140-6736(13)61611-6

Wilger, S., & Alfero, C. (2015, April). *Health professional shortage areas.* Alexandria, VA: National Rural Health Association. Retrieved from http://www.ruralhealthweb.org/index.cfm?objectid=A23C5B6E-CEA1-C8C0-ADE130F39C10E382

World Health Organization. (2002). The world health report 2002: Reducing risks, promoting healthy life. Retrieved from http://www.who.int/whr/2002/en/whr02_en.pdf?ua=1

World Health Organization. (2003). *Investing in mental health.* Geneva, Switzerland: WHO. Retrieved from http://www.who.int/mental_health/media/investing_mnh.pdf

World Health Organization. (2011, April). *Global status report on non-communicable diseases 2010: Description of the global burden of NCDs, their risk factors and determinants.* Geneva, Switzerland: WHO. Retrieved from http://whqlibdoc.who.int/publications/2011/9789240686458_eng.pdf?ua=1

World Health Organization. (2014, October). *Mental disorders* (Fact sheet N°396). Geneva, Switzerland: World Health Organization. Retrieved from http://www.who.int/mediacentre/factsheets/fs396/en/

World Health Organization, & Public Health Agency of Canada. (2005). *Preventing chronic diseases: A vital investment.* Geneva; Switzerland; Ottawa, Toronto: World Health Organization; Public Health Agency of Canada. Retrieved from http://www.who.int/entity/chp/chronic_disease_report/full_report.pdf?ua=1

Yager, J., Kunkle, R., Fochtmann, L. J., Reid, S. M., Plovnick, R., Nininger, J. E., ... Vergare, M. J. (2014). Who's your expert? Use of an expert opinion survey to inform development of American Psychiatric Association practice guidelines. *Academic Psychiatry, 38*(3), 376–382. doi:10.1007/s40596-014-0046-6

Young, K., Garfield, R., Musumeci, M., Clemans-Cope, L., & Lawton, E. (2013). *Medicaid's role for dual eligible beneficiaries* (The Kaiser Commission on Medicaid and the Uninsured Issue Brief). Menlo Park, CA: Henry J. Kaiser Family Foundation. Retrieved from https://kaiserfamilyfoundation.files.wordpress.com/2013/08/7846-04-medicaids-role-for-dual-eligible-beneficiaries.pdf

CHAPTER

12

Home Care

William W. McCloskey

Case Scenario

Mary is a 70-year-old woman with osteomyelitis of the left foot who is referred to your home care service for continuation of intravenous (IV) antibiotic therapy upon discharge from a local hospital. Her physician has prescribed cefazolin 2 g every 8 hours for 4 weeks. Mary received her first three doses of cefazolin before leaving the hospital, although the nurse had a difficult time establishing a peripheral IV line. In addition to her infection, Mary has a history of hypertension, insulin-dependent diabetes, osteoarthritis, and an allergy to oxycodone.

The case manager states that Mary is scheduled to leave the hospital today. She lives alone, but her daughter is willing to help, and she can visit her mother each day after work. Mary's insurance is provided by a health maintenance organization (HMO) that has contracted with the home care service in the past. This HMO expects the home care provider to service Mary in the least expensive way. The company sales representative is excited because he has been trying to get business from this case manager for the past month.

LEARNING OBJECTIVES

Upon completion of this chapter, the student shall be able to:

- Explain what home care is.
- Describe the various types of home care industries.
- Describe the various types of therapies provided by home infusion therapy providers.
- Explain the major factors influencing the home care industry.
- Explain the role of the pharmacist in providing home care services.

CHAPTER QUESTIONS

1. What is home care?
2. What are the primary industries that provide home care?
3. What factors influence the home care industry?
4. What is the role of the pharmacist in home care?

INTRODUCTION

The home healthcare industry is very broad in scope, encompassing a variety of products and services. Three home care industries—home health services, home infusion therapy, and home medical equipment (HME)—provide the majority of these products and services. Each of these industries is influenced by government legislation, regulatory agencies, reimbursement policies, and technological developments. Home care services are generally initiated when a patient is unable to provide for self-care due to illness, and they are intended to restore and maintain the patient's optimal level of well-being in a familiar environment (Council on Scientific Affairs, 1990).

The growth of home care is a result of many factors including an aging patient population, increases in chronic diseases, technological enhancements, consumer preference, and rapidly rising healthcare costs (Landers, 2010). The first homecare agencies were established in the 1880s, and today around 33,000 home care providers deliver care to nearly 12 million people in the United States (National Association of Home Care & Hospice, 2010). In 2013, U.S. expenditures for home healthcare services were estimated to be nearly $80 billion, and nearly 80% of home healthcare spending was related to Medicaid and Medicare (Centers for Medicare and Medicaid Services, 2014). In contrast, private insurance payers generally limit home care coverage to only a small percentage of their overall budgets (Levine, Boal, & Boling, 2003).

Because of the large role that home care plays in today's healthcare system, pharmacists must understand the diverse nature of the products and services offered by the home care industry and the factors that influence their provision. Armed with this knowledge, the pharmacist can more effectively work with other healthcare professionals to manage the clinical and financial needs of a home care patient.

This chapter presents an overview of home care by describing the products and services offered by members of each industry, the factors that affect the delivery of those products and services, and the role of the home care pharmacist.

HOME CARE INDUSTRIES

Home Health Services

Home health services are usually associated with nursing care that is provided through a home health agency. Nursing care, however, is only one type of service offered by these agencies. Additional services may include speech therapy, physical therapy, or other types of rehabilitation therapies; homemaker services; social services; and hospice care. Home health agencies employ specially trained staffs who provide a variety of services with multiple levels of complexity. These professionals work with other home care providers to obtain additional products, such as medical equipment, medication, and surgical supplies, needed to care for the patient. Home health providers perform a vital role in home care by coordinating the patient's care with family caregivers and other healthcare professionals. Effective communication between the home health provider and everyone involved with the patient's care is essential to the success of a patient's therapy. The following are some examples of home health services.

Nursing Services

Nursing services are also referred to as "skilled nursing services." Patients in the home may require the insertion and maintenance of an intravenous (IV) line, the application of dressings for wound care, assistance with disease management, or self-care education. Skilled services need to be performed by a licensed nurse to ensure patient safety and therapy effectiveness. Based on the information in the chapter-opening case scenario, Mary would most likely require a nurse to help maintain and reestablish her IV site as necessary.

With the advent of high-tech home IV therapy, the role of the home care nurse has become more diverse and sophisticated. Consequently, it is desirable for nurses to have experience in critical care nursing, IV therapy, and the administration of blood products. The introduction of new therapies often requires that the nurse undergo training in the use of complex infusion devices and access methods.

Home care nurses may be employed by a variety of organizations, including the Visiting Nurse Association of America. The Visiting Nurse Association of America is a nonprofit entity that coordinates and provides a variety of nursing services in the home. In addition, nursing services may be available through home care companies and pharmacies that provide home care products and services. Some nurses may even practice as independent contractors.

Hospice Services

Hospice services help manage the end-of-life process for terminally ill patients and their families. These services address the clinical, emotional, and spiritual needs of the patient. Support is extended to family members to help them cope with the end-of-life and bereavement processes. In 2013, approximately 1.5 to 1.6 million individuals obtained hospice services, a majority receiving these services at their place of residence (National Hospice and Palliative Care Organization, 2015). The focus of hospice is on maintaining quality of life for terminally ill patients. Hospice care aims to make patients as comfortable as possible. Hospice organizations care for patients using a team approach, which usually includes healthcare professionals, clergy, homemakers, and volunteers who work together to manage the many different aspects of patient care.

Pharmacists are important members of the hospice team. As therapeutic drug experts, they recommend appropriate medications and dosage regimens, especially concerning pain control, while monitoring for side effects and drug–drug interactions.

Speech and Physical Therapy

Rehabilitative services such as speech therapy and physical therapy are commonly offered by home healthcare agencies. Speech therapy, for example, may be provided to stroke patients who are suffering from aphasia, a condition resulting in the loss of ability to speak or to understand spoken or written communication. Physical therapy may be provided to postoperative orthopedic patients or accident victims. Given Mary's foot infection and history of osteoarthritis, she may require the services of a physical therapist. The opportunity to have these traditionally hospital-based services provided at home is particularly convenient for patients who have difficulty with transportation.

Social Services

Social workers have an important role in facilitating the transition of a patient from a hospital or long-term care facility to home and coordinating the provision of required home care services. Social services include support with both economic issues (e.g., dealing with the insurance company and assisting with paperwork) and social issues (e.g., coordinating activities with a senior center)

(Gill, 1991). Although Mary's daughter may be willing to be a caregiver, she may need the support of a social worker to deal with the complexities that home care entails, especially for older people.

Homemaker Services

With the growing elderly population in the United States, the need for homemaker services has increased rapidly since 2000. Employment of home health aides is expected to grow much more rapidly than the average for all occupations through 2022 (U.S. Department of Labor, 2014). Many elderly individuals require assistance with at least one of their activities of daily living or instrumental activities of daily living. Activities of daily living include personal care activities, such as the provision of meals and bathing. Instrumental activities of daily living include house cleaning and grocery shopping. Agencies exist that provide support for elders like Mary who may be unable to complete one or more of these activities.

One of the most well-known homemaker services is the Meals on Wheels program. Meals on Wheels ensures that low-income elderly individuals receive at least one well-balanced meal a day at minimal or no cost. These meals may be served in a congregate setting (e.g., an adult day care center or senior center) or in the senior's home.

Home Infusion Therapy

The home infusion therapy market in the United States is currently estimated to be between $9 and $11 billion per year, and is provided by over 1,500 infusion pharmacies (National Home Infusion Association, 2015). Home infusion therapy refers to the parenteral and enteral administration of drugs, solutions, and nutrition to patients in their homes. In the past, infusion therapies required hospitalization because of their complexity. As healthcare providers gained more clinical knowledge about infusion therapies, however, they were able to develop clinical policies and procedures to ensure their safe administration in the home setting. Home infusion therapy is generally a more cost-effective alternative to hospitalization and is preferred by most patients. In many cases, caregivers or patients may be taught to administer infusion therapies at home. For example, Mary's daughter could be trained to administer her antibiotic therapy. The acceptance of home infusion therapy has reduced the length of hospitalizations and allowed patients to continue active lives.

The following are the primary types of infusion therapies that are administered in the home: nutrition, anti-infective therapy, pain management therapy, chemotherapy, biologics and related plasma-derived therapies, and miscellaneous therapies.

Nutrition

Parenteral nutrition refers to the IV administration of either all (total parenteral nutrition) or some (partial parenteral nutrition) of a patient's daily nutritional requirements. Parenteral nutrition may be considered the grandfather of home infusion therapies. Home parenteral nutrition has been used for more than two decades (Howard et al., 1993) because healthcare providers quickly recognized that most patients requiring chronic therapy did not need to be hospitalized to receive IV feedings.

Home parenteral nutrition is usually administered to home care patients via a central venous catheter or a peripherally inserted central catheter. The choice of venous access is primarily dictated by the concentration of dextrose in the solution to be administered. High concentrations of dextrose (generally greater than 10%) must be administered centrally through a large vein, such as the superior vena cava, to allow for rapid dilution by the blood so as to avoid vascular irritation. In addition to dextrose (as a source of carbohydrates), parenteral nutrition solutions contain amino acids (a source of protein), electrolytes, vitamins, and trace elements. They may also contain fat emulsion (a source of lipids), heparin, insulin, or other compatible medications.

Although enteral nutrition is not a parenteral therapy, patients requiring long-term enteral feedings are often serviced by home infusion providers. Many of these patients have special feeding tubes through which enteral feedings are delivered directly into the stomach (G-tube) or jejunum (J-tube). Consequently, home care therapy providers need to have the expertise to maintain these devices.

Anti-Infective Therapy

Anti-infective therapy was one of the earliest nonnutritive therapies offered at home (Bennett & Allen, 1990), and it remains the most common home infusion therapy. Anti-infective therapy is generally used to manage infections that require relatively long-term IV administration (2 weeks or longer), such as osteomyelitis, cellulitis, Lyme disease, and respiratory infections in cystic fibrosis patients. Even some serious infections, including endocarditis, can be treated in the home setting.

Pain Management Therapy

The hospice movement and the desire of many patients with a terminal illness (and their families) not to be hospitalized in the final days of life have led to the need for the home infusion of narcotic analgesics. Morphine, hydromorphone, fentanyl, and (less commonly) other opiates are administered via continuous infusion to provide chronic pain relief while allowing the patient to remain alert. Ambulatory infusion devices can be programmed to enable patients to self-administer bolus doses of medication on demand for breakthrough pain. Pharmacists are often consulted to convert an oral or transdermal dose of analgesic medication to an appropriate infusion dose.

Chemotherapy

The administration of potent antineoplastic medications in the home setting may be considered for certain patients. Clinician acceptance of this type of home care has increased as the understanding of how to manage the complications of chemotherapy has improved (Bennett & Allen, 1990). Moreover, physicians may not have facilities adequate for the safe preparation (e.g., vertical laminar flow containment hood) of cytotoxic agents or lack USP 797 compliance, so they may utilize the services of a home infusion therapy provider. In addition, changes in the reimbursement structure for administering chemotherapy in the outpatient setting have changed the demand for treatment in the home care setting. Agents that are administered over several days (e.g., 5-fluorouracil) are the antineoplastic medications most commonly administered at home.

Biologics and Related Plasma-Derived Therapies

With the advances that we have seen in biotechnology, a number of drugs have been utilized in home infusion for treatment of diseases that would otherwise be treated in a more controlled setting. Some examples include growth hormone (for treatment of growth hormone deficiency in children), and rare enzyme deficiency diseases such as Gaucher's disease (manifested by mental effects and musculoskeletal effects and treated with alglucerase). Rheumatoid arthritis is another disease that is commonly treated in the home setting with infliximab, adalimumab, and etanercept. Patients with multiple sclerosis may receive injections of interferon beta-1A, interferon beta 1-B and etanercept in their home. As more become available, it is likely that additional biotechnology-derived agents will be suitable for administration in the home environment. Biologic agents have additional complications that may be somewhat unique to the group. Some of these agents require extensive infusion periods of up to 6 hours, which must be monitored throughout by nursing staff. Other problems are incurred if any of the drugs are utilized for a non-FDA approved indication. This off-label use is impacted by medico-legal and reimbursement risk.

Miscellaneous Therapies

Several other infusion therapies have also been delivered in the home, including hydration for such conditions as hyperemesis and inflammatory bowel disease; inotropic therapy for the treatment of refractory congestive heart failure; and blood products for hemotherapy. As more of these therapies emerge, it is anticipated that they will find roles in the management of patients in their homes.

Home Medical Equipment

The HME industry provides medical equipment and disposable supplies to treat patients at home. For example, medical equipment is used to facilitate patients' breathing, improve their mobility, and perform diagnostic testing. Such equipment often requires the use of disposable supplies by the patient. Home health providers also use surgical supplies for wound care dressings and diagnostic strips to check sugar levels in blood.

The following are examples of products and services that are provided by the HME industry.

Durable Medical Equipment

Durable medical equipment is reusable medical equipment that patients have an option to lease or purchase. Examples include wheelchairs, bathroom safety supplies, hospital beds, and ambulatory aids such as canes, crutches, and walkers. Providing durable medical equipment was one of the original home care services delivered by pharmacists.

One of the specialized categories of durable medical equipment is infusion pumps. Mary, in our case example, is to receive cefazolin every 8 hours. The drug must be administered at an equal interval of 8 hours, not three times per day. This type of administration may become problematic in the home and require a programmable pump. The pump is attached to the patient for the entire 24 hours and administers the dose at the programmed 8-hour interval. Thus, the patient does not have to be concerned about being awake for the dose at the time of administration. Infusion may be particularly important if the patient is to receive a drug at a frequency of every 4 or 6 hours. The pumps may also be used for pain management medication administration. The unique characteristic of this type of therapy is that the patient, in addition to receiving a baseline infusion, may also be allowed bolus dosing on a limited basis. The programmable pumps accommodate this type of administration quite well, by allowing for the bolus dosing and providing a limit on the total number of bolus doses a patient may self-administer within a prescribed time period. The programming feature also limits the frequency of self-administered bolus doses.

Respiratory Therapy and Supplies

Many patients suffering from chronic pulmonary conditions, who previously required hospitalization, may now receive respiratory therapy at home. Respiratory therapies include oxygen, aerosolized medications, continuous positive airway pressure, and ventilators. All of these therapies require special monitoring and patient education by a licensed respiratory therapist.

Oxygen therapy represents the largest portion of the respiratory market. Oxygen can be delivered to a patient via a concentrator, a machine that concentrates room oxygen to a higher level of purity; cylinders; compressed gas in tanks; or a liberator, a vessel that stores liquid oxygen. Providers evaluate the individual needs of the patient to determine the best method of delivery. Providing oxygen therapy is extremely profitable for HME providers.

Many patients are able to treat their respiratory conditions by administering medications via nebulization at home. In addition, some providers have developed specialty programs to treat conditions such as asthma. Once a patient is enrolled in such a program, the provider will deliver bronchodilators on a recurring basis and monitor patient compliance. The outcome of the patient's therapy is then reported to the patient's insurance carrier for review.

Miscellaneous Supplies

Miscellaneous products provided by HME dealers and pharmacies allow patients to care for themselves at home. Patients with diabetes (such as Mary) can monitor their blood glucose levels using portable monitors. A wide variety of appliances and skin care products are readily available to ostomy patients to care for their condition. The urinary incontinence market has expanded rapidly and provides home care patients, particularly the elderly, with many options. Wound care and surgical supplies are available to treat bedridden and postsurgical patients.

FACTORS THAT INFLUENCE THE HOME CARE INDUSTRY

Financial and regulatory issues present difficult challenges to the home care industry. One of the toughest challenges facing home care providers is the ability to provide patients with high-quality care given payers' reimbursement rates. The cost of caring for patients at home is increasing because home care providers are increasingly treating sicker patients with more complex therapies. Home care providers must also satisfy the requirements of statutory laws, regulations, and professional standards. These requirements improve patient care, but they also increase the cost of providing therapy.

Whereas the cost of providing therapy is on the rise, many insurance carriers are reducing reimbursement rates. To do more for less, home care providers will need to take advantage of advances in technology and changes in business practices to survive. The following sections explain some of the significant factors affecting the home care industry.

Reimbursement Issues

Insurance carriers or third-party payers exert a strong influence on the home care industry because they reimburse providers for home care products and services that are provided to patients. Many types of third-party payers exist, including government, managed care organizations (MCOs), and private insurance. Each payer determines its own levels of coverage, billing rules, and reimbursement rates. This inconsistency makes it difficult for home care providers to be reimbursed quickly and easily for the services they provide.

Government Insurance

The Centers for Medicare and Medicaid Services is the federal agency that oversees the Medicare and Medicaid programs in the United States. This agency was formerly called the Health Care Financing Administration. The Medicare program provides coverage to over 50 million people (Centers for Medicare and Medicaid Services, 2014), and Medicaid provides coverage to approximately 70 million (Kaiser Family Foundation, 2015a).

Medicare Medicare is a national health insurance program for patients with end-stage kidney disease, elderly patients, and selected patients with disabilities. It is divided into four components known as Parts A, B, C, and D. Part A refers to hospital insurance, and Part B provides medical (physician) insurance. Medicare Part A covers inpatient hospital services, skilled nursing facilities, home health services, and hospice care; Medicare Part B helps pay for the cost of physician services, outpatient hospital services, medical equipment, and supplies (Centers for Medicare and Medicaid Services, 2015b). Beneficiaries were given another option in 1997 under Medicare Part C, called Medicare Advantage (originally called Medicare + Choice). This program allows the patient to choose benefits through risk-based plans such as an HMO or other managed care plan or a private fee-for-service plan. Under Part C, beneficiaries must pay monthly Part B premiums in addition to those for the private insurance. In January 2006, Medicare Part D was implemented. This program expanded coverage to include prescription drugs.

Mary was eligible for Medicare once she reached the age of 65. She chose a Medicare Advantage HMO option.

Unfortunately, Medicare does not generally cover home infusion therapies. Only a small number of therapies that are administered using an electronic infusion device are covered, such as antiviral therapies, some chemotherapies, and dobutamine. For most other therapies, patients need to have alternative insurance coverage.

Medicaid Medicaid is a health insurance program for low-income and needy people. Unlike Medicare, which is entirely a federal program, Medicaid is actually administered by the states within federal guidelines. Medicaid is more comprehensive than Medicare, and it provides home care coverage as part of its required benefits. Many Medicaid programs also offer outpatient prescription drug coverage, although they are not required to do so. Even when prescription drugs are covered, however, infusion medications may not be. Managed Medicaid plans that provide for shared risk on the part of the Medicaid plan and the private insurer that contracts with the state to provide coverage for the patient have emerged. The private contracted insurer would offer a plan that is specifically designed to control costs by limiting the drug formulary and the services covered.

Managed Care Organizations

The goal of MCOs is to balance the delivery of high-quality health care with cost controls. MCOs control their expenditures by limiting coverage for healthcare products and services based on the needs of their patients. An HMO (like the one that covers Mary) is an example of an MCO. HMOs contract with multiple healthcare providers to meet the needs of individual groups. Employers and patients pay an HMO a set fee to manage their healthcare needs.

As large numbers of patients joined MCOs, these payers were able to negotiate sharp reductions in reimbursement rates from home care providers. Managed care principles decreased the costs of health care, but made many providers unprofitable. In response, a number of providers closed or merged with other providers. Home care providers now try to negotiate prices with MCOs. If the reimbursement levels are not favorable, providers may choose not to work with the organization. Managed care contracts can be successful only if they are beneficial to both provider and payer.

The process that a home infusion provider must go through in order to get paid for services, as provided to Mary in our case, generates risk for the provider. During the intake process, the provider may be required to obtain prior authorization for services. Once this is obtained, the provider must realize that it is not a guarantee of payment. The payer may decide that the therapy is not medically indicated or that the use of the drug is off label (a non-FDA approved indication). When this occurs, the provider is not paid, even though it may have a confirmed prior authorization.

Private Sector

Many private third-party payers exist, and some large corporations may be self-insured. These payers reimburse for many home care services in an effort to reduce their costs. The rationale for this coverage is simple: by eliminating the cost of a hospitalization, the care is less expensive. As with many other payers, the private sector may use managed care principles to contain the rising costs of health care.

Legal, Regulatory, and Professional Standards

The Balanced Budget Act of 1997

The Balanced Budget Act of 1997 introduced legislation that significantly affected the home care industry. Congress passed this act to control healthcare spending and reduce fraud within the Medicare system. The act required the institution of a prospective payment system for home health services, reductions in reimbursement rates for HME, and implementation of competitive bidding processes. Under a prospective payer system, the home health agency is paid a flat rate to care for a Medicare recipient. This rate reimburses the home health agency for all labor and medical supplies needed to care for the patient during a 60-day episode. Even though it has been in effect for some time, the overall impact of this legislation on the home care industry remains unclear, but it is expected that there will be changes in how home care providers conduct business so that they can remain profitable.

The Health Insurance Portability and Accountability Act of 1996

The Health Insurance Portability and Accountability Act (HIPAA) was enacted as a direct result of consumer demand. HIPAA is best known for its mandating confidentiality of protected health information, which affects how pharmacies and other providers handle a patient's healthcare information. However, HIPAA regulations are complex, and two other provisions of this act affect the home care industry, including (1) insurance reform and (2) administrative simplification.

The insurance reform provision of HIPAA improves insurance coverage when an individual changes employment or health plans. Exclusion from a health plan for preexisting conditions is now subject to strict limitations, which should expand the number of patients who are eligible for home care services.

The administrative simplification provision of HIPAA requires standardization of electronic claims submission. Such standardization will improve operational efficiency and payment cycles for home care providers.

Regulatory Agencies

Many federal and state agencies regulate the home care industry. It is the responsibility of home care providers to understand the legal and regulatory processes that must be followed where they practice. Home health services may be monitored by the state's department of public health. Pharmacies are monitored by the Drug Enforcement Administration and the Food and Drug Administration (FDA). HME providers may be monitored by the Department of Transportation. Providers may also be accountable to their state board of professional registration. These boards may license the facility as well as the pharmacists, nurses, respiratory therapists, and other healthcare professionals who work there.

Accrediting Organizations

Accrediting organizations are not federal or state agencies, but rather independent organizations that develop standards of practice for home care providers. Standards address issues such as clinical care, business management, and staff competency. By winning a seal of approval from these organizations, home care providers prove the quality of care that they provide to insurance carriers and patients. Providers are required to achieve accreditation by most third-party payers to be eligible for reimbursement.

The Joint Commission is perhaps the best-recognized accrediting agency. Other home care accrediting agencies include the Accreditation Commission for Health Care and the Community Health and Preventative Services Organization.

Advances in Technology

The delivery of many parenteral medications to patients in their homes has been greatly improved by advances in technology. Infusion pumps are a good example of advanced technology that has improved the care delivered by the home care industry. Once heavy and bulky, infusion pumps have evolved to be ambulatory, lightweight, and inconspicuous. The latest ambulatory models have the ability to infuse multiple therapies. Taken collectively, these advances provide both clinical advantages and cost savings.

Advances in Internet and wireless communications have enabled home care providers to readily share patient data with other healthcare professionals. Using point-of-care devices, palm-sized computers, and voice recognition software, pharmacists, nurses, physicians, and other healthcare professionals can transfer patient data quickly and securely. For more than a decade, telemedicine (i.e., transmission of medical data from a remote site to a central location) has been employed to help monitor patients with chronic conditions such as congestive heart failure, diabetes, and chronic obstructive lung disease as well as patients with acute infections (Eron, King, Marineau, & Yonehara, 2004). Home care providers can also communicate with insurance carriers to approve benefits and submit claims. The latest drug and healthcare information is also available online. Important sites include those operated by the Centers for Medicare and Medicaid Services (www.cms.hhs.gov) and the Food and Drug Administration (www.fda.gov). Easy access to information and increased communication can reduce costs and improve patient care. In addition, there are numerous subscription services that provide both drug and disease information.

Information technology systems have developed more slowly in the home infusion industry due to the small size of the industry. The market that software vendors are selling to is limited, and thus it limits the total profits available to invest in the further evolution of the software. As a result, the rate of sophistication development of the software is behind the overall medical software industry.

THE ROLE OF THE HOME CARE PHARMACIST

Pharmacists working in home care may do so through a community pharmacy, home care company, or hospital outpatient setting. In all home care organizations, the pharmacist must act as a vital member of a healthcare team that cares for the patient. This team may include nurses, physicians, caregivers, and the patient. The team members work together to develop a plan of care that will achieve the desired outcome for the patient's therapy.

Pharmacists are relied on for their pharmaceutical expertise, but they must also be competent in other areas to fulfill their role as a member of a healthcare team. A pharmacist may be responsible for the following roles when providing home care services.

Selection of Home Care Patients: Criteria Evaluation

Although Mary was discharged home to finish her course of IV antibiotic therapy, not all patients are appropriate candidates for home care. The decision to treat a patient at home is generally made jointly by nursing and pharmacy staff, in conjunction with the patient's physician. Patients must be clinically stable, have adequate support systems (e.g., telephone, family), and must be willing to accept responsibility for their own care. Given the current financial climate, patients must also have the ability to pay for home care either independently or through a third party.

Insurance

With the exception of IV medications, the major public-sector insurance programs (Medicare and Medicaid) provide good coverage for general home care services. The advent of Medicare Part D coverage in 2008 provided partial or full coverage of home care medications. Likewise, most private third-party payers provide reasonable coverage for home care. As discussed previously, the incentive to cover home care services is linked to the notion that it is less expensive than hospitalization.

Nevertheless, the patient's ability to pay is a component of the assessment process conducted before his or her discharge. Patients who meet medical and social criteria for home care may not qualify financially. Unlike many nonprofit hospitals, for-profit home care companies are not required to provide free care. Some home care companies accept a percentage of no-pay patients if they believe that this action will generate additional business with a specific physician, group practice, or hospital. It is the responsibility of the patient care coordinator or reimbursement specialist to verify a patient's insurance coverage before a patient such as Mary is considered eligible for home care.

Social Factors

Social factors play a crucial role in the decision to treat a patient at home. Patients should have family members who are willing and able to support or administer care, because 24-hour nursing care is not cost effective. Generally, patients and family members are taught to administer therapy without the assistance of a nurse or another healthcare professional. Further, patients must be positive about receiving their therapy at home for it to be successful. Some patients are reluctant to be discharged from a hospital for fear that they will lose the support a hospital offers (Bennett & Allen, 1990). Fortunately, the support that Mary's daughter provides and Mary's own willingness to be discharged will help with her transition to home care.

Other social factors are also important. For example, the physical condition of the home, its cleanliness, and the availability of refrigeration, running water, and electricity must be considered before providing complex therapies at home. Less invasive treatments such as rehabilitation services are possible without the presence of these conditions.

Another potential hazard is the presence in the home of a family member or others who may be abusing illicit substances. Home infusion therapy patients are supplied with needles and syringes to administer their treatment. Some may receive narcotic analgesics. A careful evaluation and monitoring of the home environment for substance abuse is therefore important.

Development of a Patient Plan of Care

Once a patient is discharged to the home, clear objectives must be developed as part of the patient's plan of care. These objectives include the selection of therapy, nature and frequency of monitoring parameters, including laboratory results, and desired therapeutic outcomes. The development of a care plan that outlines the individual care for a given patient will help reduce the possibility of a drug-related misadventure, including the situation in which the patient does not respond to therapy. Specific patient problems should be identified and associated with goals. Detailed interventions should then be designed to ensure the resolution of the problems. The patient care plan should include all of the patient's medical problems, not just the one requiring immediate attention. For example, in addition to her osteomyelitis, Mary's care plan should address her hypertension, diabetes, arthritis, drug allergy, and current medications. Home care accrediting bodies require the development of such a care plan.

Selection of Therapy

The choice of drug therapy is even more critical in the home than in an institutional setting. The usual safeguards (24-hour nursing and physician availability and emergency equipment) that are standard procedure in institutions may be absent in the home. As a result, several safety and convenience factors should be considered when selecting a therapy for the home care patient.

For example, because of the potential risks of allergy associated with some medications (such as antibiotics), the first dose should be administered in a controlled setting such as a hospital or clinic. If the first dose is administered at home, it should be done under medical supervision with careful screening of associated allergy history and with the presence of anaphylaxis medications. Other considerations include frequency and ease of administration. Drugs that can be administered once daily are more suitable for home care. In Mary's case, the pharmacist might recommend an alternative antibiotic that could be dosed less frequently than every 8 hours. Medications that are less likely to cause phlebitis (inflammation of the vein) and that do not require administration of large volumes of fluid are also more appropriate for home delivery.

Compounding Issues

A number of pharmaceutical compounding issues are unique to home care. These include drug/solution stability, packaging, infusion devices, and delivery schedules.

Drug/Solution Stability

In the past, most manufacturer-generated stability data were predicated on patients receiving medications in a hospital setting. As a result, expiration dating has traditionally been limited to 24 hours after product preparation. To deliver medications in a cost-effective manner at home, pharmacists need to extend stability data often for more than a week, depending on the product. Manufacturers realize that if they can demonstrate that their product is stable for more than 24 hours, it is feasible to use in the home setting; thus longer range stability data are now available.

It is important to distinguish between sterility and stability. Unless strict aseptic technique is adhered to, microbial contamination may potentially compromise the integrity of the product—regardless of its chemical stability. Consequently, all home infusion providers should have specially designed, environmentally controlled areas (such as clean rooms and laminar flow hoods) for preparation of sterile products. Home infusion companies and any organization that compounds sterile products must now be in compliance with new standards described in USP Chapter <797>. These standards define how sterile products should be prepared based on three risk levels: low, medium, and high. Risk level is determined by factors such as how many manipulations are involved in preparing the product and whether the final product is prepared from sterile or nonsterile ingredients (United States Pharmacopeial Convention, 2004).

Packaging

In institutional settings, both glass and plastic IV containers are used. However, because of the risk of breakage and potential for patient injury, plastic is generally used at home. Some products may be available or stable only in glass. In such instances, glass containers are used but with appropriate cautions to patients and caregivers.

Infusion Devices

Two major changes have occurred in IV infusion devices as a result of the growth of home care. First, the size and weight of infusion devices have decreased dramatically. These changes have allowed some patients to receive their medication while going to work or school. The devices are simply placed in a pouch, which may be concealed under the patient's clothing. Second, manufacturers have introduced disposable infusion devices, which are designed to deliver one or more doses of medication and be discarded after use. Pharmacists must be able to choose the appropriate device based on the drug therapy and the patient's needs. The selection and use of the device should be incorporated into the patient's plan of care.

Delivery Schedules

Frequency of drug administration is an important consideration when selecting parenteral medications to be used in the home. Drugs that may be administered once or twice per day are more suitable than those that must be administered four to six times per day. Pharmacists should advise prescribers who are discharging patients to the home about alternative medications that may be more suitable for home use.

Monitoring Drug Therapy

Because home care patients lack the support systems available to hospital patients, monitoring drug therapy for efficacy and for adverse drug events is critical to successful patient management. The pharmacist plays an important role in establishing and coordinating monitoring parameters such as serum drug levels and blood chemistries. The pharmacist needs to ensure that the proper tests are ordered from the time the patient is accepted for care at home until the time the therapy is completed. The pharmacist also communicates the results of these tests to the prescriber and recommends changes as appropriate.

Communication With Physicians, Nurses, Patients, and Others

Good communication among members of the healthcare team is essential for the successful care of home patients. Because the home lacks institutional safeguards, poor communication can quickly result in an adverse event for the patient. Adverse events may result in rehospitalization, which negates any benefits afforded by an early discharge.

The pharmacist has an even greater opportunity to affect patient care in the home than in an institutional setting. This impact, however, is predicated on the pharmacist's ability to communicate effectively with all members of the patient's healthcare team. For example, a pharmacist might receive laboratory data regarding Mary that may require a dosage adjustment in her antibiotic. The pharmacist must first communicate with the prescriber to effect a dosage change and then ensure that Mary's nurse is aware of the modification in therapy and the reasons for it.

Drug Information

Home care pharmacists must have adequate information resources to support the care of the patient. As a result, access to a drug information center—or, at the very least, to drug information services—is vital. The pharmacist must have the information necessary to determine whether a medication typically administered in an institutional setting can be safely delivered at home. Pharmacists should have ready access to stability and compatibility information, administration modalities, and potential complications.

American Society of Health-System Pharmacists Guidelines on Home Infusion Pharmacy Services

The American Society of Health-System Pharmacists is a professional organization that has established standards for a number of activities pertaining to pharmacy practice, including home infusion therapy (American Society of Health-System Pharmacists, 2014). These guidelines establish the role of the pharmacist and outline a minimum level of pharmacy services within the home environment and cover a number of areas including the following:

- Practice management (e.g., mission and goals, accreditation)
- Human resources (e.g., staffing, training)
- Financial management (e.g., budget, contracts, reimbursement)
- Medication use and drug information services (e.g., medication use policy development, selection of medication)
- Drug procurement and management (e.g., inventory, recalls, shortages, stability, and compatibility issues)
- Patient care (e.g., assessment, medication reconciliation, care plan, and patient education)
- Performance improvement activities (e.g., benchmarking medication error, and adverse drug reaction reporting)
- Operations (e.g., hours of operation, emergency preparedness)
- Facilities (e.g., space, storage area, and compounding area)

Education/Training

Many pharmacists who practice in home care do not have additional training beyond their entry-level degree (BS or PharmD). Curricula in U.S. colleges of pharmacy typically provide either required or elective coursework in sterile product preparation or parapharmaceuticals such as ostomy supplies and durable medical equipment, which may help better prepare practitioners for a career in home care. Some colleges of pharmacy may offer a course or component of a course that addresses home care, issues of reimbursement, and business management. It is anticipated that as home care pharmacy practice grows, pharmacy programs will incorporate more home care–related courses into their curricula.

Practice Experiences

A number of colleges of pharmacy, in conjunction with home care companies, are offering experiential training in the form of introductory and advanced practice experiences in home care. Introductory practice experiences provide students with opportunities to gain initial exposure to home care as a career option early in the professional pharmacy curriculum. Advanced practice experiences are more extended, with a focus on patient care, and occur during the final year of the curriculum.

Residency Programs

At this time, only a very limited number of postgraduate, practice-based training programs—that is, residencies—exist in home care. These programs are available to pharmacists who wish to gain additional skills in home care practice. Expansion of such programs may remain somewhat restricted given the proprietary nature of home care businesses. In particular, concerns exist about training pharmacists who will eventually work for the competition.

CONCLUSION

Home care encompasses the provision of many healthcare products and services to patients. To care for themselves, home care patients like Mary rely on home health agencies, home infusion providers, and HME dealers to provide products, service, and training.

The provision of home care is influenced by a number of factors such as reimbursement issues, regulatory requirements, and advances in technology. To ensure proper care, each provider must account for these factors when developing a patient's plan of care.

Pharmacists must maintain their competency to fulfill their roles as home care providers. As advances in technology result in new therapies and methods of delivery, the importance of the pharmacist's role in home care will continue to grow.

QUESTIONS FOR FURTHER DISCUSSION

1. Will the expansion of managed care affect the growth and development of home care? How?
2. What opportunities are available for other players (e.g., hospitals) in the healthcare delivery system in home care?
3. How do you believe the role of the home care pharmacist will change in the future?

KEY TOPICS AND TERMS

Accrediting agency
Balanced Budget Act
Health Insurance Portability and Accountability Act (HIPAA)
Home care
Home care standards for pharmacists
Home health services
Home infusion therapy
Managed care
Medicaid
Medicare
Regulatory agency
Technology

REFERENCES

American Society of Health-System Pharmacists. (2014). ASHP guidelines on home infusion pharmacy services. *American Journal of Health-System Pharmacy, 71,* 325–341.

Bennett, M. A., & Allen, R. D. (1990). High-technology home pharmacotherapy. I: An overview of anti-infective and antineoplastic therapies. *Journal of Pharmacy Practices, 3*(1), 34–39.

Centers for Medicare and Medicaid Services. (2014). *National health care expenditures 2013 highlights.* Retrieved from https://www.cms.gov/Research-Statistics-Data-and-Systems/Statistics-Trends-and-Reports/NationalHealthExpendData/downloads/highlights.pdf

Centers for Medicare and Medicaid Services. (2015a). Medicare enrollment reports. Retrieved from https://www.cms.gov/Research-Statistics-Data-and-Systems/Statistics-Trends-and-Reports/CMSProgramStatistics/Dashboard.html

Centers for Medicare and Medicaid Services. (2015b). What Medicare covers. Retrieved from http://www.medicare.gov/what-medicare-covers/index.html

Council on Scientific Affairs, American Medical Association. (1990). Home care in the 1990s. *Journal of the American Medical Association, 263*(9), 1241–1244.

Eron, L., King, P., Marineau, M., & Yonehara, C. (2004). Treating acute infections by telemedicine in the home. *Clinical Infectious Diseases, 39*, 1175–1181.

Gill, G. M. (1991). Social work intervention with stroke patients and their families. *Journal of Home Health Care Practice, 4*(1), 57–62.

Howard, L., Alger, S., Michalek, A., Heaphey, L., Aftahi, S., & Johnston, K. R. (1993). Home parenteral nutrition in adults. In J. L. Rombeau & M. D. Caldwell (Eds.), *Clinical nutrition: Parenteral nutrition* (2nd ed., pp. 814–839). Philadelphia, PA: W. B. Saunders.

Kaiser Family Foundation. (2015). Medicaid moving forward. Retrieved from http://kff.org/health-reform/issue-brief/medicaid-moving-forward/

Landers, S.H. (2010). Why health care is going home. *New England Journal of Medicine, 363*, 1690-1691.

Levine, S. A., Boal, J. B., & Boling, P. A. (2003). Home care. *Journal of the American Medical Association, 290*(9), 1203–1207.

National Association of Home Care & Hospice. (2010). Basic statistics about home care. Retrieved from http://www.nahc.org/assets/1/7/10hc_stats.pdf

National Home Infusion Association. (2015). Infusion FAQs. Retrieved from http://w.nhia.org/faqs.cfm

National Hospice and Palliative Care Organization (2015). Who receives hospice care? Retrieved from http://www.nhpco.org/sites/default/files/public/Statistics_Research/2015_Facts_Figures.pdf

United States Pharmacopeial Convention. (2004). Pharmaceutical considerations—sterile preparations (general information chapter 797). In *The United States Pharmacopeia/National Formulary* (22nd ed., 26th rev., pp. 2350–2370). Rockville, MD: U.S. Pharmacopeial Convention, Inc.

U.S. Department of Labor, Bureau of Labor Statistics. (2014). Home health aides. Retrieved from http://www.bls.gov/ooh/healthcare/home-health-aides.htm

CHAPTER

13

Government Involvement in Health Care

William G. Lang IV

Case Scenario

Biomedical innovation is a hallmark of American academic, business, and government research and development activities. The public is deeply committed to research and development that provides life-saving drugs and medical devices to individuals suffering life-threatening illness. The federal government, while supporting and engaging in biomedical research itself, also has a role in the oversight of research. Through its regulatory structures, the Food and Drug Administration (FDA) is the key federal agency with significant control of biomedical research, particularly in regard to the safety and efficacy of drugs and medical devices. During the summer of 2015, the House of Representatives passed the 21st Century Cures Act (Congress.gov, 2015a). This legislation was immediately hailed by organizations representing a wide range of individuals suffering from chronic and life-threatening illness, some of which impact a small percentage of Americans, as essential to speeding up the development of cures from the laboratory to the medicine cabinet.

The intent of this chapter is to provide the reader with an understanding of how our federal government operates, how that operation is open to influence and manipulation through three interlinked components that comprise our government, and how health care is both compliant and resistant to control through the actions of these components: citizens, Congress and the Administration.

LEARNING OBJECTIVES

Upon completion of this chapter, the student shall be able to:

- Describe how the federal government is involved in health care.
- Identify the congressional committees that have health care as a part of their jurisdiction.
- Evaluate the activities of federal agencies for their alignment with Presidential priorities.
- Describe how state action provided context for the creation of the Patient Protection and Affordable Care Act.
- Analyze public policy issues, especially health care, for the influence of any or all components of the "Iron Triangle."

CHAPTER QUESTIONS

1. Given the extent of government involvement in health care, what is the government's interest in this involvement?
2. Given the extent of government involvement in health care, how well is this involvement improving the health of our nation?
3. How would a special interest group of your choosing describe the impact of the federal government on improving health care?
4. What are the major goals of the Patient Protection and Affordable Care Act? How are federal agencies working to meet these goals?
5. The three sides of the Iron Triangle are themselves each comprised of a number of stakeholders. For any one side, who makes up the group of stakeholders? Are all these stakeholders in agreement on all issues? If not, how are differences presented in the media?

INTRODUCTION

Philosophers of the 17th and 18th centuries and their ideas and concepts about free-will and the innate goodness of humankind laid the foundation for the representative democracy here in the United States (Herman, 2002). These concepts were ground-breaking in a world dominated by monarchies, where individuals were subjects of and responsible to an individual or family whose authority was said to be a divine right. That humans are born good and not in need of intercessory assistance to become good was contrary to the existing religious philosophy of the period. This enlightened thought allowed individuals the opportunity to imagine a life free of monarchical, divine, or religious control. Due in large to the ethnic and cultural backgrounds of our nation's founding fathers, our Declaration of Independence reflects the concepts of philosophers such as Locke, Rousseau, Hutcheson and Hume, and others linked to the Western Enlightenment. Importantly, the Declaration of Independence uses these philosophies to establish the role of the individual as an essential element in the development and success of a government not lead by a monarchy and separate from religious influence (Declaration of Independence, n.d.). Inherent in the philosophical underpinnings of our Declaration is the responsibility of one individual to another. The actual meaning of the words used to describe an individual's natural or unalienable rights may be open for debate, yet "life, liberty and the pursuit of happiness," place a significant responsibility on the individual. This responsibility or benevolence is what actually makes us happy and that life and liberty are further enjoyed when we care for others.

The pursuit of happiness and its inference of caring for others supports and strengthens the role of the individual citizen as the foundation of the federal government in the United States. The first three words of the opening sentence of the United States Constitution, "We the people...," establishes this foundation (United States Constitution, n.d.). Our form of government, a representative democracy, requires the engagement of individuals who will seek elected office, elect individuals to office, and to serve within the federal administration not out of self-interest, but for the benefit of the whole. The rights that our government is required to recognize and be responsive to are listed in the amendments to the Constitution. Many of these rights are a direct response to the grievances listed in the Declaration of Independence. The importance of the individual citizen and that citizen's right to pursue not just their individual happiness, but that which ensures the happiness of the whole, creates many of the public policy approaches that our nation has and will continue to grapple with. This chapter attempts to build upon this concept as a way to understand and analyze the role of government in health care.

Along with listing our several rights as citizens, our Constitution also lays out the structure of our government. Within this structure are the three branches of federal government: legislative,

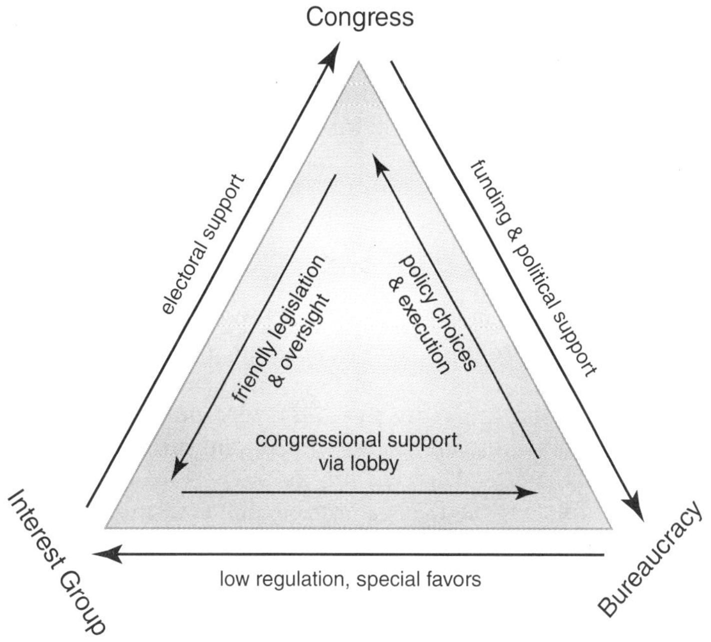

Figure 13-1 The Iron Triangle

https://commons.wikimedia.org/wiki/File:Irontriangle.PNG.

executive, and the judicial. By understanding the structure of our government a citizen advocate can gain a better appreciation of how and when to engage with the other two corners of the iron triangle, see **Figure 13-1**. The philosophical rationale for citizen advocacy has been offered above. The next portion of this chapter will provide the reader with an overview of both of the other two corners of the iron triangle, their role in healthcare policy and the opportunities for an advocate to engage with either corner.

The Legislative branch

The legislative branch consists of the House of Representatives and the Senate. The membership of the House of Representatives is based on the proportional representation of a state's total population. The membership of the Senate is comprised of two individuals from each state. Members of both the House and Senate are supported by a personal staff. The number of individuals that make up any members personal staff is decision of the individual member. Most offices include at least a Chief of Staff, a Legislative Director, Communications and Administrative staff (United States House of Representatives [U.S. House], n.d.a), (United States Senate [U.S. Senate], n.d.a).

COMMITTEES

Both House and Senate members are appointed by their respective leadership to the several committees responsible for the formulation and discussion of legislation. Each committee has a specific, although sometimes expansive, jurisdiction. Committees in the House and Senate are responsible for one of three primary functions: (1) the authorization of federal programs, (2) the funding of those authorized programs, and (3) the creation of new laws to be implemented by the executive branch. Members of committees are supported in their activities by personal staff with responsibility for the issues under the jurisdiction of the committee and by professional staff that are subject matter experts on issues relevant to the work of the committee.

The appropriations committees of the House and Senate are responsible for establishing the funding level of federal agencies and programs. Total funding for the federal government is established through a budget resolution. This nonbinding piece of legislation is not signed by the President. It establishes a target for funding allocations of federal programs within the jurisdiction of the subcommittees that comprise the full appropriations committee. When the Congress is unable to agree on the parameters of a budget resolution appropriators are allowed to establish the total funding allocations, usually in collaboration with their respective chamber leadership. Authorizing committees are traditionally responsible for the creation of legislation that authorizes a new agency or program or reauthorizes an existing agency or program. The authorizing committee is also responsible for the congressional oversight of the agency or program within their jurisdiction and this oversight responsibility frequently leads to the creation of legislation that impacts how an agency or program fulfills its mission. Any member of Congress is able to introduce legislation. Based on the purpose of the introduced legislation the respective leadership of the House or Senate determines the committee that has jurisdiction over the intended purpose of the proposed legislation.

Healthcare-Related Committees

The committees of the House of Representatives and the Senate include those whose jurisdiction includes a wide range of healthcare-related issues. Health care is a broad issue area, which is influenced by a number of other issue areas including insurance, healthcare professionals, education of those professionals, direct delivery of care, creation of programs to support healthcare improvements, and the discovery, translation, and implementation of new knowledge. The list of committees below includes those that have healthcare issues as a primary aspect of their jurisdiction. The rules of the House and Senate include complete information on committee jurisdictions (United States Senate, 2013), (United States House of Representatives, 2015). There are other committees that have a tangential relationship to issues included in anyone's definition of health care. Both House and Senate websites include a list of all their respective committees (U.S. Senate, n.d.b), (U.S. House, n.d.b).

House and Senate Judiciary Committees

Legal issues, such as tort claims arising from medical malpractice and product liability, interstate commerce, protections of intellectual property resulting from biomedical research and other issues arising from delivery and payment of health care are part of the jurisdiction of the House of Representatives Judiciary Committee and the Senate Committee on the Judiciary. Both these committees have oversight for the U.S. Department of Justice (House Judiciary Committee, n.d.), (Senate Committee on the Judiciary, n.d.).

House Ways and Means and Senate Finance Committees

The Medicare program provides insurance coverage to older adults who are 65 years or older and individuals with disabilities. This insurance program is funded through a legislatively authorized trust fund within the Social Security Act. The Medicare Trust Fund is funded through a payroll tax. Any federal revenue mechanism, including taxes, falls under the jurisdiction of the House Committee on Ways and Means and the Senate Committee on Finance (House Committee on Ways and Means, n.d.), (Senate Committee on Finance, n.d.). Any legislation related to the Medicare program, including the payment of services to providers, will fall under the jurisdiction of the Ways and Means and Finance Committees. The Medicaid program and maternal and child health programs, amendments to the Social Security Act, also fall under the jurisdiction of the Senate Finance committee.

House Committee on Energy and Commerce

The Medicare program is funded through a trust fund supported by a payroll tax as well as payments for the cost of insurance coverage for services provided by physicians and a number of other healthcare professionals. Payment of services to Medicare beneficiaries from authorized providers (Medicare Part B) is part of the jurisdiction of the House of Representatives Committee on Energy and Commerce. The Medicaid program, unlike Part A of Medicare, is not paid for through a payroll tax, and therefore it is under the jurisdiction of the Energy and Commerce Committee. The Energy and Commerce Committee also has jurisdiction over the federal agencies that are responsible for most of the federal healthcare responsibilities. These agencies include the Agency for Healthcare Research and Quality (AHRQ), Food and Drug Administration (FDA), Health Resources and Services Administration (HRSA), Indian Health Service (IHS), and National Institutes of Health (NIH) and the Substance Abuse and Mental Health Services Agency (SAMHSA) which are all part of the cabinet-level Department of Health and Human Services (HHS).

Senate Committee on Health, Education, Labor, and Pensions (HELP)

The jurisdiction of the Senate Committee on Health, Education, Labor, and Pensions is very broad and includes many of the issue areas and agencies we recognize as healthcare related (Senate Committee on Health, Education, Labor and Pensions, n.d.). These areas and the agencies that administer them are very similar to the House Energy and Commerce Committee and include the AHRQ, FDA, HRSA, IHS, SAMHSA, which are all part of the cabinet-level Department of Health and Human Services.

Senate Committee on Armed Services and the House Armed Services Committee

The United States Departments of the Army, Navy, and Air Force are part of the jurisdiction of the Senate and House Committees on Armed Services (Senate Committee on Armed Services, n.d.), (House Armed Services Committee, n.d.). These two committees are also responsible for the review and oversight of military research and development. Research undertaken by the military and their grantees provides substantial new knowledge for the pubic especially in the areas of trauma care and rehabilitation. Members of the armed services receive healthcare insurance through TRICARE (TRICARE, n.d.a).

Senate Committee on Veterans' Affairs and House Committee on Veterans' Affairs

The provision of healthcare services to U.S. veterans' is within the jurisdiction of the Senate and House Committees on Veterans' Affairs (Senate Committee on Veterans' Affairs, n.d.), (House Committee on Veterans' Affairs, n.d.). The oversight of these committees also includes the vocational rehabilitation, medical and prosthetic research that the Department of Veterans Affairs supports.

FEDERAL AGENCIES

Congress is responsible for the creation of legislation that authorizes the establishment of any federal agency, the continued existence of those agencies through reauthorization and the annual funding of those agencies. The President is responsible for the administration of the agencies authorized by Congress. The administration of federal agencies by nonelected individuals can be referred to as the bureaucracy (*Merriam-Webster,* 2015). The heads of some agencies are members of the President's cabinet (White House, n.d.). Not all federal agencies have a significant part of their mission related to health care. Below will be a list of agencies that do have a significant healthcare element to their mission. The Federal Register maintains a list of all federal agencies (Federal Register, n.d.).

The Executive Office of the President includes several offices that influence certain aspects of healthcare policy. The Office of Management and Budget (OMB) is the President's financial management organization (Office of Management and Budget, n.d.). Teams of budget analysts annually review, modify, and approve agency budgets in preparation of the President's budget proposal to Congress. Traditionally, the budget developed by the OMB staff includes an overview that highlights the policy priorities of the President (Office of Management and Budget, 2015). These priorities are further expressed in the budget overviews and funding levels of the agencies (United States Department of Health and Human Services, 2015a).

The Office of Science and Technology Policy (OSTP) advises the President on issues related to advancing science and technology policy and for advocating with stakeholders the priorities of the President related to science and technology (Office of Science and Technology, n.d.). The Office of National AIDS Policy (ONAP) is responsible for the development and revision of the National HIV/AIDS Strategy and its implementation across federal agencies and within the private healthcare sector (White House, 2015a). Consider a set of policy initiatives that demonstrate the both the involvement of the federal government and the role of the iron triangle related to AIDS research. In February of 2014, amfAR, the Foundation for AIDS Research, an advocacy organization, announced the "Countdown to a Cure for HIV/AIDS (amfAR, The Foundation for AIDS Research [amfAR], 2014a). The amfAR initiative proposes raising $100 million to support research that will lead to a cure by 2020. In July of that year, the ONAP released a fact sheet that outlined several areas in which National HIV/AIDS Strategy was impacting federal, state, and local actions related to HIV/AIDS care, identification, and legal issues (amfAR, 2014b). The fact sheet also includes information describing the development of a better-coordinated national response that included work with state and local governments and expanding HIV/AIDS research at the NIH. In July of 2015, the House Appropriations Committee reiterated its support for coordination across federal agencies yet recommended maintaining funding at FY2015 levels for federal agencies with HIV/AIDS—related programs (Congress.gov, 2015b). On August 12, 2015 the Director of the NIH released a statement that reflects the reinvigoration of research, the need for improved coordination among researchers, and the realities of stagnant funding (Collins, 2015).

FEDERAL AGENCIES WITH HEALTHCARE-RELATED MISSIONS

Department of Agriculture

When you think about the United States Department of Agriculture (USDA), government involvement in health care may not be your first thought. Like so many federal agencies, using a very broad definition of health increases the chances that an agency has some role within that broad definition. The World Health Organization defines health as "a state of complete physical, mental and social well-being and not merely the absence of disease or infirmity (World Health Organization, 1946)." Using this definition you gain an appreciation of the involvement of the Department of Agriculture, a federal agency, in health. The mission of the USDA does not include the word health, but many of the activities listed in the mission impact health. The USDA is responsible for inspections of agricultural products, producers and production systems (United States Department of Agriculture, n.d.). Originally established to improve and support the agricultural pursuits of residents of rural communities the Cooperative Extension program now shares the research of faculty at land-grant universities with both rural and urban populations. A large part of this research is focused on food safety, nutrition, healthy living among its "wide range of human, plant, and animal needs in both urban and rural areas." Research and the evidence base it establishes play a significant role in the USDA's development of dietary guidelines. In partnership with the U.S.

Department of Health and Human Services the USDA establishes recommended nutrition goals for the nation (HHS, 2015b).

As popular as many of the USDA programs such as the Cooperative Extension are, the programs of the USDA, like any federal agency, administers programs that set the Iron Triangle into action. Currently, USDA and HHS are developing the 2015 Dietary Guidelines. In February of 2015, The Dietary Guideline Advisory Group submitted its report to the Secretary of HHS and the Secretary of Agriculture. This group reviewed the nutrition research developed since the 2010 was published to make its evidence-based recommendations (Dietary Guideline Advisory Group, 2015).

The guidelines will be released later in 2015 after agency review of the workgroup report. Response to the report by special interest groups and members of Congress was swift and pointed. Special interest groups as varied as the meat industry and school nutrition programs have stated their opposition to the recommendations of the advisory group (Hering, 2015), (Aubrey, 2015). Members of Congress oppose the advisory group recommendations as well indicating a challenge for HHS and USDA to finalize the 2015 guidelines (Maynard, 2015).

Department of Health and Human Service

When considering total funding, both discretionary and mandatory, of federal agencies the U.S. Department of Health and Human Services (HHS) ranks as number one. HHS is also the federal agency with the greatest involvement in health care. Total funding of $1.048 trillion for HHS in FY15 included $71.8 billion in discretionary funds, and $862 billion in mandatory funds for the Medicare and Medicaid programs (HHS, 2014, 2015c). The mission of HHS is "… to enhance and protect the health and well-being of all Americans." There are nearly 80,000 individuals that are employed by HHS, working within 11 divisions. Eight of these divisions can be referred to as federal public health agencies (HHS, 2015c).

The policy priorities of the President related to health care are expressed in the funding levels each of HHS's 11 divisions proposed in the President's annual budget. Through the appropriations of funding levels agreed to by Congress, the President's priorities are supported or opposed. Legislation setting federal agency funding for any fiscal year usually includes a report. This report describes the mission or operation of the agency or agencies being funded and may further explain the rationale for the committee's recommended funding level. These reports frequently include text that may express support and opposition of an agencies activities and by extension the President's priorities (Congress.gov, 2015c).

FEDERAL PUBLIC HEALTH AGENCIES

Agency for Healthcare Research and Quality

The United States continues to lead the world in total healthcare-related expenditures. For all the money we spend we do poorly in population-based outcomes such as longevity and infant mortality compared to European countries (World Bank, 2013), (Organisation for Economic Co-operation and Development, 2015), (Centers for Disease Control and Prevention [CDC], 2014a). Late in the 20th century Congressional action expressed concern about the quality of health care in the United States. Given that congressional concern was included in a section of legislation dealing with Medicare Part B, quality as it impacts individual patients and the delivery of acute care services would trump population-based interventions to improve public health. The quality of medical services delivery would be researched through a newly authorized agency, the Agency for Healthcare Policy and Research (ACHPR) (Congress.gov, 2015d). The agency had a very rocky tenure, yet it was reauthorized in 1995 as the Agency for Healthcare Research and Quality (AHRQ) (Gray, Gusmano, & Collins, 2003), (Congress.gov, 2015e).

AHRQ states its mission as follows: "The Agency for Healthcare Research and Quality's (AHRQ) mission is to produce evidence to make health care safer, higher quality, more accessible, equitable, and affordable, and to work within the U.S. Department of Health and Human Services and with other partners to make sure that the evidence is understood and used (AHRQ, 2015)." This mission allows AHRQ to support research focused on improving the quality of healthcare delivery. AHRQ also collects data through which healthcare providers, health systems and payers are able to improve care quality. This data collection includes the Healthcare Utilization Project (HCUP) and the Medical Expenditures Panel Survey (MEPS). The U.S. Preventive Services Task Force (USPSTF) is also housed at AHRQ and develops recommendations regarding preventive medicine through an evidence-based process. The preventive services recommended by the USPSTF are frequently used in the primary care setting (United States Preventive Services Task Force, 2013).

Even with its evidence-based mission, AHRQ continues to lack support in Congress as exemplified by its FY2016 budget being recommended for elimination by the House Appropriations Committee (Congress.gov, 2015f). Active engagement by health services researchers and organizations that employ these researchers or benefit from their research successfully kept similar action from being taken by the Senate Appropriations Committee, although the recommended funding level was 35% less than FY16 (Friends of AHRQ, 2015a), (Friends of AHRQ, 2015b), (Congress.gov, 2015g).

Administration for Community Living

The Administration for Community Living (ACL), administers a number of programs that are important to the health of the individuals they serve, but in large it is a social services agency (Administration for Community Living, 2015). The Administration on Aging (AoA) is a division of the ACL (Administration on Aging, 2014). The AoA administers programs authorized under the Older Americans Act (Congress.gov, 2015h). Some of the programs important to the health of older adults are supported through the AoA and their state and local partners. These partners include Area Agencies on Aging (AAA) which provide support for older adults and their caregivers. Nutrition services, commonly referred to as Meals on Wheels, are some of the readily identified home and community-based services offered through AAAs in their partnership with the AoA.

Centers for Disease Control and Prevention

The Centers for Disease Control and Prevention (CDC) is the largest division of HHS and is focused on population health. The mission of the CDC includes the statement "...provides health information that protects our nation against expensive and dangerous health threats, and responds when these arise (CDC, 2014b)." The provision of health information is a significant activity of the CDC. Local, state, and national health data are collected, analyzed, and shared with the public as part of the CDC's National Center for Health Statistics (NCHS) extensive survey activities (National Center for Health Statistics, 2015). The status of our nation's health is presented in the publication Morbidity and Mortality Weekly Report (Morbidity and Mortality Weekly Report, 2015).

Responding to public health emergencies is the high-profile role of the CDC, yet preventive health plays a significant role in the day-to-day activities of CDC. This preventive health role is evident in the many programs administered by CDC. Immunization schedules across the life cycle are established through the CDC's Advisory Committee on Immunization Practices (ACIP) (Advisory Committee on Immunization Practices, 2015). Evidence-based health promotion and disease prevention programs, such as the National Diabetes Prevention Program, are developed and disseminated by the CDC's National Center for Chronic Disease Prevention and Health Promotion (NCCDPHP)

(National Center for Chronic Disease Prevention and Health Promotion, 2015), (National Diabetes Prevention Program, 2015). The Guide to Preventive Services, commonly referred to as the Community Guide, is a resource to individuals searching for programs and policies that can help them improve the health of their community (Community Guide, 2015). The programs and policies available through the Community Guide are reviewed and approved by the Community Services Task Force (Community Services Task Force, 2015).

Centers for Medicare and Medicaid Services

Government involvement in health care is most often associated with the Medicare, Medicaid, and Children's Health Insurance Program (CHIP) administered by the Centers for Medicare and Medicaid Services (CMS) (Centers for Medicare and Medicaid Services [CMS], n.d.a). There were nearly 51 million individuals enrolled in either Part A or Part B of Medicare in 2012 (CMS, n.d.b). CMS reported 51 million individuals were enrolled in the Medicaid program as of January 2015 (CMS, 2015a). Nearly 72 million individuals were enrolled in Medicaid and CHIP as of May 2015 (CMS, 2015b).

The Medicare and Medicaid programs were established in 1965 through legislation amending the Social Security Act. Medicare provides insurance coverage to eligible beneficiaries for hospital care (Part A) and service delivery by physicians and other authorized providers (Part B). This same legislation created the Medicaid program (Congress.gov, 2015i). In 2003, Congress passed the Medicare Prescription Drug Improvement and Modernization Act. This legislation provides beneficiaries the opportunity to have their care insured through private managed care plans (Part C) and a prescription drug plan offered through private managed care plans or private prescription drug plans (Part D) (Congress.gov, 2015j). The Balanced Budget Act of 1997 authorized the creation of the State Children's Health Insurance Program (Congress.gov, 2015k). Both Medicaid and CHIP are partnerships between the federal and state governments.

The passage of the Patient Protection and Affordable Care Act (ACA) brought several new responsibilities to CMS to help move our current volume-based, provider-centered approach to one that is team-based, patient-centered, and quality-focused. While most of the Medicare provisions in the ACA were related to administrative improvements focused on care quality, the creation of the Center for Medicare and Medicaid Innovation (CMMI) would prove to be both lauded and controversial.

Food and Drug Administration

Controversial and yet lauded also applies to the FDA (Woodcock, 2012). Responsible for the ensuring the safety and effectiveness of drugs and medical devices and the purity of food products, the FDA has a mission that frequently exceeds the capacity of its financial and human resources (Institute of Medicine, 2006), (Woodcock, 2015). It is unlikely that you go through your day without coming in contact with, applying or ingesting something that is not under the regulation of the FDA. The breadth of the FDA mission, its successes and challenges and its impact on individual and public health are easily fodder for an entire book. Former Commissioner Margaret Hamburg, speaking at the National Press Club in March 2015 provided an excellent summary of the FDA. "... its not just the diversity of the products we oversee that some might find surprising—it is the way that we bring our enormous expertise to bear. In this age of skepticism about government, it is easy to imagine FDA regulators simply as bureaucrats focused on a narrow set of responsibilities. Yet nothing could be further from the truth. What a remarkable group of physicians, scientists, lawyers, policy analysts, and other professionals and support staff, committed to helping people get the products they need and count on (Hamburg, 2015)." Both patients and healthcare providers play a role in making sure the programs administered by the FDA are of maximum benefit to the U.S. public. One example is through the FDA's MedWatch program that allows for input about negative consequences of adverse drug events. Public monitoring of these events is an important tool for assuring the continued postmarket safety and effectiveness of FDA-approved drugs and medical devices (FDA, 2015a).

Health Resources and Services Administration

One of the federal government's oldest healthcare programs are those focused on maternal and child health which were authorized in the Social Security Act in 1935. This program is administered through the HRSA (United States Code [U.S. Code], 2015a). Several other highly-regarded programs are administered by HRSA. Most of these programs are authorized within the Public Health Service Act (PHSA) (U.S. Code, 2015b). HRSA's mission is "to improve health and achieve health equity through access to quality services, a skilled health workforce and innovative programs (Health Resources and Services Administration, n.d.)." The community health centers program, the Ryan White AIDS program, rural health programs and the National Health Service Corps are all programs administered by HRSA that enjoy broad support across Congress, the current administration and advocacy groups. Programs administered by HRSA that frequently face both congressional and administration challenges even in light of strong special interest support include the health professions education programs and the 340B drug discount program (American Association of Community Colleges, 2003), (Democratic Underground.com, 2005), (American Society of Health Systems Pharmacists, 2003).

Indian Health Service

Native American tribes recognized by the federal government are members of sovereign nations. The federal government's long and often contentious relationship with tribes is authorized by our Constitution. Since 1787, the Commerce Clause has provided the federal government the authority to enter into agreements that include the provision of healthcare services to tribes. Today this care provision is undertaken by the Indian Health Service (IHS) (Indian Health Service [IHS], n.d.).

National Institutes of Health

In 1930, legislation formally authorized the NIH with further legislative action in 1944 placing the NIH within the Public Health Service Act (National Institutes of Health [NIH], 2015a). Today the NIH is the nation's preeminent research institute with a broad mission supporting the development of new biomedical knowledge and the translation of that knowledge into improvements in health care (NIH, 2015b). Comprised of 27 Institutes and Centers, the NIH is the primary federal funder of extramural biomedical research with a FY15 budget of $30 billion. The NIH also maintains a significant intramural research portfolio administered by scientists in laboratories on the NIH campus. The Clinical Center offers world-class, cutting-edge care to patients for whom current community-based knowledge is insufficient for their medical needs.

The NIH is strongly supported by members of Congress and the public. Through the years this support has included doubling of the NIH budget through the congressional appropriations process (Congress.gov, 2015l). Even though this appropriations legislation in its final text does not include remarks related to doubling of the NIH budget, the Senate report accompanying its passed legislation included the following: "This amount maintains the goal of doubling funding for the NIH by fiscal year 2003 (Congress.gov, 2015m)" Public support for NIH continues to be strong as demonstrated by annual survey of the U.S. public by the advocacy organization Research!America. Since 1992, the public has indicated its strong support for federal clinical research (Research!America, 2015).

Substance Abuse and Mental Health Services Administration

The current epidemic of opioid pain-relief drug abuse is heightening public and policy-maker awareness and support for better integration of behavioral health services into our healthcare delivery system. The SAMHSA is poised to play its greatest role yet to meet this current challenge (Market Watch, 2015), (McGarvey, 2015). The need for improving access to behavioral health care created the support for the creation of SAMHSA in 1992 (Congress.gov, 2015n). Since that time a number of public laws have been enacted that facilitate access to behavioral services, yet even with these laws public use of these services and agreement with what these services should include remain elusive (Congress.gov, 2015o), (Wall Street Journal, 2014).

Veterans Administration

Support for federal agencies, including those mentioned in this chapter, can wax and wane overtime. The challenges of using federal funds to provide direct care are significant and are influenced by the public, the Congress and the Administration. Providing healthcare services to nearly 9 million veterans annually, the Veterans Health Administration (VHA) "is America's largest integrated health care system... (Veterans Health Administration, n.d.)." Support for our wounded soldiers has a long history in this country. According the Veterans Administration (VA) the Pilgrims passed a law requiring the colony to support the care of individuals wounded during fights with members of native tribes (Veterans Administration, 2015). The personal damage of war has only increased overtime. The research supported by the VA has led to significant benefits to veterans wounded in battle and the general public suffering acute trauma. Yet, the complexity of this care, the need for significant recovery and rehabilitation of Veterans, the growing need for the integration of behavioral health into this care system as well as an aging veteran population place huge pressure on the VA and the VHA.

The negative outcomes of that pressure were laid out in a report by the VA Office of the Inspector General in May of 2014 (Veterans Administration Office of the Inspector General Veterans, 2014). The report makes it clear that the VHA has had difficulty in the past meeting the needs of our most dedicated citizens. "Since 2005, the VA Office of Inspector General (OIG) has issued 18 reports that identified, at both the national and local levels, deficiencies in scheduling resulting in lengthy waiting times and the negative impact on patient care." Since the release of the report the OIG has published numerous reports about the management challenges at ... "America's largest healthcare system..." These challenges have created public outrage and grave concern among members of Congress. Yet, even in light of this outrage and concern, our nation's veterans are receiving services and health care within a system that is attempting to respond to the needs of its constituents in new and innovative ways (McDonald, 2015).

Through legislation passed in 2014, Congress authorized the VHA to increase access to needed care for veterans at locations other than VHA clinics and by non-VA providers (Congress.gov, 2015p). The implementation of the Veterans Access, Choice and Accountability Act of 2014 includes improvements in access that will take time to improve. The law authorizes the annual assessment of staffing shortages and the creation of additional medical residency positions. Medical residency positions are to be increased in the VA by up to 1500 over 5 years after enactment of the Act.

Increasing staff to improve access will certainly take time. Yet, the VA is engaged in another activity that could certainly improve the quality of care veterans receive. Based on the concept of using teams to improve care quality through improved care coordination, the VA has developed the Patient Aligned Care Teams program. "A PACT achieves coordinated care through collaboration. All members of your team have clearly defined roles. They meet often to talk with you and each other about your progress toward achieving your health goals. The focus is on forging trusted, personal relationships, and the result is coordination of all aspects of your health care (Veterans Administration, n.d.)."

Department of Defense

Members of the U.S. military are eligible to participate in the TRICARE insurance program. TRICARE currently provides coverage options to over 9.5 million individuals. Service coverage is offered through several plan types (TRICARE, n.d.b). Like all public and private healthcare plans there are a variety of opinions regarding the effectiveness of TRICARE. Who gets care, what care do those eligible have access to, is the quality of care reflective of the cost of that care are all concerns voiced by bureaucrats, members of Congress and the public (House Armed Services Committee, 2015), (Government Accountability Office, 2013).

Environmental Protection Agency

Air and water quality are important indicators of overall health of individuals and population health. Congress has responded in the past to public concerns about air and water quality through the creation of the Clean Air Act and the Clear Water Act (Environmental Protection Agency [EPA], n.d., 2015a). The Environmental Protection Agency (EPA) is the cabinet-level agency that is responsible for protecting "...the human health and the environment" and implementing environmental legislation (EPA, 2015b). Representing the bureaucracy, the policies of the EPA, as reflected in the rules and guidance they propose and implement, are regularly greeted with strong feelings by representatives of the other two triangle points-special interest and Congress. The Obama administration, through the EPA proposed rules related to air quality, has created a great deal of reaction from the current Congress and certain special interest groups (Eilperin & Mufson, 2014), (Bauers, 2013), (Foran, 2013), (House Committee on Natural Resources, 2015). A spill of toxic water from an abandoned mine in Colorado in August 2015 is an important example of the role the EPA plays in both the mitigation of environmental disasters and setting the expectations for preventing similar events in the future (EPA, 2015c).

State and Local Government Involvement

Many of the federal programs mentioned above are administered through state and local government agencies. Federal programs may support state and local program administration through a variety of mechanisms. The HRSA maternal and children health programs are funded through block grants. State maternal and child health programs submit annual grant applications using a specific grant formula. Block grants are a funding mechanism that offers applicants the greatest amount of flexibility. State agencies are allowed to use the block grant funds to meet broad federal guidelines for services through programs tailored specifically to meet state and local needs. State health departments are frequently the administering agencies for these programs.

Federally qualified health centers (FQHC) are able to apply for grant funding from HRSA based on funds made available through the annual federal appropriations process. Grants for FQHC funding are competitive and applicants must request funding for specific activities included in the request for grant application documents published by HRSA. Medicaid is a federal-state partnership with the federal government funding a portion of the program based on specific state demographic information. Medicaid is administered through state agencies that use the combined federal and state contributions to pay providers for the delivery of services to individuals enrolled in the program. State Medicaid agencies are responsible for administering both the mandatory or standard benefits required of every state as well as any optional benefits established through legislation at the state level (Medicaid.gov., n.d.a).

There are many other federal programs that are administered through state and local agencies. State and local agency funding is based on the various mechanisms discussed above. State and federal partnerships provide services and programs that include: rural health programs administered through state offices of rural health; assistance to Medicare beneficiaries through State Health Insurance Programs (SHIP); quality improvement programs for providers of services to Medicare beneficiaries through Quality Improvement Organizations (QIO) that may be housed in state medical organizations; inspections of facilities that provide services to Medicaid and Medicare beneficiaries through state facilities agencies; and state environmental health agencies administer the federal rules promulgated by the EPA.

The U.S. Constitution states that "The powers not delegated to the United States by the Constitution, nor prohibited by it to the States, are reserved to the States respectively, or to the people (United States Constitution, 2003)." In regard to government involvement in health, this delegation plays a significant role in the oversight of healthcare professionals. The federal government may have the authority to create programs for the delivery and payment of care, but states maintain authority of who can provide that care. State practice acts list the services that a specific professional is able to legally provide in that state. These scopes of practice authorities are a source of frequent state legislative action as various healthcare professionals attempt to influence both state and federal healthcare laws to the advantage or to the disadvantage of another profession.

ROLE OF CITIZENS IN THE IRON TRIANGLE

Citizen Advocacy

The third angle of the triangle represents the interests and concerns of the public. At the start of this chapter, the role of the individual in the successful operation of our government was presented in the context of philosophical expressions of happiness, goodness, and responsibility. Citizens of the United States have put these philosophical concepts into practice at a level that have amazed individuals that have seen our engagement up close and personally (Tocqueville & Thomas, 1981). Today, participation in the business of influencing government, regardless of the issue or your support or opposition to the issue, remains an essential activity of citizens. Establishing this civic responsibility early on is an important aspect of civics classes, yet these classes may need to be strengthened (Reiss, 2012), (Levine & Kawashima-Ginsberg, 2015).

Regardless of your personal level of civic engagement the impact of civic engagement remains essential to the health of our system of government (Cilliza, 2015). At the federal level, individuals can influence both the administration/bureaucracy and the legislative points of the triangle. The many federal agencies that are listed above include opportunities for citizen engagement. Agencies frequently provide web portals that allow individuals to access information in a variety of formats and schedules (NIH, 2015a, 2015b, 2015c), (CMS, 2015c). Some federal agencies seek the input of citizens through participation on advisory groups and committees (FDA, 2015b). The activities of agencies are frequently influenced through the input they receive during community forums that are held in areas of the country selected because of the potential or current impact of a program or activity or in anticipation of future impact (National Institute of Environmental Health Sciences, 2015), (CMS, n.d.c).

Similarly, today individual citizens have greater access to the members of Congress than ever before. The individual webpages of most if not all members include opportunities to contact them through email, follow them on Facebook and Twitter and sign up for their newsletters that are regularly sent to constituents (Congress.gov, n.d.). Members continue to seek constituent input during town hall meetings that are held in various locations within their districts or states. The best way to find out when your member schedules town hall meetings is through their newsletters or visiting their websites on a regular basis.

It is also important to recognize that civic engagement is not just associated with the federal government. State and local governments are important creators and administrators of programs that provide direct healthcare services or regulate the provision of those services. Like the federal agencies, state agencies frequently seek the input of state residents to help them develop rules and create programs that may be authorized by federal and/or state legislation and supported by federal and/or state funds. State legislatures and agencies frequently provide a time for public comment during hearings related to healthcare programs within their jurisdictions.

For almost every federal agency with a healthcare-related mission listed above there is a group that represents the interest of the programs administered by that agency. These groups are frequently referred to as "Friends of..." including Friends of AHRQ and Friends of HRSA (Friends of AHRQ, n.d.), (Friends of HRSA, n.d.). Special interest groups also support the specific programs administered by the agencies including the Health Professions and Nursing Education Coalition (HPNEC) which advocates for the health professions education programs at HRSA (Health Professions and Nursing Education Coalition, n.d.). The influence of special interest groups regarding this information sharing capacity is heightened when they join together in coalitions based on shared interest. The Coalition for Health Funding (CHF) includes members of the agency specific groups mentioned above as well as disease-specific special interest groups such as the American Heart Association (Coalition for Health Funding, 2015).

The Shifting Power of the Triangle

The nature of the Iron Triangle and its impact on health care and health policy is far from rigid as the name may indicate. The influence of the Congress, Administration, and special interest on matters related to health care in America changes over time. The shifting natures of these three interests are more frequently subtle than dramatic. The involvement of government in health care has certainly not followed a straight line trajectory from identification of need to implementation of programs that meet that need. Possibly influenced by the policy development concept of disjointed incrementalism, the examples included in this chapter attempt to illustrate the influence of the three elements of the triangle in how, when, and in what context our government involves itself in health care (The Oxford Index, 2014). Over time the influence of one element of the triangle on the others will wax and wane and there are times when all three are in concert making health care and the role of government in it a fascinating area of study.

Growing Influence of Citizens And Patients and the Affordable Care Act

As the involvement of our federal and state governments in health care grew as a result of the influence of the Iron Triangle, that same influence created increasing demands for accountability, access, and cost control across the healthcare system. The growing concern about healthcare quality lead to the Institute of Medicine (IOM) publishing a series of reports presenting the quality problem to the American public and policy makers. In the seminal report, *To Err is Human: Building a Safer Health System,* the IOM laid bare the morbidity and mortality associated with our poorly coordinated healthcare system (Institute of Medicine, 1999). It is unlikely that at the time of publication in 1999 there were a lot of people involved in healthcare provision, payment, program development, and research that were completely unaware of the negative and unintended consequences of poor quality on patients. For years prior to the IOM report, states were the "laboratories of innovation," to paraphrase Justice Brandeis, for health system improvements (North Carolina Health Planning Commission, 1994), (Oregon Health Decisions, 2015), (Minnesota Health Care Commission, 2006). The sustained impact of the recommendations or actions emanating from these efforts are not the subject of this chapter, yet the attempts were based on growing numbers of uninsured, poor individual and population health outcomes, and increasing costs.

Several states continued their reform efforts and created state-level health plans. While some of these states attempted to address their concerns through the Medicaid waiver process, the limits of Medicaid eligibility did not allow for universal access to care or coverage for state residents (Medicaid.gov., n.d.b). The state of North Carolina used the Medicaid waiver approach to create programs that culminated in Community Care of North Carolina (CCNC) (Community Care of North Carolina, 2015). Increasing patient access to primary care services is an approach to improving healthcare outcomes and controlling costs access formed the basis of the CCNC framework. Using the concepts of the primary care medical home networks of primary care providers across the state were established to provide and coordinate care for Medicaid patients. Several elements of health policy discussions relevant to improving care quality were integrated into the CCNC model. These elements include population management tools, case management and clinical support, and use of data to improve provider—patient interactions. The success of CCNC was a source of inquiry during congressional hearings focused on healthcare reform prior to the development of the Affordable Care Act (Senate Committee on Health, Education, Labor and Pensions, 2009).

States that attempted innovative, comprehensive reform efforts include Vermont and Massachusetts. In 2006, Vermont created a health plan, Catamount Health, available to uninsured state residents (The Vermont Legislature, 2006). A partnership between the state and Blue Cross and Blue Shield, enabled eligible to receive some level of premium assistance to make coverage more affordable. Individuals with preexisting conditions were eligible for coverage within certain limits. In 2011, Vermont passed additional legislation that created a single-payer health insurance program, Green Mountain Care (The Vermont Legislature, 2011).

In Massachusetts, the dynamics of increasing cost and the rising number of uninsured mirrored the concerns of other states across the nation. To address these concerns, the state legislature passed *An Act Providing Access to Affordable, Quality, Accountable Health Care* (General Court of the Commonwealth of Massachusetts, 2012). The Massachusetts legislation included provisions that addressed long-standing recommendations from health policy experts. The most significant may be the requirement that all state residents purchase health insurance. This approach, referred to as the individual mandate, responded to health policy discussions recognizing the potential cost benefit to individual premium costs when the risk pool expands to include individuals with differing healthcare needs (Cooper, 2014). Those who did not purchase healthcare insurance were subject to monetary penalties.

The Patient Protection and Affordable Care Act

Past efforts to address systemic change in a comprehensive manner at the federal level were largely unsuccessful (Oberlander, 2007), (Kaiser Family Foundation, 2011). State-level activity generated concern among state legislatures and public policy makers that state generosity could be overwhelmed if the number of individuals seeking support exceeded estimates and system capacity, referred to as the woodwork effect (Sher, 2010). Health reform efforts were tarred with accusations of socialism (Mencimer, 2010). Concerns with universal health care, warranted or not, threatened public support for comprehensive action even as public recognition of a problem increased (Hanson, 2008), (Sack & Connelley, 2009).

Congress is challenged in the writing and passage of large, comprehensive pieces of legislation. The greatest challenge is the need to bring the competing influences of the bureaucracy, special interests, and its own members to consensus. Agreement is rarely unanimous in the development of legislation. The strength of federal agency administrators can overwhelm even the best laid plans of the President. The history of cabinet secretaries challenging each other and even the President go back to George Washington. The variety of special interests in Washington and the specific nature of their constituent issues require significant management by both personal and committee staff. Congressional members themselves are essentially advocates representing the special interests of their district or state populations. These competing interests, whether for personal advantage or meeting the needs of diverse constituencies mean there is rarely homogeneous pool of ideas from which to move toward consensus and express that consensus in legislation. Congress was successful in the writing and passage of some major pieces of healthcare-related legislation in the late 1990s and in the middle of the first decade of the 21st century. In 1996, Congress passed the Health Insurance Portability and Accountability Act (HIPAA) establishing the foundation for privacy of personal health information (Congress.gov, 2015q). How that personal health information would be transmitted and shared among providers and payers was the rationale for the creation and passage of the Health Information Technology for Economic and Clinical Health Act of 2009 (Congress.gov, 2015r). These pieces of legislation, focused on specific components of health systems, were seen building blocks for more comprehensive reform (O'Harrow, 2009).

During much of 2009, the U.S. Congress was engaged in a series of hearings and legislation markups all aimed at building support for comprehensive healthcare reform (United States Senate Committee on Finance, n.d.). In early 2010, President Obama invited congressional and health care industry leaders to meetings at the White House to discuss the development of hearth reform legislation (White House, 2010a, 2010b). The hearings and meetings reflected historic concerns about the need for reform voiced by the public, policy experts, members of congress, healthcare providers, and many other special interest groups that sought improvements to healthcare insurance issuance and maintenance as well as improvements to care quality and the need to control costs. In 2009, President Obama also appointed Kathleen Sebelius as Secretary of Health and Human Services. Secretary Sebelius was the Governor of Kansas with a strong relationship with other governors, an important point since state administration of the ACA would be essential to successful implementation. As the former Insurance Commissioner of Kansas, Sebelius was well positioned to support and implement reforms focused on increasing access to health insurance and improving the quality of health care.

THE PATIENT PROTECTION AND AFFORDABLE CARE ACT OF 2010

On March 3, 2010, President Obama signed the Patient Protection and Affordable Care Act of 2010 (ACA) (Congress.gov, 2015o). Government involvement in health care reached a pinnacle. Short of universal care, it does support universal coverage. Short of overt cost controls, it supports a change in the payment of care delivery. Short of total reform, it does support reorganization of health systems. The protection provisions make healthcare insurance easier to access and keep. These insurance-related provisions make insurance coverage easier to purchase even if they have health conditions that in the past would have reduced their chances of gaining coverage. To make the access issues affordable the law requires all individuals to purchase insurance. The cost of insurance is made easier by the authorization of tax credits for qualifying individuals. Finding the policy that is right for you is facilitated through health insurance exchanges administered by either states or the federal government. The insurance provisions also include protecting individuals under the age of 26 from losing coverage by allowing them to be covered by a parents' plan.

The affordability-related provisions are focused on improving the quality of the Medicare and Medicaid programs and extending the quality of care for all Americans. The law reflects the reality that for the $3 plus trillion we spend on health care the individual and population outcomes associated with that spending lag behind many other nations. The primary focus of these affordability provisions is improving overall health, improving the individual care experience, and controlling costs. These three elements are a primary responsibility of the CMMI that was also created in the law (Center for Medicare and Medicaid Innovation [CMMI], 2015). The challenge to the CMMI is to move the care of Medicare and Medicaid patients to a value-based system from the current fee-for-service or volume-based system. With an allocation of $10 billion CMMI, through a variety of innovation grants, is attempting to find the best way to make this transition a success.

The ACA's intent to improve health is as paradigm-shattering as the entire bill itself. For the first time improving health raises the profile of health promotion and disease prevention. The incidence of chronic illness in the Medicare population makes this paradigm-shift very timely. In 2010, two-thirds of Medicare beneficiaries had two or more chronic conditions (CMS, 2012). The traditional approach to healthcare delivery here in the United States is to provide care after the patient is sick. Prevention of illness is a small component of our current system. The ACA moves prevention of disease into the forefront by requiring health insurance plans to include certain wellness and health promotion benefits. The law also authorizes the establishment of a National Prevention, Health Promotion and Public Health Council which is given the primary responsibility for the creation of a National Prevention and Health Promotion Strategy. The authorization of a Prevention and Public Health Fund provides an additional source of discretionary funding—up to $2 billion per year in 2015 and beyond—"to provide for expanded and sustained national investment in prevention and public health programs to improve health and help restrain the rate of growth in private and public sector healthcare costs."

Like any legislative action the creation and implementation of the ACA was and continues to be impacted by the Iron Triangle. The law is now under attack by some of the very special interest groups and congressional committees that raised the importance of and brought forward recommendations to its health policy underpinnings (Butler, 2012), (Abelson, 2012). The ACA has survived two Supreme Court challenges including its constitutionality (Kaiser Family Foundation, 2012), (Supreme Court of the United States, 2015). A legal challenge by the U.S. House of Representatives to the Administration's implementation of the ACA was allowed to go forward in September of 2015 (Schenker, 2015).

While the ACA continues to be controversial, public support for the law and its benefits to individuals continues to grow (Benen, 2015). The reasons for increasing public support of this landmark legislation will become clearer as the law continues to impact the lives of individuals and that impact is inevitable. There are many provisions within the law, such as gaining access to health insurance even if you have preexisting conditions that will provide benefits to the American public. One intent of the law that will likely lag in the public's eye will be the move toward a healthcare system that is patient-centered (Rickert, 2012). The individual patient will now be the most important component in the implementation of ACA provisions aimed at improving health, improving health care, and controlling costs. This move from our physician-centered system of care delivery will require a substantial change in the way healthcare providers communicate with and establish outcomes satisfactory to the patient. One way to move in the direction of patient-centered care is by improving the quality of care patients have access to and opt to receive. To accomplish this, the ACA authorized the creation of the Patient-Centered Outcomes Research Institute (PCORI). Given that many of the care options we all have access to are unlikely to be of proven benefit, PCORI will support research to close these benefit gaps (Patient Centered Outcomes Research Institute [PCORI], 2014). Of particular interest is the role of the patient view in the development of the PCORI research agenda (PCORI, 2015). Applicants for PCORI grants are required to explicitly indicate how patients and patient stakeholder groups are engaged in the proposed research and in the dissemination of the project outcomes.

The ACA contains other patient-centered provisions including the requirement that no-for-profit hospitals conduct a community needs assessment. The law requires community health needs assessment to take "into account input from persons who represent the broad interests of the community served by the hospital facility, including those with special knowledge of or expertise in public health." As a result of this patient-centered focus, patient engagement is increasingly a part of federal program development and implementation as well as the basis of congressional action related to speeding the approval of drugs and medical devices (FDA, 2015c), (Congress.gov, 2015a).

CONCLUSION

The importance of the patient involvement in a reforming healthcare system may seem new, but it reflects the importance of the individual in all aspects of our government. As government involvement continues to evolve, the engagement of the public in setting the parameters of that involvement gains greater value. Like health care in general, our government is also evolving (Office of the Speaker, 2012). The oversight of federal agencies and programs by congressional committees is increasing (Mills, Kalaf-Hughes, & MacDonald, 2015). The issues we have to grapple with, many of which are based on questionable or a lack of science, are increasingly important and relevant to our health and well-being (Carroll, 2015), (Boulanger, 2014). While it would likely take an entire book to fully describe all the ways our government is involved in health care, the important take away is that this involvement is influenced through the Iron Triangle. Whether the point of view or activity of the bureaucracy, Congress, or special interest, all three of these are comprised of individuals. The individual continues to play an essential role in how we support or oppose government involvement in health care, for together that role reflects ... "We the people..."

QUESTIONS FOR FURTHER DISCUSSION

1. Does form follow function in the government's organization of its healthcare activities? That is, are U.S. government agencies organized around healthcare activities that have similar functions, similar resource needs, or overlapping jurisdictions? What are the advantages and disadvantages of this organizational structure?
2. Based on your responses to the question above, how has the organization and the function of federal public health agencies changed over time? How has this change been impacted by each of the sides of the Iron Triangle?
3. What are the advantages and disadvantages of having different roles and responsibilities for federal, state, and local governments with regard to health care?
4. Select a current issue that presents a challenge for both federal and state governments (telemedicine, professional licensure, insurance issuance, health systems service areas). Based on your responses to the question above, describe how a state or federal legislative body, a state or federal agency, or a special interest group might influence these roles and responsibilities?

KEY TOPICS AND TERMS

Administration on aging
Administrative agencies
Agency for Healthcare Research and Quality
Centers for Disease Control and Prevention (CDC)
Centers for Medicare and Medicaid Services (CMS)
Department of Health and Human Services (DHHS)
Federal public health agencies

Food and Drug Administration (FDA)
Government Accountability Office (GAO)
Indian Health Service (IHS)
Iron Triangle
Medicaid
Medicare
National Institutes of Health (NIH)
Office of Management and Budget (OMB)
Office of the Inspector General
TriCare
Veterans administration

REFERENCES

Abelson, R. (2015, July 21). Health care tax faces united opposition from labor and employers. *The Wall Street Journal*. Retrieved from http://www.nytimes.com/2015/07/22/business/labor-and-employers-join-in-opposition-to-a-health-care-tax.html?_r=0

Administration on Aging. (2014). Retrieved from http://aoa.acl.gov/Index.aspx

Administration for Community Living. (2015). Retrieved from http://www.acl.gov/

Advisory Committee on Immunization Practices. (2015). Retrieved from www.cdc.gov/vaccines/acip

Agency for Healthcare Research and Quality. (2015). *About AHRQ mission and budget*. Retrieved from http://www.ahrq.gov/cpi/about/mission/index.html

American Association of Community Colleges. (2003). *Stop the elimination of health professions education programs*. Retrieved from http://www.aacc.nche.edu/Resources/aaccprograms/health/Documents/rollcall_ad.pdf

American Society of Health Systems Pharmacists. (2003). *HRSA reorganization could affect 340B program*. Retrieved from http://www.ashp.org/menu/News/PharmacyNews/NewsArticle.aspx?id=1246

amfAR, The Foundation for AIDS Research. (2014a). *"Countdown to a cure for HIV/AIDS" aims to invest $100 Million in HIV cure research*. Retrieved from http://www.amfar.org/amfAR-Launches-Initiative-Aimed-at-Finding-a-Cure-for-HIV-by-2020/

amfAR, the Foundation for AIDS Research. (2014b). *FACT SHEET: Progress in four years of the National HIV/AIDS Strategy*. Retrieved from https://www.whitehouse.gov/the-press-office/2014/07/15/fact-sheet-progress-four-years-national-hivaids-strategy

Aubrey, A. (2015, September 8). Lunch ladies want Healthy Hunger-FreeKids Act to lighten up. *NPR*. Retrieved from http://www.npr.org/2015/09/08/438473608/lunch-ladies-want-healthy-hunger-free-kids-act-to-lighten-up

Bauers, S. (2013, October 17). Groups support EPA rules for coal plant discharges. *Philadelphia Inquirer*. Retrieved from http://www.philly.com/philly/blogs/greenliving/Groups-support-EPA-rules-for-coal-plant-discharges.html

Benen, S. (2015, April 21). Public support shifts in ACA's favor. *MSNBC*. Retrieved from http://www.msnbc.com/rachel-maddow-show/public-support-shifts-acas-favor

Boulanger, A. (2014, November 14). Opposition to vaccines. *Healthline*. Retrieved from http://www.healthline.com/health/vaccinations/opposition#Overview1

Butler, S. (2012, February 6). Don't' Blame Heritage for Obamacare Mandate. The Heritage Foundation. Retrieved from http://www.heritage.org/research/commentary/2012/02/dont-blame-heritage-for-obamacare-mandatehttp://www.heritage.org/research/commentary/2012/02/dont-blame-heritage-for-obamacare-mandate

Carroll, A. (2015, August 24). No you do not have to drink 8 glasses of water a day. *New York Times*. Retrieved from http://www.nytimes.com/2015/08/25/upshot/no-you-do-not-have-to-drink-8-glasses-of-water-a-day.html?partner=rss&emc=rss&smid=tw-nytimes&smtyp=cur&abt=0002&abg=0

Centers for Disease Control and Prevention. (2014a). *International comparisons of infant mortality and related factors: United States and Europe, 2010*. Retrieved from http://www.cdc.gov/nchs/data/nvsr/nvsr63/nvsr63_05.pdf

Centers for Disease Control and Preventions. (2014b). *Mission, role and pledge*. Retrieved from http://www.cdc.gov/about/organization/mission.htm

Collins, F. S. (2015). *Statement on the efforts to focus research to end the AIDS pandemic*. National Institutes of Health. Retrieved from http://www.nih.gov/about/director/08122015_statement_aids_pandemic.htm

Center for Medicare and Medicaid Innovation. (2015). Retrieved from http://innovation.cms.gov/

Centers for Medicare and Medicaid Services. (n.d.a). *About CMS*. Retrieved from https://www.cms.gov/About-CMS/About-CMS.html

Centers for Medicare and Medicaid Services. (n.d.b). *Medicare enrollment —All beneficiaries as of July 2012*. Retrieved from https://www.cms.gov/Research-Statistics-Data-and-Systems/Statistics-Trends-and-Reports/MedicareEnrpts/Downloads/12All.pdf

Centers for Medicare and Medicaid Services. (n.d.c). *Stakeholder engagement*. Retrieved from https://www.cms.gov/CCIIO/Resources/Stakeholder-Engagement/index.html

Center for Medicare and Medicaid Services. (2012). *Chronic conditions among Medicare beneficiaries*. Retrieved from https://www.cms.gov/Research-Statistics-Data-and-Systems/Statistics-Trends-and-Reports/Chronic-Conditions/Downloads/2012Chartbook.pdf

Centers for Medicare and Medicaid Services. (2015a). *Total Medicaid Enrollees- VIII Group Breakout Report, January 2015*. Retrieved from http://www.medicaid.gov/medicaid-chip-program-information/program-information/downloads/cms-64-enrollment-report-jan-mar-2015.pdf

Centers for Medicare and Medicaid Services. (2015b, July 28). *Medicaid and CHIP: May 2015 monthly applications, eligibility determinations and enrollment report*. Retrieved from http:/medicaid.gov/medicaid-chip-program-information/program-information/downloads/may-2015-enrollment-report.pdf

Centers for Medicare and Medicaid Services. (2015c). *The Medicare Blog*. Retrieved from http://blog.medicare.gov/2015/08/01/pneumonia-shot/

Cilliza, C. (2015, May 6). Politics is a dirty business. It should stay that way. *Washington Post*. Retrieved from http://www.washingtonpost.com/news/the-fix/wp/2015/05/06/politics-is-a-dirty-business-it-should-stay-that-way/

Coalition for Health Funding. (2015). Retrieved from http://www.publichealthfunding.org/

Community Care of North Carolina. (2015). *A history of CCNC*. Retrieved from http://www.communitycarenc.com/about-us/history-ccnc-rev/

Community Guide. (2015). Retrieved from http://www.thecommunityguide.org/about/guide.html

Community Services Task Force. (2015). Retrieved from http://www.thecommunityguide.org/about/task-force-members.html

Congress.gov. (n.d.). *Members of the U.S. Congress*. Retrieved from https://www.congress.gov/members

Congress.gov. (2015a). *House Resolution 6. 21st Century Cures Act*. Retrieved from https://www.congress.gov/114/bills/hr6/BILLS-114hr6rfs.pdf

Congress.gov. (2015b). *House report 114-195. Departments of Labor, Health and Human Services and Education and related agencies appropriations bill, 2016*. Retrieved from https://www.congress.gov/114/crpt/hrpt195/CRPT-114hrpt195.pdf

Congress.gov. (2015c). *House Report 114-19. Departments of Labor, Health and Human Services, and Education and related agencies appropriations bill, 2016*. Retrieved from https://www.congress.gov/congressional-report/114th-congress/house-report/195/1

Congress.gov. (2015d). Public Law 101-239. (1989). *Omnibus Budget Reconciliation Act of 1989*. Retrieved from https://www.congress.gov/bill/101st-congress/house-bill/3299

Congress.gov. (2015e). Public Law 106-129. (1999). *Healthcare Research and Quality Act of 1999*. Retrieved from https://www.congress.gov/bill/106th-congress/senate-bill/580/text/pl

Congress.gov. (2015f). House Resolution 3020. *Departments of Labor, Health and Human Services, and Education and related agencies appropriations, 2016*. Retrieved from https://www.congress.gov/bill/114th-congress/house-bill/3020

Congress.gov. (2015g). Senate Bill 1695. *Departments of Labor, Health and Human Services and Education and Related Agencies Appropriations Act, 2016*. Retrieved from https://www.congress.gov/bill/114th-congress/senate-bill/1695/related-bills

Congress.gov. (2015h). Public Law 109-365. *Older Americans Act of 2006*. Retrieved from https://www.congress.gov/bill/109th-congress/house-bill/6197/text/pl

Congress.gov. (2015i). Public Law 89-97. (1965). *Social Security Act Amendments of 1965*. Retrieved from http://www.legisworks.org/GPO/STATUTE-79-Pg286.pdf

Congress.gov. (2015j). Public Law 108-173. (2003). *Medicare Prescription Drug Improvement and Modernization Act of 2003*. Retrieved from https://www.congress.gov/bill/108th-congress/house-bill/1/text/pl

Congress.gov. (2015k). Public Law 105-33. (1997). *Balanced Budget Act of 1997*. Retrieved from https://www.congress.gov/bill/105th-congress/house-bill/2015/text/pl

Congress.gov. (2015l). PL 107-116. (2002). *Departments of Labor, Health and Human Services, and Education, and related agencies appropriations act, 2002*. Retrieved from https://www.congress.gov/bill/107th-congress/house-bill/3061/text/pl

Congress.gov. (2015m). Senate Report 107-84. (2002). *Departments of Labor, Health and Human Services and Education and related agencies appropriations bill, 2002*. Retrieved from https://www.congress.gov/congressional-report/107th-congress/senate-report/84/1

Congress.gov. (2015n). Public Law 102-321. (1992). *ADAMHA Reorganization Act. PL 102-321*. Retrieved from https://www.congress.gov/bill/102nd-congress/senate-bill/1306

Congress.gov. (2015o). Public Law 113-148. (2010). *Patient Protection and Affordable Care Act*. Retrieved from https://www.congress.gov/bill/111th-congress/house-bill/3590/text/pl

Congress.gov. (2015p). Public Law 113-146. (2014). *Veterans Access Choice and Accountability Act*. Retrieved from https://www.congress.gov/bill/113th-congress/house-bill/3230/text?overview=closed

Congress.gov. (2015q). Public Law 104-191. (1996). *Health Insurance Portability and Accountability Act (HIPAA). PL 104-191*. Retrieved from https://www.congress.gov/bill/104th-congress/house-bill/3103/text/pl

Congress.gov. (2015r). Public Law 111-5. (2009). *Health Information Technology for Economic and Clinical Health Act (HITECH)*. Retrieved from https://www.congress.gov/bill/111th-congress/house-bill/1/text/pl

Cooper, M. (2014, February 12). Conservatives sowed idea of healthcare mandate, only to spurn it later. *Washington Post*. Retrieved from http://www.nytimes.com/2012/02/15/health/policy/health-care-mandate-was-first-backed-by-conservatives.html?_r=0

Declaration of Independence. (n.d.). Retrieved from http://www.loc.gov/rr/program/bib/ourdocs/DeclarInd.html

Democratic Underground.com. (2005). *"Here's the list of programs that will be cut/eliminated by budget cuts."* Retrieved from http://www.democraticunderground.com/discuss/duboard.php?az=view_all&address=104x3099226

Dietary Guideline Advisory Group. (2015). *Scientific Report of the 2015 Dietary Guidelines Advisory Committee*. Retrieved from http://health.gov/dietaryguidelines/2015-scientific-report/PDFs/Scientific-Report-of-the-2015-Dietary-Guidelines-Advisory-Committee.pdf

Eilperin, J. & Mufson, J. (2014, June 2). Everything you need to know about the EPAS's proposed rules on coal-burning power plants. *Washington Post*. Retrieved from http://www.washingtonpost.com/national/health-science/epa-will-propose-a-rule-to-cut-emissions-from-existing-coal-plants-by-up-to-30-percent/2014/06/02/f37f0a10-e81d-11e3-afc6-a1dd9407abcf_story.html

Environmental Protection Agency. (n.d.). *The plain English guide to the Clean Air Act*. Retrieved from http://www.epa.gov/air/caa/peg/

Environmental Protection Agency. (2015a). *Summary of the Clean Water Act*. Retrieved from http://www2.epa.gov/laws-regulations/summary-clean-water-act

Environmental Protection Agency. (2015b). *About EPA*. Retrieved from http://www2.epa.gov/aboutepa

Federal Register. (n.d.). *List of federal agencies*. Retrieved from https://www.federalregister.gov/agencies

Environmental Protection Agency. (2015c). *Emergency response to August 2015 release from King Gold Mine*. Retrieved from http://www2.epa.gov/goldkingmine

Food and Drug Administration. (2015a). *MedWatch: The FDA Safety and Adverse Event Reporting Program*. Retrieved from http://www.fda.gov/safety/medwatch/default.htm

Food and Drug Administration. (2015b). *FDA Advisory Committees*. Retrieved from http://www.fda.gov/AdvisoryCommittees/default.htm

Food and Drug Administration. (2015c). *About the FDA Patient Network*. Retrieved from http://www.fda.gov/forpatients/about/default.htm

Foran, C. (2013, November 13). Manchin: "There's and overreach by the EPA." *National Journal*. Retrieved from http://www.nationaljournal.com/energy/manchin-there-s-an-overreach-by-the-epa-20131113

Friends of AHRQ. (n.d.). Retrieved from http://www.academyhealth.org/Advocacy/content.cfm?ItemNumber=8316&navitemnumber=1992

Friends of AHRQ. (2015a). *Letter to House Appropriations Committee*. Retrieved from http://www.academyhealth.org/files/FoAHouseLaborHHSFY16.pdf

Friends of AHRQ. (2015b). *Letter to Senate Appropriations Committee*. Retrieved from http://www.academyhealth.org/files/FoASenateSignOnFY16.pdf

Friends of HRSA. (n.d.). Retrieved from http://friendsofhrsa.org/

General Court of the Commonwealth of Massachusetts. (2012). *An Act Providing Access to Affordable, Quality, Accountable Health Care. Chapter 58, Sessions Laws of 2006.* Retrieved from https://malegislature.gov/Laws/SessionLaws/Acts/2006/Chapter58

Government accounting Office. (2013). Defense health care: TRICARE Multiyear surveys indicate problems with access to care for nonenrolled beneficiaries. Available at http://gao.gov/products/GAO-13-364

Gray, B. H., Gusmano, M. K., & Collins, S. R. (2003, June). AHCPR and the changing politics of health services research. *Health Affairs.* Retrieved from http://content.healthaffairs.org/content/suppl/2003/12/09/hlthaff.w3.283v1.DC1

Hamburg, M. A. (2015, March 15). Lessons learned: How the FDA matters. Remarks of Margaret A. *Hamburg at the National Press Club.* Retrieved from http://www.fda.gov/NewsEvents/Speeches/ucm440315.htm

Hanson, R. (2008, January). *The hidden dangers of government health care.* Child and Family Protection Association. Retrieved from http://www.childandfamilyprotection.org/HiddenDangers080107.html

Health Professions and Nursing Education Coalition. (n.d.). Retrieved from https://www.aamc.org/advocacy/hpnec/

Health Resources and Services Administration. (n.d.). *About HRSA.* Retrieved from http://www.hrsa.gov/about/index.html

Hering, G. (2015, May 19). Meat industry has a cow over US dietary guidelines. *The Guardian.* Retrieved from http://www.theguardian.com/lifeandstyle/2015/may/19/us-dietary-guidelines-health-and-human-services-tom-vilsack

Herman, A. (2002). *How the Scots invented the modern world.* Broadway Books.

House Armed Services Committee. (n.d.). Retrieved from http://armedservices.house.gov/index.cfm/committee-rules

House Armed Services Committee. (2015, June 11). *Opening Remarks of Chairman Heck. Subcommittee on Military Personnel.* Retrieved from http://armedservices.house.gov/index.cfm/press-releases?ContentRecord_id=7A1CB532-028D-4B03-AFC5-FF9CEA137CB3

House Committee on Natural Resources. (2015). *Controversial social cost of carbon, developed behind closed doors, jeopardizes energy production & American way of life.* Retrieved from http://naturalresources.house.gov/news/documentsingle.aspx?DocumentID=399130

House Committee on Veterans' Affairs. (n.d.). Retrieved from http://veterans.house.gov/

House Committee on Ways and Means. (n.d.). Retrieved from http://waysandmeans.house.gov/

House Judiciary Committee. (n.d.). Retrieved from http://judiciary.house.gov/index.cfm/subcommittees

Indian Health Service. (n.d.). Retrieved from www.ihs.gov

Institute of Medicine. (1999). *To Err is human: Building a safer health system.* Washington, D.C: National Academy Press.

Institute of Medicine. (2006). *The Future of drug safety: Promoting and protecting the health of the public.* Retrieved from http://iom.nationalacademies.org/reports/2006/the-future-of-drug-safety-promoting-and-protecting-the-health-of-the-public.aspx

Kaiser Family Foundation. (2011). *Timeline: A history of health reform in the U.S.* Retrieved from https://kaiserfamilyfoundation.files.wordpress.com/2011/03/5-02-13-history-of-health-reform.pdf

Kaiser Family Foundation. (2012). *A Guide to the Supreme Court's decision on the ACA's Medicaid expansion.* Retrieved from https://kaiserfamilyfoundation.files.wordpress.com/2013/01/8347.pdf

Levine, P. & Kawashima-Ginsberg, K. (2015). *Civic education and deeper learning.* Retrieved from http://jff.org/publications/civic-education-and-deeper-learning

Market Watch. (2015). *Naltrexone for opioid abuse spotlighted in Vermont treatment grant.* Retrieved from http://www.marketwatch.com/story/naltrexone-for-opioid-addiction-spotlighted-in-vermont-treatment-grant-2015-08-13

Maynard, J. (2015, June 26). Fat makes a comeback as republicans oppose Obama's dietary guidelines. *Tech Times.* Retrieved from http://www.techtimes.com/articles/63986/20150626/low-fat-diets-make-comeback-republicans-oppose-obama-guidelines.htm

McDonald, B. (2015, July 30). *My VA: A Message from Secretary Bob McDonald.* Retrieved from http://www.blogs.va.gov/VAntage/21806/myva-a-message-from-sec-bob-mcdonald/

McGarvey, R. (2015, August 10). The epidemic of senior citizen drug and alcohol abuse. *Main Street.* Retrieved from https://www.mainstreet.com/article/the-epidemic-of-senior-citizen-drug-and-alcohol-abuse

Medicaid.gov. (n.d.a). *Medicaid benefits.* Retrieved from http://www.medicaid.gov/Medicaid-CHIP-Program-Information/By-Topics/Benefits/Medicaid-Benefits.html

Medicaid.gov. (n.d.b). *Medicaid waivers.* Retrieved from http://www.medicaid.gov/Medicaid-CHIP-Program-Information/By-Topics/Waivers/Waivers.html

Mencimer, S. (2010, September 19). Health care reform as socialism meme dates to Roosevelt. *Mother Jones.* Retrieved from http://www.motherjones.com/mojo/2009/09/health-care-reform-socialism-meme-dates-roosevelt

Merriam-Webster. (2015). Retrieved from http://www.merriam-webster.com/dictionary/bureaucracy

Mills, R. W., Kalaf-Hughes, N., & MacDonald, J. A. (2015). Agency policy preferences, congressional letter-marking and the allocation of distributive policy benefits. *Journal of Public Policy.* Available on CJO2015. doi:10.1017/S0143814X15000252. Retrieved from http://journals.cambridge.org/action/displayAbstract?fromPage=online&aid=9875488&fulltextType=RA&fileId=S0143814X15000252

Minnesota Health Care Commission. (2006). *Introduction.* Retrieved from http://www.health.state.mn.us/mhcc/index.htm

Morbidity and Mortality Weekly Report. (2015). Retrieved from http://www.cdc.gov/mmwr/

National Center for Chronic Disease Prevention and Health Promotion. (2015). Retrieved from http://www.cdc.gov/chronicdisease/index.htm

National Center for Health Statistics. (2015). Retrieved from http://www.cdc.gov/nchs/

National Diabetes Prevention Program. (2015). Retrieved from http://www.cdc.gov/diabetes/prevention/index.htm

National Institute of Environmental Health Sciences. (2015). *Community Forums.* Retrieved from http://www.niehs.nih.gov/about/community/communityforums/index.cfm

National Institutes of Health. (2013a). *NIH legislative almanac.* Retrieved from http://www.nih.gov/about/almanac/historical/legislative_chronology.htm

National Institutes of Health. (2013b). *Mission of the NIH.* Retrieved from http://www.nih.gov/about/mission.htm

National Institutes of Health. (2015a). *NIH Feedback.* Retrieved from http://feedback.nih.gov/

National Institutes of Health. (2015d). *NIH Health Information.* Retrieved from http://health.nih.gov/

National Institutes of Health. (2015c). *Follow the NIH Director.* Retrieved from http://www.nih.gov/about/director/index.htm

North Carolina Health Planning Commission. (1994). *North Carolina Health Planning Commission: Recommendations, 1994.* Retrieved from https://archive.org/details/healthrecommend00nort

Patient Centered Outcomes Research Institute. (2014). *Why PCORI was created.* Retrieved from http://www.pcori.org/about-us/why-pcori-was-created

Patient Centered Outcomes Research Institute. (2015). *How we evaluate key aspects of our work.* Retrieved from http://www.pcori.org/research-results/evaluating-our-work/how-we-evaluate-key-aspects-our-work

Oberlander, J. (2007, October 25). Learning from failure in health care reform. *The New England Journal of Medicine,* 2007, 357, 1677–1679.

Office of Management and Budget. (n.d.). Retrieved from https://www.whitehouse.gov/omb

Office of Management and Budget. (2015). *Fiscal year 2016 budget overview.* Retrieved from https://www.whitehouse.gov/omb/overview

Office of Science and Technology Policy. (n.d.). Retrieved from https://www.whitehouse.gov/administration/eop/ostp

Office of the Speaker. (2012, November 16). *House Republicans Renew Earmark Ban for 113th Congress. Office of the Speaker.* Retrieved from http://www.speaker.gov/general/house-republicans-renew-earmark-ban-113th-congress

O'Harrow Jr. R. (2009, May 16). The Machinery behind health-care reform. *Washington Post.* Retrieved from http://www.washingtonpost.com/wp-dyn/content/article/2009/05/15/AR2009051503667.html

Oregon Health Decisions. (2015). *Oregon Health Decisions/Background.* Retrieved from https://oregonhealth-decisions.org/about-us/background.html

Organisation for Economic Co-operation and Development. (2015). *Health at a Glance 2013: OECD Indicators.* Retrieved from http://www.oecd.org/health/health-systems/health-at-a-glance.htm

Reiss, D. (2012, October). Why teaching civics is essential. *District Administration.* Retrieved from http://www.districtadministration.com/article/why-teaching-civic-engagement-essential

Research!America. (2015). *Public Opinion Polls*. Retrieved from http://www.researchamerica.org/polls-and-publications/polls/public-opinion-polls

Rickert, J. (2012, January 24). Patient-centered care: What it means and how to get there. *Health Affairs Blog*. Retrieved from http://healthaffairs.org/blog/2012/01/24/patient-centered-care-what-it-means-and-how-to-get-there/

Sack, K. & Connelly, M. (2009, June 20). In poll, wide support for government-run health. *The New York Times*.

Schenker, L. (2015, September 9). House Republican's ACA lawsuit moves forward. *Modern Healthcare*. Retrieved from http://www.modernhealthcare.com/article/20150909/NEWS/150909879?utm_source=modernhealthcare&utm_medium=email&utm_content=externalURL&utm_campaign=am

Senate Committee on Armed Services. (n.d.). Retrieved from http://www.armed-services.senate.gov/about/history

Senate Committee on Finance. (n.d.a). Retrieved from http://www.finance.senate.gov/about/jurisdiction/

Senate Committee on Finance. (n.d.b). *Health care reform from conception to final passage*. Retrieved from http://www.finance.senate.gov/issue/?id=32be19bd-491e-4192-812f-f65215c1ba65

Senate Committee on Health, Education, Labor and Pensions. (n.d.). Retrieved from http://www.help.senate.gov/

Senate Committee on Health, Education, Labor and Pensions. (2009, January 22). Statement of Allen Dobson, CCNC. Retrieved from https://www.communitycarenc.org/media/related-downloads/dobson-testimony-to-us-senate.pdf

Senate Committee on the Judiciary. (n.d.). Retrieved from http://www.judiciary.senate.gov/about/jurisdiction

Senate Committee on Veterans' Affairs. (n.d.). Retrieved from http://www.veterans.senate.gov/about

Sher, A. (2010, April 20). Most new Tenn-Care costs involve now-eligible people state says. *Times Free Press*.

Supreme Court of the United States. (2015, June 2015). King et al v. Burwell, Secretary of Health and Human Services et al. Supreme Court of the United States- Syllabus. Retrieved from http://www.supremecourt.gov/opinions/14pdf/14-114_qol1.pdf

The Oxford Index. (2014). *Disjointed incrementalism*. Retrieved from http://oxfordindex.oup.com/view/10.1093/oi/authority.20110803095721690

Tocqueville, A. D., & Thomas B. 1981. *Democracy in America*. New York: Modern Library.

TRICARE. (n.d.a). Retrieved from http://tricare.mil/Welcome.aspx

TRICARE. (n.d.b). Retrieved from http://tricare.mil/

United States Code. (2015a). *Social Security Ac*. Retrieved from http://uscode.house.gov/browse/prelim@title42/chapter7&edition=prelim

United States Code. (2015b). *Public Health Service Act*. Retrieved from http://uscode.house.gov/view.xhtml?path=/prelim@title42/chapter6A&edition=prelim

United States Constitution. (n.d.). Retrieved from http://www.archives.gov/exhibits/charters/constitution.html

United States Constitution. (2003). Amendment X. *United States Constitution* (23rd ed.). Washington, DC: Government Printing Office.

United States Department of Agriculture. (n.d.). *About the USDA*. Retrieved from http://www.usda.gov/wps/portal/usda/usdahome?navid=ABOUT_USDA

United States Department of Health and Human Services. (2014). *HHS FY2015 budget in brief*. Retrieved from http://www.hhs.gov/about/budget/fy2015/budget-in-brief/overview-tables/index.html#a2

United States Department of Health and Human Services. (2015a). *Highlights of the President's HHS FY2016 budget*. Retrieved from http://www.hhs.gov/about/budget/budget-factsheet/index.html

United States Department of Health and Human Services. (2015b). *U.S. dietary guidelines, 2010*. Retrieved from http://health.gov/dietaryguidelines/

United States Department of Health and Human Services. (2015c). *Operating Divisions*. Retrieved from http://www.hhs.gov/about/agencies/operating-divisions/index.html

United States House of Representatives. (n.d.a). *The House explained*. Retrieved from http://www.house.gov/content/learn/

United States House of Representatives. (n.d.b). Retrieved from www.house.gov

United States House of Representatives. (2015a.). *Rules of the United States House of Representatives*. Retrieved from http://clerk.house.gov/legislative/house-rules.pdf

United States Preventive Services Task Force. (2013). *USPSTF overview*. Available http://www.uspreventiveservicestaskforce.org/Page/Name/task-force-101-resources

United States Senate. (n.d.a). *Learn about the Senate*. Retrieved from http://www.senate.gov/reference/Index/Learning_About_Senate.htm

United States Senate. (n.d.b). Retrieved from www.senate.gov

United States Senate. (2013). *Rules of the United States Senate*. Retrieved from http://www.rules.senate.gov/public/index.cfm?p=RuleXXV

The Vermont Legislature. (2006). *Legislative Action on Health Care*. Retrieved from http://www.leg.state.vt.us/HealthCare/2006LegAction.htm

The Vermont Legislature. (2011). *An act relating to a universal and unified health system. Public Act 48*. Retrieved from http://www.leg.state.vt.us/docs/2012/Acts/ACT048.pdf

Veterans Administration. (n.d.). *Patient Aligned Care Teams*. Retrieved from http://www.va.gov/health/services/primarycare/pact/index.asp

Veterans Administration. (2015). *About VA, History*. Retrieved from http://www.va.gov/about_va/vahistory.asp

Veterans Administration Office of the Inspector General Veterans. (2014). *Review of patient wait times, scheduling practices and alleged patient deaths at the Phoenix Health Care System*. Retrieved from https://www.documentcloud.org/documents/1174886-vaoig-14-02603-178.html

Veterans Health Administration.(n.d.). Retrieved from http://www.va.gov/health/

Wall Street Journal. (2014). *The definition of insanity*. Retrieved from http://files.www.cmhnetwork.org/media-center/morning-zen/WSJ-editorial-SAMHSA/The-definition-of-insanity.pdf

White House. (n.d.). *The President's Cabinet*. Retrieved from https://www.whitehouse.gov/photos-and-video/video/inside-white-house-cabinet

White House. (2010a, February 25). *Discussion of Cost Containment at Bipartisan Meeting On Health Care Reform*. Retrieved from https://www.whitehouse.gov/the-press-office/discussion-cost-containment-bipartisan-meeting-health-care-reform

White House. (2010b, March 5). *White House Forum on Health Reform*. Retrieved from https://www.whitehouse.gov/assets/documents/White_House_Forum_on_Health_Reform_Report.pdf

White House. (2015a). *National HIV/AIDS strategy: Updated to 2020*. Retrieved from https://www.whitehouse.gov/sites/default/files/docs/national_hiv_aids_strategy_update_2020.pdf

White House. (2015b). *Budget of the United States government, Fiscal Year 2016.Historical tables. Table 5.2, Budget Authority by Agency 1976-2020*. Retrieved from https://www.whitehouse.gov/omb/budget/Historicals

Woodcock, J. (2012, May). *Todays' biomedical innovation: Lost in translation?* Lecture at the UCSF California Institute for Quantitative Biosciences. Retrieved from http://www.ucsf.edu/news/2012/05/11991/fda-official-says-drug-advances-could-get-boost-academic-medical-centers

Woodcock, J. (2015). *Transcript: Director's Corner Podcast-Looking back and moving forward*. Retrieved from http://www.fda.gov/Drugs/NewsEvents/ucm433971.htm

World Bank. (2013). *Health Expenditure, total (% GDP), 2013*. Retrieved from http://data.worldbank.org/indicator/SH.XPD.TOTL.ZS/

World Health Organization. (1946). Preamble to the Constitution of the World Health Organization as adopted by the International Health Conference, New York, 19–22 June, 1946; signed on 22 July 1946 by the representatives of 61 States (Official Records of the World Health Organization, no. 2, p. 100) and entered into force on 7 April 1948. http://www.who.int/governance/eb/who_constitution_en.pdf

PART

III

ECONOMIC ASPECTS OF HEALTHCARE DELIVERY

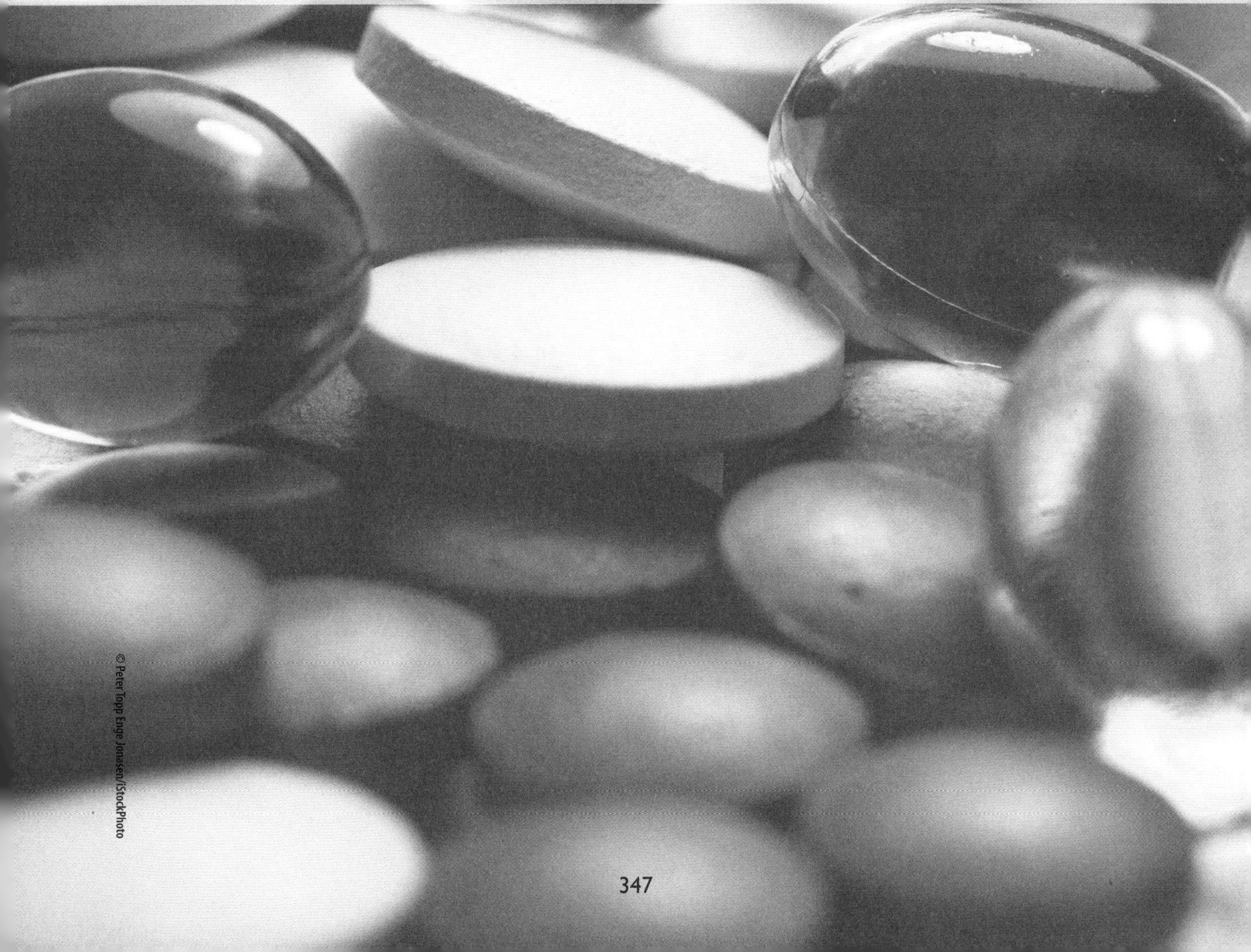

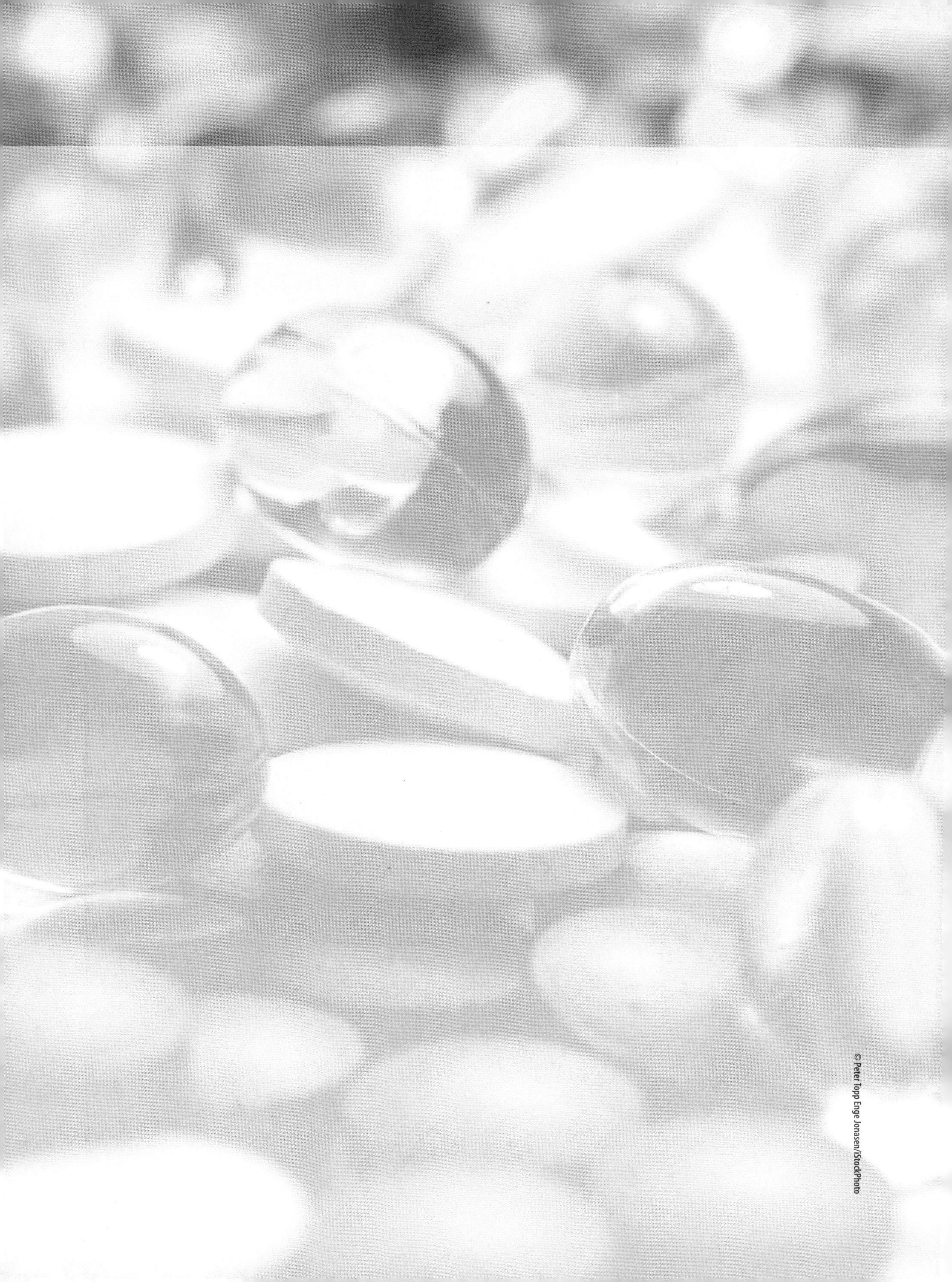

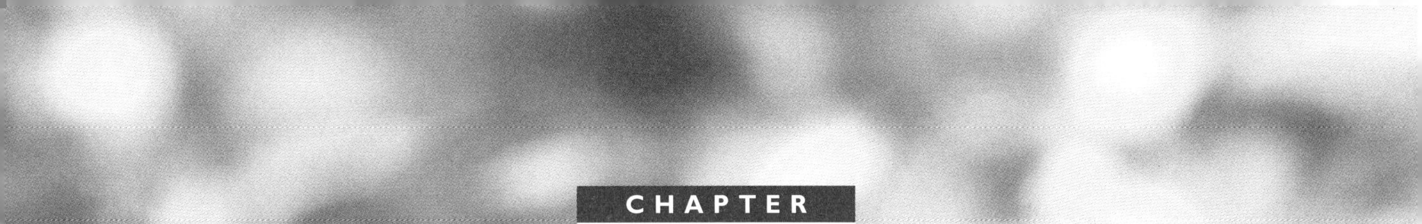

CHAPTER

14

Basic Economic Principles Affecting Health Care

Kenneth W. Schafermeyer and Scott K. Griggs

Case Scenario

Angie Plasty, a recent pharmacy graduate, is trying to determine the reasons for a 15% increase in prescription drug expenditures for a large managed care organization. Angie attributes some of the increased expenditures to the growing number of high-priced specialty medications, increases in the prices of some generic medications, as well as manufacturers' price increases. While modest price increases for some commodities can result in large decreases in quantity demanded and, therefore, a decrease in total expenditures, Angie knows that this is not true for most healthcare services, including prescription drugs. Of even greater concern to Angie, however, is that the prescription drug program experienced a large increase in prescription utilization rates.

Before she can suggest any solutions, Angie must first know the factors that contributed to an increase in demand for prescription drugs. She also needs to know why the quantity of prescription drugs demanded continues to increase even while prices are increasing.

What recommendations could Angie make to try to control the increases in prescription drug expenditures? To answer these questions adequately, one needs to understand some of the basic economic principles affecting health care.

LEARNING OBJECTIVES

Upon completion of this chapter, the student shall be able to:

- Define the basic economic concepts of utility, demand, supply, equilibrium price, the price system, price discrimination, and elasticity of demand.
- Explain the factors that cause a change in the demand or supply of a product or service.
- Determine the impact that a change in demand or supply will have on the equilibrium price and equilibrium quantity of a product or service.
- Explain how elasticity of demand influences the effect that a change in price will have on the total revenue earned by a firm.

CHAPTER QUESTIONS

1. What factors cause changes in the supply or demand of a product or service?
2. How does a change in the supply or demand of a commodity affect its price and the quantity sold?
3. Under what circumstances will an increase in the price of a company's product result in either an increase or a decrease in the total revenue earned by the firm?
4. What factors cause consumers to be more sensitive to changes in price?

INTRODUCTION

Economics is involved in nearly all contemporary issues facing health care, such as the growing demand for healthcare products and services, prices for pharmaceuticals, competition and consolidation among healthcare organizations, and remuneration for healthcare professionals. Economics encompasses an understanding of value, efficiency, opportunities, trade-offs, elasticity, and incentives, as well as how consumers (e.g., patients) and producers react to changing conditions. In essence, economics investigates how people utilize their limited resources to most efficiently meet their needs. Maybe you're asking yourself, "Why is understanding economics important to me and my future as a healthcare professional?" To assist in answering that question, let's consider a few economic questions:

General:

- How does a company determine what to sell...and who to hire?
- How do you determine what you will buy, to achieve the best value, given your limited resources (money)?
- How does an economic boom (or recession) affect consumer demand for varying products and services?
- How would an economic boom (or recession) alter a person's decision to go to college or graduate school?
- What are the economic incentives (or disincentives) to seeking full-time versus part-time employment regarding issues such as insurance, childcare, and quality of life?
- What is the result of a price increase (or decrease) on the number of items that an individual will purchase?

Health care:

- How would a shortage (or surplus) of nurses/pharmacists/physicians affect their salaries?
- How does increasing health insurance coverage (e.g., due to the Affordable Care Act) affect healthcare demand?
- How does the use of automated prescription dispensing systems (or mail order prescription dispensing) affect pharmacists, pharmacy, and health care?
- With an aging population that is also living longer, how will the healthcare market (and the pharmacy market) adjust to meet this increase in demand?
- If a product or service is subsidized (such as a government subsidy for health insurance premiums) or taxed, how will the quantity demanded of the product or service be changed?
- If patients anticipate there will be a shortage of a product or service (such as the flu vaccination), will either supply or demand be affected and how?
- As healthcare resources are limited, does the system distribute these goods and services equitably...or efficiently? If not, why?

These questions highlight the importance of economics from a personal as well as a professional perspective. As you will discover through this and future chapters, economics will significantly affect your career in health care and pharmacy, but understanding economics will also impact your understanding of society, business, politics, and the world. In a broad sense, economics can inform healthcare professionals and policy makers as to how health care can be both organized and financed in the United States as well as in other countries around the world. As a healthcare professional and manager, economics gives you a rational decision-making framework to focus on critical issues and recognize how consumers (i.e., patients) perceive value. In a more personal sense, economics can assist each of us in making better value-based decisions, given limited resources, about what, when, and how much to purchase, such as at the grocery store. A lack of understanding of basic economic principles, however, contributes to faulty decision making—people form opinions on issues based on emotions and feelings rather than on sound economic principles.

Using real-world examples, this chapter examines the fundamental economic principles that govern how the price system allocates resources in various industries, especially health care. It describes the concepts of utility, demand, supply, and equilibrium price; the causes of shortages and surpluses, the price system, price discrimination, and the effect of elasticity of demand on a firm's pricing decisions and total revenue. Knowledge of basic economic principles will help students and practitioners understand and respond to the economic forces shaping the healthcare market.

ECONOMIC CONCEPTS IN INDIVIDUAL CONSUMER DECISION MAKING

Consumers' wants may be considered limitless. Our society has never had enough resources to meet the demands of everyone. Because of this scarcity of resources, the science of economics has been developed. Economists have defined economics as "the study of how individuals and societies allocate their limited resources in attempts to satisfy their unlimited wants." The study of economics seeks to answer three important questions:

1. What shall we produce with society's limited resources?
2. How shall they (resources) be used in production?
3. Who shall receive the resulting goods and services?

Utility is the economic term for satisfaction obtained from purchasing a particular good or service. Utility is difficult to measure. For example, if a person eats a pizza, he or she would receive some satisfaction, but the amount of satisfaction could be described only in hypothetical terms. We may conclude with confidence, however, that the pizza provided some utility. Economics assumes that an individual's behavior reflects rational self-interest. People therefore allocate their time, energy, and money to maximize their utility. Their decisions, weighing both costs and the benefits, are purposeful (not random) with a desired outcome in mind. Therefore, people continually try to maximize their utility, usually within their budget constraints. Generally speaking, if the utility of a good is greater than its cost, people will buy more of that good. Conversely, when the cost exceeds a good's utility, they will not purchase it.

As stated previously, we have an economic system for only one reason: resources are scarce relative to human wants. Our three basic resources are (1) land, including all natural resources; (2) labor; and (3) capital, including physical resources produced by labor. Economists refer to these resources as factors of production because they are used to produce those things that people desire, which are called commodities. Commodities may be divided into goods and services. Pharmacists provide both goods and services, although when a transaction involves both, they typically receive reimbursement only for the product. However, as pharmacists learn to market cognitive services separately from products, they are beginning to find ways to be reimbursed for these services.

Cost originates from constraints on our resources. With unlimited resources, every good would be free, like air. In reality, we live in a state of economic scarcity. Economic resources, therefore, are allocated according to the price system. Most goods and services are obtained only by those individuals who are willing and able to pay for them.

If no limits existed on resources, goods would have no monetary value because we would use them until totally satisfied. Also, the marginal utility of any good would be zero because the value of any commodity is determined by its marginal utility. Value, then, originates from our personal desires and oftentimes changes over time.

Marginal is the economic term for "extra." Thus the value of a good is measured by its marginal utility. For example, the marginal utility of purchasing one pair of tennis shoes may be high if you currently do not have any tennis shoes, but the marginal utility of purchasing a second pair of tennis shoes at the same time would be lower.

When someone decides to make a purchase, he or she is, in a sense, deciding to forgo some other use of that money. This trade-off is known as an opportunity cost, the value of the best forgone use of a given resource. For example, if a person has enough money for only one pair of shoes, the shoes he or she buys will not only cost the money he or she pays for them, but also the satisfaction (utility) that he or she gives up by not being able to spend that money on something else, such as a new pair of pants. An example that every college student understands is that the true economic cost of going to school full time is more than just the cost of tuition, books, and other direct expenditures; it also includes the loss of the income that could have been earned had the student decided to work rather than go to school. Although this lost income is not a direct expenditure, it certainly is an opportunity cost.

LAW OF DIMINISHING MARGINAL UTILITY

The *law of diminishing marginal utility* states that the value of any additional goods declines as one consumes more of it. In other words, the more we have of a good, the less we desire more of it. A person who likes pizza will receive some utility if he or she eats a piece of pizza for lunch. If the same person eats a second piece, it provides less utility than the first one. A third piece of pizza would provide still less utility. Eventually, the cost of a pizza would exceed its marginal utility, and the person would not purchase more (**Table 14-1**).

Table 14-1 Illustration of the Law of Diminishing Marginal Utility

Quantity consumed	Total utility	Marginal utility
0	0	—
1	3	3
2	5	2
3	6	1
4	6	0

THE LAW OF DEMAND

The two most important economic concepts are demand and supply. The theories of supply and demand explain how millions of individual consumer and supplier decisions interact to determine market prices for available goods and services. Buyers exert a market force on prices by the amount of goods and services they demand, and suppliers exert a market force based on their ability and willingness to supply products for consumption.

A demand schedule shows the various amounts of a commodity consumers are willing and able to purchase at each specific price in a set of possible prices during some specified period of time. Note that demand is not synonymous with "need" or "want." As the term is used in economics, for a person to have a demand, he or she must have both the ability and willingness to pay. Merely wanting a given commodity that he or she cannot afford or is not willing to buy does not constitute a demand for that commodity.

Table 14-2 shows a hypothetical demand schedule for pizza. Two variables exist: (1) the price charged (independent variable) and (2) the quantity demanded at each given price (dependent variable). It is assumed, for the sake of simplicity, that all other variables are held constant—this simplification of limiting economic models to only two variables is known by the Latin phrase, *ceteris paribus*, literally meaning "all else being equal." According to the table, as the price of pizza increases, less of it is purchased. This illustrates the *law of demand:* As price falls, the corresponding quantity demanded rises; alternatively, as price increases, the corresponding quantity demanded falls. In short, an inverse relationship exists between price and quantity demanded.

The Demand Curve

The law of demand can be illustrated by drawing a demand curve. **Figure 14-1** represents the demand curve for the demand schedule shown in Table 14-2. Readers who have not been exposed to economics before may notice two unusual things about Figure 14-1. First, the relationship between the two variables is often illustrated as a straight line, even though we still call it a "curve." Second, the independent variable (the price charged for the commodity) is plotted on the Y-axis rather than the more conventional way of plotting it on the X-axis. Demand curves slope downward and to the right. This graphic illustration of the data in Table 14-2 shows the inverse relationship between the price of pizzas and the quantity demanded.

Table 14-2 Demand Schedule for Pizza

Price per pizza	Pizzas purchased per week
$6	80
$8	64
$10	48
$12	32
$14	16

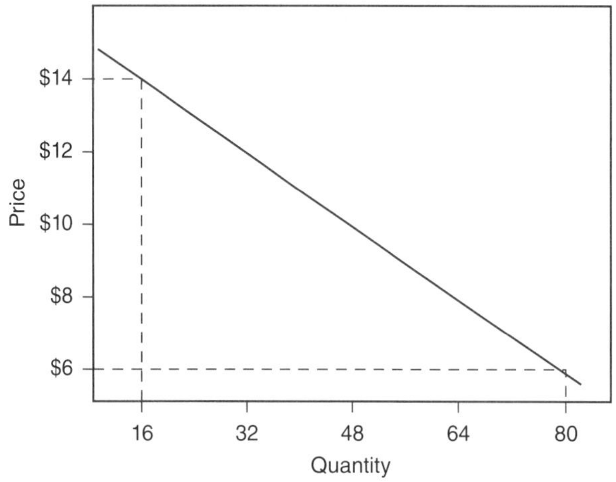

Figure 14-1 A Demand Curve for Pizza.

Changes in Demand

It is important to distinguish between the terms "change in quantity demanded" and "change in demand." A change in quantity demanded refers to movement along a given demand curve. In Figure 14-1, for example, a decrease in the price of a pizza from $10 to $8 results in an increase in the quantity demanded, from 48 to 64 pizzas. This increase is referred to as a change in the quantity demanded.

Some factors can result in an entire demand curve shifting; this movement is referred to as a change in demand. **Figure 14-2** shows that demand curve *D* has moved to the right toward demand curve D_1, representing what is meant by a change in demand. Since the demand curve has shifted to the right, the demand has increased. A movement from right to left would mean demand has decreased.

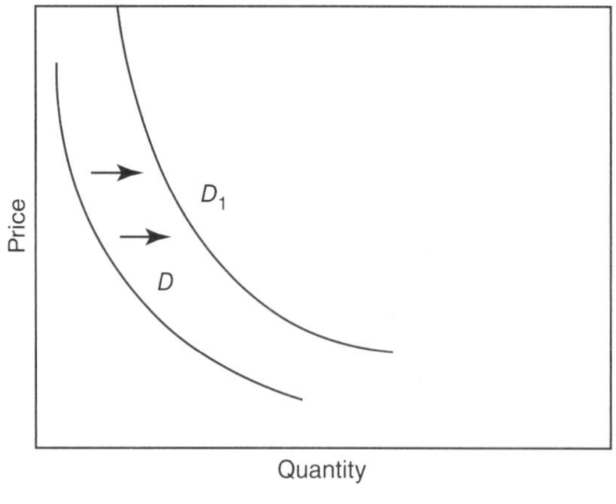

Figure 14-2 Illustration of a Change in Demand.

Changes in one or more of five factors can cause consumers to change their demand for a good:

- Prices of related goods
- Money income of the consumer
- Number of consumers in the market
- Attitudes, tastes, and preferences of the consumer
- Consumer expectations with respect to future prices and incomes

Prices of Related Goods

When the price of one good and the demand for another good are directly related, the pair are called substitute goods. An example is the relationship between beef and chicken. As the price of beef increases, the demand for chicken increases (assuming the chicken was reasonably priced), all else being equal. As another example, increases in coffee prices cause the demand for tea to increase. To some degree, many drugs or drug classes may be substitutes for each other (e.g., aspirin, acetaminophen, nonsteroidal anti-inflammatory drugs [NSAIDs], and now COX-2 inhibitors).

When the price of one good and the demand for another good are inversely related, the two products are referred to as complementary goods. In this case, an increase in the price of one good may cause a decrease in the demand for another good. An example would be the relationship between computer printers and printer cartridges. As the price of computer printers decreases, more people will purchase them, thus causing an increase in the demand for printer cartridges. Additional examples of complementary goods might include peanut butter and jelly, lettuce and salad dressing, or ice cream and ice cream toppings. In the prescription market, potassium supplements are often complements of potassium-depleting diuretics. For some patients taking NSAIDs, antacids, H_2 antagonists, or proton pump inhibitors may be complementary products.

Money Income of the Consumer

Commodities whose demand increases with an increase in consumer income are called superior or normal goods. Examples include sirloin steak, new sports cars, and summer homes. Because the demand for healthcare services increases as consumers' incomes rise, health care is a normal good. (Poor people may have as much need for health care, of course, but their demand—their ability and willingness to pay—is less than that of wealthier individuals. This helps to explain why a higher concentration of hospitals and physicians exists in high-income areas than in the inner city.)

If the demand for a good decreases as income increases, it is known as an inferior good. Examples include used cars and generic liquor or film. An example of an inferior good related to pharmacy could be the inexpensive prescription medication, promethazine, often used for morning sickness versus the superior but much more expensive prescription medication, ondansetron, a 5-HT_3 receptor antagonist.

Number of Consumers in the Market

If a manufacturer is able to attract new customers to a market, demand naturally increases (the demand curve shifts to the right). For example, the U.S. Postal Service discovered that it could increase the number of stamp collectors (and increase its revenue) by creating stamps that are more appealing to children (e.g., cartoon characters rather than historical events or "old dead guys"). Likewise, breweries and cigarette companies have allegedly increased demand for their products by attracting newer, younger customers with advertising featuring cartoon characters.

Manufacturers also use a variety of strategies to increase the number of consumers who are willing to purchase a particular type of pharmaceutical product. That explains why aspirin products are promoted as treatments for minor arthritis, and arthritis products are promoted as treatments for headaches and assorted pains. By finding new indications for prescription drugs, for example, the number of customers (and consequently, demand) for these products will increase. One example is the use of calcium-channel blockers (originally used for treatment of angina) for prevention of migraine headaches. Another example is minoxidil, which was originally marketed as Loniten for treatment of hypertension, but reformulated as Rogaine for hair growth applications.

Attitudes, Tastes, and Preferences of the Consumer

Consumer attitudes, tastes, and preferences are affected greatly by advertising or by fashion changes. The manufacturer of NyQuil liquid cold medicine, for example, created a demand for its product by marketing it as a medication that works while a person is sleeping. This appeal, combined with the distinguishing characteristic that the medication was a liquid rather than a tablet or capsule, resulted in an increased demand for the product, and NyQuil's sales skyrocketed. Conversely, the environmental concerns associated with polystyrene containers for fast food decreased demand for products that use such materials.

Consumer Expectations

A good example of how consumer expectations of future prices and personal incomes affect demand was seen in the demand for oranges. Newspapers published articles reporting that Florida's orange crop had been badly damaged by freezing weather, and suggested this shortage of oranges would cause orange juice prices to rise in the United States. Consumers responded by immediately buying several cans of frozen orange juice concentrate to have on hand when orange juice prices were high. The grocers understood economics and had read the same newspaper articles, so they immediately raised the price of orange juice.

As another example, consider the housing market. Despite tremendous increases in the cost of building a home, the number of houses being built has tended to increase over the years. Two reasons underlie this increase: (1) Economists predicted that housing costs would continue to rise, so people are deciding to build now before costs go any higher; and (2) people anticipated a continual growth in their incomes, so they built homes based on what they expected to earn.

In summary, an increase in the demand for Product X can be caused by any of the following:

- An increase in the price of Product Y if it is a substitute for Product X
- A decrease in the price of Product Y if it is a complement to Product X
- A rise in one's income if Product X is a normal good
- A decrease in one's income if Product X is an inferior good
- An increase in the number of buyers for Product X in the market
- A favorable change in the consumer tastes for Product X
- Consumer expectation that the price of Product X will increase in the future

The case scenario at the beginning of this chapter described an increase in the demand for prescription drugs. This increase in demand could have been due to several factors: (1) an increase in enrollment in health plans, (2) an increase in the average age of enrollees, (3) an increase in the cost of alternative therapies such as surgery, or (4) an increase in physicians' and patients' tastes and preferences in response to the increase in drug advertising aimed directly at consumers. Examples of factors that can affect the demand for healthcare services are shown in **Table 14-3**.

Table 14-3 Factors that Affect Demand for Healthcare Services

Cause for change in demand	Explanation	Examples
Prices of related goods 1) Substitutes 2) Complements	Assuming: A is a substitute for B and X is a complement of Y 1) ↑ price of product A = ↑ demand for B 2) ↑ price of product X = ↓ demand for Y	1) ↑ price of brand-name products = ↑ demand for generics 2) ↑ price of NSAIDs = ↓ demand for antacid
Consumers' incomes	↑ income = ↑ demand	↓ income = ↑ self treatment ↑ income = ↑ demand for physician visits and elective surgery
Number of consumers	↑ population = ↑ demand	New indications for old drugs = ↑ demand Aging of population = ↑ drug use
Attitudes, tastes, and preferences	↑ preferences = ↑ demand	↑ advertising of prescription drugs = ↑ drug use
Expectations	Expected shortage or price increase in future = ↑ demand	Fear of flu vaccine shortage = ↑ demand for flu vaccine

EXERCISE 1: CHANGE IN DEMAND

A rightward shift in the demand curve for a commodity means that:

a. Consumers' incomes may have fallen.
b. Supply conditions are more favorable.
c. Consumers are willing to buy more of the good at each price than previously.
d. The price of the commodity has decreased.

Answer

Answer "a" is incorrect because a drop in buyers' incomes would decrease their ability and willingness to pay and, therefore, decrease their demand, which would be represented by a leftward shift of the demand curve.

Answer "b" is incorrect because a change in supply does not cause a change in demand. Supply and demand are affected by different sets of factors.

Answer "c" is correct because a rightward shift in the demand curve represents an increase in demand. Because of this increase in demand, consumers are willing to buy more at each given price.

Answer "d" is incorrect because a change in price causes a change in the quantity demanded, not a change in demand. In other words, a given demand curve represents the various quantities that would be demanded by consumers for each of the prices that may be charged by the seller. A change in price simply moves you up and down the curve; it does not change the curve itself.

EXERCISE 2: CHANGE IN DEMAND

If the price of Product A decreases, what is the effect on Product B (a substitute)?

a. The quantity demanded for Product B increases.
b. The quantity demanded for Product B decreases.
c. The demand increases for Product B.
d. The demand decreases for Product B.
e. The supply increases.
f. The supply decreases.

Answer

Answers "a" and "b" are incorrect because a change in price of a product causes a change in the demand of a substitute product, not a change in quantity demanded. In other words, the demand curve itself is changed; you do not just move up and down the curve.

Answer "c" is incorrect because a decrease in the price of Product A means that more consumers will switch from B to A, thereby decreasing the amount of B that people buy at a given price.

Answer "d" is correct for the same reason.

Answers "e" and "f" are incorrect because a change in the price of Product A changes the demand but has no effect on the supply curves. A change in demand does not cause a change in supply. Supply and demand are affected by independent factors.

THE LAW OF SUPPLY

Supply, like demand, can be depicted as a schedule. A supply schedule shows the number of goods or services offered for sale at specific prices during some specified period of time. **Table 14-4** shows a hypothetical supply schedule for a producer of pizza. Again, only two variables are considered; all others are assumed to be held constant. The independent variable in this case is the price that consumers are willing to pay. Notice that there is a subtle difference between this variable and the independent variable for the demand schedule. For the demand schedule, the independent variable is the price charged; for the supply schedule, the independent variable is the price customers are willing to pay.

The dependent variable for the supply schedule is the quantity that sellers are willing to supply at each given price. As shown in Table 14-4, as the price that consumers are willing to pay increases, more pizzas are produced. This illustrates the *law of supply,* which states that as the price that people are willing to pay rises, the corresponding quantity supplied also increases. In short, a direct relationship exists between price and quantity supplied.

Table 14-4 Supply Schedule for Pizza

Price per pizza	Pizzas produced per week
$6	24
$8	36
$10	48
$12	60
$14	72

The Supply Curve

Just as the law of demand was illustrated by drawing a demand curve, so the law of supply can be illustrated with a supply curve. **Figure 14-3** illustrates the supply curve for the supply schedule given in Table 14-4. Supply curves slope upward to the right, in this case illustrating a direct relationship between the price that people are willing to pay for pizza and the quantity supplied to consumers.

Changes in Supply

The terms "change in quantity supplied" and "change in supply" are used similarly to those discussed under demand. Whereas changes in the quantity supplied are caused only by changes in prices people are willing to pay, changes in several factors can bring about a change in supply:

- Techniques of production, including technology
- Number of sellers in the market

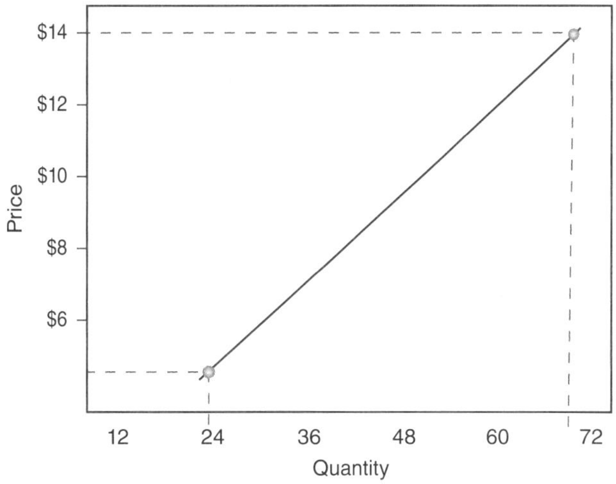

Figure 14-3 A Supply Curve for Pizza.

- Resource costs (e.g., materials, wages, taxes)
- Prices for related goods
- Sellers' expectations

Note that a change in supply is NOT caused by a change in demand; supply and demand are independent.

Techniques of Production

When technology advances, the costs of production usually decrease. At a given price, suppliers will make more profits and, consequently, are willing to produce more. Technological advances could include equipment (e.g., more efficient tractors), supplies (e.g., genetically engineered seeds), methods of production (e.g., crop rotation), or management techniques (e.g., using the advice of agricultural experts).

Number of Sellers in the Market

More producers create more output. Therefore, as the number of sellers in a market increases, supply also increases. This outcome is represented by a rightward shift in the supply curve.

Resource Costs

As the costs of resources (e.g., materials, labor, rents, interest rates) increase, sellers cannot make as much profit at a given price. Companies, therefore, have less incentive to produce when input costs increase. However, a decrease in resource costs will cause supply to increase. Lower fertilizer prices, for example, can lead to an increase in agricultural production that will encourage farmers to produce more. Some employers have used this same principle to predict that increases in the minimum wage would hurt production levels. If sellers incur an additional expense, in the form of a tax increase, then the cost of producing that good or service has increased and thus reduces supply. Conversely, if a seller receives a subsidy, say from the government, then the production cost would be lowered and supply increased.

Prices for Related Goods

Producers recognize two types of related goods: (1) substitute products and (2) joint products. Substitute products are those that are produced with the same, or similar, inputs. If the price of one product increases, it will affect the supply of another product. For example, if the price of wheat increases, farmers will start growing less corn and more wheat. Therefore, the price of wheat affects the supply of corn.

Goods that are almost always produced together are known as joint products. Leather and beef, for example, are joint products because they cannot be produced separately. An increase in the price of beef will induce a greater quantity of beef supplied; consequently, the supply of leather will increase even if the price of leather falls.

Seller Expectations

If sellers expect prices to increase in the near future, they may increase production now or withhold some product from the market. This happens in agriculture when farmers try to time their sales to obtain favorable prices.

Examples of factors that affect the supply of healthcare services are shown in **Table 14-5**.

Table 14-5 Factors that Affect Supply of Healthcare Services

Cause for change in supply	Explanation	Examples
Prices of related goods 1) Substitutes 2) Joint products	Assuming: A = substitute for B and W = joint product with Z 1) ↑ price of product A = ↓ supply of B 2) ↑ price of product W = ↑ supply for Z	1) ↑ reimbursement for generic substitutes = ↓ brand-name drugs supplied 2) ↑ reimbursement for teaching hospitals = ↑ amount of medical education
Resource costs	↑ production cost = ↓ supply	↑ wages = ↓ personnel hours
Production technology	↑ technology = ↓ production cost = ↑ supply	↑ department automation = ↓ cost to dispense a prescription and ↑ willingness to supply prescriptions
Number of sellers	↑ number of sellers = ↑ supply and ↓ price	↑ number of generic companies = ↑ number of generic products supplied and ↓ price for generic products

EQUILIBRIUM PRICE

The price system—the interaction of supply and demand—determines how economic resources are allocated. Because buyers in any market always want to demand more units of a good at a lower price and sellers always want to supply more units of that good at a higher price, a market equilibrium price can be achieved, which creates economic efficiency by exactly balancing these competing market forces. This market equilibrium price represents the point where the supply and demand curves intersect, as illustrated in **Figure 14-4**.

In this case, market equilibrium occurs when pizza is priced at $10. At that price, the quantity demanded equals the quantity supplied. At the equilibrium price of $10, both the seller and the buyer are satisfied with the price. At any price other than $10, economic forces will attempt to change the price. These economic forces can be illustrated with two cases.

Case 1: Price increases to $12. At a price of $12, pizza sellers produce 60 pizzas, whereas consumers want to buy only 32 pizzas. Thus a surplus (excess supply) of pizza exists. What happens? Consumers buy only 32 pizzas. Eventually, one pizza seller will lower the price to get rid of unsold pizza, which will increase the quantity demanded for the product. Other sellers also lower their prices until at $10 the demands of the consumers equal what the sellers are willing to produce at that price.

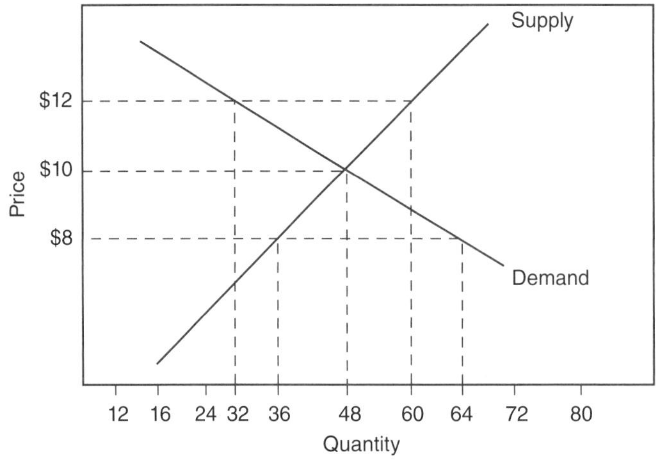

Figure 14-4 Supply and Demand Curve for Pizza.

Case 2: Price decreases to $8. At a price of $8, pizza sellers produce 36 pizzas, whereas consumers want to buy 64. Thus a shortage (excess demand) for pizza exists. What happens? Consumers order a pizza, but the seller is sold out. The seller notices that each day every pizza produced is sold. Consumers might even be calling the seller to say they will pay extra if a pizza is saved for them. This increased demand and the opportunity to increase the price serve as incentives for the seller to produce more pizza. When the price reaches $10, both the seller and the buyer are satisfied. Everyone who wants to buy a pizza does, and the seller does not have any unsold pizza remaining.

EXERCISE 3: CHANGE IN EQUILIBRIUM DUE TO AN INCREASE IN SUPPLY

When supply increases in a competitive market:

a. Equilibrium price will fall.
b. Demand will fall.
c. Shortages will emerge.
d. Quantities sold will decrease.

Answer

Answer "a" is correct because the new supply curve will shift to the right and intersect with the demand curve at a new point that represents both a decrease in equilibrium price and an increase in equilibrium quantity (**Figure 14-5**).

Answer "b" is incorrect because a change in supply does not cause a change in demand. Supply and demand are affected by independent factors.

Answer "c" is incorrect because an increase in supply will result in a temporary surplus, which will be corrected when prices drop to a new equilibrium point. At this new equilibrium point, the quantity demanded will equal the quantity supplied.

Answer "d" is incorrect for the same reason given for answer "a."

Note that the equilibrium would also change when there is a change in demand. The increased demand for prescription drugs discussed in the case scenario at the beginning of this chapter, for example, resulted in increases in both the price and the quantity of prescription drugs dispensed.

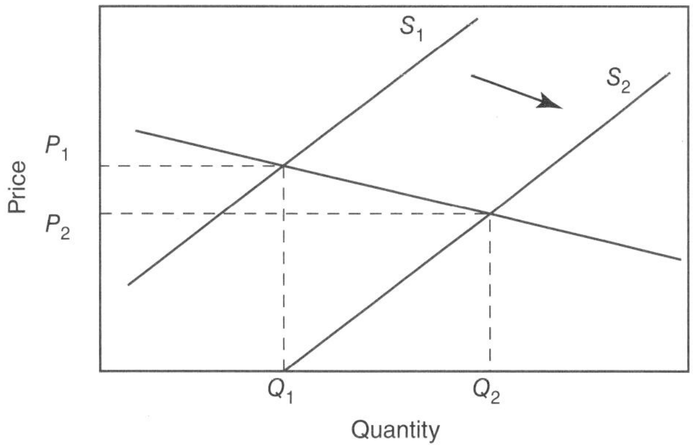

Figure 14-5 Change in Equilibrium for a Product with an Elastic Demand.

ELASTICITY OF DEMAND

Elasticity is a widely used economic concept that measures the responsiveness (or sensitivity) of consumer demands to a change in price. As stated previously, the demand curve slopes downward because as the price of a commodity decreases, the quantity demanded increases. However, the degree (or angle) of this downward slope varies with different types of goods. Depending on the slope, a commodity is said to have an elastic demand, an inelastic demand, or a unitary demand.

The producers (or sellers) of any good typically can charge whatever price they desire. Naturally, they will try to sell the good at a price that maximizes their profits. If they think they can make more money by lowering the price, they will do so. Likewise, if they think they can make more money by raising the price, they will do so. The key factor in such an analysis is not the good's selling price, but rather the total revenue the producer receives. This total revenue equals the selling price multiplied by the quantity sold. Whether a change in the selling price will result in an increase or a decrease in total revenue depends on the elasticity of demand for the particular good.

Elastic Demand

Suppose a producer is faced with the demand schedule shown in **Table 14-6** for one of its goods. As the price of the good increases, the producer's total revenue decreases. This relationship

Table 14-6 Demand Schedule for an Elastic Good

Price	Expected number to be sold	Total revenue
$2	56	$112
$3	36	$108
$4	26	$104
$5	20	$100

characterizes a good with an elastic demand. Demand is elastic if an increase in price causes the quantity demanded to decrease enough to result in a decrease in total revenue. Conversely, a decrease in price causes the quantity to increase enough to result in an increase in total revenue. Thus, when a good has an elastic demand, the quantity demanded is sensitive to the price.

Many consumer goods that have substitutes have an elastic demand. As long as chicken is seen as a substitute for beef, the demand for beef will be relatively elastic. For example, if the price of beef were to double, consumption of beef would decrease significantly because consumers could easily find substitutes that would satisfy them.

Another example of a good with an elastic demand is a brand of gasoline. If a Shell Oil gas station proprietor lowered his or her price below the competitor's price, sales likely would increase so much that total revenue would increase. The opposite outcome will occur if prices are raised above other brands. That is why gasoline prices are often standardized within a community; the demand for any brand of gasoline is extremely sensitive to price. (Note that gasoline is narrowly and specifically defined here as a particular brand of gasoline at a particular station, and it is understood that this station's gasoline has interchangeable substitutes at many competing stations. When we look at prices for gasoline in general, rather than prices at particular stations, demand is more inelastic.)

Inelastic Demand

Suppose a producer is faced with a demand schedule like the one shown in **Table 14-7** for one of its goods. As the price of the good increases, total revenue increases. This relationship characterizes a good with an inelastic demand. With inelastic demand, an increase in price causes only a slight decrease in the quantity demanded, resulting in an increase in total revenue. Conversely, a decrease in price causes the quantity demanded to increase, but the increase is so small that the result is a decrease in total revenue. Thus, when a good has an inelastic demand, the quantity demanded is relatively insensitive to price.

Note that when graphing demand curves, those with an inelastic demand curve will be steeper or more vertical than those with an elastic demand, which will tend to be flatter and more horizontal.

An example of a good with an inelastic demand is gasoline (when broadly defined as noted in the preceding section). An automobile will not operate without gasoline, so when the price of gasoline increases, people will buy a little less, but they will still buy enough to give the gas station proprietor an increase in total revenue. Thus gasoline has a relatively inelastic demand. Although the

Table 14-7 Demand Schedule for an Inelastic Good

Price	Expected number to be sold	Total revenue
$2	45	$90
$3	31	$93
$4	24	$96
$5	20	$100

Table 14-8 Demand Schedule for a Unitary Good

Price	Expected number to be sold	Total revenue
$2	50	$100
$2.50	40	$100
$4	25	$100
$5	20	$100

quantity of gasoline demanded by consumers does not tend to depend too much on price (inelastic demand), the quantity purchased at a particular station does depend on how prices at that station compare with the competitors' prices (elastic demand).

As described in the case scenario at the beginning of this chapter, studies show that the demand for healthcare services, including prescription drugs, is inelastic. People with true emergencies (such as a broken arm or a heart attack) will seek treatment without regard to the cost. Nevertheless, high prices may create an elastic demand for treatment of routine problems or minor ailments. This explains the rationale behind patient cost-sharing mechanisms, which are designed to discourage unnecessary use of services while not inhibiting demand for truly necessary services.

A logical question to ask at this point is this: If total revenue increases every time the price of an inelastic good increases, what keeps the price from rising to infinity? Usually competition keeps prices in check or, in the case where not much competition exists (such as public utilities), government intervention may be needed to regulate prices. Although managed care organizations in the United States have controlled costs by facilitating competition among some pharmaceutical products through generic and therapeutic substitution, government agencies in Canada and Europe control costs by regulating pharmaceutical manufacturers' prices.

Unitary Demand

Suppose a producer is faced with a demand schedule like the one shown in **Table 14-8** for one of its goods. As the price of the good increases or decreases, the producer's total revenue remains the same. This relationship characterizes a good with a unitary demand. Unitary demand is not common in the actual marketplace; instead, products tend to have either an elastic or inelastic demand.

EXERCISE 4: ELASTICITY OF DEMAND

If demand is price elastic, an increase in supply will cause a relatively

a. Large decrease in quantity demanded.
b. Large increase in quantity demanded.
c. Small decrease in quantity demanded.
d. Small increase in quantity demanded.

Answer

Answers "a" and "c" are incorrect because an increase in supply will result in an increase in quantity demanded.

Answer "b" is correct because an elastic demand curve, by definition, means that consumers are sensitive to changes in price and any change in price will result in a proportionately greater change in quantity demanded. Therefore, an increase in the supply of a product with an elastic demand curve will result in a large increase in quantity demanded (**Figure 14-5**).

Answer "d" is incorrect for the reason explained for answer "c."

DETERMINANTS OF ELASTICITY OF DEMAND

What makes the demand for a particular good or service elastic or inelastic in the short run? To differentiate between the terms "short run" and "long run," consider that a consumer has two resources when shopping: money and time. In other words, a person can purchase a demanded good with money now or wait until a later time when more money is available, when the price of the demanded commodity decreases, or when the consumer's demand may change to favor another commodity. Elasticity of demand for a given commodity changes when one talks about the short run versus the long run because a longer time span allows people to pursue more alternatives (substitutes).

For example, when the price of gasoline increases, automobile owners continue to buy gas in the short run because they need their cars for business or other important purposes. In the long run, alternative means of transportation such as buses, commuter trains, or carpools may be sought as companies continue to work on developing a car that operates on some form of energy other than gasoline. The desired result, of course, is eventually to decrease one's need for—and thus one's demand for—gasoline.

Three additional determinants of elasticity exist: (1) the availability of substitutes for the commodity, (2) the price of a commodity relative to consumers' incomes, and (3) the degree to which a commodity is a necessity or a luxury.

The Availability of Substitutes

When the price of one good and the demand for another good are directly related, the two products are substitute goods, like beef and chicken. The greater the number of substitute goods available for a particular commodity, the more elastic the demand for that commodity.

The more narrowly and specifically a commodity can be described, the more substitutes it will have. Consequently, the demand for such a commodity will be more elastic. For example, when a person is suffering from athlete's foot, he or she probably has a strong desire for an antifungal. Because no other kinds of over-the-counter (OTC) drugs will help relieve athlete's foot, the demand for antifungals is inelastic. Because numerous antifungal products are available, however, the demand for any particular brand of antifungal is elastic.

Sellers have found that some customers have more substitutes available than other customers. For example, business travelers are not as flexible in their plans as individuals planning vacations. Therefore, vacation travelers have a more elastic demand for air travel and can obtain less expensive airfares.

Segregating customers and charging prices according to customers' elasticity of demand is known as differential pricing (also known as price discrimination). Because hospitals and managed care organizations use formularies (and consequently have more substitutes available), they can obtain larger discounts or rebates from pharmaceutical manufacturers. Another example of differential pricing is the higher long-distance telephone rates charged during working hours as opposed to weekends and evenings. For price discrimination to work, it must be difficult for buyers to resell to one another. Price differences reflecting actual production cost differences, such as volume discounts, do not represent true price discrimination.

The Price Relative to Consumers' Incomes

The demand for commodities that account for a large portion of a person's income will be more elastic than the demand for purchases that are relatively inexpensive. For example, most managers are more price conscious when they are shopping for a computer than when shopping for envelopes or paper clips. Because envelopes and paper clips account for a negligible fraction of a company's budget, changes in price likely will have little effect on the quantity demanded. Thus the demand for these products is relatively inelastic.

Necessity versus Luxury

The greater degree to which a good is regarded as a "necessary" item as compared to a "luxury" item, the more inelastic the demand. A consumer will be less sensitive to the price of a necessary good, for example, insulin for a diabetic patient, electricity for a house/apartment, or gasoline for a car. Luxury items, such as chocolate, expensive food, vacation travel, entertainment, and jewelry, are much easier to reduce or eliminate when money is tight. While the necessary goods are relatively price inelastic, luxury items have much higher price elasticity.

EXERCISE 5: DETERMINANTS OF ELASTICITY OF DEMAND

Elasticity of demand will increase as the

a. Number of available substitutes decreases.
b. Price of the good relative to income decreases.
c. Time horizon increases.

Answer

Answer "a" is incorrect because the greater the number of substitute goods available for a particular commodity, the more elastic the demand for that commodity.

Answer "b" is incorrect because those commodities that account for a large portion of a person's income will have a more elastic demand than those purchases that are relatively inexpensive.

Answer "c" is correct because the longer time frame allows consumers to consider more alternatives and find more substitutes for a product in the long run.

ELASTICITY OF DEMAND FOR PRESCRIPTION DRUGS

The three determinants of elasticity can be applied to prescription drugs. First, when a physician writes a prescription order for a specific drug for an ambulatory patient, usually no substitute goods are involved. The patient has the choice of having the prescription filled. If he or she decides to have the prescription filled, the patient often has no choice as to which drug will be dispensed by the pharmacist. Product selection legislation gives the patient some choices in the case of a prescription with generic alternatives, so the demand for generic drugs is relatively elastic while the demand for drugs without generic equivalents is relatively inelastic. This situation is altered to some degree by the adoption of formularies and the practice of therapeutic selection. As described in more detail in the chapter on managed health care, two drug products in the same therapeutic class that are different chemical entities are more likely to be considered substitutes for each other within a hospital formulary system than in a community setting. Therefore, the elasticity of demand for these drug products would be higher within a hospital pharmacy setting than in a community pharmacy setting.

Second, prescription drugs usually (but not always) take up a relatively small portion of most people's income.

Third, prescription drugs are typically considered necessities. An antidepressant or an antiviral medication may be necessary to return the patient back to normal mental or physical health.

In summary, many prescription drugs have few—if any—substitutes; they take a relatively small portion of one's income (particularly if the patient pays only a copayment); and they are usually considered necessary. Thus a prescription drug has an inelastic demand. As described in the case scenario at the beginning of this chapter, the quantity demanded is relatively insensitive to changes in price.

Three additional factors unique to the pharmaceutical industry contribute to the inelasticity of demand for prescription drugs. First, the decision maker (the physician) is not the payer (the patient and/or prescription benefit plan); consequently, price is not usually the primary consideration when prescribing a particular drug. Second, the industry promotes product differentiation between drug products, reducing the importance of price in selecting a particular drug to prescribe. Third, having a third-party plan pay all or part of the cost of a person's prescription drugs significantly increases the inelasticity of demand for those drugs. These last three issues are described in more detail in the next chapter describing some of the unique aspects of health economics.

CONCLUSION

This chapter introduced some basic economic concepts, such as supply, demand, equilibrium price, the price system, price discrimination, and elasticity of demand. The next chapter discusses how economic forces in the healthcare marketplace compare with those of other industries and how health care can be influenced by competition.

Healthcare professionals should understand and use economic principles to work effectively with healthcare organizations and health benefit programs. By understanding these basic principles, one can begin to appreciate the factors affecting the economics of the healthcare industry.

QUESTIONS FOR FURTHER DISCUSSION

1. For most products, when substitutes appear in the market, the innovator must usually decrease its price to be competitive. Why don't the prices of brand-name prescription drugs tend to decline when generic substitutes become available?

2. What steps can be taken to control the rapid increase in the quantity demanded for prescription drugs?
3. A demand for a product or service exists only if the potential customers have the ability and willingness to pay for it. What would pharmacists have to do to be reimbursed for nondispensing services?
4. If many healthcare products and services have inelastic demand, how might companies compete with one another to increase their market shares?
5. Give examples of healthcare products or services that have an elastic demand. Do competitors compete on price?

KEY TOPICS AND TERMS

Changes in demand
Change in quantity demanded
Change in quantity supplied
Change in supply
Complements
Demand
Demand curve
Demand schedule
Economic resources
Economics
Elastic demand
Elasticity
Equilibrium point
Equilibrium price
Equilibrium quantity
Law of demand
Law of diminishing marginal utility
Law of supply
Marginal utility
Shortage
Substitutes
Supply
Supply curve
Supply schedule
Surplus
Utility

CHAPTER

15

Unique Aspects of Health Economics

Kenneth W. Schafermeyer

Case Scenario

There has been a great deal of controversy and debate over how to control rapidly rising healthcare costs and expand healthcare services to the millions of Americans who do not currently have health insurance. Some observers believe that these problems can be resolved by encouraging more competition into the healthcare system. Others believe that health care is such a unique industry that more competition will not necessarily create efficiencies that will reduce costs and improve access. Some members of the latter group also question the morality of using the price system to allocate healthcare resources.

Using your knowledge of economics and the healthcare system, what do you think are some of the arguments that would be used by both sides in this debate?

LEARNING OBJECTIVES

Upon completion of this chapter, the student shall be able to:

- Give examples of how basic economic principles apply to contemporary healthcare issues.
- Compare and contrast the various types of market structures: perfect competition, monopolistic competition, oligopoly, and monopoly.
- Explain how the economics of health care is different from the economics of other industries.
- Describe how economic performance of the healthcare system could be improved.
- Explain the factors that can cause healthcare costs to increase.
- Describe how various forms of reimbursement can create different incentives to control utilization of health care.

CHAPTER QUESTIONS

1. To what extent is health care a competitive industry? Does competition always result in decreases in price?
2. How is the economics of health care different from the economics of other industries?
3. What factors can cause healthcare costs to increase?
4. How do various forms of reimbursement create different incentives to control utilization of health care?

INTRODUCTION

This chapter is designed to help students and practitioners understand and respond to the economic forces shaping the healthcare market. The previous chapter presented the basic economic concepts of supply, demand, equilibrium price, the price system, price discrimination, and elasticity of demand. This chapter discusses some of the factors that influence supply and demand for healthcare services and describes how economic forces in the healthcare marketplace compare with those of other industries.

In recent years, there has been renewed interest in reforming the healthcare system through the use of market forces rather than government regulations. One example of such a "market-based policy" is the provision of subsidies to low-income patients for the purchase of health insurance rather than direct payments for healthcare services. Another example is the increased use of higher cost-sharing levels (Rice, 1997). The critical question, and the one discussed in this chapter, is this: Is the healthcare market a competitive market?

PERFECTLY COMPETITIVE INDUSTRIES

To describe the unique aspects of the healthcare market, it is helpful to compare it with the four basic types of market structures: (1) perfect competition, (2) monopolistic competition, (3) monopoly, and (4) oligopoly. First, this chapter describes a market structure known as perfect competition. Next, it contrasts the perfectly competitive market with the other types of market structures and discusses how the healthcare industry may or may not resemble one or more of these basic structures.

Perfect competition has the following characteristics:

- Many buyers and sellers
- Freedom of entry and exit
- Standardized products
- Full and free information
- No collusion

Many Buyers and Many Sellers

In perfect competition, the number of buyers and sellers has to be large enough so that the entry (or exit) of one firm or one customer into (or out of) the marketplace does not affect market prices. Companies in a perfectly competitive industry do not set prices; instead, prices are set by the market. These firms are referred to as "price takers, not price makers." The demand curve for a company's product is horizontal and referred to as perfectly elastic. In other words, if a single company increased its price, customers would not demand the product from that company—they would just switch to another company.

Freedom of Entry and Exit

Most industries have barriers to entry or exit. Entry barriers may consist of patents, licenses, zoning, environmental regulations, or large investments in technology, training, inventories, or fixed assets such as buildings, specialized equipment, or research and development. Exit barriers exist when a firm's fixed assets cannot be transferred to another use, thereby preventing a company from easily switching to a more profitable industry. Low barriers to entry into and exit from an industry stimulate competition; high barriers inhibit it. In perfect competition, there are no barriers to entry or exit.

Standardized Products

By "standardized products," we mean all products are similar and interchangeable and, therefore, many substitutes exist. Clothing, building materials, gasoline, tires, and many other products have standard sizes or grades, so consumers can easily identify substitutes. In perfect competition, products are perfectly substitutable for each other.

Full and Free Information

In perfect competition, customers have complete information on the prices of goods and services and can compare the prices offered by competing sellers. Equally important, consumers can identify and compare the quality of these goods and services.

No Collusion

In perfect competition, companies in a given industry compete with each other rather than colluding or getting together to set prices. Collusion is more likely to be successful when there are few sellers, because the competitors know each other well and can easily retaliate against each other if the agreement is broken. Because of its anticompetitive nature, collusion is illegal in the United States. Collusion does occur in international trade, where it is referred to as a cartel. The most famous cartel is the Organization of Petroleum Exporting Countries (OPEC).

Although no industries fit the perfectly competitive model exactly, agriculture is usually cited as the industry that most closely matches this description. Although farmers can transfer their resources to producing different crops, they cannot usually do so in the short run. Also, products are fairly standardized, although some differentiation exists by grade and by production method (e.g., organically grown or genetically engineered). Most industries, however, can be categorized into one of the other market structures.

OTHER MARKET STRUCTURES

Monopolistic Competition

The market structure closest to perfect competition is known as monopolistic competition. Despite its somewhat confusing name, monopolistic competition is similar to perfect competition except that it does not have standardized and interchangeable products. In most cases, firms in this industry rely heavily on product differentiation. They minimize price competition by differentiating their products from those of their competitors by promoting perceived or real advantages in style, image, quality, or other attributes. The automobile industry is an example of monopolistic competition.

Monopoly

At the opposite extreme is a market structure known as monopoly, which features only one seller of a product that has no close substitutes. To maximize income, monopolists do not have to produce as much output as possible; they can accomplish this same purpose by producing less and charging higher prices. Some monopolies are formed by controlling the supply source. Barriers that prevent other firms from entering a market, such as legal restrictions (e.g., licenses, government approval, or patents), can also create monopolies. By granting patents, the government allows temporary monopolies to encourage research and innovation. According to Folland, Goodman, and Stano (1997), pharmaceutical firms that control patents for certain drugs that lack close substitutes may be considered monopolists during the life of the patent. With managed care formularies, however, competition can be created between some patented drugs and other therapeutic alternatives.

Other monopolies exist because the required infrastructure for the industry is so expensive that the presence of competing firms would increase—rather than decrease—prices. The prime example of these natural monopolies is utilities. To ensure adequate output at reasonable prices, natural monopolies are usually regulated by government agencies such as public service commissions.

Although a monopoly consists of only one seller, situations exist in which there is only one buyer. In this situation, which is known as a monopsony, the buyer sets the price. The federal government is often a monopsony for military hardware and for healthcare services for Medicare and Medicaid patients. Unlike private businesses, however, the government is sometimes unable to fully exploit its market power to set prices because it is subject to political pressure and due process.

Oligopoly

Between perfect competition and monopoly is a market structure known as oligopoly, which consists of a few sellers and many buyers. Firms in oligopolies are often interdependent, and a dominant firm can exert influence through price leadership. Although this situation falls short of meeting the definition for collusion, the pricing practices of the oligopolists tend to coincide, with one firm usually taking a leadership role. Oligopolists know that the firms in the industry will not benefit if all of them decrease their prices. However, a single firm that increases its price may lose business if the other firms do not follow suit. This factor usually restricts the ability of smaller companies to change prices unilaterally. If a dominant firm increases prices, however, the other competitors usually follow.

Cereal manufacturers constitute a well-known oligopoly: four major companies have at least 80% of the market share for cereal. In medium-sized urban areas, hospitals may represent an oligopoly. Certain drug classes with market share concentrated among a few manufacturers may also be oligopolies.

Although an oligopoly consists of few sellers and many buyers, a market structure in which there are many sellers but only a few buyers is known as an oligopsony. To the extent that three large national pharmacy benefit managers (to be discussed in Chapter 17) pay for the large majority of prescriptions, they are considered by some to be an example of an oligopsony. As one might expect, oligopsonists are interdependent to the extent that they tend to offer similar products or services, copy each other's ideas, and take into account competitors' pricing structures when setting their own.

THE HEALTHCARE MARKET

Having just described the characteristics of the various market structures, we now consider whether the healthcare market fits these characteristics. As pointed out in the case scenario at the beginning of this chapter, this remains a highly debated issue in economic circles. In a survey of health economists, 50% thought the competitive model could apply to the healthcare industry, whereas 50% did not (Feldman & Morrisey, 1990). Those who did not believe that health care qualifies as a competitive market cited the following factors:

- Numbers of buyers and sellers
- Entry to and exit from the market
- Variation in products, services, and quality
- Full and free information
- Inelastic demand
- Universal demand
- Unpredictability of illness
- Health care as a "right"
- Supplier-induced demand
- Third-party insurance and patient-induced demand

Numbers of Buyers and Sellers

A maldistribution in the supply of healthcare services exists by geographic and specialty area. Although some healthcare markets are served by large numbers of sellers (e.g., retail pharmacies), some communities have a shortage of healthcare providers or healthcare facilities. In addition, although the United States as a whole has a sufficient supply of physicians, a shortage of primary care physicians (and an oversupply of specialists) exists. In some cases, the shortage exists because the market size is just too small to support enough hospitals or providers in each specialty to create a competitive market (e.g., transplant services).

Further, consolidation among buyers and sellers is occurring. The number of sole practitioners and small group practices is shrinking, while large medical groups are growing larger. Likewise, health maintenance organizations (HMOs), pharmacy benefit managers, pharmaceutical manufacturers, and drug wholesalers are merging into fewer, but larger organizations. Employer groups have also pooled their purchasing power in many cities by forming employer health coalitions to negotiate better rates for healthcare services. Retail pharmacies have also participated in this trend through consolidation of chain pharmacies and by independent pharmacies forming volume purchasing alliances and cooperatives.

By consolidating, buyers and sellers find they can lower costs and have more market power to negotiate favorable prices. The concern is that too much consolidation could reduce competition. In some cases, the Federal Trade Commission has intervened to restrict or prevent acquisitions and mergers that it believed would unduly inhibit competition.

Entry to and Exit from the Market

High barriers to entry exist for suppliers of health care, whether they are individual providers or institutions. To pursue a career as a healthcare provider, one must apply to a limited number of schools and seek out one of a limited number of positions. Becoming a healthcare professional can require a great deal of education and compulsory licensure. These entry barriers effectively limit the number of new healthcare professionals who can be added to the labor force at any one time. Healthcare facilities must also be licensed, certified, and inspected and often require large capital investments. Pharmaceutical manufacturers face extremely large financial barriers to get new drugs approved by the Food and Drug Administration. These same barriers, however, can also inhibit potential competitors.

Because healthcare resources are not easily transferred to producing other products and services, exit barriers are also formidable. For example, closing a hospital is difficult in part because it is not always possible to convert the building and equipment to other uses.

Variation in Products, Services, and Quality

Instead of producing standardized products and services, health care is usually customized for individual patients. Well-documented variations exist in patterns of medical care. Quality, although hard to measure, also varies; that is why requesting a second opinion is common. For all these reasons, it can be difficult to identify true substitutes for a particular product or service.

Full and Free Information

Most healthcare services require specialized knowledge. Although patients have more sources of information available today than ever before, they nevertheless may have incomplete information about the prices and quality of healthcare services. Patients and other healthcare purchasers often do not know what constitutes good physician care or pharmaceutical care and cannot often tell when they are getting accurate information.

Inelastic Demand

In perfect competition, even small price increases may result in significant loss of quantity demanded and, therefore, losses in revenue; thus demand is relatively elastic. Demand for healthcare services, however, is relatively inelastic. In other words, patients who need healthcare services are usually not price sensitive, especially in emergency situations. In part because of this sensitivity, prices for healthcare services increase more rapidly than the prices for most consumer goods and services. According to the Bureau of Labor Statistics, the Consumer Price Index for Urban Consumers (CPI-U) has increased during the past decade at nearly twice the rate for medical care (49.5%) as it has for all items (28.4%). Demand, however, has not decreased. Per capita prescription utilization for non-Medicaid patients enrolled in HMOs has increased from 5.7 prescriptions per person per year in 1990 to 8.5 in 2004. Per capita prescription utilization for Medicare beneficiaries enrolled in HMOs increased from 16.5 prescriptions per year in 1994 to 21.3 prescriptions per year in 2004 (Aventis, 2001, 2005).

Universal Demand

Many products and services offered for sale in the United States are used by only part of the potential market (e.g., rollerblades, cordless power tools, high-adventure vacations). Healthcare products and services, however, are used by nearly everyone. Not only is demand universal, but it is also nearly insatiable. Because of the lack of complete knowledge, many people demand healthcare services that are of questionable value. Even those services that are usually helpful are sometimes used in inappropriate ways that produce little or no value (e.g., antibiotics for the common cold or heroic efforts to prolong the life of a patient who is in the last stages of a terminal illness). In some cases, too many services may produce net losses in value (e.g., antibiotic resistance, addiction, iatrogenic disease, or unnecessary pain and suffering).

Unpredictability of Illness

Given a large enough group of people, we can predict with some certainty the number of individuals who will need trauma care in the emergency department during a given time. We cannot, however, predict exactly which individuals will need this care. Because consumers are often unable to time their healthcare purchases, they are typically not in a negotiating position when they need services. An obvious implication of this unpredictability is the need to pool risk through health insurance, especially if done so through a managed care organization that is in a position to negotiate discounts before services are actually needed.

Health Care as a "Right"

Many people view health care as a "right" because it is a prerequisite for individuals to become useful, productive members of society (much like public education). Those who espouse this viewpoint also believe that the allocation of scarce resources should not be determined by people's ability and willingness to pay, as is the case with most goods and services in the United States; instead, some level of health care should be provided to everyone. This position holds, therefore, that the price system should not be the sole determining factor in deciding who will receive healthcare products and services.

Supplier-Induced Demand

Physicians are in the unique position of controlling both the supply of and the demand for healthcare services. Although patients do not usually gain financially from illness or injury, their physicians often do. Acting as the patients' agents, physicians can create demand for their services and, at the same time, supply the services. This potential conflict of interest is an inherent element of health care under fee-for-service reimbursement and is difficult to prevent completely. Many managed care organizations, however, have restricted physicians' abilities to create self-referrals for laboratory, radiology, and other healthcare services.

Chapter 14 illustrated that an increase in the supply of most goods and services will result in an increase in the equilibrium quantity and a decrease in the equilibrium price. However, this is not necessarily the case in health care. Studies conducted in 1959 and 1961 first illustrated the effect of what is now called supplier-induced demand by showing a close correlation between the number of hospital beds per 1,000 people and rates of utilization measured as hospital days per 1,000 people (Roemer, 1961; Shain & Roemer, 1959). This led to an observation known as Roemer's Law: "A bed built is a bed filled."

The effect of supplier-induced demand has also been demonstrated by the increases in utilization that often accompany attempts to impose controls on physician fees (Folland et al., 1997). Other studies have shown that physicians' clinical decisions can be influenced by financial incentives (Hemenway, Killen, Cashman, Parks, & Bicknell, 1990; Hillman, Pauly, & Kerstein, 1989). This may explain, in part, why increases in the supply of physicians during the 1980s and 1990s were accompanied by acceleration—rather than moderation—in the growth of healthcare costs. However, increases in the supply of healthcare services may be favorable if they allow more people to access care or if they lead to improvements in quality.

Third-Party Insurance and Patient-Induced Demand

The availability of insurance creates a form of induced demand that is initiated by patients. As discussed in Chapter 14, when the price of a product or service decreases, the quantity demanded tends to increase. By decreasing patients' out-of-pocket expenses, health insurance has encouraged patients to consume more healthcare services than they would if they had to bear the full cost of the product or service (Torrens & Williams, 1993). One concern with expanding Medicare coverage for outpatient prescription drugs, therefore, is the potential for growth in prescription drug utilization resulting from induced demand. A potential solution is patient cost sharing that—if structured properly—can reduce unnecessary utilization without decreasing the quality of care (Manning et al., 1987).

The open-ended nature of most health insurance coverage leads to a situation that economists call "moral hazard," where people overconsume health care. For health insurance plan enrollees, the out-of-pocket costs for healthcare services are generally much less than the actual cost for providing those services. At some point, the additional health benefits achieved from consuming additional health services are not really worth their full costs; nevertheless, because the enrollees are paying only a fraction of the costs, they still want to use these services. Overconsumption of health services from moral hazard increases total health expenditures and insurance premiums.

Not all induced demand is undesirable, of course. In some cases, reducing financial barriers to health care may encourage patients to seek healthcare services earlier, thereby avoiding more expensive health expenditures in the future, particularly for lower-income and more severely ill persons.

IMPROVING ECONOMIC PERFORMANCE OF THE HEALTHCARE SYSTEM

Using Market Forces

From the preceding discussion, it should be clear why many observers feel that the economic aspects of health care are unique. Strategies that successfully reduce costs in most industries (e.g., promoting an increase in supply or an increase in competition) are often not seen as effective in the healthcare industry. Some individuals and groups, however, believe that health care is more monopolistic than competitive, and consequently, advocate that healthcare services should be considered a public utility and regulated accordingly. Many industrialized nations have already adopted this stance and regulate both provider fees and manufacturers' prices for pharmaceuticals.

Recognizing that health care is unique, many public policy leaders and payers for healthcare services advocate instead that the healthcare industry be managed in a way that allows market forces to work more effectively. Some of the more common approaches are described next.

First, patients can be made aware of and sensitive to healthcare costs. For example, patients can be given itemized receipts showing the actual costs paid by their insurance programs. They can also be required to pay more through patient cost sharing, especially through tiered copayments, which allow lower copayments for preferred products, such as generic drugs, and require higher copayments for nonpreferred drugs, such as expensive brand-name products.

Second, healthcare providers can be given feedback about variations in the cost, quantity, and quality of healthcare services through performance reports and academic detailing.

Third, managed care organizations can design physician and hospital reimbursement so as to create incentives for reducing costs. Because costs are a function of price and quantity, both factors need to be considered. Price (i.e., cost per unit) increases are attributable to inflation and can be controlled to some extent through contracting and competitive bidding. Increased utilization, by contrast, is a function of three separate components (as illustrated in **Table 15-1**): population effects, duration of treatment, and intensity of services.

Creating Incentives

As discussed in Chapter 17, managed healthcare plans have designed reimbursement methods that seek to reduce unnecessary hospital admissions, decrease hospital length of stay, and decrease the intensity of services provided to hospitalized patients. Similar steps have been implemented to control the cost and utilization of ambulatory services.

Healthcare providers, like everyone else, usually respond to incentives. **Table 15-2** shows the incentives created by each of the various types of hospital reimbursement. Discounted fee-for-service reimbursement (i.e., retrospective reimbursement based on a negotiated fee schedule), for

Table 15-1 Examples of Utilization Measurements for Various Types of Healthcare Services

	Hospital	Physician	Pharmacy
Population effects	Number of admissions	Number of new patients	Number of new prescriptions
Duration	Length of stay	Episode of care	Number of prescription drug refills
Intensity	Number and types of diagnostic tests	Number and types of treatments ordered	Relative expense of prescription drug or mix of brands versus generics

example, creates incentives to increase admissions (population), length of stay (duration), and intensity of services. Per diem reimbursement (i.e., prospective reimbursement of a flat rate per day without regard to actual cost), the most common form of managed care reimbursement for hospitals (Kongstvedt, 1997), creates incentives for hospitals to increase admissions and length of stay but decrease the intensity of services. Prospective reimbursement of a flat rate based on the patient's admission diagnosis, known as diagnosis-related group (DRG) reimbursement, creates incentives to increase admissions but minimize length of stay and intensity of services. Capitation (i.e., prospective reimbursement of a fixed amount each month for each enrolled patient, regardless of the amount of healthcare services actually provided) creates incentives to minimize all three utilization measures.

Physicians and pharmacies that are paid under discounted fee-for-service systems have the same incentives to increase utilization as do hospitals. Per diems, however, are difficult to apply to outpatient care services. Capitation reimbursement can also be applied to outpatient services in the form of case management (or disease state management). As under DRGs, prospective payments for outpatient services are based on diagnosis but are known as ambulatory patient groups

Table 15-2 Incentives under Various Forms of Hospital Reimbursement

	Number of admissions	Length of stay	Intensity of services
Discounted fee-for-service	↑	↑	↑
Per diem	↑	↑	↓
DRGs	↑	↓	↓
Capitation	↓	↓	↓

(APGs). Although these programs continue to evolve, they are expected to work best for chronic conditions with a wide range of costs. Again, healthcare providers in the outpatient setting would have the same types of incentives as would hospitals under prospective (APG) and capitation reimbursement.

Balancing Cost and Value

Another approach to improving the economic performance of the healthcare system is balancing the cost of healthcare services with the value received. As described in Chapter 14, most consumers make purchases only when the marginal value of those services meets or exceeds the marginal cost. However, this principle does not always apply in the healthcare industry. To illustrate, assume that the quantity of medical services (*M*) provided to a patient is compared with the patient's resulting health status (*H*) as shown in **Figure 15-1.** The curve in Figure 15-1 illustrates a variation of the law of diminishing marginal utility discussed in Chapter 14—marginal increases in the number of resources consumed result in ever smaller marginal increases in utility. Providing initial medical care services causes health status to improve rapidly at first; as more medical care is provided, however, health status increases more slowly. At some point we will reach the "flat of the curve," where additional healthcare expenditures produce very little incremental benefit (Jacobs, 1991, 1996).

When patients are isolated from costs, they often demand additional services, even though these services may provide limited or no benefits. It is important to consider the marginal benefit of additional medical services and to determine whether increases in services will produce proportional increases in benefits. If a great deal must be spent to produce a small incremental benefit, this usage may be a waste of limited health care resources.

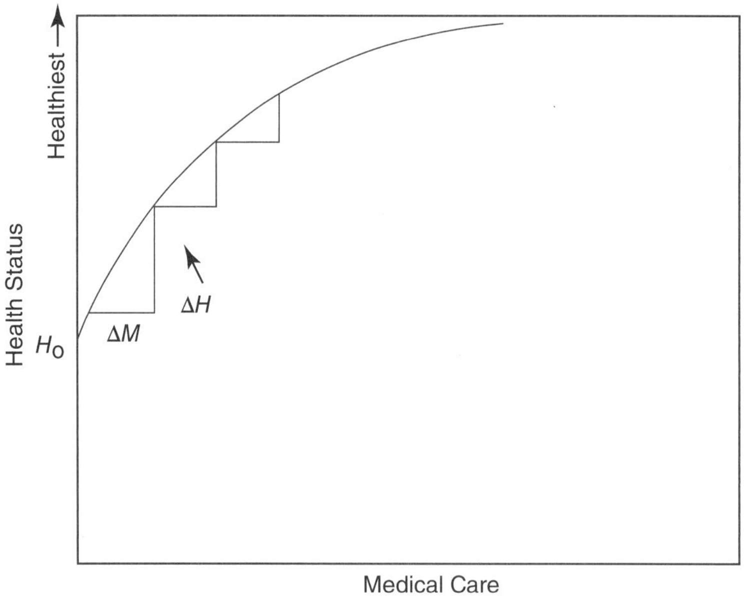

Figure 15-1 Hypothesized Relationship Between Health and Medical Care. In this representation, additional doses of medical care have diminishing impacts on health; eventually, a situation of low medical productivity, termed "flat of the curve medicine," is reached.

Reprinted from The Economics of Health and Medical Care, Fourth Edition, by P. Jacobs, p. 12, 1996, Jones and Bartlett Publishers.

This concept was used by the state of Oregon when it faced a shortage of funds for its Medicaid program and needed to reform its healthcare system. Use of limited funds for some services meant that opportunities to help other patients had to be forgone. To minimize these opportunity costs, Oregon wanted to allocate resources in a manner that would maximize marginal outcomes. A decision was made to provide coverage for those treatments that provided the greatest benefits compared with the cost of services. By not covering procedures such as removal of benign skin cancer, removal of benign tumors in the gastrointestinal system, and liver transplants for liver cancer patients, the state expanded basic services to approximately 120,000 more uninsured patients (Clewer & Perkins, 1998).

Although Oregon's experience has not been widely adopted, many other examples exist where this principle is applied to some degree. Managed care organizations are giving more attention to pharmacoeconomic considerations (e.g., cost-effectiveness, cost-benefit, and cost-utility analyses). Formulary decisions, step care protocols, and disease management, for example, all consider the incremental costs and outcomes of healthcare services. More attention will be given in the future to ways in which scarce healthcare resources can be applied more efficiently and effectively.

CONCLUSION

This chapter described some of the unique aspects of health economics and ways to enhance the economic performance of the healthcare system. Healthcare practitioners should understand and use these economic principles to work effectively with or for healthcare institutions and insurance programs. Because of the unique nature of the healthcare industry, payers are still investigating how they might better control healthcare costs and improve quality so that patients can receive more benefits from the limited resources available.

QUESTIONS FOR FURTHER DISCUSSION

1. To what extent is health care a monopoly or oligopoly?
2. What can be done to enhance competition in the healthcare industry? Are there cases where competition will not decrease prices?
3. If pharmacists are able to charge for nondispensing services, how might payers act to prevent or minimize potential supplier-induced demand?
4. In addition to the healthcare services listed in the text, what other types of healthcare services might be considered for elimination from health insurance coverage because their marginal cost is likely to exceed their marginal benefits?
5. Which disease states would lend themselves best to pharmacy reimbursement on a capitation basis through ambulatory patient groups (APGs)? Why?

KEY TOPICS AND TERMS

Ambulatory patient groups (APGs)
Capitation
Diagnosis-related group (DRG)
Discounted fee-for-service
Duration of treatment
Flat of the curve
Intensity of services
Market structure

Monopolistic competition
Monopoly
Monopsony
Oligopoly
Oligopsony
Patient-induced demand
Per diem
Perfect competition
Population effects
Roemer's Law
Supplier-induced demand
Tiered co-payments

REFERENCES

Aventis. (2001). *Managed care digest series, 2001.* Bridgewater, NJ: Aventis Pharmaceuticals, Inc.

Aventis. (2005). *Managed care digest series, 2005.* Bridgewater, NJ: Aventis Pharmaceuticals, Inc.

Clewer, A., & Perkins, D. (1998). *Economics for health care management.* Hertfordshire, UK: Prentice Hall Europe.

Feldman, R., & Morrisey, M. A. (1990). Health economics: A report on the field. *Journal of Health Politics, Policy and Law, 15,* 627–646.

Folland, S., Goodman, A. C., & Stano, M. (1997). *The economics of health and health care* (2nd ed.). Upper Saddle River, NJ: Prentice Hall.

Hemenway, D., Killen, A., Cashman, S. B., Parks, C. L., & Bicknell, W. J. (1990). Physicians' responses to financial incentives: Evidence from a for-profit ambulatory center. *New England Journal of Medicine, 322,* 1059–1063.

Hillman, A. L., Pauly, M. V., & Kerstein, J. J. (1989). How do financial incentives affect physicians' clinical decisions and the financial performance of health maintenance organizations? *New England Journal of Medicine, 321,* 86–92.

Jacobs, P. (1991). *The economics of health and medical care* (3rd ed.). Gaithersburg, MD: Aspen.

Jacobs, P. (1996). *The economics of health and medical care* (4th ed.). Sudbury, MA: Jones and Bartlett.

Kongstvedt, P. R. (1997). Negotiating and contracting with hospitals and institutions. In P. R. Kongstvedt (Ed.), *Essentials of managed health care* (2nd ed.). Gaithersburg, MD: Aspen.

Manning, W. G., Newhouse, J. P., Duan, N., Keeler, E. B., & Leibowitz, A. (1987). Health insurance and the demand for medical care. *American Economic Review, 77,* 251–277.

Rice, T. (1997). Can markets give us the health system we want? *Journal of Health Politics, Policy and Law, 22,* 383–426.

Roemer, M. I. (1961). Bed supply and hospital utilization: A national experiment. *Hospitals, Journal of the American Hospital Association, 35,* 988–993.

Shain, M., & Roemer, M. I. (1959). Hospital costs relate to the supply of beds. *Modern Hospital, 92,* 71–73.

Torrens, P. R., & Williams, S. J. (1993). Understanding the present, planning for the future: The dynamics of health care in the United States in the 1990s. In S. J. Williams and P. R. Torrens (Eds.), *Introduction to health services* (4th ed., pp. 421–429). Albany, NY: Delmar.

ACKNOWLEDGMENT

Adapted with permission from the Academy of Managed Care Pharmacy.

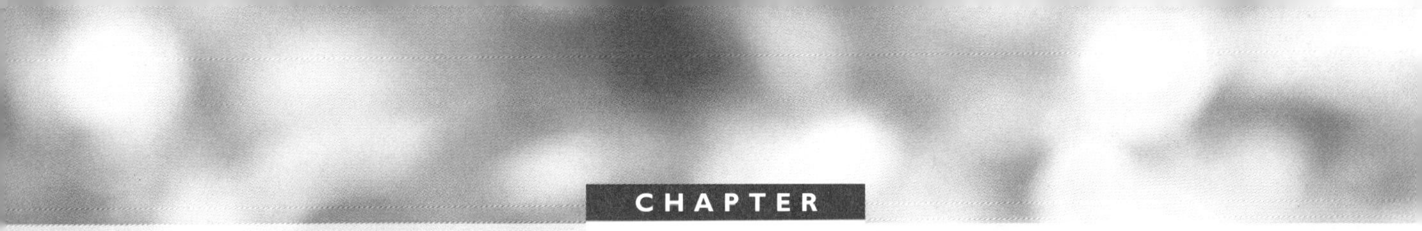

CHAPTER

16

Private Health Insurance

Kenneth W. Schafermeyer and Taehwan Park*

Case Scenario

Barb Ital recently graduated from pharmacy school and is considering a job offer from a large pharmacy chain. As part of her benefits package, the company will pay one half of the premium for Barb's health insurance coverage. Barb knows that this is a good deal. Even if she paid 100% of the premium, the group policy would be much less expensive than a policy that she could buy on her own. Barb also knows that if she does not elect to participate in the plan when she begins her employment, she will have to wait until next year before she can join the plan during another open enrollment period. Also, if she joins later, there will be an elimination period; she will have to wait a specified period of months before any preexisting health conditions are covered. Upon reading the policy, Barb discovers that she is required to pay part of the cost for most healthcare services and that some healthcare procedures, such as cosmetic surgery, are not covered.

Questions

1. Why are group policies less expensive than individual policies?
2. What is the purpose of the open enrollment period and the elimination period?
3. Why are patients required to pay part of the cost of most healthcare services?
4. Why are some procedures not covered?

LEARNING OBJECTIVES

Upon completion of this chapter, the student shall be able to:

- Identify the factors that determine whether an event is insurable.
- Describe the original purpose of health insurance.
- List and define the various parties involved in the health insurance industry.

*The authors wish to express appreciation to Brenda R. Motheral and Evan S. Schnur for their contributions to this chapter.

- Explain how prepaid prescription programs are inconsistent with the principles of health insurance.
- Explain why health insurance plans cover prescriptions despite their incompatibility with some risk management principles.
- Outline the advantages and disadvantages of the U.S. practice of offering health insurance as an employee benefit.
- Describe the potential risk management problems faced by health insurance programs, and explain how insurance companies try to minimize these risks.
- Describe the impact of managed care on pharmacy.
- Describe the purpose of pharmacy benefit managers and the types of services they provide to control prescription cost and quality.
- Given a third-party plan's reimbursement formula, the pharmacy's actual acquisition cost, and the pharmacy's cost of dispensing the prescription, calculate the pharmacy's earned discount, gross margin, and net profit for that prescription when reimbursed by the third-party plan.
- Describe how private health insurance has affected pharmacy practice.

CHAPTER QUESTIONS

1. What determines whether an event is insurable or uninsurable?
2. What was the original purpose of health insurance?
3. How are prepaid prescription programs inconsistent with the principles of health insurance?
4. Why do health insurance plans cover prescriptions despite their incompatibility with some risk management principles?
5. Why are most private health insurance policies offered through employers?
6. What can insurance programs do to reduce their risk?

INTRODUCTION

The last half of the 20th century witnessed dramatic changes in the way health care is provided, paralleled by equally profound transformations in the way health care is financed. Although health insurance has preserved financial security and improved access to health care for millions of Americans, it has also ensured payment for healthcare providers and fueled the growth of hospitals and the development of new health services. Without health insurance, many Americans could not afford the services they need to stay healthy and to continue working as productive members of society.

Health insurance is a vital component of the U.S. healthcare system, and yet, many individuals—including both healthcare providers and consumers—do not have a clear understanding of how it works. The difficulty of understanding health insurance may be due in part to a number of interesting paradoxes, such as:

- Health insurance ensures payment for healthcare providers, yet it restricts provider reimbursement.
- Health insurance improves patient access to healthcare services by reducing financial barriers, yet it restricts utilization of those services.
- Healthcare providers supply services, yet they also create the demand for these services—an inherent conflict of interest that can drive up healthcare costs.
- Health insurance increases access to health care, yet it can encourage unnecessary use of healthcare services.

- Groups of patients who were once thought of as uninsurable (the poor, the disabled, and the elderly) are now covered through Medicaid and Medicare, yet millions of working poor and their families remain uninsured.
- Individuals with chronic or expensive health problems have the greatest need for health insurance, yet they have the most difficulty obtaining it.

Health insurance has been roundly maligned because of these problems, especially by pharmacists and other healthcare providers who depend on health insurance for payment for services rendered. These paradoxes do make sense, however, when one understands the basic principles of insurance and the needs of the insurance industry. This chapter dispels some of the mystery of health insurance by explaining some of the principles of insuring risk. First, the chapter discusses the variables that affect health insurance (i.e., access, cost, and quality) and then explains the evolution and structure of the health insurance industry, especially as it relates to prescription drug programs. Next, it outlines the basic principles of insurance and highlights the tools that insurers use to manage risk. The impact of health insurance on pharmacy and strategies for working with insurance programs are also discussed.

IRON TRIANGLE OF HEALTH CARE

Figure 16-1 shows the *Iron Triangle of Health Care*, which consists of three essential components of healthcare systems: cost, access, and quality (Kissick, 1994). The figure demonstrates the reciprocal trade-offs among these components. For example, changes in healthcare costs affect access to care, which in turn impact the quality of care. This chapter focuses on how private health insurance affects access to care and affects healthcare costs. Initiatives designed to control the quality of care will be discussed in the chapter on managed health care.

Access to Care

In 2013, 42 million Americans (13.4% of the population) lacked health insurance—about 600,000 less people than in 2012 (Smith & Medalia, 2014). These uninsured individuals face greater barriers to receiving health care, are generally in poorer health, and have shorter life expectancies than do individuals with health insurance coverage.

Catastrophic medical bills also are a major cause of personal bankruptcies in the United States, accounting for about 62.1% of these filings in 2007 (Himmelstein, Thorne, Warren, & Woolhandler, 2009). Financial difficulties resulting from such healthcare expenses affect not only the uninsured, but also individuals with inadequate insurance coverage. The demographic groups most likely to be financially devastated by noncovered medical expenses are the elderly, women, and families headed by single women.

Surprisingly, the individuals most likely to be uninsured are not the groups that were traditionally considered uninsurable—the impoverished, the disabled, and the elderly. These groups are

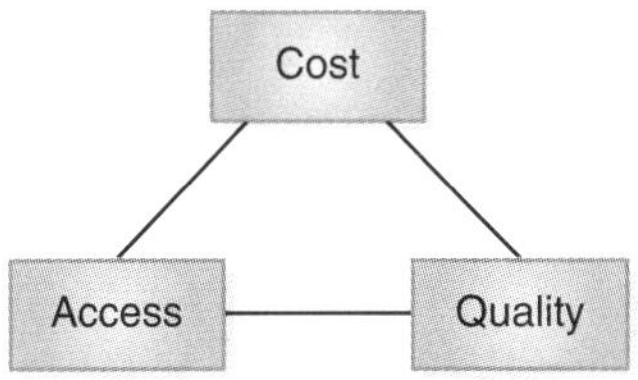

Figure 16-1 The Iron Triangle of Health Care.

provided some protection by the public sector through Medicare and Medicaid (discussed in the chapter on Medicare and Medicaid). Who, then, are the uninsured? Following are some of the highlights from a U.S. Census Bureau report shown in **Table 16-1** (Smith & Medalia, 2014):

- Among adults, the largest group of uninsured comprises the working poor—individuals who are working in low-paying jobs that either do not offer health insurance benefits or require workers to pay premiums that are unaffordable.
- Foreign-born U.S. residents are about 2.5 times as likely as U.S.-born individuals to be uninsured (27.7% vs. 11.2%). The highest rate of uninsured status is found among foreign-born Hispanics. This finding has serious public health implications for areas of the country with large numbers of immigrants (Thamer, Richard, Casebeer, & Ray, 1997).
- Almost one-fourth (22.6%) of young adults between the ages of 19 and 25 are uninsured (about twice the rate of the general population). Because of the Affordable Care Act's dependent coverage provision, individuals aged 19 to 25 years may be eligible to be a dependent on a parent's health insurance plan. About one-fourth of adults between the ages of 26 and 34 are also uninsured.
- As might be expected, the proportion of individuals with health insurance increases with household income; only 7.1% of individuals living in households with incomes greater than $75,000 lack health insurance.

Removing financial barriers by providing universal health insurance coverage will not, by itself, eliminate all of the barriers to receiving high-quality health care. For example, insurance coverage was not found to be an independent predictor of vaccination in a study of preschool children (Santoli et al., 2004). An earlier study showed that the barriers to immunization reported by middle/upper income parents are similar to those reported by lower income parents. Only about one-third identify cost and lack of insurance coverage as problems (Salsberry, Nickel, & Mitch, 1994). Greater health problems faced by low-income people are attributable not only to lack of adequate insurance coverage but also to organizational barriers, such as a lack of flexibility in scheduling, long waiting times, and personal barriers such as a lack of reliable transportation, chaotic home environments, and employment conflicts. Other obstacles include lack of knowledge of healthcare needs and misperceptions about the safety of healthcare services (Lannon et al., 1995). Although attempts to reform health care in the United States must focus first on providing adequate insurance coverage, other barriers, such as education and transportation, must be addressed as well. More discussion about covering the uninsured and reforming the healthcare system is included in the chapter on healthcare reform.

As for-profit entities, private health insurance companies would find it unprofitable to provide insurance coverage to certain high-risk groups (e.g., the elderly, mentally ill, and disabled people) and to certain groups unable to pay premiums (e.g., the impoverished or "medically indigent"). Certain governmental programs, such as Medicare and Medicaid, therefore, are designed to cover so-called "uninsurable" patients who would find it difficult or impossible to obtain private health insurance. Even with these "safety net" programs, there are still millions of Americans without health insurance coverage. (See the chapters on Medicare and Medicaid and healthcare reform for more information.)

Cost of Care

In 2013, U.S. health care spending was estimated $2.9 trillion—an increase from $1.4 trillion in 2000 (**Figure 16-2**). Expenditures covered by public health insurance, which accounted for 39% of national health spending, grew 4.4% to $1.1 trillion in 2013, an acceleration from 3.8% growth in 2012. Expenditures covered by private health insurance (33% of national health spending)

Table 16-1 People Without Health Insurance Coverage by Selected Characteristic, 2008 and 2013

Category	Percentage 2008	Percentage 2013
Total population	15.4	13.4
Race		
White	10.8	12.8
Black	19.1	15.9
Asian	17.6	14.5
Hispanic	30.7	24.3
Age		
Under 19 years*	9.9	7.6
19–25 years*	28.6	22.6
26–34 years	26.5	23.5
35–44 years	19.4	19.0
45–64 years	14.4	14.5
65 years or older	1.7	1.6
Nativity		
Native born	12.9	11.2
Foreign born	33.5	27.7
Region		
Northeast	11.6	9.9
Midwest	11.6	11.3
South	18.2	17.4
West	17.4	16.5
Household income		
Less than $25,000	24.5	21.6
$25,000–$49,999	21.4	18.7
$50,000–$74,999	14.0	13.1
$75,000 or more	8.2	7.1

*These age groups are special interest because of the Affordable Care Act of 2010. Children under the age of 19 are eligible for Medicaid/CHIP, and individuals aged 19–25 may be a dependent on a parent's health plan.

Source: Data from U.S. Census Bureau, 2014 current population survey annual social and economic supplements. From *Health Insurance Coverage in the United States: 2013*.

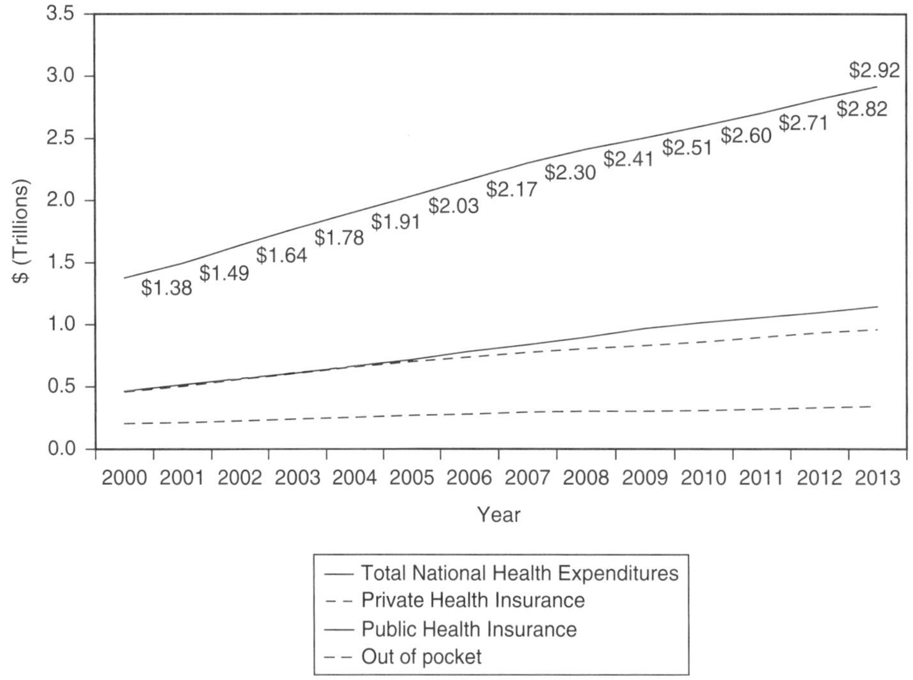

Figure 16-2 National Health Expenditures.

Data from Centers for Medicare & Medicaid Services, national health expenditure data. Retrieved from https://www.cms.gov/Research-Statistics-Data-and-Systems/Statistics-Trends-and-Reports/NationalHealthExpendData/NHE-Fact-Sheet.html

grew 2.8% to $961.7 billion, slower than the 4% growth in 2012. In 2000, there was relatively no large difference in public spending ($461.2 billion) and private spending ($459.8 billion), representing 33.5% and 33.4% of national health spending, respectively. Out-of-pocket spending, which represented 12% of national health spending in 2013, reached $339.4 billion and increased by 3.2%—a slower rate of growth than the 3.6% in 2012. Because of the rapid growth in healthcare costs, there is a need to increase cost-control efforts. The cost controls are discussed in more detail in the chapter on managed health care.

HISTORY OF HEALTH INSURANCE

Early Health Insurance Programs

Health insurance has a long history in the United States, beginning with the federal Marine Hospital Service, which was first authorized in 1798. Starting in the mid-19th century, accident insurance and life insurance companies began entering the field of health insurance. The Massachusetts Health Insurance Company of Boston was incorporated in 1847, and several health insurance plans were offered for California gold rush workers in 1849 and for railroad workers in 1860 (Campbell & Newsome, 1995).

Most early health insurance plans were really disability insurance—that is, they did not cover health expenses, but instead protected individuals from the loss of income resulting from illness. At first, only specified diseases such as diabetes, diphtheria, scarlet fever, and typhus were covered. Coverage was later expanded to include more diseases and to reimburse individuals for certain out-of-pocket health expenses. The emphasis, however, remained on protecting income.

Hospital Insurance

In 1929, Baylor University Hospital offered hospital care to a group of Dallas teachers on a prepaid basis. The plan collected premiums from each covered person and then reallocated those funds to the small portion of the group that had hospital expenses. With fewer financial barriers to hospital care, the demand for hospital services eventually increased. As hospitals experienced empty beds and declining revenues during the Great Depression, the increased revenue and financial stability promised by insurance became increasingly attractive. One problem, however, was that these plans restricted care to a particular hospital. This problem was resolved when the American Hospital Association expanded the prepayment concept by establishing statewide Blue Cross hospital insurance plans allowing free choice of hospitals. These plans did not pay hospitals directly; instead, patients were expected to pay their bills and then were reimbursed by the plan for 80% of the first 21 days of hospital expenses. It should be noted that this insurance program was designed to increase the *demand* for healthcare services (i.e., the ability and willingness of consumers to pay); it did not address the issue of *supply* (i.e., the extent to which healthcare services were available).

Medical Insurance

At the same time that Blue Cross was being created, a medical group practice in Los Angeles organized a similar program to cover medical services. Not only did this plan create insurance for physician services, but it also organized physicians into a large group practice—a unique arrangement at the time that became a model for today's medical foundations and health maintenance organizations (Pharmaceutical Manufacturers Association, 1973). In 1939, the California Medical Association established the first Blue Shield plan to facilitate payment for medical services. Like Blue Cross, Blue Shield focused on reimbursing patients for a portion of their medical expenses, not on organizing or providing health services directly.

The rapid adoption of health insurance occurred in the 1940s, fueled by government policy. Health insurance benefits became an important part of labor negotiations during World War II; the reason being that government wage and price controls prohibited wage increases during the war, so companies that wanted to attract workers began offering additional benefits, especially health insurance. Before World War II, health insurance was an occasional employee benefit, covering about 5% of the U.S. population; in just a few years; however, it became commonplace, covering more than 50% of the population (Institute of Medicine, 1993).

Health insurance remains a standard employee benefit today, with 90% of workers in manufacturing jobs covered; it is less common in the service sector (75%) and in agriculture (70%) (Lee, Soffel, & Luft, 1992). Evidence suggests, however, that the percentage of workers covered by employment-based health insurance is declining because of decreased unionization, the trend toward using part-time workers, and the decreased percentage of employers sponsoring health insurance plans (Fronstin & Snider, 1996).

Major Medical Insurance

With the merger of Blue Cross and Blue Shield and the formation of several other commercial insurance companies, hospital coverage and medical coverage were combined into more comprehensive insurance plans. By the early 1950s, most employee health benefit plans took the form of major medical insurance. These policies were designed to help offset expenses incurred because of catastrophic illness or injury. Until major medical insurance was developed, insurance policies generally limited coverage to a specific dollar amount that was relatively modest and/or limited coverage to specific types of services. Also in the 1950s, the health insurance industry came full circle by reemphasizing income replacement through long-term disability insurance policies.

Indemnity versus Service Benefit Insurance

Blue Cross, Blue Shield, and other health insurers initially reimbursed subscribers—not providers—for a portion (usually 80%) of their medical expenses. These plans, which were known as indemnity insurance, represented the dominant form of health insurance for decades because they were simple and effective in achieving their objectives—to protect both patients and healthcare providers from financial loss and bankruptcy. Indemnity plans, however, also presented some problems. Patients found it inconvenient to collect receipts and complete claim forms. In turn, insurance companies found the individual claims submitted by thousands of policyholders expensive to process. Premiums for these plans increased rapidly because insurance companies reimbursed on a fee-for-service basis and, consequently, were relatively ineffective at controlling expenditures for reasons discussed later in this chapter. Today, the term *indemnity* is used loosely to refer to any health insurance program reimbursing on a fee-for-service basis with few cost controls.

Most health insurance programs have discontinued the indemnity approach in favor of service benefit programs, in which healthcare providers submit claims and are paid directly by the insurance plan. This arrangement allows standardization and automation of claims processing and better control of costs through contractual agreements between the insurance plans and healthcare providers.

Current Trends

Private health insurance has primarily supported and reinforced existing patterns of health services rather than address gaps in care. Those areas that were neglected by the private sector—prevention, control of communicable diseases, and care for segments of society that have the highest incidence of disease and the greatest need for care (persons who are poor, disabled, chronically ill, mentally ill, retarded, and elderly)—have become the responsibility of the public sector (Litman, 1994). This problem was addressed in 1965 when the Social Security Act was amended to provide government-sponsored health insurance coverage for the poor (Medicaid) and for older and disabled persons (Medicare). Medicare and Medicaid are discussed in more detail in Chapter 18.

Because early health insurance programs, such as Blue Cross and Blue Shield, were controlled by hospitals and physicians, the primary goal was to protect providers—not patients—from financial loss. The form of insurance preferred by these indemnity plans guaranteed that reimbursement would be generous and that little attention would be given to controlling costs (Starr, 1982). Until recently, most healthcare providers have been reimbursed on a fee-for-service basis—that is, they received a fee for each service performed. This system offered little financial incentive to control utilization, reduce costs, or enhance quality of care.

As healthcare costs increased rapidly during the 1970s, employer groups that paid for health benefits demanded that health insurance programs control costs and change their governing bodies to reduce the extent of provider control. Health insurance companies responded by restricting reimbursement to providers and by controlling the use of healthcare services. However, until more recently, there was little desire or perceived need to improve quality or ensure positive outcomes—ordinary management functions for most businesses. In other words, healthcare services were not managed.

In the past few decades, traditional health insurance programs have evolved into managed healthcare plans through the implementation of extensive cost controls and through the use of patient information and claims databases to improve the quality of healthcare services in an attempt to enhance patient outcomes. Managed care is discussed in more detail in the chapter on managed health care.

Evolution of Prepaid Prescription Drug Programs

Until the early 1970s, most insurance coverage for prescription drugs was offered through major medical insurance programs. The first program to focus primarily on prepayment of prescription drug expenses was the Green Shield plan offered in Ontario, Canada, in the 1950s. Outpatient coverage of prescription drugs through insurance programs other than major medical plans grew slowly in the United States, however, for several reasons. First, other healthcare services, such as hospital and medical services, historically accounted for a much larger portion of health expenditures; prescription drug coverage, therefore, was a much lower priority. Second, because prescriptions result in a large number of small claims, prescription coverage is not consistent with some of the principles of insurance and risk management. (This point is discussed later in this chapter.) Third, antitrust laws prohibit U.S. pharmacists from doing what Canadian pharmacists had done—working together to negotiate fees.

After the United Auto Workers Union negotiated a prescription drug plan administered by Blue Cross in 1969, labor unions became the major catalyst driving the growth of prepaid prescription plans. In response to this trend, a new industry of fiscal intermediaries was created in the early 1970s to help employer groups provide these prescription benefit programs to their employees. These fiscal intermediaries, which are described in more detail in the next section of this chapter, made it easier for employee benefit plans to include prescription drug coverage.

Private insurance coverage for prescription drugs has continued to grow and represented 39% of all prescription expenditures in 2013. Public insurance programs (e.g., Medicare and Medicaid) covered about 51% of prescription expenditures, and the remaining 10% were paid by patients out of pocket, commonly as a part of a patient cost-sharing requirement (West, 2014).

THE HEALTH INSURANCE INDUSTRY

Structure of the Industry

Although the term *third party* implies that only three individuals or companies are involved in a transaction (in this case, the patient, the healthcare provider, and the payer), the health insurance industry actually includes many different participants, each with its own specific function. To work successfully with third-party programs, healthcare providers need to understand the structure of the industry and the objectives of each of the participants.

Figure 16-3 outlines the most important participants in employer-sponsored group health insurance. At the top of the diagram is the patient—either an employee of a company that sponsors the health insurance plan or a family member of the covered employee. Sometimes employees are represented by labor unions that negotiate benefits on their behalf. The labor contract may specify the type of health care and prescription coverage that employees and their families receive.

As shown in Figure 16-3, patients often have to pay a portion of the cost of health services received. This patient cost sharing is designed to control utilization of health services by making patients more cost conscious. As discussed later in this chapter, patient cost sharing can take one of the following three forms: a copayment, a deductible, or coinsurance. Most plans use patient cost sharing as a financial incentive to avoid using unnecessary healthcare services. To be effective, however, patient cost-sharing provisions should not be so high as to discourage use of truly necessary health services.

Figure 16-3 also shows the sponsor of the insurance program—usually an employer that assumes responsibility for obtaining coverage and pays some or all of the premiums. Because healthcare costs for small groups (several hundred persons or fewer) can be unpredictable, and the payment

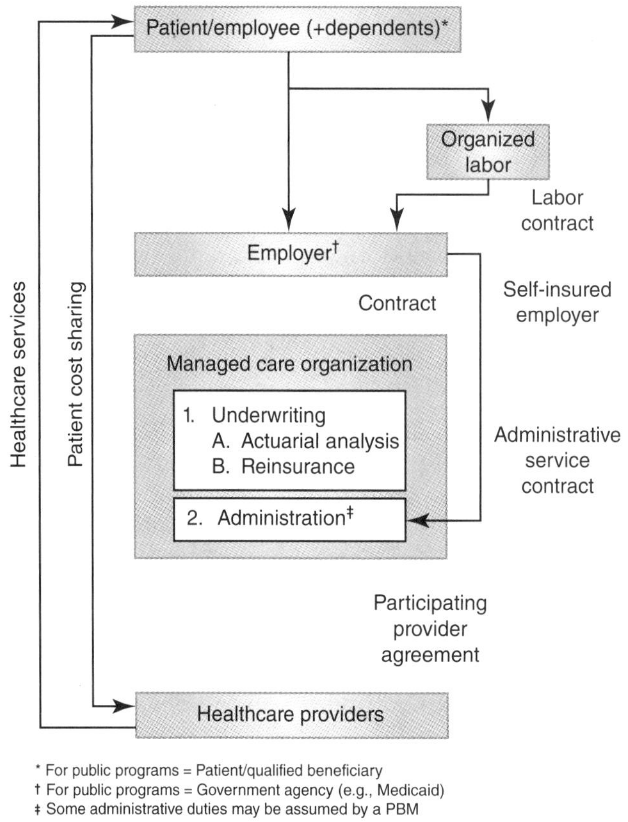

Figure 16-3 The Third-Party Prescription Industry.

Source: Data from Schafermeyer, K. W. (1996). Third-party prescription program evaluation. In *Effective Pharmacy Management,* 8th ed., p. 322. Alexandria, VA: National Community Pharmacists Association.

of claims for health expenditures is complex, most employer groups seek professional help from fiscal intermediaries—companies that provide underwriting and/or administrative services.

Underwriting is the process of insuring someone. The underwriter assumes the financial risk for health services in return for premiums paid by an individual or by an employer for a group of employees. To limit their own risk, most insurance companies purchase reinsurance to cover losses that exceed a specified amount. For health insurance programs, this means that both underwriters and reinsurance companies must agree that a health insurance program is designed properly with minimum expenses (referred to as losses). Consequently, insurance programs tend to limit the types of claims that may be billed by providers unless they determine them to be necessary or that they will reduce costs elsewhere in the program. Estimating the amount of risk assumed by an insurance company is known as actuarial analysis. An actuary conducts a statistical analysis of the population served and estimates the income (premiums) that must be earned to cover the estimated expenses, usually expressed as cost per member per month. An actuary estimates these three expenses: (1) the cost for each type of service; (2) the projected number of services that will be received by the group as a whole (the utilization rate); and (3) the administrative expenses that the fiscal intermediary incurs by insuring and administering the healthcare benefit program. Actuaries may then adjust their estimates based on the insurance company's overall expenses for a specific geographic area during the previous year (community rating) or adjust the rates for a specific subset of insured individuals—usually an employer group—based on the group's experience for the previous year (experience rating). These adjustments affect premiums for the next year, depending on whether the claims expenses were higher or lower than the actuary's estimate.

Sometimes a large corporation decides that it is unnecessary to use an insurance company to underwrite a health benefit program and decides to self-insure instead. Laws in most states require employers that self-insure healthcare benefits to place a large sum of money aside into a restricted account that can be used only to pay for employees' health benefits. This restricted account (reserve pool) must be large enough to pay any unexpected future health benefit claims. Because self-insurance is a risky strategy and ties up a considerable amount of cash, most small employers prefer to use the underwriting services of an insurance company.

Some fiscal intermediaries specialize in providing only underwriting services; others provide only administrative services, meaning that they do not take on the risk. Some fiscal intermediaries, such as Blue Cross/Blue Shield, provide both underwriting and administrative services. Because healthcare providers and administrators are linked through contractual arrangements, administrators are the component of the healthcare industry that is most visible to healthcare providers. The elements of this contractual arrangement are discussed later in this chapter.

Viewpoints of the Participants

The various groups involved in the health insurance industry often have competing goals. Employees are interested primarily in having convenient access to healthcare providers, quality services, and reduced out-of-pocket costs. Employers want healthy, satisfied employees but also want to reduce or control the amount they spend on health benefits. Administrators need to satisfy their customers—employer groups—by maintaining an adequate network of participating healthcare providers and helping employers manage their health benefit programs at a reasonable cost.

Healthcare providers, however, often see third-party programs as an unnecessary and unwelcome intrusion into the provider–patient relationship and as an unfair market force that controls their practice and limits their earnings. Individual providers do not like to be viewed as commodities to be purchased at the lowest price. Although providers express concern that cost-containment efforts are frequently imposed at the expense of quality, this concern is difficult to document.

BASIC PRINCIPLES AND STRATEGIES OF HEALTH INSURANCE

Principles of Risk Management

To understand insurance and its effect on the provision of health care in the United States, it is helpful to first understand the principle of risk and how it can be managed. The purpose of insurance is to help individuals and businesses manage certain types of unanticipated risk. Death, for example, is inevitable; because it can be sudden or unexpected (unanticipated); however, it is insurable. Most accidents and many other perils are also unanticipated and, therefore, insurable. In contrast, risk that can be anticipated is not insurable (e.g., spoilage of products, depreciation of buildings and equipment, or expiration of drugs).

Risk can be described as pure or speculative. Pure risk occurs in situations where a person faces the possibility of loss but no gain. Illness, fires, or storms are unpredictable perils and are often unavoidable. Because these events can cause significant loss but seldom result in any type of gain, they are referred to as pure risk. Speculative risk involves a chance of gain as well as a chance for loss. Gambling is a classic example of speculative risk. Pursuing a business venture also involves speculative risk because an individual accepts the risk of losing money while pursuing the chance of making profits. Speculative risk cannot be insured because risk takers can usually choose the amount of risk they are willing to assume; removing the risk would encourage overspending or careless behavior.

Insurance is designed to help people to reduce pure risk, not speculative risk. Pure risk becomes an insurable hazard when all six of the following elements are present:

1. The probability of a peril occurring in a population can be accurately determined. We can predict with reasonable certainty, for example, the percentage of 60-year-old women who will develop breast cancer in a given year and the percentage of 19-year-old men who will have traffic accidents during a given year.
2. The peril is an irregular event on an individual basis. Although we can predict approximately how many breast cancer cases or traffic accidents will occur in a population, we cannot determine to whom these events will occur.
3. The loss must be accidental. For example, arson committed by the insured party is not covered by insurance; neither is murder by a beneficiary of a life insurance policy. This requirement is essential to avoid creating profit-making incentives for purchasing insurance.
4. The event must result in a substantial loss. Insurance is designed to protect a person's financial security. Although most people can sustain small losses, insurance is needed to cover the large, unexpected losses that can overwhelm an individual's income stream or wipe out a family's accumulated resources.
5. The loss must be measurable. For a loss to be measurable, the following two conditions must be met: the loss must be attributable to a specific event, and the monetary value of the loss must be relatively easy to determine. For example, normal wear and tear for an automobile does not come from a specific event. In contrast, the loss from a theft or a hailstorm is the result of a specific incident and, therefore, can be insured. Insurance policies state the basis under which the amount of loss will be measured. For personal property, insurance coverage is set at either market value (the amount for which the item could have been sold before it was damaged) or replacement value (the amount it would cost to fix or replace the item). Insurance companies may also establish schedules stipulating the amount they will pay for various services. The intrinsic value of a lost heirloom or a favorite photograph, however, cannot be measured in monetary terms and, therefore, is difficult to insure.
6. The individual must have an insurable interest. Because insurance is designed to compensate for loss, an individual who does not suffer the loss personally usually cannot receive insurance compensation. A person cannot, for example, be reimbursed when a neighbor's house burns down. Likewise, whereas people can purchase life insurance for family members or business partners (with their permission), they cannot purchase insurance on an acquaintance who is a poor driver, thereby speculating that they can cash in when the acquaintance finally has an accident.

Purchasing insurance involves incurring a small, certain loss (prepayment of an annual or monthly premium) in exchange for the possibility of a large, unpredictable loss. Trading uncertainty for certainty reduces risk. Insurance has several other equally valuable benefits; it reduces worry, it makes it easier to borrow money, and it frees up capital for investment.

Insurance does not make risk disappear, but rather transfers some or all of the risk from individuals to the insurance company for a fee. The insurance company then pools the risk with that assumed from many other insurance policyholders. Transfer of risk and risk pooling are based on *the law of large numbers*; the larger the number of insured persons, the more accurate the predictions regarding losses. When losses are more predictable, the risk related to uncertainty actually decreases, which is important because the underwriter estimates the predicted amount of loss and sets premiums accordingly.

Premiums are based on the claims experience of the policyholders who make up the risk pool. If claims are higher than anticipated, next year's premiums will increase to make up for this loss. In these experience-rated pools, each insurance subscriber is affected by the aggregate claims experience of the group. A large amount of bad risk that results in a high number of claims leads to large premium increases; good risk with fewer claims results in lower premium levels.

Prescription Coverage: An Exception to the Principles of Risk Management

The need for health insurance is obvious. Unexpected injury or hospitalization costing tens of thousands of dollars (or more) can quickly exceed a family's annual income or accumulated savings. Most families consider the financial security provided by health insurance to be a necessity. Insurance coverage for pharmaceuticals, however, is not consistent with all of the requirements of an insurable hazard as described previously. Compared with other health expenditures, the cost of a prescription usually does not represent a substantial loss, the most common exceptions being some biotechnology drugs and specialty medications. In addition, for some medications, such as oral contraceptives, the prescriptions do not represent an accidental or unpredictable hazard. Also, because prescriptions represent a large number of relatively small claims, administrative costs represent a significant portion of total expenditures.

If prescription coverage is inconsistent with some of the basic principles of insurance, why, then, are prescriptions covered by most health insurance programs? One explanation is that drug therapy is often preventive in nature and is less expensive than other medical alternatives, such as surgery. If medications can keep patients out of the hospital, it is theorized, encouraging proper use of medications may reduce overall healthcare costs. Another explanation is that the growth in prescription coverage may have been driven by an entitlement mentality of employees as well as a lack of understanding of the insurability of pharmaceuticals on the part of corporations' employee benefit managers. However, rising prescription expenditures are starting to make prescription drugs more of an insurable risk for some groups of patients, especially older persons and those with rare, chronic conditions that require specialty medications.

Potential Risk Management Problems

Theoretically, the law of large numbers allows accurate prediction of losses for insured populations. A number of potential risk management problems, however, can make it difficult for insurance companies to predict losses accurately. These risk management problems include catastrophic hazard, adverse selection, supplier-induced demand, and moral hazard.

Catastrophic Hazard

One of the most important risks to avoid is catastrophic hazard. Most insurance policies exclude coverage for widespread, catastrophic events that, if covered, would exceed the company's ability to pay and could, consequently, bankrupt the company. Property insurance policies, for example, exclude coverage for damages caused by earthquakes. Earthquakes are, however, sometimes covered under special addenda (riders) to homeowners' policies. As another example, both health insurance and casualty insurance policies exclude catastrophic losses caused by acts of war.

Adverse Selection

If individuals could predict future losses accurately, they would be more likely to purchase insurance coverage only when they knew they were going to need it and to drop coverage when they did not need it. The situation in which individuals or companies purchase insurance because they expect a loss is known as adverse selection. This practice, of course, makes it difficult for insurers to raise enough premium income from individuals who do not have losses to cover those who do. Adverse selection inevitably results in premium increases for future policyholders.

Flood insurance is notorious for being subject to adverse selection; only policyholders residing in flood plains buy it. Therefore, premiums would be extremely high, and flood insurance probably would not be available without federal subsidies. Adverse selection is also a problem inherent in health insurance; older or sicker individuals are more likely to use insurance and, therefore, more likely to purchase it. Because large, employer-sponsored groups usually include many healthy individuals, adverse selection is not likely to be a problem if all employees are covered, and, consequently, premiums for group policies are usually less expensive than individual policies. Dental insurance is also subject to adverse selection because individuals, theoretically, could obtain coverage only when they know they will need it.

For the benefit of insurance companies and policyholders, it is important to avoid adverse selection. Many restrictions in insurance policy contracts (discussed later in this chapter) are aimed at avoiding the problems associated with adverse selection.

Incentives to Create Losses and Supplier-Induced Demand

A third potential risk management problem occurs when an individual actually gains from an apparent loss. For example, insuring a car for more than its value could give the policyholder an incentive to destroy the car. Insurers try to prevent this kind of profiteering by limiting the amount of insurance coverage to the market value of the insured item. For health insurance, however, it is more difficult to avoid incentives to incur losses (i.e., medical claims). Physicians, who serve as the patients' agents, can always create a demand for the same services that they supply. This potential conflict of interest, known as supplier-induced demand, is an inherent element of health care under fee-for-service reimbursement and is difficult to avoid completely.

Moral Hazard

In theory, some forms of insurance may enable insured individuals to take more risk. For example, a person with automobile insurance or health insurance may feel less need to wear seat belts. Likewise, individuals with health insurance may be more inclined to participate in extreme sports. Health insurance is often subject to a problem known as moral hazard, where people overconsume health care when they have health insurance. By decreasing patients' financial risk for out-of-pocket healthcare expenses, health insurance may have encouraged patients to use services that they might not seek out otherwise (Torrens & Williams, 1993).

If a person has health insurance coverage, then his or her out-of-pocket costs are generally much less than the true cost of providing the individual's health care. At some point, the benefits of additional health services in terms of improving one's health are not really worth their full costs. Overconsumption of health services can drive up health expenses and health insurance premiums for everyone. As presented in the case scenario at the beginning of this chapter, insurers often mandate cost sharing (deductibles, coinsurance, or copayments) as a means to decrease unnecessary demand.

Strategies for Avoiding Risk Management Problems

Insurers must be careful to avoid the problems discussed previously. Failure to do so may result in large increases in premiums or—even worse—make insurance coverage difficult or impossible for individuals or even groups to obtain. Fortunately, insurance companies have developed a variety of strategies to overcome potential risk management problems and to limit their own risks.

Group Policies

To avoid adverse selection, insurance companies use group policies, which are usually sponsored by employer groups and provided to employees and their dependents. As highlighted in the case scenario at the beginning of this chapter, group policies are usually less expensive than individual policies for two reasons. They are less prone to adverse selection, and they are less expensive to sell and administer. Employer groups assume many of the administrative costs associated with enrolling policyholders and explaining the plan's benefits. Selling costs are lower because the insurance company only has to negotiate a master contract with the employer group; it does not have to sign individual contracts with each insured person. Obviously, for a group policy to be cost effective for the insurer, enough policyholders must be in the risk pool so that the law of large numbers allows accurate prediction of losses.

Employer-sponsored group health insurance is popular with workers because it reduces their tax liability; if the amount paid in premiums had been given to employees as salary instead, the workers would have paid income tax and Social Security tax on this income first and then purchased premiums out of their own pockets. Employers also benefit because their payroll taxes, such as the employers' Social Security matching payments and federal and state unemployment taxes, are not paid on the amount of compensation given as employee benefits.

Elimination Period

As introduced in the case scenario at the beginning of this chapter, another contract restriction aimed at avoiding adverse selection is the elimination period (also known as an exclusionary period), in which preexisting health problems are not covered by a new health insurance policy until after the policyholder has been covered for a given period of time. Expenses related to pregnancy and childbirth, for example, may not be covered for the first nine months of a new policy. Elimination periods are often waived for a short period of time after new employees begin their employment. Thereafter, many policies either impose an elimination period for preexisting health problems or require a health test to demonstrate that the patient does not have preexisting health problems that would result in adverse selection.

Coverage Limitations

Even when a given service is covered, the insurance contract will restrict losses by limiting the amount paid for certain covered expenditures and/or what services are covered. Health insurance policies commonly limit payments for physician office visits or prescriptions.

Insurance companies carefully restrict the perils covered to reduce costs and, more importantly, to avoid adverse selection. This is why health insurance policies, such as the one described in the chapter-opening case scenario, often exclude elective treatments such as cosmetic surgery, fertility treatment, abortion, childbirth, and dental care. Mental health and drug and alcohol rehabilitation were commonly excluded until many states adopted laws requiring insurers to cover these services. The perils associated with some injury-prone activities, such as contact sports, aviation, and military service, are also commonly excluded from coverage.

Coordination of Benefits

Occasionally individuals have overlapping coverage from two insurance policies, and questions may arise about which insurance company should be responsible for payment. This can happen, for example, when a person with health insurance is injured in an auto accident or on the job. In these cases, medical expenses may also be covered by the auto insurance policy or by the employer's workers' compensation policy. To avoid the case in which multiple payments are made for the same care, insurance policies usually include a coordination of benefits provision that limits total reimbursement of all insurance to the amount of loss. An insurance policy's subrogation provision states which company pays first. In the examples cited previously, health insurance policies usually pay after auto, homeowner's, or workers' compensation insurance policies have paid their portion.

Other Strategies

The risk management techniques discussed previously are designed to prevent some of the most common risk management problems and are aimed primarily at policyholders. Reducing risk is extremely important because it is a prerequisite for achieving the basic financial objective of all insurance companies—generating revenues in excess of expenses. (Even nonprofit companies need to avoid losses and build reserves.)

Risk can also be reduced by controlling underwriting—avoiding bad risks by refusing coverage to those individuals who are most likely to incur high costs. In the past, some insurance companies have canceled or refused to renew policies for policyholders who incurred major healthcare expenses. Most states now prohibit this practice. Insurance companies have also refused new coverage to people with certain preexisting health problems; this practice makes it difficult for some workers to change jobs because they cannot afford to lose their health insurance coverage. Some of these problems were addressed by the Health Insurance Portability and Accountability Act (HIPAA), discussed in the chapter on healthcare reform.

The facts that health insurance premiums have increased faster than the cost of other goods and services in the United States and that more than 37 million Americans still do not have health insurance (Huffington Post, 2015) are evidence that risk management is a complex endeavor and risk management problems are difficult to overcome.

ADMINISTRATION OF PRESCRIPTION DRUG PROGRAMS

Pharmacy Benefit Manager

Given that the administration of prepaid pharmacy programs is complex and requires a large prescription volume to be conducted efficiently, third parties often separate (or carve out) prescription programs from other health benefits and contract with a type of administrator known as a pharmacy benefit manager (PBM) to manage them. Using a PBM isolates cost centers and concentrates a workforce of prescription benefit experts to manage the prescription program. The administrative services provided by PBMs usually include the following:

- Contracting with healthcare providers to supply specified services
- Communicating with both patients and providers to explain and update administrative policies
- Providing reports to plan sponsors
- Identifying eligible beneficiaries
- Maintaining formulary systems
- Conducting drug utilization reviews
- Processing claims submitted by providers
- Reimbursing providers
- Auditing providers
- Controlling costs
- Controlling utilization
- Ensuring program quality

Participating Pharmacy Agreement

Even health insurance contracts that are carefully crafted to minimize risk management problems include provisions to control healthcare expenditures by reducing the costs per claim and the overall number of claims. Many cost-control provisions for prescription drug programs are specified in participating pharmacy agreements—contracts that stipulate the services to be provided by contracting pharmacies in exchange for a specified reimbursement. (These contracting pharmacies are sometimes referred to as "participating pharmacies" or "network pharmacies." If only a selected group of pharmacies is allowed to contract, these entities are known as "preferred pharmacies" or "preferred providers.")

Plan administrators recruit healthcare providers who are willing to sign participating provider agreements. A clear understanding of the terms of these contracts is important for pharmacy managers and other key employees. Following is a description of some of the most important elements of the participating pharmacy agreement.

Reimbursement

The participating pharmacy agreement specifies the amount and frequency of payment. For pharmacies that dispense large numbers of third-party prescriptions, timely reimbursement is vital. Even more important is the amount of reimbursement. Prescription reimbursement consists of three components: the PBM's cost for the drug ingredients, the dispensing fee, and the amount paid by the patient in the form of copayments, coinsurance, or deductibles. These factors are shown in **Equation 16-1**.

$$\text{Rx payment} = \text{ingredient cost} + \text{dispensing fee} - \text{patient cost sharing} \qquad (16\text{-}1)$$

Ingredient Costs Ingredient costs (also known as the cost of goods sold) represents between 75% and 80% of the cost of the average prescription. Pharmacy reimbursement for drug ingredient costs has traditionally been based on the average wholesale price (AWP)—that is, the list price established by the manufacturer. The AWP is higher than the actual acquisition cost (AAC) that pharmacies pay for drug products. As shown in **Equation 16-2**, the difference between the AWP and the pharmacy's AAC is known as the earned discount.

$$\text{AWP} - \text{AAC} = \text{earned discount} \qquad (16\text{-}2)$$

As shown in **Equation 16-3**, the amount of the pharmacy's earned discount varies depending on the pharmacy's purchasing volume (volume discount), its ability to pay early (cash discount), and special deals and promotions the pharmacy is able to take advantage of (trade discounts).

$$\text{Earned discount} = \text{volume discount} + \text{cash discount} + \text{trade discount} \qquad (16\text{-}3)$$

Earned discounts are very important because they decrease the pharmacy's AAC. A lower AAC, of course, results in a higher gross margin (the difference between the selling price and the cost to the pharmacy for the product that was sold; see **Equation 16-4**). By supplementing low dispensing fees, earned discounts allow pharmacies to participate in managed care plans that would otherwise have been unprofitable.

$$\text{Gross margin} = \text{reimbursement} - \text{AAC} \qquad (16\text{-}4)$$

Because earned discounts vary among pharmacies and even for the same pharmacy from time to time, managed care plans usually do not reimburse pharmacies for their AAC. Instead, the participating pharmacy agreement usually specifies that reimbursement for drug ingredient costs will be based on an estimated acquisition cost, which is usually calculated as a percentage of the AWP (**Equation 16-5**).

$$\text{Estimated acquisition cost} = \text{AWP} - (x\% \text{ of AWP}) \quad (16\text{-}5)$$

Of course, because AWP is a reference price rather than a transaction price, payers are looking for a better way to estimate AACs. Instead of calculating the estimated acquisition cost as a percentage of the AWP, some payers have begun using alternative methods of calculating estimated acquisition cost such as wholesale acquisition cost (WAC). WAC is defined in federal statutes as "The manufacturer's list price for the drug ... to wholesalers or direct purchasers in the United States, not including prompt pay or other discounts, rebates or reductions in price ... as reported in wholesale price guides or other publications of drug ... pricing data" (CCH Health Law Editorial Staff, 2004). Estimated acquisition cost (EAC) is often calculated as WAC plus a specified percentage, as shown in **Equation 16-6**.

$$\text{EAC} = \text{WAC} + X\% \quad (16\text{-}6)$$

When a drug product has chemically equivalent generics, managed care plans often limit reimbursement to the price of a commonly used generic product, referred to as the maximum allowable cost (MAC). Each managed care plan creates its own MAC list. On those occasions when a physician requires the pharmacy to dispense the brand-name version of a multiple-source product, some managed care plans allow full reimbursement for the higher-cost branded product if the pharmacist indicates that the physician specified that the prescription was a dispense-as-written order. Medicaid also sets upper limits for reimbursement of multiple-source drugs but uses the term *federal upper limit* (FUL) instead of MAC.

Dispensing Fees The second part of the reimbursement for a managed care prescription (Equation 16-1) is the dispensing fee paid to the pharmacy. It is a fixed amount that is paid to the pharmacy for each prescription dispensed. PBMs, of course, try to keep total reimbursement for ingredient costs and dispensing fees as low as possible while still maintaining an adequate provider network.

Patient Cost Sharing The third component of the reimbursement for a managed care prescription (Equation 16-1) is patient cost sharing. Patient cost sharing effectively decreases managed care organizations' prescription costs by shifting some responsibility for payment directly to the patient. This practice is designed to not only decrease prescription costs, but to also decrease the utilization rates. Patient cost sharing can take one of three forms:

(1) a copayment, (2) a deductible, or (3) coinsurance. Cost-sharing provisions may also include out-of-pocket limits (i.e., a stop-loss provision) or maximum benefit limits.

Under a copayment system, patients pay a specified dollar amount every time a service is received (e.g., \$50 per hospital admission or \$5 per prescription). Copayments are the most common form of patient cost sharing for prescription benefits.

A deductible requires patients to cover their own healthcare expenses until a specified dollar amount has been paid out of pocket during a given period of time, usually a year. (For example, the insurance company might begin paying health expenses once a patient has paid \$200 of out-of-pocket healthcare expenses during the policy year.) Because patients may receive health services from several different providers, in the past it has sometimes been difficult to determine exactly when the deductible requirement has been met. The expansion of online computerized claims processing makes it easier to keep track of expenses, encouraging more plans to use deductibles in their programs.

The third form of patient cost sharing, coinsurance, requires the patient to pay a specified percentage (often 20%) of the cost of the service; the plan pays the remainder. Although copayments are the most common type of patient cost sharing, the use of coinsurance increased over the last decade and was used by about 18% of plans in 2007. (*The Takeda Prescription Drug Benefit Cost and Plan Design Survey Report,* 2009). Copayment levels have been increasing significantly since the mid-1990s to reflect rising drug prices; coinsurance levels, by contrast, have not changed because the actual dollar amount paid by patients automatically increases as the price of prescriptions increases. Deductibles, on the other hand, have increased significantly (from an average of $303 for single coverage in 2006 to $1,007 in 2015), reflecting a trend of employer-sponsored health insurance plans to shift more medical costs to employees (Kaiser Family Foundation, 2015).

To encourage patients to ask for generic prescriptions, many prescription plans require patients to pay a tiered copayment, which is a relatively low copayment for generic drugs, a higher copayment for preferred brand-name drugs, and an even higher copayment for nonpreferred brand-name products. A small number of employers have created a fourth tier for certain "lifestyle" drugs (e.g., Viagra) that are subject to very high copayments or 50% coinsurance. A fifth tier is sometimes reserved for nonformulary products, euphemistically referred to as a "100% copayment." Multitiered cost-sharing levels are often coordinated with formulary systems to encourage patients to request that their physicians prescribe lower cost medications.

Plans without patient cost-sharing offer first-dollar coverage. Although first-dollar coverage once was common, most plans now see patient cost sharing as a financial incentive that encourages enrollees to avoid using unnecessary healthcare services (i.e., moral hazard). To be effective, however, patient cost-sharing provisions should not be so high as to discourage use of truly necessary health services.

Payment

To be adequate, the total reimbursement should cover the cost of drug ingredients dispensed (the cost of goods sold or AAC) plus the overhead cost incurred by the pharmacy in dispensing the prescription (the cost of dispensing) and a reasonable return on the pharmacy's investment (the net profit); see **Equation 16-7**. If reimbursement covers only the pharmacy's cost without any profit, then it pays at the break-even point. The gross margin is the portion of the reimbursement that exceeds the pharmacy's AAC for drug ingredients.

$$\text{Rx payment} = \overbrace{\underbrace{\text{drug ingredient cost}}_{\text{Cost of goods sold}} + \text{cost of dispensing}}^{\text{Breakeven cost}} + \text{net profit} \tag{16-7}$$

(Gross margin = cost of dispensing + net profit)

For most plans, total reimbursement for a managed care prescription will not exceed the pharmacy's usual and customary price (i.e., the price charged most commonly to private-pay patients). Third-party pharmacy contracts typically state that pharmacy reimbursement is usually the lower of

1. The specified estimated acquisition cost plus the dispensing fee
2. The specified maximum allowable cost plus the dispensing fee
3. The pharmacy's usual and customary charge

Other Contract Provisions

The participating pharmacy agreement tells the pharmacy how to determine whether a person is eligible for benefits. Usually, eligible beneficiaries receive some form of identification card. Because cardholders often change jobs or insurance plans, the card itself may not be a guarantee of payment; pharmacies typically confirm eligibility through a computerized eligibility verification system.

The participating pharmacy contract also specifies how pharmacies are to submit claims for reimbursement. In most cases, this step involves submitting electronic claims through the pharmacy's computer at the time the prescription is dispensed. Such an online adjudication system is a major improvement over the old paper claims system because it is faster and less expensive and tells the pharmacy immediately whether the claim will be accepted, the amount of copayment that should be collected, and the amount that the plan will reimburse for the prescription.

Not all third-party programs cover the same products. A section of the contract titled "limitations" or "exclusions" specifies what is not covered. Some common exclusions are nonprescription drugs (other than insulin), compounded prescriptions, devices (such as syringes), and products used for cosmetic purposes (such as hair growth or wrinkle removal). There may be a maximum quantity that can be dispensed for some products (e.g., a 30-day supply). However, some contracts specify a minimum quantity (such as a 3-month supply) that may be dispensed for certain maintenance medications used for chronic conditions.

Almost all contracts reserve the right to audit the pharmacy's records as a deterrent to fraudulent claims. Preferably, the contract specifies the auditing procedures that will be used.

IMPACT OF HEALTH INSURANCE ON PHARMACY

Health insurance covered approximately 90% of all prescriptions in 2013; the remaining 10% was paid out-of-pocket (i.e., directly by patients). Private health insurance covered 39%, whereas public insurance covered 51% (Medicare covered 34%, whereas Medicaid covered 17%) (West, 2014). Health insurance has profoundly affected the profitability of pharmacies. In the past decade, dispensing fees have declined while inventory costs have increased. This has contributed to a decline in the average pharmacy's gross margin from 32.2% of sales in 1986 to 23.3% of sales in 2013—a drop of about 9 percentage points (West, 2014). As shown in **Table 16-2**, those pharmacies that have survived have maintained net profits at around 3% of sales. They have done so by becoming more efficient and by decreasing their expenses. These efficiencies have been achieved primarily through aggregation of buying power, automation, and increased use of pharmacy technicians.

Why do pharmacies participate in third-party plans that offer low reimbursement? The answer to this question is not simple and varies from pharmacy to pharmacy. Some pharmacies accept third-party plans because they are reluctant to lose customers who may be buying over-the-counter products and other goods from the front of the store. For others, as long as reimbursement covers the variable costs of the dispensed prescription, fixed expenses can be spread among the larger percentage of private-pay prescriptions. However, this strategy is effective only as long as third-party prescriptions represent a minority portion of a pharmacy's business. Given that the majority of prescriptions are now paid for by third parties, such cost shifting will not be feasible as a long-term strategy.

To survive or prosper in the managed care environment, all community pharmacies—both chains and independents—need to be run by good managers. Community pharmacy managers must know their costs and lower them to the greatest extent possible by managing their operations efficiently, and they must be familiar with the prescription benefit plans sponsored by major employer groups. Pharmacists in all settings should also be prepared to document the value of their services.

Table 16-2 Changes in Pharmacy Operations, 1986–2013

	1986 (%)	1996 (%)	2006 (%)	2013 (%)	Change 1986–2013 (%)
Sales	100.0	100.0	100.0	100.0	+0.0
Cost of goods sold	67.8	74.4	77.2	76.7	+8.9
Gross margin	32.2	25.6	22.8	23.3	–8.9
Expenses	29.5	22.5	20.0	20.2	–9.3
Net profit	2.7	3.1	2.8	3.1	+0.4

Source: Data from Dankmeyer, T. (Ed.). (1997). *1997 NCPA-Searle Digest.* Alexandria, VA: National Community Pharmacists Association and West, D. S. (Ed.). (2014). *2014 NCPA Digest.* Alexandria, VA: National Community Pharmacists Association.

Pharmacists have tried to work together through a variety of pharmacy organizations, such as volume purchasing groups and pharmacy associations to help pharmacists succeed in this environment. (There is a limit, however, to the extent to which pharmacies can work together. Because of antitrust laws, they cannot collectively boycott undesirable plans, nor can they collectively negotiate fees with third parties.) Above all, pharmacy managers must understand the healthcare marketplace and the roles of the various participants in the health insurance industry. Without this knowledge, even the best manager will be unprepared to work effectively in today's rapidly changing healthcare environment.

CONCLUSION

Health insurance has profoundly changed how health care is financed and delivered in the United States. The health insurance industry has grown rapidly during the last century and will continue to evolve toward managed care. Although health insurance presents some formidable challenges for pharmacists and other healthcare providers, it also presents some promising opportunities. All pharmacists—whether staff or managers, community or institutional—must understand the principles and dynamics of the health insurance industry to be effective in their position. Those pharmacists who strive to genuinely understand the needs and perspectives of insurance plan sponsors, underwriters, and administrators and are able to identify new opportunities for pharmacists and pharmacies will help determine the profession's future success.

QUESTIONS FOR FURTHER DISCUSSION

1. What is the difference between controlling costs and managing care? What are some examples of each?
2. How can experience rating decrease premiums and at the same time increase the number of uninsured?
3. How can health insurance companies reduce or prevent problems associated with adverse selection and moral hazard?
4. What is the traditional role of public insurance programs? How might this role change in the future?

KEY TOPICS AND TERMS

Actual acquisition cost (AAC)
Actuary
Adjudication
Adverse selection
Average manufacturer's price (AMP)
Average wholesale price (AWP)
Catastrophic hazard
Coinsurance
Community rating
Coordination of benefits
Copayment
Deductible
Dispense as written (DAW)
Earned discount
Elimination period
Estimated acquisition cost
Experience rating
First-dollar coverage
Fiscal intermediary
Gross margin
Group policies
Health Insurance Portability and Accountability Act (HIPAA)
Indemnity
Induced demand
Insurable hazard
Insurable interest
Law of large numbers
Major medical insurance
Maximum allowable cost
Moral hazard
Open enrollment period
Participating pharmacy agreement
Patient cost sharing
Pharmacy benefit manager (PBM)
Pure risk
Reinsurance
Risk pool
Service benefit
Speculative risk
Subrogation
Supplier-induced demand
Underwriting
Wholesale acquisition cost (WAC)

REFERENCES

Campbell, W. H., & Newsome, L. A. (1995). The evolution of managed care and practice settings. In S. M. Ito & S. Blackburn (Eds.), *A pharmacist's guide to principles and practices of managed care pharmacy* (pp. 1–14). Alexandria, VA: Foundation for Managed Care Pharmacy.

CCH Health Law Editorial Staff. (2004). *Medicare Prescription Drug, Improvement, and Modernization Act of 2003: Law and Explanation* (2nd ed.). Chicago, IL: CCH, p. 178.

Fronstin, P., & Snider, S. C. (1996). An examination of the decline in employment-based health insurance between 1988 and 1993. *Inquiry, 33,* 317–325.

Himmelstein, D. U., Thorne, D., Warren, E., & Woolhandler, S. (2009). Medical bankruptcy in the United States, 2007: Results of a national study. *American Journal of Medicine, 122*(8), 741–746.

Institute of Medicine. (1993). *Employment and health benefits: A connection at risk.* Washington, DC: National Academy Press.

Kaiser Family Foundation. (2015). *Benchmark employer survey: Family premiums rise modest 4 percent to $17,545.* Retrieved from http://kff.org/health-costs/press-release/employer-family-health-premiums-rise-4-percent-to-17545-in-2015-extending-a-decade-long-trend-of-relatively-moderate-increases

Kissick, W. (1994). *Medicines dilemmas.* New Haven and New London, CT: Yale University Press.

Kreling, D. H., Mott, D. A., & Wiederholt, J. B. (2001, November). *Prescription drug trends—A chartbook update.* Kaiser Family Foundation, p. 56.

Lannon, C., Brack, V., Stuart, J., Caplow, M., NcNeill, A., Bordley, W. C., & Margolis, P. (1995). What mothers say about why poor children fall behind on immunizations. A summary of focus groups in North Carolina. *Archives of Pediatric Adolescent Medicine, 149*, 1070–1075.

Lee, P. R., Soffel, D., & Luft, H. S. (1992). Costs and coverage: Pressures toward health care reform. *Western Journal of Medicine, 157*, 576–583.

Litman, T. L. (1994). Government and health: The political aspects of health care—A sociopolitical overview. In P. R. Lee & C. L. Estes (Eds.), *The nation's health* (4th ed., pp. 107–120). Sudbury, MA: Jones and Bartlett.

Pharmaceutical Manufacturers Association. (1973). *Pharmaceutical payment programs: An overview.* Washington, DC: Pharmaceutical Manufacturers Association.

Salsberry, P. J., Nickel, J. T., & Mitch, R. (1994). Immunization status of 2-year-olds in middle/upper- and lower income populations: A community survey. *Public Health Nurse, 11*, 17–23.

Santoli, J. M., Huet, N. J., Smith, P. J., Barker, L. E., Rodenwald, L. E., Inkelas, M., ... Halfon, N. (2004). Insurance status and vaccination coverage among U.S. preschool children. *Pediatrics, 113*, 1959–1964.

Smith, J. C., & Medalia, C. (2014). *Health insurance coverage in the United States: 2013. Current population reports.* Washington, DC: U.S. Government Printing Office.

Starr, P. (1982). *The social transformation of American medicine.* New York, NY: Basic Books.

The Takeda prescription drug benefit cost and plan design survey report. (2009). Scottsdale, AZ: The Pharmacy Benefit Management Institute.

Thamer, M., Richard, C., Casebeer, A. W., & Ray, N. F. (1997). Health insurance coverage among foreign-born U.S. residents: The impact of race, ethnicity, and length of residence. *American Journal of Public Health, 87*, 96–102.

Torrens, P. R., & Williams, S. J. (1993). Understanding the present, planning for the future: The dynamics of health care in the United States in the 1990s. In S. J. Williams & P. R. Torrens (Eds.), *Introduction to health services* (4th ed., pp. 421–429). Albany, NY: Delmar.

West, D. S. (Ed.). (2011). *2011 NCPA Digest.* Alexandria, VA: National Community Pharmacists Association.

West, D. S. (Ed.). (2014). *2014 NCPA Digest.* Alexandria, VA: National Community Pharmacists Association.

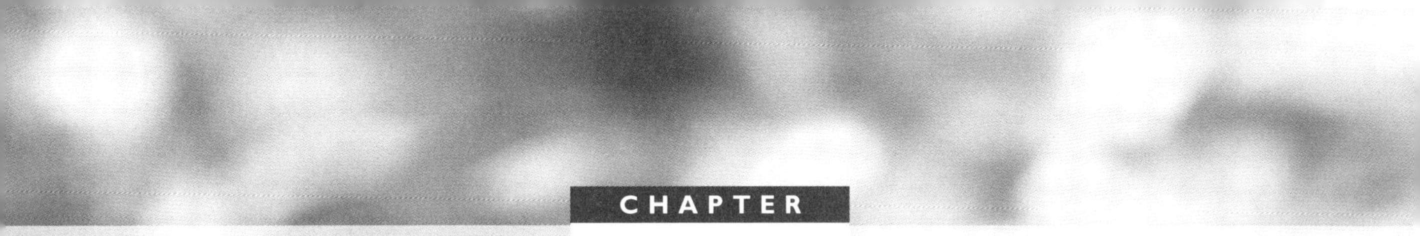

CHAPTER

17

Managed Health Care

Kenneth W. Schafermeyer and Taehwan Park*

Case Scenario

Sovaldi®, which was approved by the Food and Drug Administration in 2013, is indicated for the treatment of hepatitis C virus (HCV) infection. According to FDA, Sovaldi® is the first drug that showed safety and efficacy to treat certain types of HCV infection without the need for coadministration of interferon. In the first year of its introduction, this drug was on pace to become the biggest blockbuster medication in the last 10 years. In 2014, it was the best-selling prescription drug with sales of $7.8 billion, which was primarily driven by its expensive costs of $1,000 per one tablet and $84,000 per person over the three-month treatment (Lindsley, 2015).

Notably, patients' access to Sovaldi® varies state by state because of differences in coverage among the various state Medicaid programs. Some states list Sovaldi® as a preferred drug and impose few restrictions on access. Other states require prior authorization (PA) before patients can receive treatment with Sovaldi®. These PA provisions sometimes require prospective patients to meet a set of clinical or clinical-related criteria. Some states also place frequency, quantity, and duration limits on the dispensing of Sovaldi®.

Suppose you work for a pharmacy benefit manager and clients are asking about your company's recommendation concerning Sovaldi® coverage. What are the key ethical, political, clinical, financial, and equity issues to consider in deciding whether to cover Sovaldi®? What is your recommendation and why?

How would your recommendation change, if at all, if the client already covers other medications for the treatment of hepatitis C infection?

One client has decided to cover Sovaldi® but has indicated that it does not want the drug's utilization, and hence its costs, to skyrocket out of control. What plan design recommendations would you suggest for Sovaldi® (e.g., prior authorization, quantity limits, and cost-sharing levels)?

*The authors wish to express appreciation to Brenda R. Motheral and Evan S. Schnur for their contributions to this chapter.

LEARNING OBJECTIVES

Upon completion of this chapter, the student shall be able to:

- Describe the objectives of managed health care (i.e., access, quality, and cost).
- Differentiate between insuring health and managing health care.
- Differentiate between retrospective and prospective payment for services.
- Compare and contrast fee-for-service and capitation reimbursement.
- Describe and differentiate among the major types of managed care organizations (MCOs).
- Describe the market power of MCOs.
- List the functions of a pharmacy benefit manager.
- Describe MCO tools used to control costs and enhance quality.
- Define third-party and managed care terminology.
- Describe outcomes of consumer-driven health plans (CDHPs).
- Define the organizations and methods used to accredit MCOs.

CHAPTER QUESTIONS

1. What factors have encouraged or hindered the growth of managed care?
2. How do staff-, group-, network-, and independent practice association–model health maintenance organizations (HMOs) differ?
3. Since 1980, what have the enrollment trends been for the four basic types of HMOs?
4. What are the characteristics of the four major tools used to manage the pharmacy benefit?
5. What measures are considered in National Committee for Quality Assurance accreditation?

INTRODUCTION

Managed care has profoundly affected the way in which medical care is delivered, consumed, and perceived. While there is no universally accepted definition of managed care, most would agree that any movement away from strict payment of services and toward governing of the provision of medical services is a form of managed care. Managed care organizations (MCOs) provide healthcare services, including prescriptions, to defined populations such as employer groups on a prepaid basis. Because MCOs assume financial risk for expenditures, they have strong incentives to control costs and utilization of healthcare services. A major challenge facing MCOs continues to be the need to balance advocacy for patient care against the efficient allocation of scarce resources.

THE HISTORY OF MANAGED CARE

Managed care's roots can be traced to the lodges, fraternal orders, and benevolent societies established in the 1800s by European immigrants to care for their sick and disabled. The first organized health delivery services were offered to recruit employees to work in isolated areas such as pineapple plantations in Hawaii, lumber camps in Michigan, iron ranges in northern Minnesota, and railroads in isolated pockets across the country. Physicians were usually on contract or salary because the best way to recruit physicians was to provide them with a guaranteed income. Hospital beds were either owned or under contract (Friedman, 1996).

The American Medical Association (AMA) did not object to these plans in the rural areas, considering them an economic necessity. However, the AMA continued to object to any other form of organized medicine that involved a third-party intermediary (Jecker, 1994). By the 1920s, the AMA had established the solo practitioner with a fee-for-service (FFS) reimbursement (where a fee was paid for each service performed) as the predominant model of medical practice (Miller & Luft, 1994). Despite the AMA's opposition, numerous state courts ruled that medical societies could not take actions against physicians who participated in prepaid plans (plans in which patients paid in advance of receiving service for the cost of predetermined benefits) (Jecker, 1994).

The availability of prepaid plans expanded during World War II. Many of the plans formed during that era still exist today (such as Group Health Cooperative of Puget Sound and Kaiser Permanente), but in the early years they generally had some advantage that allowed them to survive in the antimanaged care environment that prevailed at the time (Miller & Luft, 1994).

Perhaps the most famous MCO was, and is, Kaiser Permanente. Henry J. Kaiser, an industrial contractor, called upon Dr. Sidney Garfield to develop a system for providing medical care to his 15,000 workers and dependents who were building the Grand Coulee Dam in Washington. The Kaiser Company financed everything from hospital equipment to nurses and staff for outpatient clinics, thereby creating an entire medical delivery system. Kaiser covered workers' industrial injuries and illnesses, and employees had the option of contributing 50 cents per week for themselves, 50 cents per week for each adult dependent, and 25 cents per week for each child to cover nonindustrial injuries and illnesses (Campbell & Newsome, 1995).

The passage in 1973 of the Health Maintenance Organization Act was a major catalyst in the growth of managed care (Davis, Collins, & Morris, 1994). The legislation supported start-up grants and loans for health maintenance organizations (HMOs), a type of MCO, and required employers with 25 or more employees to provide HMO enrollment as an alternative to traditional indemnity insurance for their employees where it was available (see Chapter 16 for a description of indemnity insurance). These factors, taken collectively, had a tremendous effect on the growth of managed care. In 1970, there were 3 million enrollees in HMOs; in 1980, there were 9 million HMO members (Miller & Luft, 1994). In 1989, HMO enrollment had grown to 35 million enrollees; by 1998, the number had tripled to 105.3 million participants (Hoechst Marion Roussel, 1999). Since the early 2000s, HMO popularity has declined significantly. In 2012, there were only 81 million Americans enrolled in HMO plans (Sanofi-Aventis, 2013). This decline may be a reflection of employers' growing inability to afford the state-mandated comprehensive healthcare benefits that are typical of HMO offerings. While employers still use many of the principles and tools conceived in early managed care, they have more flexibility in cost sharing and service coverage by steering away from the heavily regulated HMO offerings with higher premiums.

TYPES OF MANAGED CARE ORGANIZATIONS

While the term *managed care* can be defined in many ways and is constantly evolving to meet the demands of the healthcare market, the differentiating feature of managed care relative to FFS plans is the use of provider networks (Miller & Luft, 1994). A network is a defined group of providers, typically linked through contractual arrangements, who supply a full range of primary and acute healthcare services (Medicom International, n.d.). Managed care enrollees who use providers outside the network may receive reduced coverage or even no coverage. Four characteristics differentiate the various managed care plans (**Table 17-1**):

- *Risk bearing* refers to the amount of risk borne by the providers, which can range from full risk to no risk.
- *Physician type* refers to the relationship between the MCO and the physician(s).
- *Relationship exclusivity* addresses whether the physician provides care to patients from one MCO only or to patients from multiple MCOs.
- *Out-of-network coverage* identifies whether care received from a provider who is not in the MCO's network is a covered benefit. Types of MCOs are discussed below in terms of these distinguishing characteristics (see Miller & Luft, 1994, for a thorough discussion).

Table 17-1 Characteristics of Managed Care Plans

Type	Physician risk bearing	Physician type	Exclusivity of relationship with physician	Out-of-network coverage
HMO				
Staff	No	Staff	Yes	No
Group	Yes	Large group	Yes	No
Network	Yes	Large group	No	No
IPA	Yes	Solo/small group	No	No
PPO	No	Solo or group	No	Yes
EPO	No	Solo or group	No	No
POS	Varies	Varies	Varies	Yes

HMO—health maintenance organization
IPA—independent practice association
PPO—preferred provider organization
EPO—exclusive provider organization
POS—point of service

Source: Reproduced with permission of *Annual Review of Public Health*, Volume 15(1), © 1994, by Annual Reviews, Inc., http://www.annualreviews.org.

Health Maintenance Organizations

The distinguishing characteristics of HMOs are that they place providers at risk, either directly or indirectly, and generally do not provide coverage for medical care that is received out of network. The risk arrangement can take many forms. In capitation, costs of care for a given population are estimated for some time span (typically 1 year), and physicians are prospectively paid this set amount of money to provide agreed-upon services (Rognehaugh, 1996). The provider keeps the capitation payment, regardless of whether a patient actually receives any services during the year. The provider is, however, obligated to provide any services—no matter how many—needed by the patient. Thus, the physician is taking the risk that the capitation rate will be sufficient to cover all the costs of care for the population. In this way, the provider assumes risk that traditionally was underwritten by the insurance company.

Risk pools, in which a portion of payments for services rendered (i.e., a withhold) is placed in a pool as a source for any subsequent claims that exceed projections (Rognehaugh, 1996), have been implemented for hospitals and other high-risk services. In these schemes, the physician and the HMO share the surplus or loss from the risk pool at the end of the year (Mack, 1993). The use of this strategy peaked in 2003 with 32.1% of plans using risk pools, then the usage rate declined to 28.9% in 2010. The rate rebounded and reached 35.7% in 2012 (Sanofi-Aventis, 2013).

The gatekeeper is a central component of most HMOs. Gatekeepers, who are typically primary care physicians, must coordinate and authorize all medical services, including laboratory services, specialty referrals, and hospitalizations (Medicom International, n.d.). In many gatekeeper systems, a patient must receive a referral from his or her primary care physician to receive coverage for a specialist's care. The rationale behind this approach is that it avoids unnecessary and often expensive referrals to specialists. The gatekeeper may be financially at risk—not only for the services that he or she provides, but also for the medical services provided by specialists to whom a patient is referred.

Traditionally, HMOs were classified into four major types:

1. *Staff-model HMO:* a type of HMO characterized by direct ownership of healthcare facilities and direct employment physicians. Physicians in a staff-model HMO typically bear no direct risk, but the HMO can influence the care given by the physicians through utilization review (the review of the necessity and efficiency of patients' utilization patterns). In addition, because the HMO pays most or all of the physicians' salaries, these providers risk termination of their contracts if their treatment patterns do not meet administrators' expectations.
2. *Group-model HMO:* a type of HMO characterized by contracts with large, multispecialty medical groups offering services exclusively to the HMO on a capitated basis.
3. *Network-model HMO:* a type of HMO characterized by nonexclusive contracts with large medical groups. While networks typically bear risk, the nonexclusivity of the arrangement reduces the influence of the risk on the physician's behavior.
4. *Independent practice association (IPA)-model HMO:* a type of HMO in which physicians form a separate legal entity, usually a corporation or partnership, that then contracts with the MCO. The IPA usually shares risk with the MCO, and then individual providers are paid by the IPA for services provided to enrolled patients for a negotiated fee. The IPA may reimburse physicians on a discounted FFS basis or may share some risk with them. These physicians typically maintain their own private practices and are allowed to provide services to patients enrolled in other MCOs.

While these four models represent the traditional categories into which HMOs are classified, recent innovations in plan designs have blurred the distinctions among these models. Plans can have elements of two or more of these categories and, therefore, be difficult to classify as fitting into any single model.

Preferred Provider Organizations

Preferred provider organizations (PPOs) are affiliations of providers that seek contracts with insurance plans. The physicians are usually from solo or small-group practices and have nonexclusive arrangements with the PPO. Under a PPO plan, individuals are free to see any provider they choose but have a financial incentive (i.e., lower out-of-pocket expenses) to receive care from providers in the preferred network. PPOs generally do not capitate physicians who are members of their network. Rather, physicians accept discounted FFS payment in exchange for increased patient volume and a quick turnaround on claims payment. Because physicians bear no risk, plan administrators emphasize fee reduction and case-by-case utilization management to control costs. PPOs have proved more popular than HMOs with sponsors, providers, and patients because they are perceived to be less restrictive, with enrollment at nearly 152 million people in 2012 (Sanofi-Aventis, 2013). Nevertheless, the number of operating PPO plans has decreased since 1998 (Sanofi-Aventis, 2013).

Exclusive provider organizations (EPOs) are similar to PPOs in their structure, administration, and operation. However, EPOs strictly limit the number of providers and enrollees typically receive no reimbursement for using healthcare services from out-of-network providers.

Hybrid Plans and Categorical Limitations

Many plans combine two or more of the previously described organizational models and, accordingly, are referred to as hybrid plans. An example of a hybrid plan is a point-of-service (POS) plan. POS plans allow patients to select providers at the time a service is needed rather than when they join the plan. As with PPOs, when care is received from a provider outside the network, partial coverage is provided. As with HMOs, physicians may be at risk or contract exclusively with the plan.

With the rapidly changing healthcare market and much creative plan design, the categorization of the various types of MCOs becomes more difficult. As HMOs provide more diversified products, the lines of distinction become blurred. For example, mixed-model HMOs, which contract with more than one type of physician organization, are becoming more prevalent as the arrangements among the organizations grow increasingly complex (Miller & Luft, 1994).

Growth and Composition of Managed Care Plans

Early on, managed care plans were predominantly not-for-profit, operating as either staff- or group-model HMOs. IPAs and network-model HMOs appeared in the 1950s in response to physicians' feeling threatened by the staff and group models (Davis et al., 1994). Since then, growth in this market has been greatest in IPA models and slowest in staff and group models. In recent years, however, both the number of HMOs and HMO enrollment have declined. For example, in 1998, there were 902 HMOs licensed in the United States; by 2012, the number dropped to 430. Although IPAs are still the predominant HMO model—accounting for 46% of all HMOs in 2012—the number of plans declined from 606 in 1998 to 197 in 2012 (Aventis, 2002; Sanofi-Aventis, 2014). Group and staff models remain the least popular options, accounting for 10% and 3% of all HMOs in 2012, respectively (Sanofi-Aventis, 2014).

In 2001, 31.7% of the U.S. population was enrolled in some kind of HMO; by 2012, that percentage had dropped to 25.7%. There were, however, some significant regional differences in acceptance of HMOs. The highest enrollment is in Hawaii, California, and Utah; in these states, more than 40% of patients belong to an HMO. By contrast, the following 10 states posted HMO penetration rates of less than 10%: Alabama, Alaska, Arkansas, Idaho, Mississippi, Montana, North Dakota, Nebraska, South Dakota, and Wyoming (Aventis, 2002; Sanofi-Aventis, 2013).

Managed health care continues to evolve rapidly. While HMO enrollment has declined in recent years, enrollment in other types of MCOs has increased. Managed health care has also shifted from being predominantly a not-for-profit industry to a for-profit sector (Davis et al., 1994). Concurrently, there has been a marked expansion of managed care to the Medicaid and Medicare populations.

CONSUMER-DRIVEN HEALTH PLANS

During the past several years, consumer-driven health plans (CDHPs) have become popular.

The CDHP enrollment has increased from 4% in 2006 to 20% in 2014 among the workers covered by employer-sponsored insurance (Kaiser Family Foundation, 2014). A CDHP refers to a health insurance plan which combines high-deductible insurance coverage with a personal health savings account such as a health savings account (HSA) or a health reimbursement arrangement (HRA). The CDHP enrollees pay all their health care expenditures with funds from their health savings account. When health savings account funds are exhausted, they begin to pay with out-of-pocket funds before reaching the deductible limit. Once the deductible limit is met, coinsurance-based health insurance coverage begins. Because any unused balance remaining at year's end can be rolled over to the next year in an HSA, a CDHP provides consumers with discretionary management responsibility for their health care expenditures. Cost-conscious CDHP enrollees would try to reduce unnecessary costs from unneeded medications and seek better care, which can result in cost savings and improvement in quality of care.

MANAGING THE PHARMACY BENEFIT

Much emphasis is placed on managing the pharmacy benefit in MCOs, given the large expenditure growth in this sector over the last 15 years. Companies that manage the pharmacy benefit may offer performance guarantees. If they do not achieve a certain level of performance, they are subject to financial penalties. Performance guarantees can relate to cost savings (e.g., generic substitution rates), customer service (e.g., wait time on calls to customer service), or client reporting (Lipton, Kreling, Collins, & Hertz, 1999).

Pharmacies are rarely reimbursed on a capitation basis because it is physicians—not pharmacists—who have the greatest influence over prescription utilization and costs. Physicians, therefore, are more likely to be held responsible for prescription costs. An effective way to influence prescribing practices is to give physicians financial incentives to control drug costs. Traditionally, these incentives took the form of performance bonuses or withholds and risk pools. While physicians are most commonly reimbursed retrospectively on a discounted FFS basis, prospective payment methods that encourage cost control (e.g., capitation) are gaining more acceptance among PPOs (Sanofi-Aventis, 2010).

Because managed care prescription programs reimburse pharmacies on an FFS basis, health plans' cost-containment efforts are directed to the following three types of costs incurred whenever a prescription is dispensed:

1. *Unit cost,* which refers to the amount paid for each prescription, consists of reimbursement for drug ingredient costs and a dispensing fee.
2. *Utilization rate,* which refers to the number of prescriptions dispensed per patient.

3. *Administrative costs,* which are the charges for processing a claim and managing the prescription benefit program. These costs are greatly reduced by having pharmacies submit claims for reimbursement electronically, thereby eliminating most, if not all, paperwork. While administrative costs are commonly paid on a per-claim-processed basis, some are paid on a per-enrollee basis.

Pharmacy Benefit Managers

In 2013, approximately 90% of retail prescription claims were paid for by a third party rather than by individual patients (West, 2014). Most often, the payer was a specialized organization known as a pharmacy benefit manager (PBM). Even the largest MCOs commonly outsource management of the pharmacy benefit to a PBM. As explained in Chapter 16, PBMs administer the prescription drug part of health insurance plans on behalf of plan sponsors, which could be HMOs, self-insured employers, PPOs, or indemnity insurers.

While not always considered a type of MCO, PBMs have many of the characteristics of managed care, including having a provider network of pharmacies. Typically, PBMs contract with existing community pharmacies to create a network of pharmacies from which patients can receive prescriptions at the rate established by the plan sponsor. PBMs negotiate with network pharmacies for decreased product reimbursement prices in exchange for an increased volume of prescriptions to be dispensed through their pharmacies.

Because the administration of pharmacy programs is rather complex and requires a claims-processing system and large prescription volume to be handled efficiently, PBMs typically can offer lower costs and patient access to a greater number of pharmacies than can an individual plan sponsor. Services offered by most PBMs include pharmacy network development, claims processing, eligibility maintenance, client reporting, rebate contracting, generic use programs, formulary management, therapeutic interchange, mail service, drug utilization review (DUR), patient and provider education, step therapy, and medication adherence programs. The following sections describe some of these tools.

Limited Networks

As previously mentioned, PBMs contract with community pharmacies to create a network of pharmacies from which patients can receive prescriptions. In selecting a network, considerations include location, cost, and quality, which are interrelated (Sterler & Stephens, 1999). For example, plans can simultaneously reduce administrative expenses and negotiate greater fee reductions by contracting with fewer pharmacies in return for increased prescription volume. Location is a key consideration in network development because it determines the ease with which patients can access a pharmacy. When developing a network, the PBM will model the average distance between pharmacies and patients in the area using geographic information systems that are based on the pharmacies' and the patients' ZIP codes. An example of a common target is that a pharmacy provider be located within 1 to 5 miles of each enrollee's home in metropolitan areas, within 5 miles in suburban areas, and within 10 miles in rural areas (Sterler & Stephens, 1999).

Cost is the second critical element in network development and requires negotiation of multiple reimbursement rates for the various types of medications dispensed. Pharmacy benefit managers often lack data on actual pharmacy drug costs and, instead, determine an estimated acquisition cost (EAC) based on a discount from published pricing data such as the average wholesale price (AWP). AWP is a published reference price from which pharmacies obtain significant discounts; it is not based on actual selling prices. Studies have shown actual acquisition cost for brand-name drugs to be about 79% of AWP (Myers & Stauffer, 2007), and pharmacies are typically reimbursed by private plans for brand medications in the range of AWP minus 14% to 18%.

Wholesale acquisition cost (WAC) is a more accurate estimate of prices charged by wholesalers for brand-name drugs before applying certain discounts based on volume and prompt payment; it is not, however, a uniformly accurate estimate of generic prices.

Rather, the vast majority of plans use maximum allowable cost (MAC) in setting generic prices. MAC is a maximum ingredient cost that will be paid for a drug, independent of the manufacturer's AWP. The use of MAC incentivizes retail pharmacies to purchase from lower-cost generic providers as there are typically multiple manufacturers of generics, and price competition can be significant. Regardless of the discount that is stipulated for brands and generics, most contracts require that the payment be the lowest of the following three measures:

1. The contract rate—usually stated as an EAC plus a dispensing fee
2. The MAC plus a dispensing fee
3. The usual and customary price charged to a cash-paying customer

Thus, in those cases where the pharmacy's usual and customary price is less than the contract rate, the pharmacy is paid the lower usual and customary price.

Once a network has been established, ongoing network communication and provider performance (i.e., quality) are key issues. The PBM can use a variety of methods to communicate with network providers, including newsletters, online communications, and Internet websites (Sterler & Stephens, 1999). Audits are a key tool that is used in pharmacy network performance. While online adjudication systems help minimize fraud and abuse problems, audits serve as an additional quality control technique. Electronic audits (i.e., automated algorithms that look for outlier patterns of prescription utilization that may be indicative of potential fraud problems) are very common. An electronic audit may trigger an on-site audit in which the auditor visits the pharmacy and examines its prescription records (Sterler & Stephens, 1999). On-site audits may result in no action, termination from the network, a request for reimbursement for select claims, or other actions.

Claims Adjudication

PBMs use online electronic claims submission systems to adjudicate claims for prescriptions dispensed by network pharmacies. This electronic data interchange has been standardized and is maintained by the National Council for Prescription Drug Programs. Electronic claims systems can carry out distinct administrative functions, including eligibility verification and claims adjudication. The pharmacy is notified of the formulary status of the prescribed medication, and any limits on medication quantities or refills are addressed. The amount to be remitted to the pharmacy and the patient's copayment are also determined.

In addition, electronic claims systems can review the prescribing, dispensing, and usage patterns for given patients or drug products and suggest improvements (see "Drug Utilization Review" later in this chapter). They may also suggest therapeutic alternatives and provide information regarding physician network status and various patient and provider characteristics.

A transaction can be rejected by the PBM during adjudication if the pharmacy violates a clinical or administrative requirement. An online dispensing message that can be overridden by the pharmacist is known as a soft-edit message; a hard-edit message cannot be overridden without approval of the plan/PBM or an appropriate change to one or more components of the submitted claim. Under the latest National Council for Prescription Drug Programs guidelines, intervention/outcome codes allow pharmacists to override certain edits by indicating which intervention took place to address the identified issue (e.g., the pharmacist called the doctor to notify him or her about a potentially serious drug–drug interaction).

Mail Service

Most PBMs offer mail service pharmacies—either through their own mail-order facility or by contracting with one. As a result of their large prescription volumes, these mail service pharmacies are able to negotiate discounts on product costs and achieve economies of scale that reduce their dispensing costs. Because of the scale advantage, mail service pharmacies usually provide deeper discounts (when measured as cost per dose) to plan sponsors than retail pharmacies can, and they also represent the greatest profitability per prescription for PBMs. Accordingly, with the approval of the plan sponsor, PBMs may require members to use only a mail service pharmacy for certain prescriptions (usually refills of maintenance medications for chronic conditions), or at least give incentives, such as discounted copayments, to encourage patients to use the mail service pharmacy. As a result of the continued focus on mail order by PBMs, its use has continued to grow over the last decade. However, the growth has been slowing recently as economic advantage of using mail service is diminishing (Fein, 2011). Community pharmacies are now allowed to fill 90-day prescriptions for maintenance medications, which reduces retail reimbursement and shrinks the cost gap between mail and community pharmacy for consumers and third-party payers. Mail prescriptions represent about 15% of all prescriptions as of 2013 (Fein, 2014).

Generic Promotion, Formularies, and Prior Authorization

Plan sponsors use a variety of tools to promote use of lower-cost generic and brand medications and to reduce unnecessary use of medications. Generics have represented one of the greatest opportunities for savings in the pharmacy benefit over the last decade as the number of generic alternatives has grown. Generic fill rates are calculated as: (number of generic claims) ÷ (number of generic claims + number of brand claims). PBMs frequently report that 50% to 60% of prescriptions reimbursed are for generic drug products; some closed-model plans report rates of 70% or more (Navarro & Hailey, 2009). To promote use of generics, PBMs recommend lower copayments for generics than brands and offer a variety of educational tools to help promote generics, such as online tools that identify generic alternatives to brand medications, letter- or telephone-based outreach programs that identify generic alternatives to brand medications that a patient is currently taking, and physician education programs aimed at increasing the writing of prescriptions for generic alternatives.

The use of lower-cost brand medications also represents a significant savings opportunity for plan sponsors, which is typically achieved through the use of a formulary. PBMs generate significant savings from the rebates received from pharmaceutical manufacturers in return for placing specific drugs on the formulary or giving these drugs preferred status. The amount of these rebates may be based on the plan sponsor's benefit design (e.g., open, three-tier, or closed formulary and number of drugs on formulary) or strictly on market share (i.e., the percentage of all prescriptions within a given therapeutic class that are dispensed for the company's product) relative to national market share. When a PBM is administering the plan sponsor's pharmacy benefit, the rebate may be shared between the PBM and the plan sponsor or may be awarded solely to one party, depending on the contract between the plan sponsor and the PBM. Due to a greater push for transparency in PBM pricing, rebates are generally passed on to clients or are used to reduce pharmacy program costs (Navarro & Hailey, 2009). As described in the case scenario at the beginning of this chapter, formulary development and management is a core function of PBMs. Formularies can be described as open, closed, or incented, and plan sponsors choose which type of formulary design they want to offer. In an open formulary, all drugs are covered, regardless of their formulary status. In a closed formulary, drugs not on the formulary are not covered by the health plan. In an incented formulary, patients are provided with financial incentives (i.e., lower copayments) to use preferred drugs; coverage is also provided for nonpreferred products, albeit at higher copayments.

Incented formularies are often referred to as multiple-tiered formularies or described as having tiered copayments. (Tiered copayments are discussed in more detail in the "Cost Sharing" section of this chapter.) In recent years, traditional open or closed formularies have been replaced for the most part by incented formularies.

As in the Sovaldi® case scenario at the beginning of this chapter, plan administrators have debated whether they should cover clinically beneficial, but very expensive drugs and, if so, whether they should be subject to higher copayments or require approval from the PBM.

Plan sponsors often exclude specific classes of drugs from coverage, such as the following:

- Nonprescription drugs (other than insulin)
- Parenteral products (other than insulin)
- Compounded prescriptions
- Devices (e.g., syringes, blood glucose monitors, blood pressure machines, and glucose test strips)
- Appetite suppressants
- Products for smoking cessation
- Drugs for erectile dysfunction
- Oral contraceptives
- Growth hormone
- Fertility agents
- Products used for cosmetic purposes (such as hair growth or wrinkle removal) (Takeda Pharmaceuticals, 2007)

In addition to benefit exclusions, plan sponsors frequently ask PBMs to employ utilization management tools such as limiting the quantity of a particular prescription or the number of refills, to mitigate fraud and waste. Quantity may be limited to a specified number of dosage units or, more commonly, to a specified day's supply. Usually the day's supply is limited to 30 days. Early refills may not be allowed unless the PBM gives authorization to do so (e.g., if the patient is going on vacation). Some plan sponsors, however, specify a minimum quantity (such as a 3-month supply) that may be dispensed for certain maintenance medications used for chronic conditions.

Most plans incorporate a prior authorization (PA) program, another type of utilization management tool, into their pharmacy benefit. A PA program, which allows a patient's physician to request coverage of nonpreferred or noncovered medications such as those listed previously, provides access to certain drugs when they are needed without covering the drug for the general population. A variation on the formulary and PA is step therapy. With step therapy, the use of the more expensive agent is reserved for second-line treatment if treatment with the less expensive agent, commonly a generic, proves unsuccessful. For example, a patient with heartburn might be required to try a generic proton pump inhibitor (PPI) before a more expensive brand-name PPI will be covered. Some staff- and group-model HMOs authorize pharmacists to dispense therapeutic alternatives in accordance with previously established formulary guidelines to promote either generic or lower-cost brand alternatives. This practice, known as therapeutic interchange, is used by some PBMs for the following two reasons: (1) therapeutic categories are becoming more crowded with very similar drugs and generic alternatives, and (2) there is growing pressure to increase the market share of particular products so that the payer can receive manufacturer rebates.

Outside of these tightly managed environments, the term *therapeutic interchange* takes on a somewhat different meaning because the pharmacist contacts the physician to request approval for a switch in medication. Depending on the particular plan, the pharmacist may also contact the patient to get his or her permission before making the switch. Such programs, which are also called therapeutic conversion, therapeutic substitution, or switch programs, have been more commonly administered in mail-service pharmacies than in the retail networks because of the efficiencies that can be achieved in the mail-order setting (Kreling, Lipton, Collins, & Hertz, 1996). However, controversy surrounds these therapeutic conversion programs. Opponents argue that these programs have negative effects on patients' health and are motivated by rebate revenues; proponents advocate their use as a way to control the growth in drug costs without compromising quality of care as promoted alternatives must be therapeutically equivalent. Research is beginning to emerge on these programs. For example, Cheetham and colleagues found in 2005 that patients converted from simvastatin to generic lovastatin had an improvement in their lipid profile without evidence of hepatic or muscle enzyme elevations (Cheetham et al., 2005). Despite claims in some published editorials expressing concern about the interchangeability of generic drugs, Kesselheim and colleagues found that there was little evidence of important clinical differences between brand name and generic drugs in cardiovascular disease (Kesselheim et al., 2008).

Drug Utilization Review

The review of physician prescribing, pharmacist dispensing, and patient use of drugs is known as DUR (Palumbo & Ober, 1995). The goal of DUR is to ensure that drugs are used appropriately, safely, and effectively.

Reviews based on claims data for prescriptions that have already been dispensed are known as retrospective DUR. The primary goal of a retrospective DUR is educational—to find ways in which drug therapy can be improved and inform prescribers and dispensers about these findings. Retrospective DUR may focus on physicians' prescribing patterns, individual patients' patterns, or patterns of use for certain therapeutic categories—especially for drugs that may be subject to abuse.

Prospective DUR is conducted at the time the prescription is dispensed via the electronic claims adjudication system. Patients' medication records are reviewed during the dispensing process to determine whether the prescriptions are appropriate. If a problem is identified, a message describing the problem is returned to the pharmacy through the computer system before the prescription is dispensed. Examples of reviews performed by these systems include appropriateness of dose, drug interactions, duplication of therapy, and drug–allergy interactions. Online prospective DUR programs may duplicate pharmacists' reviews of their own records but have the added benefit of screening prescription claims from other pharmacies that may have filled prescriptions for the same patient.

Cost Sharing

Cost sharing requires the patient to share in the cost of a medication based on some predetermined rate schedule established by the plan sponsor. It tries to optimize utilization by requiring patients to consider the cost of the medication (at least part of the cost), just as they would in any other purchasing transaction. Cost sharing can take many forms, including copayments, coinsurance, deductibles, out-of-pocket limits, or maximum benefits. Many health plans use a combination of deductibles and copayments or coinsurance when designing their pharmacy benefits. These techniques are fully described in the chapter on private health insurance.

PBMs commonly use tiered co-payments to promote utilization of lower-cost alternatives in place of high-cost brand-name medications. In the very common three-tier pharmacy benefit, generic drugs are placed on the first tier of the formulary and have the lowest copayment; preferred brand-name drugs are placed on the second tier with a higher copayment; and nonpreferred brand-name drugs are placed on the third tier and have the highest copayment. Some plans specify four-tier copayments, with certain lifestyle drugs (e.g., drug products for erectile dysfunction) or nonformulary drugs appearing on the fourth tier. This fourth tier often has a coinsurance requirement ranging from 50% to 100%.

Provider Education

Physician profiling is a tool for comparing the practice patterns of providers on cost and quality dimensions. Measures are generally expressed as a rate over a specific period of time within the physician's patient population (e.g., the average dollars spent per patient per month). Report cards are then provided to individual physicians. These reports show not only the specific physician's practice patterns but also the average practice patterns of their physician counterparts, thereby providing a benchmark for comparison. The information on a report card typically includes healthcare and prescription costs per patient per month, number of prescriptions per patient per month, percentage of brand-name versus generic prescriptions, compliance with formulary guidelines, and prescribing patterns for selected prescription drugs.

As a follow-up to physician profiling, some health plans and PBMs provide counterdetailing (also known as academic detailing). Plans monitor physicians' prescribing patterns to identify those physicians who are prescribing inappropriately as viewed by the health plan. A health plan representative (or the contracting PBM) then visits targeted physicians to provide information regarding the most cost-effective use of selected drugs and to encourage physicians to prescribe in ways that will reduce overall costs while maintaining program quality. The targeted physicians are usually identified by the practice profiling program as ones with higher than average costs or unusual prescribing patterns. As discussed previously, the ability to influence providers' behavior depends greatly on how much of the contracted provider's business the organization controls.

Patient Education

With the growing emphasis on consumerism in health care, patient education is becoming more prevalent in PBMs and health plans. The goal of these programs is to produce voluntary changes in patients' behavior that will improve their health. Such efforts take a variety of forms, from passive educational mailing to more active educational efforts through telephone call centers. More encompassing patient education programs are sometimes referred to as disease management programs. The idea behind disease management is to take a broad view of a disease, focusing on how it is treated across the continuum of care. Often disease management programs target high-cost or high-prevalence diseases for which pharmaceutical therapy plays a central role, with the goal of improving how patients and physicians manage the disease. Examples include asthma, diabetes, heart disease, and depression.

PBMs are now focusing efforts on increasing medication adherence with the supposition that better adherence will lead to improved health outcomes. These efforts to improve patient adherence include contacting patients by mail, email, phone calls from nurses, text messages, auto-dial messaging, etc. There is some evidence indicating that these programs are successful at increasing medication adherence; whether these programs actually improve patient health outcomes still remains to be seen (Allen, 2014).

ETHICAL ISSUES IN MANAGED CARE

Managed care takes an active approach to managing health, and this approach frequently intervenes in the physician–patient relationship. Considering the historical perspective discussed at the beginning of the chapter (see "The History of Managed Care"), it should not be surprising that the growth of managed care has fueled many ethics debates almost since its inception

(Jecker, 1994). Ethical concerns related to managed care revolve around four central themes: the sanctity of the physician–patient relationship, the ethics of medicine, the quality of care, and freedom of choice for patients and providers (**Table 17-2**). The challenge for managed care is to balance these concerns against the limited amount of resources that can be devoted to medical care spending.

Table 17-2 Summary of the Ethical Issues in Managed Care

Anti-managed care position	Pro-managed care position
The financial incentives of managed care threaten the role of physician as the patient advocate, undermining the patient's trust and jeopardizing the oath of doing good while avoiding harm.	The financial incentives of FFS resulted in overtreatment of patients, which can also be detrimental to the patient.
The ethics of medicine will be replaced with the ethics of business.	The ethics of medicine are not as superior as perhaps believed. Physicians do not take vows of poverty. In addition, businesses are increasingly being held to ethical standards. By considering medicine to be both a profession and a business, society will not overlook the ethical issues that can arise as a result of these conflicting agendas.
Physicians' autonomy is removed, which will eventually harm patients.	Physicians did not have complete autonomy under FFS. Nonetheless, reducing physician autonomy is not necessarily a bad thing. Who is to say that physicians are the experts or have special authority about the ethical values that should be considered in making resource allocation decisions? Further, empirical evidence does not show that managed care results in a lower quality of care. Rather, it can provide numerous benefits, such as an emphasis on preventive care.
Patients' freedom to choose providers and obtain medical services is limited, resulting in decreased patient satisfaction.	Patients have limits under FFS. Further, as managed care grows, a greater number of providers will be included in managed care, increasing patients' choice of providers.

Source: This article was published in *Clinics in Geriatric Medicine,* Vol 10(3), N. S. Jecker, "Managed Competition and Managed Care: What are the Ethical Issues,?" pp. 527–540, Copyright Elsevier 1994.

QUALITY IN MANAGED CARE

Background

While much of the interest in managed care has traditionally focused on controlling costs, today there is a growing emphasis on ensuring the quality of care. A major difficulty facing those who attempt to measure quality is that there is no universally agreed-upon definition of quality. Which variables should be measured, and how should they be weighed? Donabedian (1978) identified the following three measures for the assessment of quality that are still used today: structure, process, and outcomes.

Structure refers to the personnel and other resources used to provide care as well as the policies and procedures that govern the use of resources and providers' decision making. Examples include availability of X-ray equipment, the type of information system used, the number of physicians and their credentials, and the policy for receiving PA for noncovered services. Structural criteria are generally easy to measure and document, but their relationship to other measures of quality is not always clear.

Process refers to the interactions that occur between practitioners and patients or what was done to the patient. Examples in a community pharmacy include the percentage of patients counseled per day and the number of dispensing errors as a percentage of prescriptions dispensed. For a PBM, a process measure may include the number of patients switched to a preferred medication.

Outcomes are the end results of medical care—that is, what happened to the patient. Examples of outcomes include stroke, death, quality of life, and patient satisfaction. While most would agree that outcomes are the best indicators of quality, quality assessment efforts often focus on the structure and process of care because they are much easier to measure and interpret.

Oversight and Accreditation

Oversight is the process of reviewing and monitoring MCOs to determine whether they meet specified structure, process, and/or outcome criteria. Government agencies, such as state insurance departments, are responsible for ensuring compliance with state laws and regulations regarding issues such as financial solvency, enrollment procedures, and patient rights. Accreditation, by contrast, is a voluntary form of oversight involving independent, nonprofit, nongovernment entities. Accreditation goes beyond oversight in that it evaluates and reports on the quality and performance of MCOs, thereby enabling purchasers and consumers of managed health care to make comparisons and more informed healthcare purchasing decisions. Accreditation, therefore, serves as a seal of approval that is relied upon by employers, patients, and, sometimes, government agencies (Kongstvedt, 2007).

There are three major accreditation agencies in the United States, which include:

1. The National Committee for Quality Assurance (NCQA)
2. The Joint Commission for the Accreditation of Healthcare Organizations (JCAHO)
3. The Utilization Review Accreditation Commission (URAC)

The majority of HMOs voluntarily submit to accreditation—more than any other type of MCO. NCQA is the dominant accreditation agency for HMOs. Accreditation of PPOs is increasing but still is not as common as for HMOs. URAC is the main accreditation agency for PPOs; and more recently, URAC has also begun to accredit PBMs. Generally speaking, the accreditation process looks at utilization management, patient satisfaction, access, financial performance, provider credentialing, treatment of specific diseases and outcomes achieved, and other measures (Kongstvedt, 2007). The accreditation survey process involves both on- and off-site components that are assessed by a team of reviewers.

In addition to accrediting HMOs, NCQA promotes performance standards, quality assurance, and review standards. It has also developed the Healthcare Effectiveness Data and Information Set (HEDIS), a group of measures that gives plan sponsors objective information that they can use to evaluate MCOs. The NCQA claims that over 90% of America's health plans use HEDIS to evaluate performance on important dimensions of care and service. Customers can use HEDIS data to compare the quality of care in different health plans and select an appropriate health plan for their needs. Health plans use HEDIS results to track year-to-year performance and make improvements in their quality of care and service. The HEDIS 2015 consists of 81 measures across five domains of care as described in **Table 17-3** (National Committee for Quality Assurance, 2015). Examples of healthcare areas measured by HEDIS include immunization rates, cancer screening, mental health services, and treatment of diabetes, asthma, and heart attacks. Measures are revised, added, or deleted in every year. Some recently added measures in HEDIS 2015, for example, focus on areas such as antipsychotic medications in children and adolescents and nonrecommended PSA-based screening in older men.

The HEDIS measures were sometimes criticized because compliance with the measures was not always associated with better health outcomes (Berger et al., 2004; Lim et al., 2008). However, the HEDIS measures are still widely adopted because of their usefulness to evaluate the quality of care in health plans.

Table 17-3 Major Categories of HEDIS Measures

Area measured	Examples
Effectiveness of care	Childhood immunization rates Mammography rates Annual monitoring for patients on persistent medications
Access/availability of care	Adults' access to preventive/ambulatory health services Call answer timeliness
Experience of care	Times visited doctor's office or clinic Difficulty understanding doctor's explanation Rating of all health care
Utilization and relative resource use	Mental health utilization Well-child visits Frequency of selected procedures
Health plan descriptive information	Board certification Race/ethnicity diversity of membership Language diversity of membership

CREATING INCENTIVES

Managed healthcare plans have designed reimbursement methods that seek to reduce unnecessary hospital admissions, decrease hospital length of stay, and decrease the intensity of services provided to hospitalized patients. Similar steps have been implemented to control the cost and utilization of ambulatory services.

Healthcare providers, like everyone else, usually respond to incentives. **Table 17-4** shows the incentives created by each of the various types of hospital reimbursement. Discounted FFS reimbursement (i.e., retrospective reimbursement based on a negotiated fee schedule), for example, creates incentives to increase admissions (population), length of stay (duration), and intensity of services. *Per diem* reimbursement (i.e., prospective reimbursement of a flat rate per day without regard to actual cost), the most common form of managed care reimbursement for hospitals (Kongstvedt, 1997), creates incentives for hospitals to increase admissions and length of stay but decrease the intensity of services. Prospective reimbursement of a flat rate based on the patient's admission diagnosis, known as diagnosis-related group (DRG) reimbursement, creates incentives to increase admissions but minimize length of stay and intensity of services. Capitation (i.e., prospective reimbursement of a fixed amount each month for each enrolled patient, regardless of the amount of healthcare services actually provided) creates incentives to minimize all three utilization measures.

Physicians and pharmacies that are paid under discounted FFS systems have the same incentives to increase utilization as do hospitals. *Per diems*, however, are difficult to apply to outpatient care services. Capitation reimbursement can also be applied to outpatient services in the form of case management (or disease state management). As under DRGs, prospective payments for outpatient services are based on diagnosis but are known as ambulatory patient groups (APGs). Although these programs continue to evolve, they are expected to work best for chronic conditions with a wide range of costs. Again, healthcare providers in the outpatient setting would have the same types of incentives as would hospitals under prospective (APG) and capitation reimbursement.

IMPACT OF MANAGED CARE ON PHARMACISTS

As discussed in the chapter on private health insurance, the growth of health insurance coverage for prescription drugs has resulted in extra work (e.g., PA, online prospective DUR, and formulary restrictions) and reduced reimbursement for pharmacists. Nevertheless, the concept of

Table 17-4 Incentives under Various Forms of Hospital Reimbursement

	Number of admissions	Length of stay	Intensity of services
Discounted fee-for-service	↑	↑	↑
Per diem	↑	↑	↓
DRGs	↑	↓	↓
Capitation	↓	↓	↓

pharmaceutical care is consistent with the goals of managed care. Changes in pharmacy education are preparing pharmacists to manage care and affect positive patient outcomes. Taking a broader perspective, greater focus on patient outcomes and cost-effectiveness will encourage pharmacists, physicians, and other healthcare providers to collaborate for the benefit of the patient to realize the goal of optimally managed health care.

Managed care has also expanded the roles played by pharmacists. New opportunities include roles as formulary managers, DURers, clinical specialists in disease management programs, outcomes researchers, and numerous other positions that combine the clinical and business aspects of pharmacy benefit management.

CONCLUSION

MCOs continue to evolve in response to consumer and payer preferences and regulatory initiatives, and it is expected that they will continue to invest in data management and experiment with benefit designs that will enhance quality and cost controls. Plan sponsors can customize managed care benefits by designing the scope of coverage, provider incentives, and the various quality and cost-control options that they want to implement. When plan benefits are designed optimally, managed healthcare plans can contribute to better clinical outcomes and reduce healthcare costs.

QUESTIONS FOR FURTHER DISCUSSION

1. Bad publicity continues to plague managed care. To what extent is the current trashing of managed care an unavoidable cost of bringing change to the U.S. medical system? How much, if any, are the media to blame?
2. What are the strengths and limitations of prospective DUR systems from the perspectives of the PBM and the retail pharmacist? Given your explanation, what could be done to improve prospective DUR?
3. Describe some of the new and innovative career opportunities that have developed for pharmacists as managed care enrollment has grown.

KEY TOPICS AND TERMS

Academic detailing (counterdetailing)
Capitation
Cost sharing
Consumer-driven health plan (CDHP)
Diagnosis-related group (DRG)
Drug utilization review (DUR)
Fee-for-service (FFS)
Formularies
Gatekeeper
Group-model HMO
Health maintenance organization (HMO)
Healthcare effectiveness data and information set (HEDIS)
Independent practice association (IPA)-model HMO
Managed care organization (MCO)
National Committee for Quality Assurance (NCQA)
Network
Network-model HMO
Per diem
Pharmacy benefit manager (PBM)
Point-of-service (POS) plan
Preferred provider organization (PPO)
Prior authorization (PA)
Prospective drug utilization review

Rebates
Report cards
Retrospective drug utilization review
Risk bearing
Risk pool
Staff-model HMO
Tiered copayments

REFERENCES

Allen, J. (2014). Bringing the patient back into adherence. *Express Scripts.* Retrieved from http://lab.express-scripts.com/insights/adherence/bringing-the-patient-back-into-adherence

Aventis. (2002). *Managed care digest series.* Bridgewater, NJ: Aventis Pharmaceuticals.

Berger, W. E., Legorreta, A. P., Blaiss, M. S., Schneider, E. C., Luskin, A. T., Stempel, D. A., ... Weiss, K. B. (2004). The utility of the health plan employer data and information set (HEDIS) asthma measure to predict asthma-related outcomes. *Annals of Allergy, Asthma & Immunology, 93,* 538–545.

Campbell, W. H., & Newsome, L. A. (1995). The evolution of managed care and practice settings. In S. M. Ito & S. Blackburn (Eds.), *A pharmacist's guide to principles and practices of managed care pharmacy* (pp. 1–14). Alexandria, VA: Foundation for Managed Care Pharmacy.

Cheetham T. C., Chan, J., Benson, V., Richmond, C., Levin, E., & Campen, D. (2005). Successful conversion of patients with hypercholesterolemia from a brand name to a generic cholesterol-lowering drug. *American Journal of Managed Care, 11,* 546–552. Retrieved from http://www.ajmc.com/issue/managed-care/2005/2005-09-vol11-n9/Sep05-2126p546-552

Davis, K., Collins, K. S., & Morris, C. (1994, Fall). Managed care: Promise and concerns. *Health Affairs, 13*(4), 178–185.

Donabedian, A. (1978). The quality of medical care. *Science, 200*(4344), 856–864.

Fein, A. (2011). Retail and mail pharmacy economics start converging. *Drug Channels.* Retrieved from http://www.drugchannels.net/2011/10/retail-and-mail-pharmacy-economics.html

Fein, A. (2014). 2013 Pharmacy market analysis: Chains up, mail down. *Drug Channels.* Retrieved from http://www.drugchannels.net/2014/05/2013-pharmacy-market-analysis-chains-up.html

Friedman, E. (1996). Capitation, integration, and managed care lessons from early experiments. *Journal of the American Medical Association, 275*(12), 957–962.

Hoechst Marion Roussel. (1999). *HMO-PPO/Medicare–Medicaid digest.* Kansas City, MO: Hoechst Marion Roussel.

Jecker, N. S. (1994). Managed competition and managed care: What are the ethical issues? *Clinics in Geriatric Medicine, 10*(3), 527–540.

Kaiser Family Foundation. (2014). *Employer health benefits survey.* Retrieved from http://kff.org/report-section/ehbs-2014-summary-of-findings

Kesselheim, A. S., Misono, A. S., Lee, J. L., Stedman, M. R., Brookhart, M. A., Choudhry, N. K., Shrank, W. H. (2008). Clinical equivalence of generic and brand-name drugs used in cardiovascular disease: A systematic review and meta-analysis. *The Journal of the American Medical Association, 300*(21), 2514–2526.

Kongstvedt, P. R. (1997). Negotiating and contracting with hospitals and institutions. In P. R. Kongstvedt (Ed), *Essentials of managed health care* (2nd ed.). Gaithersburg, MD: Aspen.

Kongstvedt, P. R. (2007). *Essentials of managed health care* (5th ed., pp. 521–551). Sudbury, MA: Jones and Bartlett.

Kreling, D. H., Lipton, H. L., Collins, T. C., & Hertz, K. C. (1996). *Assessment of the impact of pharmacy benefit managers: Final report to the Health Care Financing Administration* (Pub. No. PB97-103683). Springfield, VA: National Technical Information Service.

Lim, K. G., Patel, A. M., Naessens, J. M., Li, J. T., Volcheck, G. W., Wagie, A. E., ... Beebe, T. J. (2008). *American Journal of Managed Care, 14,* 487–494.

Lindsley, C. W. (2015). 2014 Prescription medications in the United States: Tremendous growth, specialty/orphan drug expansion, and dispensed prescriptions continue to increase. *ACS Chemical Neuroscience, 6*(6), 811–812.

Lipton, H. L., Kreling, D. H., Collins, T., & Hertz, K. C. (1999). Pharmacy benefit management companies: Dimensions of performance. *Annual Review of Public Health, 20,* 361–401.

Mack, J. M. (1993). Managed care relationships from the physician's perspective. *Topics in Health Care Financing, 20*(2), 38–52.

Medicom International. (n.d.). *Medical interface. A thru Z. Managed care terms.* Bronxville, NY: Medicom International.

Miller, R. H., & Luft, H. S. (1994). Managed care plans: Characteristics, growth, and premium performance. *Annual Review of Public Health, 15*, 437–459.

Myers & Stauffer. (2007). *Survey of dispensing and acquisition costs of pharmaceuticals in the state of California.* California Department of Health Services, pp. 39–40.

National Committee for Quality Assurance. (2015). *What is HEDIS?* Retrieved from http://www.ncqa.org

Navarro, R. P., & Hailey, R. (2009). Overview of prescription drug benefits in managed care. In R. P. Navarro (Ed.), *Managed care pharmacy practice* (2nd ed., pp. 17–45). Sudbury, MA: Jones and Bartlett.

Palumbo, F. B., & Ober, J. (1995). Drug use evaluation. In S. M. Ito & S. Blackburn (Eds.), *A pharmacist's guide to principles and practices of managed care pharmacy* (pp. 51–59). Arlington, VA: Foundation for Managed Care Pharmacy.

Rognehaugh, R. (1996). *The managed health care dictionary.* Gaithersburg, MD: Aspen.

Sanofi-Aventis. (2013). *Managed care digest series.* Bridgewater, NJ: Sanofi-Aventis Pharmaceuticals. Retrieved from http://www.managedcaredigest.com/hmo/default.aspx

Sanofi-Aventis. (2014). *Managed care digest series.* Bridgewater, NJ: Sanofi-Aventis Pharmaceuticals. Retrieved from http://www.managedcaredigest.com/hmo/default.aspx

Sterler, L. T., & Stephens, D. (1999). Pharmacy distribution systems and network management. In R. P. Navarro (Ed.), *Managed care pharmacy practice* (pp. 89–123). Sudbury, MA: Jones and Bartlett.

Takeda Pharmaceuticals of North America, Inc. (2007). *The prescription drug benefit cost and plan design survey report.* Retrieved from https://www.pbmi.com/shop-category/reports/prescription-drug-benefit-cost-and-plan-design-reports/page/2/

West, D. S. (2014). *NCPA–Digest.* Alexandria, VA: National Community Pharmacists Association.

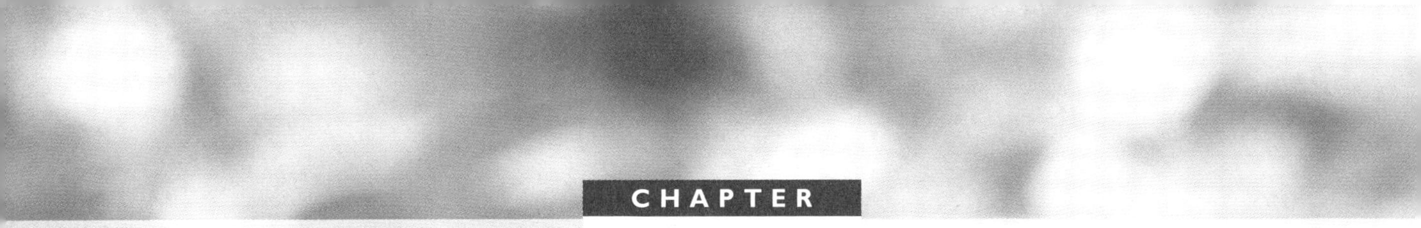

CHAPTER

18

Medicare and Medicaid

Scott K. Griggs, Taehwan Park, and Kenneth W. Schafermeyer*

Case Scenario: Medicare

Helen is a retired bank teller, 67 years of age, who was recently afflicted with a serious illness. After spending 10 days in the hospital, she spent 4 weeks in a skilled nursing facility (SNF) before being discharged to her home. During her recuperation, Helen often reflected on how lucky she was to be enrolled in Medicare. Because of her limited income, it was reassuring to know that Medicare would take care of her substantial healthcare expenses. Helen was shocked, however, when she began receiving bills that Medicare did not pay. Adding up the bills from the hospital, SNF, pharmacy, and her physician, she owed more than $2,500! Helen could not understand how she could owe so much money when she had health insurance through Medicare.

LEARNING OBJECTIVES

Upon completion of this chapter, the student shall be able to:

- Explain the eligibility requirements of the Medicare program.
- Describe the sources of funding for Medicare.
- Describe the benefits provided under Medicare Parts A and B.
- Describe the types of cost sharing required for Medicare patients.
- Explain the concepts of approved charges and assignment.
- Explain the benefits provided under Medicare Part C.
- Describe the major provisions of the Medicare Part D prescription drug benefit.
- Describe the magnitude of Medicare enrollment and spending.
- Explain the need for and types of Medicare supplement policies.
- Describe the three broad groups of people who may be eligible for Medicaid.
- Describe the roles of state and federal governments in financing and administering Medicaid.

*The authors wish to express appreciation to Alan P. Wolfgang, who authored a previous edition of this chapter.

- Describe the mandatory and optional benefits provided under Medicaid.
- Describe the types of cost sharing required for Medicaid patients.
- Describe the magnitude of Medicaid enrollment and spending.
- Explain the role of waivers in encouraging innovation in Medicaid programs.
- Describe the purpose of the Medicare Star Ratings.

CHAPTER QUESTIONS: MEDICARE

1. Which groups of people are eligible to be covered by Medicare?
2. How is Medicare financed?
3. What services are covered by Parts A and B of Medicare?
4. What types of cost sharing are imposed on Medicare beneficiaries?
5. What is *assignment*, and why is it important to Medicare beneficiaries?
6. What is a Medicare supplement insurance policy?

CHAPTER QUESTIONS: MEDICAID

1. What are the characteristics of the persons mandated categorically needy, optionally eligible, and medically needy?
2. What are the roles of federal and state governments in financing and administering Medicaid?
3. Which services must be covered by state Medicaid programs?
4. What are examples of optional services in Medicaid programs?
5. What types of cost sharing are imposed on Medicaid beneficiaries?
6. How have waivers been used by states to test innovative Medicaid programs?

MEDICARE: LEGISLATIVE HISTORY

The development of the Medicare program can be traced back to the 1935 Social Security Act (SSA). Although Medicare was not enacted at that time, this landmark legislation marked the beginning of the federal government's central role in the area of social insurance (Longest, 1994). Passed by Congress during President Franklin Roosevelt's first term, the SSA was designed to provide for the material needs of Americans (Hellman & Hellman, 1991). Title XVIII of the SSA, "Health Insurance for the Aged and Disabled," was established as part of the Social Security Amendments of 1965. More commonly known as Medicare, Title XVIII launched a health insurance program that complemented the SSA's retirement, survivors, and disability insurance benefits (Medicare and Medicaid Statistical Supplement, 1995).

The concept of Medicare was introduced early in 1952 during the Harry Truman administration. Abandoning his advocacy of a universal health program, President Truman suggested a more limited health insurance plan that would cover all Social Security beneficiaries (Ball, 1995). However, Truman's plan received little serious consideration. Fein (1989) believes that the introduction of a bill by Representative Aimee Forand of Rhode Island in August 1957 initiated the legislative activity that led to the enactment of Medicare. This bill, which proposed a social insurance program of health insurance for the aged, and its legislative successors received sustained attention in Congress for the next 8 years. Hearings on the bill held in 1959 helped build a consensus for the belief that many aged Americans faced severe difficulties in obtaining health insurance and that federal action in this arena was necessary.

Health insurance for the elderly was at the top of the federal legislative agenda in 1965 following the reelection of Lyndon Johnson as president in November 1964. During the early months of 1965,

Representative Wilbur Mills of Arkansas, chairman of the House Ways and Means Committee, designed a compromise that encompassed three major proposals that were under consideration at that time: (1) a compulsory health insurance program for the elderly, which was to be financed by payroll taxes; (2) a voluntary insurance program for physician services, which was to be subsidized with general tax revenues; and (3) a means-tested health insurance program for the poor, which was to be administered by the states (Ginsburg, 1988). The first two proposals were combined in the Mills compromise to form the Medicare program; the third proposal was addressed through development of the Medicaid program.

After many years of often acrimonious debate about the government's responsibility for ensuring Americans' access to health services, passage of the 1965 SSA amendments was made possible by Johnson's landslide victory in the 1964 election and the accompanying large Democratic majority in Congress (Longest, 1994). If not for these unique circumstances that existed in 1965, it is unlikely that Medicare could have mustered the votes necessary for passage (Ball, 1995). In fact, some have argued that this comprehensive program could not have been enacted at any time except in 1965. The legislation was signed into law by President Johnson on July 30, 1965, with Medicare's implementation set for July 1, 1966 (Fein, 1989).

PROGRAM STRUCTURE

Medicare was traditionally a two-part insurance program. Part A, also known as Hospital Insurance, pays for care provided to patients in hospitals, skilled nursing facilities, hospices, and home healthcare programs. Part B, or Supplementary Medical Insurance, provides coverage for physicians' services, outpatient hospital care, and a variety of other medical services not covered under Part A (Centers for Medicare and Medicaid Services, 2010). Part C, which was added in 1997, was originally known as the Medicare + Choice program, but now is called Medicare Advantage. It expanded beneficiaries' ability to participate in a wide variety of private health plans, including health maintenance organizations (HMOs) and preferred provider organizations (PPOs). The Medicare Prescription Drug, Improvement, and Modernization Act of 2003 established a new prescription drug benefit, also known as Part D (Centers for Medicare and Medicaid Services, 2005a; Henry J. Kaiser Family Foundation, 2003).

ELIGIBILITY

Part A

In 2015, approximately 55 million people were enrolled in Medicare (Cubanski et al., 2015). Most of these people qualify for Medicare by virtue of the fact that they or their spouse worked for at least 10 years in Medicare-covered employment, they are citizens or permanent residents of the United States, and they are at least 65 years old. Persons who are 65 or older are entitled to receive Part A automatically without paying any premium if they (1) are receiving or are eligible to receive retirement benefits from either Social Security or the Railroad Retirement Board, or (2) had Medicare-covered government employment. People age 65 or older who do not meet these criteria can purchase Part A by paying a monthly premium (Health Care Financing Administration, 1996, 1998; Medicare and Medicaid Statistical Supplement, 1995). This premium, which varies based on an individual's length of Medicare-covered employment, ranged between \$226 and \$411 per month in 2016 (Centers for Medicare and Medicaid Services, 2015a).

Two groups of people younger than age 65 can receive Part A without paying a monthly premium: (1) individuals who have received disability benefits from Social Security or the Railroad Retirement Board for at least 24 months, and (2) patients with end-stage renal disease who require dialysis or a kidney transplant (Health Care Financing Administration, 1996; Medicare and Medicaid Statistical Supplement, 1995). Legislation enacted in 2000 allows persons with amyotrophic lateral sclerosis (also known as Lou Gehrig's disease) to waive the 24-month waiting period for Part A coverage. Overall, the nonelderly account for about 16% of the Medicare population (Centers for Medicare and Medicaid Services, 2015b).

Part B

Although most Medicare patients do not pay a premium for Part A coverage, everyone who wishes to be covered by Part B is charged a monthly premium, and for most individuals this amount is deducted from the monthly Social Security benefit checks. For 2015, the standard Part B was set at $104.90 per month. However, there is a "hold-harmless" provision that can alter the premium rate for certain enrollees. This provision prohibits states from increasing the standard Part B premium to an amount that exceeds an individual's Social Security cost-of-living adjustment. Since there was no cost-of-living adjustment in 2015, this meant that enrollees' Part B had to remain at the same level as the previous year. Certain individuals, such as first-time enrollees and those whose Part B is paid by a state Medicaid program, are not protected by the hold-harmless provision and thus were charged the higher Part B premium. Approximately 93% of the Medicare population voluntarily enrolls in Part B (Centers for Medicare and Medicaid Services, 2009a). Individuals who would have to pay a premium for Medicare Part A can purchase Part B even if they do not enroll in Part A.

Beginning in 2007, higher-income Medicare beneficiaries began paying a higher, income-related Part B premium. For 2014, the higher premium was triggered when annual income exceeded $85,000 for an individual or $170,000 for a couple, with the minimum premium being $104.90 per month. The premium increases on a sliding scale, with the maximum premium of $335.70 per month being paid when income exceeded $214,000 for an individual or $428,000 for a couple. Higher-income beneficiaries are not protected by the hold-harmless provision described above (Klees, Wolfe, & Curtis, 2014). It is estimated that 5% of Medicare beneficiaries (2.4 million) paid this income-related Part B premium in 2013 (Cubanski, Neuman, & Jacobson, 2014).

FINANCING

The expenses of providing the benefits and administration of Parts A and B are paid from separate trust funds. Part A expenses are paid from the hospital insurance trust fund, which is financed primarily through payroll taxes paid by employees, employers, and self-employed individuals. At present, employees and employers each contribute 1.45% of earnings to the trust fund; self-employed individuals pay 2.9% of earnings. Additional funding is provided by beneficiary cost-sharing mechanisms (such as premiums, deductibles, and coinsurance) that are required for most Part A and B services (Centers for Medicare and Medicaid Services, 2009a; Davis & Burner, 1995; Medicare and Medicaid Statistical Supplement, 1995). Approximately 25% of the contributions to the hospital insurance fund come from beneficiary cost sharing. Most of the income for the supplementary medical insurance trust fund is provided from general revenues of the federal government (Davis & Burner, 1995; Zarabozo, Taylor, & Hicks, 1996).

ADMINISTRATION

Administration of the Medicare program is the responsibility of the U.S. Department of Health and Human Services. Within the Department of Health and Human Services, Medicare eligibility and enrollment are the responsibility of the Social Security Administration. The Centers for Medicare and Medicaid Services (CMS), formerly the Health Care Financing Administration, is charged with carrying out most other duties pertaining to Medicare, including developing operational policies and guidelines, formulating conditions of participation for providers, maintaining and reviewing utilization records, and overseeing general financing of the program. The U.S. Department of the Treasury manages the hospital insurance and supplementary medical insurance trust funds (Medicare and Medicaid Statistical Supplement, 1992, 1995).

To be reimbursed for providing services to Medicare patients, healthcare providers must comply with the program's conditions of participation, which are requirements relating to the health and safety of Medicare beneficiaries. Agencies of state governments assist CMS in the certification process by surveying and inspecting potential providers (Medicare and Medicaid Statistical Supplement, 1995).

Providers are paid for services delivered to Medicare patients after they file claims with designated administrators (such as Blue Cross/Blue Shield associations and commercial insurers), which are organizations that contract with CMS to administer Part A and B claims. These administrators determine reasonable charges for covered services, make payments to providers, and guard against unnecessary utilization of services. Providers are required to file claims with the administrators on patients' behalf (Medicare and Medicaid Statistical Supplement, 1995).

MEDICARE SERVICES AND COST SHARING

Part A

Inpatient Hospital Care

Services for inpatient hospital care are based on the concept of a benefit period. A benefit period begins on the day an individual enters the hospital and ends when that person has not been a patient in either a hospital or skilled nursing facility (SNF) for 60 consecutive days. It also ends if the person resides in a nursing home for 60 consecutive days without receiving skilled care. A Medicare beneficiary can have several benefit periods during a given year, and there is no lifetime limit on the number of benefit periods available to individuals (Centers for Medicare and Medicaid Services, 2003a).

Part A covers 90 days of medically necessary inpatient hospital care per benefit period. Each patient also has a lifetime reserve of 60 days that can be used if he or she needs to be hospitalized for more than 90 days in one benefit period. This lifetime reserve is not renewed at the beginning of each benefit period. The services that Medicare covers for hospital inpatients include a semiprivate room, meals, nursing care, operating and recovery room, drugs, laboratory tests, and X-rays. Medicare does not cover extra charges such as those for a private room or the cost of amenities such as a television or telephone.

A separate limit applies to inpatient services received in psychiatric hospitals; each Medicare beneficiary is entitled to just 190 days of inpatient psychiatric care during his or her lifetime. Psychiatric care provided in a general hospital does not count toward this 190-day limit (Centers for Medicare and Medicaid Services, 2003a).

Hospitalized Medicare patients are subject to a schedule of deductibles and copayments, the amount of which changes each year. For days 1 through 60 of hospitalization during a benefit period, the patient is responsible for paying a deductible ($1,260 in 2015). Regardless of how many times a person might be admitted to the hospital, as long as he or she has not received more than 60 days of care within the benefit period, he or she pays only this deductible. The patient is not required to pay for any other portion of the costs of covered services during that time period. If, however, a patient is hospitalized for more than 60 days in a benefit period, further cost sharing is required in the form of daily copayments. For days 61 through 90 of a benefit period, the copayment amount ($315 per day in 2015) equals one-fourth of the inpatient hospital deductible; for the lifetime reserve days, the copayment ($630 per day in 2015) is one half of that deductible (Cubanski et al., 2015).

The other form of cost sharing that may be imposed on hospitalized Medicare patients is the blood deductible. Patients are required to pay for or replace (either by themselves or another person on their behalf) the first three pints of blood used each year. Both Parts A and B cover blood. Thus, to the extent that the blood deductible is met under one part of Medicare, it does not have to be met under the other part (Centers for Medicare and Medicaid Services, 2003a).

Skilled Nursing Facility Care

Medicare patients are entitled to 100 days of care in a SNF per benefit period. During stays in such facilities, covered services include a semiprivate room, nursing care, meals, drugs, medical supplies and equipment, and rehabilitation services (such as physical therapy and speech therapy). A number of criteria must be met before a Medicare patient can qualify for these services. Perhaps most important is the requirement that the patient require daily skilled nursing or rehabilitation services that can be provided only in a SNF. Because this benefit is intended to serve acutely ill patients who can be cured or improved by short-term, daily, skilled services, Medicare will not cover SNF care for patients who need only custodial care (such as assistance with eating, toileting, or taking medication). In addition to the requirement regarding level of care, admission to an SNF must be preceded by a hospital stay of at least 3 days, and it typically must occur within 30 days of hospital discharge (Centers for Medicare and Medicaid Services, 2003a; Hellman & Hellman, 1991).

There is no charge to the patient for the first 20 days of care in an SNF. For days 21 through 100 of care within a benefit period, however, Medicare patients are responsible for a daily copayment. This copayment ($157.50 per day in 2015) is set at one eighth of the inpatient hospital deductible (Cubanski et al., 2015).

Home Health Care

Like the skilled nursing care benefit, Medicare's home healthcare coverage is designed to help people recover from illnesses through the provision of skilled services—not to provide long-term, unskilled care. Part A and Part B actually share responsibility for home healthcare services. Part A covers a maximum of 100 home health visits following a hospital or SNF stay of at least 3 days. Thereafter, visits are covered by Part B, as is home health care not associated with a hospital or SNF stay. Homebound patients may continue to receive home healthcare benefits as long as they require intermittent skilled nursing care, physical therapy, occupational therapy, or speech therapy. If a patient receives any of those services, he or she is entitled to a variety of other services, including home health aide services, medical social services, medical supplies (such as bandages or incontinence pads), and durable medical equipment (such as wheelchairs and walkers). Services not covered include meal preparation and delivery and full-time nursing care.

Medicare Part A pays the entire bill for most covered services provided by approved home health agencies without requiring any patient cost sharing. The one exception concerns durable medical equipment, for which the patient must pay a 20% coinsurance (Centers for Medicare and Medicaid Services, 2003a, 2005a; Hellman & Hellman, 1991).

Hospice Care

The hospice benefit provides care to patients who have life expectancies of 6 months or less (as certified by a physician) and who voluntarily waive their right to traditional treatment of their terminal illnesses (such as cancer chemotherapy). Hospice services, which primarily are delivered in a home setting, can include relief of pain and other symptoms (such as nausea or diarrhea), physician services, nursing care, counseling, and homemaker services. Short-term respite care in a nursing home or hospital, which provides temporary relief for the family members who regularly assist with home care, is also covered for a maximum of 5 consecutive days. If a hospice patient requires care for conditions not related to his or her terminal illness, these services may be covered under the standard Medicare plan (Centers for Medicare and Medicaid Services, 2003a; Hellman & Hellman, 1991).

Very little patient cost sharing is required for covered services provided under the hospice benefit. Patients pay small coinsurance amounts for outpatient prescription drugs and inpatient respite care (Centers for Medicare and Medicaid Services, 2005a).

Other Services

Medicare Part A covers emergency services received in all hospitals, even those that do not participate in the Medicare program, including hospitals in Canada and Mexico under some circumstances. In general, Medicare does not pay for healthcare services received outside the United States and its territories (Centers for Medicare and Medicaid Services, 2003a). Therefore, elderly patients are advised to obtain other health insurance when they travel outside the country.

Part B

Services Covered

Part B covers services provided by physicians in a wide variety of settings, including hospitals, physicians' offices, nursing homes, and patients' homes. Thus, when a Medicare patient undergoes an inpatient surgical procedure, Part A pays the hospital charges and Part B pays for the surgeon's services. Also covered are services provided by nonphysician providers such as physician assistants, nurse practitioners, and certified registered nurse anesthetists (Centers for Medicare and Medicaid Services, 2009a).

Other services covered under Part B include outpatient hospital services, X-rays and laboratory tests, physical and occupational therapy, home health care (if not covered under Part A), drugs that are usually not self-administered, immunosuppressive drugs subsequent to a transplant, kidney dialysis, durable medical equipment, and ambulance transportation. A variety of other preventive services are covered under Part B, including bone mass measurements, colorectal cancer screenings, diabetes screening and supplies, mammograms, Pap tests, and prostate cancer screenings. Limited coverage is available for services provided by chiropractors, podiatrists, optometrists, and dental surgeons (Centers for Medicare and Medicaid Services, 2009a, 2010).

Although a wide variety of physician and outpatient services are covered by Part B, many services are not covered. Services not covered by Medicare Part B include routine physical examinations, routine vision and hearing tests, hearing aids, routine dental care, homemaker services, and most healthcare services received while traveling outside the United States (Centers for Medicare and Medicaid Services, 2003a; Hellman & Hellman, 1991).

Cost Sharing

Each calendar year, Medicare patients pay a deductible ($147 in 2015) for Part B services. After that deductible has been met, Medicare typically pays 80% of the approved charge for most services; this approved charge may be lower than the amount actually billed by the healthcare provider. The patient is responsible for paying the other 20% of approved charges and may be financially responsible for the difference between Medicare's approved charge and the provider's actual charge, depending on whether the provider accepts assignment (Centers for Medicare and Medicaid Services, 2013).

When a provider accepts assignment, it means that his or her actual charge will equal Medicare's approved charge (i.e., no balance billing). In such cases, Medicare patients are assured that they will be billed only for 20% of the approved charge. However, when patients receive services from providers who do not accept assignment, they can also be billed for the difference between actual and approved charges. The amount of this balance billing is limited, as federal law prevents providers who do not accept assignment from charging Medicare patients more than 115% of Medicare's approved charges (Centers for Medicare and Medicaid Services, 2003a). States may place even further restrictions on providers' ability to balance bill.

Physicians can agree on an annual basis to accept assignment for all services provided to Medicare beneficiaries; they are then referred to as Medicare participating physicians. To encourage physicians to sign up for this program, payments for participating physicians are set approximately 5% higher than payments for nonparticipating physicians (Coleman, 1990). Averaged across all states, about 93% of nonpediatric physicians accept Medicare—about the same percentage (94%) that accepts private health insurance. (Boccuti et al., 2015; Centers for Medicare and Medicaid Services, 2015c).

Part C

One solution to controlling Medicare spending might be to implement the types of managed care innovations that appear to have been successful in constraining healthcare costs in the private sector. Encouraging more Medicare enrollees to obtain their healthcare services through managed care organizations might allow the federal government to maintain—if not improve—the level of service provided to older Americans while assisting in its efforts to control expenditures. Even though Medicare does not require its beneficiaries to enroll in managed care plans, Medicare managed care enrollment nevertheless increased tremendously beginning in the latter half of the 1990s. The number of Medicare beneficiaries in HMOs increased from fewer than 2 million in 1995 to 10.75 million (19.5% of all Medicare beneficiaries) in 2015 (Henry J. Kaiser Family Foundation, 2015a).

Enrollment in traditional HMOs was the only managed care option available to Medicare beneficiaries from 1985 until implementation of the Balanced Budget Act of 1997. Under the new Part C (Medicare Advantage) program, an expanded set of options for the delivery of healthcare services became available to Medicare beneficiaries, including PPOs and other types of managed care plans. The addition of these new managed care options made the variety of plans available under Medicare similar to those available to non-Medicare patients. In 2015, 31% of Medicare beneficiaries were enrolled in Medicare Advantage plans (Henry J. Kaiser Family Foundation, 2015a).

Medicare Advantage plans are required to provide a benefit package that is actuarially equivalent to traditional Medicare. If plan costs are lower than Medicare payments, plans are required either to pass those savings along to beneficiaries in the form of lower premiums, reduced cost sharing, and/or additional benefits (e.g., preventive dental care, eyeglasses, hearing aids), or to return the excess payments to Medicare. In 2010, 90% of Medicare Advantage plans imposed no cost sharing for preventive services, almost 80% limited out-of-pocket spending for covered services, and more than 90% provided unlimited days of inpatient hospital care (Henry J. Kaiser Family Foundation, 2010a). It has been estimated that the value of these enhanced benefits, for the average enrollee, is $79 per month (Medicare Payment Advisory Commission, 2009).

Part D

Since January 1, 2006, prescription drug coverage has been available to Medicare beneficiaries through voluntary enrollment in Part D. Individuals obtain this coverage in one of two ways: (1) by enrolling in a freestanding prescription drug plan while getting other Medicare benefits through the traditional fee-for-service program or (2) by joining a Medicare Advantage plan that covers all Medicare benefits, including prescription drugs. Beneficiaries will pay an additional premium for Part D benefits. This premium, estimated to have averaged about $32 per month in 2015, varies across plans and regions, with a low of $11.40 and a high of $174.70 per month. An additional monthly premium surcharge is assessed for higher-income Part D enrollees (>$85,000/individual or $170,000/couple), ranging from $12.70 to $72.90 for 2016. Other sources of funding for Part D include contributions from the general fund of the U.S. Treasury and payments from states, which must offset some of the cost of prescription drugs for Medicaid beneficiaries who also are enrolled in Medicare (Centers for Medicare and Medicaid Services, 2005a, 2009a; Henry J. Kaiser Family Foundation, 2005a, 2015a, 2015b, 2015d).

Under the Part D standard benefit, beneficiaries pay a $360 deductible for prescription drugs in 2016, after which they pay 25% of the next $2,950 of drug costs. Thus, in total, patients pay $1,098 of the first $3,310 in prescription drug costs. At that point, there is a coverage gap (or "doughnut hole") in Medicare coverage that requires Medicare patients to pay a larger share of their total drug costs until they have paid a total of $4,850 in prescription drug costs out of their own pockets. After beneficiaries have spent this amount out of pocket, Medicare's catastrophic coverage kicked in; beneficiaries then pay the greater of either a 5% coinsurance charge or copayments of $2.95 for generic or preferred multisource drugs and $7.40 for other drugs. The annual deductible, benefit limits, and catastrophic threshold are indexed to rise with Part D spending and, with the exception of 2014, have increased each year since 2006 (Henry J. Kaiser Family Foundation, 2015b).

As long as their designs are at least actuarially equivalent to this standard benefit, prescription drug plans are given the flexibility to offer alternative benefit designs. For example, in 2010 only 36% of stand-alone prescription drug plans charged a $310 deductible, and another 40% of those plans charged no deductible at all. Similarly, only 11% of plans utilized the standard 25% coinsurance; the vast majority used a tiered cost-sharing structure instead (Henry J. Kaiser Family Foundation, 2009a).

Part D coverage includes most FDA-approved prescription drugs (drugs currently covered under Parts A and B are still covered by these Medicare components). However, although they must provide a broad range of drugs, plans are allowed to have formularies under Part D. Likewise, plans can use tiered cost sharing, prior authorization, and other cost-containment tools, so long as they are not deemed unduly restrictive. While the law that created Part D prevents Medicare from negotiating drug prices with manufacturers, individual drug plans can use such tactics to produce savings in their drug expenditures (Centers for Medicare and Medicaid Services, 2005a; Henry J. Kaiser Family Foundation, 2005b). Because formularies and cost-containment strategies differ among drug plans, as do premiums and cost-sharing requirements, patients' actual out-of-pocket expenses can vary considerably among plans, and it is important for Medicare beneficiaries to shop wisely when selecting plans.

Medicare provides a variety of subsidies for low-income beneficiaries who enroll in Part D. For example, individuals with both Medicare and Medicaid (those who are "dual eligibles") pay no monthly premium or deductible, and their copayments for prescription drugs are fairly nominal and vary according to income with those for generic drugs being less than for brand-name drugs. Dual eligibles in nursing homes have no copayments. Numerous other groups of

Medicare beneficiaries with limited incomes and resources also qualify for some type of assistance with Part D premiums, deductibles, and copayments. In 2009, more than one third of Medicare Part D enrollees received some form of low-income subsidy (Henry J. Kaiser Family Foundation, 2009b).

The Patient Protection and Affordable Care Act (known informally as the healthcare reform act) enacted in March 2010 brought important changes to the Part D drug benefit. This healthcare reform law provided for a $250 rebate to Part D enrollees to cover spending in the coverage gap during 2010. Additional subsidies in the coverage gap will be phased in for generic drugs beginning in 2011 and for brand-name drugs beginning in 2013, eventually reducing the coinsurance rate in that gap from 100% to 25% by 2020. The law also reduces the level of out-of-pocket spending required for catastrophic coverage between 2014 and 2019 (Henry J. Kaiser Family Foundation, 2010b).

Part D was not launched without its share of problems. Most notably, widespread eligibility verification problems frustrated both Medicare patients and the community pharmacists who served them (Pharmacy Times, 2006; Ukens, 2006). Despite what many viewed as a rough start, however, enrollment has continued to increase, and by 2009 almost 27 million Medicare beneficiaries were enrolled in Medicare Part D plans. Combined with another 14 million individuals who had drug coverage through retiree health plans or systems such as the Indian Health Service or Veterans Affairs, approximately 90% of Medicare beneficiaries had some form of prescription drug coverage (Henry J. Kaiser Family Foundation, 2009c).

EXPENDITURES

Growth in Medicare Spending

Medicare has witnessed tremendous growth since its inception. When this program was first implemented, Medicare served some 19 million enrollees; by 2015, some 55 million Americans were enrolled in Medicare (Cubanski et al., 2015).

Accompanying this expansion in the Medicare population has been rapid growth in Medicare program spending. Between 1968 and 2014, expenditures increased from $6 billion to more than $597 billion. The important role of this program in the American healthcare system is illustrated by the fact that Medicare accounts for 22% of all national personal healthcare expenditures in 2013 (Cubanski et al., 2015).

SPENDING BY TYPE OF SERVICE

Inpatient hospital services and physician services are two of the largest individual components of total Medicare payments (**Table 18-1**), but the proportion of Medicare spending attributable to these two types of services has decreased markedly over time due to various payment reforms and cost-containment efforts. While inpatient hospital services and physician services accounted for more than 90% of Medicare payments in 1967, they accounted for just 35% of such payments in 2014. Conversely, the proportion of payments attributable to home health care and other outpatient benefits has increased substantially since 1967, and managed care, which was virtually nonexistent in 1967, accounted for more than one quarter of Medicare payments (Cubanski, Neuman, & Jacobson, 2014; Medicare and Medicaid Statistical Supplement, 2001).

Table 18-1 Estimated Medicare Expenditures by Service, 2014

Service	% of expenditures
Managed care	26
Inpatient hospital	23
*Other services	14
Physician payments	12
Outpatient prescription drugs	11
Hospital outpatient care	7
Skilled nursing	5
Home health	3

*Includes hospice, durable medical equipment, Part B drugs, outpatient dialysis, ambulance, laboratory services, and other services.

Source: Data from Congressional Budget Office, March 2015.

MEDICARE SUPPLEMENT (MEDIGAP) INSURANCE

Need for Supplemental Insurance

Although some Medicare beneficiaries, such as Helen in the case scenario at the beginning of this chapter, may be under the impression that Medicare will pay for all of their healthcare bills, it does not. Medicare pays less than half of the average beneficiary's medical expenses (Noel-Miller, 2015). Substantial patient cost sharing is required in the form of deductibles, copayments, coinsurance, and premiums. As an extreme example, a seriously ill Medicare patient who stayed 150 consecutive days in the hospital during 2016 would have been responsible for more than $42,000 in hospital deductibles and copayments. But even relatively healthy Medicare enrollees who visit their physicians a few times per year will be liable for the premiums, deductibles, and coinsurance associated with Part B, as well as the full cost of services that are not covered by Medicare. Medicare beneficiaries paid 18.1% of their incomes for out-of-pocket healthcare expenses in 2011 (Noel-Miller, 2015). Several options are available to help Medicare beneficiaries meet these cost-sharing requirements, aside from paying these expenses out of their own pockets. First, some patients might have additional retiree health insurance through a former employer or union. Second, they might be poor enough to qualify for assistance from Medicaid, which would help pay for their care. Third, they might enroll in a Medicare Advantage plan that covers more services than does traditional Medicare. Lastly, Medicare beneficiaries can purchase additional private insurance, known as Medicare supplement or Medigap insurance, which is designed to pay for many of the charges for Medicare-covered services for which the beneficiary is responsible (Centers for Medicare and Medicaid Services, 2016).

Types of Medigap Policies

Most states have adopted regulations designed to make it easier for consumers to comparison shop for a Medigap policy. Standardized policies, which were developed by the National Association of Insurance Commissioners and incorporated into state and federal laws, are assigned letter designations from A through N. To further enhance comparison shopping, insurers must use the same format, language, and definitions in describing their plans. In accordance with federal regulations, each state must allow the sale of Plan A, the most basic type, and all Medigap insurers must offer Plan A. Beyond this requirement, states may restrict the number of other plans that may be sold, and insurers are not obligated to sell any other Medigap plans (Center for the Study of Services, 1995; Centers for Medicare and Medicaid Services, 2016).

Plan A consists of five basic benefits, which cover:

1. Part A coinsurance hospital costs up to an additional 365 days after Medicare benefits are used up
2. Part B coinsurance or copayment
3. Part A hospice care coinsurance or copayment
4. Three-pint blood deductible
5. Preventive care Part B coinsurance

Other plans offer combinations of other benefits in addition to those provided in Plan A. These additional benefits can include coverage of the SNF copayment, the Part A hospital deductible, the Part B deductible, and foreign travel emergency care. Two plans, K and L, include an annual limit on beneficiaries' out-of-pocket spending; once it is met, the plan pays for 100% of covered services for the rest of the calendar year (Centers for Medicare and Medicaid Services, 2016).

Case Scenario: Medicaid

Charlotte is a single parent of two children younger than age 6, and her annual income is about 10% above the federal poverty level for a family of three. She and her children receive health insurance through her state's Medicaid program.

In a nearby state, Ed and Teresa are married and have an infant daughter. Ed and Teresa both work at low-wage jobs, providing a family income equal to the federal poverty level, but neither of their employers offers a health insurance benefit. While their daughter is covered by the state's Medicaid program, Ed and Teresa have no health insurance.

In yet another state, Jack is an agricultural worker with an annual income that is less than half the federal poverty level. Despite his extremely low income, Jack does not qualify for health insurance through his state's Medicaid program.

How can some, but not all, of these people be covered by Medicaid? Why is Medicaid eligibility not uniform across the United States?

MEDICAID: LEGISLATIVE HISTORY

In addition to initiating the Medicare program, the 1965 amendments to SSA established a program popularly known as Medicaid. Officially designated as Title XIX of the SSA, Grants to the States for Medical Assistance Programs, Medicaid was designed to provide medical assistance to eligible needy Americans and is now the largest source of funding for the provision of health-related services to the United States' poorest people (Medicare and Medicaid Statistical Supplement, 1995).

Medicaid remained a rider on the Medicare bill until late in the 1965 legislative debate, when it became a separate title at the last minute. For this reason, Medicaid has been referred to as Medicare's "kid brother." Some have suggested that no one knew enough in 1965 to predict accurately how large the Medicaid program would become. Of course, Medicaid proponents may have also provided unrealistically low estimates of the program's cost and eligibility to ensure its passage in Congress (Friedman, 1987). Many people viewed the legislation that created Medicaid and Medicare as a stopgap measure. Democrats assumed that either Lyndon Johnson or Hubert Humphrey would be elected president in 1968 and that a universal health plan for all Americans would become a reality soon thereafter. After Richard Nixon's election, however, movement toward a universal health plan stalled and these temporary measures became permanent fixtures in the U.S. healthcare market (Friedman, 1990).

ELIGIBILITY

Three broad groups of people may be covered by a state's Medicaid program: the mandated categorically needy, the optionally categorically needy, and the medically needy (Oberg & Polich, 1988). Because Medicaid is a joint state–federal program, states have some flexibility in determining criteria for Medicaid eligibility. States establish their own criteria within federal guidelines, so eligibility for each of these groups may vary considerably from state to state.

Mandated Categorically Needy

If a state has a Medicaid program and wishes to receive matching federal funding, it must provide coverage for several groups of people. Federal welfare reform legislation enacted in the latter half of the 1990s made a major change with respect to individuals who must be provided Medicaid coverage. Prior to enactment of the Personal Responsibility and Work Opportunities Act of 1996, individuals who received cash assistance (welfare) through Aid to Families with Dependent Children (AFDC) were automatically eligible for Medicaid. The 1996 welfare reform act, however, cut the link between Medicaid and cash welfare by replacing the AFDC program with the Temporary Assistance for Needy Families (TANF) program, which provides block grants to states to be used for time-limited cash assistance. TANF generally allows a family to receive cash welfare (income maintenance) benefits for no more than 5 years and allows states to impose other requirements related to employment. Even if they are not receiving welfare, families are still eligible for Medicaid if they meet the AFDC eligibility criteria that were put in place in July 1996 (Centers for Medicare and Medicaid Services, 2009a; Centers for Medicare and Medicaid Services, 2012).

While those eligible for Medicaid must fall below income and financial resources thresholds, Medicaid is not designed to provide assistance to all poor Americans. Even for very poor individuals, Medicaid covers healthcare services only if they fall into certain categories. Several eligibility groups of families and children are considered to be mandatory categorically needy, including the following:

- Low-income families with children, with limits on income and resources determined by individual states.
- Children under age 6 and pregnant women whose family income is below 133% of the federal poverty level (FPL).
- Children under age 19 in families with incomes below the FPL (Centers for Medicare and Medicaid Services, 2009a: Kaiser Commission on Medicaid and the Uninsured, 2009).

A second mandatory group of individuals qualifies for Medicaid because they receive government cash assistance through the Supplemental Security Income program (Centers for Medicare and Medicaid Services, 2009a). This program provides assistance to persons who are poor and either elderly, blind, or disabled. As with TANF, eligibility for the Supplemental Security Income program is based on income and asset limits.

States must also provide limited Medicaid coverage to certain groups of low-income Medicare enrollees. Medicare-eligible individuals with incomes below the FPL and limited assets are known as qualified Medicare beneficiaries. Medicaid must pay the premiums and other cost-sharing expenses (such as deductibles and coinsurance) incurred with Part A and Part B of Medicare for qualified Medicare beneficiaries. For low-income Medicare beneficiaries with incomes between 100% and 120% of the FPL, Medicaid must pay only the Part B premiums. Individuals who have lost their Medicare disability benefits because they returned to work but are allowed to purchase Medicare coverage (called qualified disabled and working individuals) can qualify to have Medicaid pay their Medicare Part A premiums if their incomes are less than twice the FPL (Centers for Medicare and Medicaid Services, 2009a).

One provision of the Patient Protection and Affordable Care Act would have expanded Medicaid coverage to all non-Medicare eligible individuals under age 65 with incomes up to 133% of the federal poverty level, effective January 1, 2014. To assist with financing for these newly eligible Medicaid recipients, states will receive 100% federal funding for these individuals for 2014 through 2016. This percentage will decline thereafter and stabilize at 90% federal financing for 2020 and subsequent years (Henry J. Kaiser Family Foundation, 2010c). However, the Supreme Court ruled that states may opt out of Medicaid expansion and, as of 2015, 20 states have refused to expand Medicaid coverage (National Academy for State Health Policy, 2015).

Optional Eligibility Groups

States have the option of providing coverage for other groups of needy individuals who do not meet the requirements for mandated coverage, although they may share certain characteristics with people in the aforementioned categories. Many of those considered optionally eligible are children or pregnant women. For example, states may cover infants up to one year of age and pregnant women in families not qualifying for mandated coverage but with incomes below 185% of the FPL. Likewise, children younger than age 21 who meet the income and asset requirements for TANF, but not the family status requirements, can be covered by state Medicaid programs (Centers for Medicare and Medicaid Services, 2005a). Another example of an optional eligibility group is persons with tuberculosis who would be financially eligible for Medicaid if they were in a Medicaid-covered category; their coverage is limited to tuberculosis-related services (Centers for Medicare and Medicaid Services, 2009a). If a state program does include the optionally categorically needy, it must provide these individuals with the same Medicaid benefits as those provided to people in the mandatory categories (Oberg & Polich, 1988).

Medically Needy Groups

At their option, state Medicaid programs may elect to cover a group known as the medically needy. These individuals include people who would be eligible for Medicaid under one of the mandated or optional groups, except for the fact that their income and/or assets are higher than allowed by the state. Such individuals become Medicaid eligible under the medically needy provision if their medical expenses reduce their net income to the Medicaid eligibility threshold or less. Thus, the medically needy consist of families and children, or elderly, blind, or disabled individuals, who spend down to Medicaid eligibility by incurring high out-of-pocket medical expenses (Medicare and Medicaid Statistical Supplement, 1995). This spending-down process is especially important for granting Medicaid eligibility to institutionalized persons who incur extremely large medical expenses (Medicare and Medicaid Statistical Supplement, 1992).

Thirty-four states and the District of Columbia cover medically eligible persons in their Medicaid programs. When a state chooses to have a program for the medically needy, it must cover certain groups of people (e.g., children younger than age 19 and pregnant women who are medically needy) and services (e.g., prenatal and delivery care for pregnant women). States may include other groups and may offer different benefits to different groups under the medically needy option (Centers for Medicare and Medicaid Services, 2009a).

FINANCING AND ADMINISTRATION

Because Medicaid is funded by both federal and state governments, these entities share responsibility for administering this program. Through the CMS, the federal government establishes broad guidelines under which states must design and operate their individual programs. At the state level, a single agency must be designated as responsible for the Medicaid program. Within the federal guidelines, states have responsibility for establishing eligibility criteria, determining the type and scope of services to be covered, setting rates of payment for services, and administering their programs. Because states differ in exactly how they carry out these responsibilities, Medicaid programs vary considerably from state to state. A person who is Medicaid eligible in one state may not be eligible in nearby states, and the services provided may differ considerably between states (Centers for Medicare and Medicaid Services, 2009a; Medicare and Medicaid Statistical Supplement, 1995). Thus, while one may speak of Medicare as a program that is essentially uniform across the entire United States, there are actually 56 different Medicaid programs (one for each state, territory, and the District of Columbia).

Medicaid is entirely optional in the sense that the federal government does not require any state to have a Medicaid program. All 50 states do have Medicaid programs, of course, but they do so at their own discretion. Medicaid does not provide healthcare services for all poor Americans. Even in states with the broadest eligibility provisions, as illustrated by the case scenario presented above, Medicaid is unlikely to provide care for poor individuals unless they are children, parents, pregnant, elderly, blind, or disabled. As a consequence, it is important to recall that low income is only one criterion determining Medicaid eligibility (Centers for Medicare and Medicaid Services, 2003b).

The portion of Medicaid program costs that is paid by the federal government for provider services is known as the Federal Medical Assistance Percentage (FMAP). Each state's FMAP is determined annually through the use of a formula that compares a given state's average per capita income to the national average. By law, the FMAP can be no greater than 83% and no less than 50% for any given state. States that are wealthier in terms of average per capita income have a smaller share of their Medicaid costs paid by the federal government than do relatively poorer states. In 2016, the FMAP ranged from a high of about 74% in Mississippi to 50% in 13 states (Department of Health & Human Services, 2016). There are some exceptions to the FMAP rules. For example, the federal government reimburses states at a higher rate for family planning services and for healthcare services provided through Indian Health Service facilities. Most administrative costs are matched at 50%, but higher than normal matching rates are allowed for certain activities and functions, such as the costs of developing mechanized claims processing systems (Centers for Medicare and Medicaid Services, 2009a).

The total amount of money that the federal government spends on Medicaid has no set limit. It must match state government spending at the percentages established by law (Centers for Medicare and Medicaid Services, 2005b, 2009a). Thus, as state spending on Medicaid has escalated over time, so has the amount of money that the federal government contributes to the program.

State programs make payments directly to participating healthcare providers for services delivered to Medicaid patients. These providers must accept the amount of Medicaid reimbursement as payment in full; they may not bill patients for any difference between actual charges and Medicaid's approved charges (i.e., no balance billing). Payment levels are subject to federally mandated conditions to which states must adhere. For example, payments must be high enough to attract sufficient numbers of providers so that services will be available to Medicaid recipients to the same extent that those services are available to the general population in a given geographic area. As another example of the conditions that must be met, Medicaid payments for institutional services may not exceed the amounts that would be paid by Medicare (Medicare and Medicaid Statistical Supplement, 1995).

MEDICAID SERVICES AND COST SHARING

Services Covered

To receive federal matching funds, state Medicaid programs are required to offer a specified list of services to the mandatory and optional categorically needy groups. These required services include the following:

- Inpatient hospital services
- Outpatient hospital services
- Physician services
- Rural health clinic services
- Federally qualified health center services
- Laboratory and X-ray services
- Nursing facility services for individuals age 21 or older
- Early and periodic screening, diagnosis, and treatment services for individuals younger than 21 years of age
- Family planning services and supplies
- Home health services for persons eligible for skilled nursing services
- Nurse-midwife services
- Pediatric nurse practitioner and certified family nurse practitioner services
- Pregnancy-related services (Centers for Medicare and Medicaid Services, 2009a)

States also may receive federal funding for provision of a variety of optional services. States are under no obligation to cover any of these additional services, and the number of optional services provided by Medicaid programs varies widely. Outpatient prescription drugs are an optional service, for example, although they are covered by Medicaid programs in all 50 states. The following are examples of other optional services that are commonly covered:

- Prosthetic devices
- Physical and rehabilitative therapy
- Optometrist services and eyeglasses
- Services in an intermediate care facility for the mentally retarded
- Transportation services
- Hospice care
- Dental services (age 21 and older)
- Home and community-based care for certain persons with chronic impairments (Centers for Medicare and Medicaid Services, 2009a)

Cost Sharing

States have broad discretion in determining reimbursement methodologies and payment rates within federal guidelines. Many states require Medicaid recipients to contribute to the cost of their health care in the form of deductibles, copayments, or coinsurance (Centers for Medicare and Medicaid Services, 2009a). However, the magnitude of this cost sharing cannot be so great that it would present a serious barrier to receiving needed services. For example, in 2008, 80% of states imposed copayments on outpatient Medicaid prescriptions, but most ranged between $0.50 and $3.00 (Kaiser Commission on Medicaid and the Uninsured, 2008). Likewise, nursing home patients are expected to contribute most of their income to help pay for their care. There are certain services, however, for which cost sharing cannot be required (e.g., emergency care, family planning services, pregnancy-related services, and services provided to children younger than age 18) (Centers for Medicare and Medicaid Services, 2009a).

EXPENDITURES

Growth in Medicaid Enrollment and Spending

In terms of both the number of beneficiaries and total expenditures, Medicaid has experienced tremendous growth since its inception. In 1972, Medicaid covered 17.6 million poor Americans, about 8.5% of the U.S. population, with total expenditures of less than $10 billion (National Center for Health Statistics, 1993). By 2010, the Medicaid program covered about 60 million persons, almost 20% of the population, and expended more than $400 billion annually (Centers for Medicare and Medicaid Services, 2009a; Truffer et al., 2010).

Spending by Eligibility Group

There are considerable differences between the proportion of beneficiaries and the proportion of expenditures accounted for by the major enrollment groups. Although 52% of all Medicaid beneficiaries in 2006 were children, less than 20% of Medicaid spending went to provide care for children. By comparison, the elderly represented only 8% of Medicaid beneficiaries but accounted for more than 22% of total spending. Similarly, blind and disabled persons made up just 16% of recipients, but they were responsible for 45% of expenditures. This disparity is explained by the fact that average Medicaid payments for children, the elderly, and the disabled were $1,752, $12,712, and $13,409, respectively (Centers for Medicare and Medicaid Services, 2009a).

Spending by Type of Service

Medicaid spending also varies by type of healthcare service. Substantial portions of Medicaid payments are associated with managed care, inpatient hospitals, nursing homes, and home health care (see **Table 18-2**). These proportions have changed considerably for some services since the mid-1970s. Inpatient services (e.g., those delivered in inpatient hospitals, nursing homes, and intermediate care facilities for the mentally retarded) accounted for 66% of all Medicaid payments in 1975 but only about 33% in 2008. Similarly, payments for physician services declined from 10% to about 4% over the same period. Prescription drugs accounted for less than 5% of Medicaid spending in 2008, a reduction from previous years due to enactment of Medicare Part D. The greatest change has been in managed care, which was essentially nonexistent in Medicaid in 1975 but now accounts for about 31% of Medicaid expenditures. Like Medicare, Medicaid has become a vital part of the U.S. healthcare system, accounting for 16% of all personal healthcare spending and 42% of nursing home expenditures (Centers for Medicare and Medicaid Services, 2009a, 2009b; Paradise, 2015; Henry J. Kaiser Family Foundation, 2010d).

Table 18-2 Medicaid Expenditures by Service, 2013

Service	% of expenditures
Managed care	31.1
Inpatient hospital	13.5
Home health	12.9
Nursing homes	11.6
Outpatient care	6.2
Physician/laboratory/X-ray	3.0
ICF/MR*	2.8
Prescription drugs	1.5
Other	17.4

*ICF/MR = intermediate care facility/mentally retarded.

Source: Data from Henry J. Kaiser Family Foundation, 2013.

STATE FLEXIBILITY

General Requirements for Medicaid Programs

State Medicaid programs must operate within broad guidelines established by the federal government. In addition to meeting the eligibility and services restrictions already described, the 1965 legislation required that states adhere to three other general requirements:

1. *Statewideness*. A state's Medicaid plan must be in effect across the entire state; the services covered in one part of a state generally cannot differ from those covered in another part of the state.
2. *Freedom of choice*. Medicaid recipients must be allowed to obtain covered services from any qualified participating provider.
3. *Comparability of services*. The amount, duration, and scope of services must be equal for all persons in the mandatory and optional eligibility categories (Medicare and Medicaid Statistical Supplement, 1992).

Section 1115 and 1915b Waivers

Under the SSA, CMS is given the power to grant two types of waivers of these requirements: (1) Section 1115 waivers, which allow statewide demonstration projects aimed at covering additional uninsured individuals and testing new budget-neutral delivery systems, and (2) Section 1915b waivers, which allow states to implement innovative delivery and reimbursement systems. These waivers were extremely important in allowing states to begin experimenting with managed care options for their Medicaid beneficiaries. The Balanced Budget Act of 1997 eliminated the need for states to request a waiver to implement Medicaid managed care programs (Centers for Medicare and Medicaid Services, 2009a; Muirhead, 1996).

Managed Care

As evidenced by these waiver programs, many of the efforts aimed at reforming Medicaid have involved greater utilization of managed care organizations for delivery of healthcare services. As a result of a number of factors, including the need for cost containment in light of Medicaid's cost explosion, the proliferation of managed care in the private sector, and changes in federal policy that have promoted the expansion of Medicaid-managed care through the waiver process, there has been tremendous growth in the number of Medicaid beneficiaries who are enrolled in managed care programs (Kaiser Commission on the Future of Medicaid, 1995). By 2008, almost 71% of Medicaid beneficiaries were enrolled in some form of managed care (Centers for Medicare and Medicaid Services, 2009a).

COMPARISON OF MEDICARE AND MEDICAID

Medicare and Medicaid are similar in the sense that both are health insurance programs financed and administered by government entities, and that both are roughly equivalent in terms of the number of beneficiaries and total expenditures. In many ways, however, Medicare and Medicaid are very different. Philosophically, Medicare is a social insurance policy for which beneficiaries have paid through taxes; Medicaid is based on a welfare concept of redistributing wealth among citizens of the United States. There also are differences between the two programs with respect to financing, administration, eligibility, and benefits. Thus, these two government programs actually represent two very different mechanisms for delivering healthcare benefits to selected segments of American society, thereby providing a vital safety net for many of the nation's most vulnerable citizens.

PAY FOR PERFORMANCE

Also known as "P4P," pay for performance is a payment model that rewards healthcare providers or managed care organizations for meeting quality and efficiency performance measures. The U.S. healthcare system continues to move toward value-based or value-driven healthcare, balancing both costs and quality (Henry J. Kaiser Family Foundation, 2015c; Hutchison, 2008; Institute of Medicine, 2007). While rewards may be given for meeting or exceeding performance standards or benchmarks, providers are penalized for poor outcomes, errors, or increased costs. For example, a state Medicaid program that contracts with a managed care organization may withhold a portion of the payment until the managed care organization establishes that they can meet the standard; conversely, bonus payments can be made for demonstrating high performance in comparison to a benchmark (Henry J. Kaiser Family Foundation, 2015c). The purpose of P4P, in addition to incentivizing provider performance and patient outcomes while reducing (or maintaining) costs, is to coordinate and align processes and systems of care for ongoing improvement and innovation to achieve healthcare value now and into the future (Institute of Medicine, 2007).

MEDICARE'S HOSPITAL READMISSIONS REDUCTION PROGRAM

The Affordable Care Act of 2010 established the hospital readmissions reduction program, which became effective on October 1, 2012. This program was designed to provide incentives for hospitals to reduce the number of unnecessary hospital readmissions by coordinating transitions of care and improving the quality of care delivered to Medicare recipients. The incentives are imposing penalties for hospitals with "high readmission rates" within 30 days of a discharge from the same or another hospital if the condition for the initial hospital inpatient admission is acute myocardial infarction, heart failure, pneumonia, chronic obstructive pulmonary disease (COPD), and hip/knee replacement. Hospitals are compared with a national average readmission rate and then the excess readmission ratio is determined after adjustment for clinical factors. For hospitals that exceeded the average readmission ratio, a penalty is determined and applied to Medicare payments. Therefore, hospitals implement various strategies to reduce the readmission rates. Although the 30-day hospital readmission rate was steady around 19% from 2007 to 2011, this rate dropped to 18.5% in 2012 and below 18% in 2013 (American College of Emergency Physicians, 2015).

MEDICARE STAR RATINGS

Medicare star ratings, a performance standard for pharmacies similar to product ratings by *Consumer Reports*, measure how well Medicare Part D (prescription) and Advantage plans perform on a scale of one to five stars, with one being the lowest and five being the highest. The Medicare star ratings scores are determined from several categories: there are five categories for Medicare health plans (staying healthy, managing chronic conditions, member experience/satisfaction with the health plan, member complaints, and customer service) and four categories for Medicare drug plans (customer service, member complaints, member experience/satisfaction with the drug plan, and drug safety and pricing) (Medicare.gov, 2015). There is a summary star rating for the overall performance of a plan as well as separate star ratings for each individual category. The overall star rating allows for comparisons between plans; however, the star ratings are updated each year in the fall. Attaining a higher star rating has marketing advantages for the health plan as well as financial incentives in the form of bonuses. A 2-year lag exists between the service year and the star ratings reporting year; for example, drug claims from 2013 are used for 2015 star ratings.

The Pharmacy Quality Alliance (PQA), established in 2006, is a consensus-based, multistakeholder, nonprofit alliance that creates quality medication performance measures for pharmacy services as well as drug plans. CMS uses these PQA-endorsed measures in their Part D star ratings (Pharmacy Quality Alliance, 2015; O'Neill, 2015). In 2014, five measures from PQA (out of 15 individual measures) accounted for 48% of the Part D summary rating due to a higher weighting of the clinical measures; these measures included two medication safety measures and three medication adherence measures. Additional Part D "display" measures are not part of the star rating calculation but allow for benchmarking and feedback to the plans. A higher star rating, such as a four or five star, can yield a bonus via a pay for performance incentive program (described previously) (Henry J. Kaiser Family Foundation, 2011).

QUESTIONS FOR FURTHER DISCUSSION

1. If Medicare did not exist today, do you believe such a program would be enacted by Congress? Why or why not?
2. If you were speaking to a group of senior citizens, how would you explain the importance of Medicare supplemental insurance?
3. What do you see as the advantages and disadvantages of delivering services to Medicare beneficiaries through managed care plans?
4. What do you believe are the primary strengths and weaknesses of the Part D prescription drug coverage?
5. Should Medicaid be expanded to cover more low-income people? Why or why not?
6. Do you believe Medicaid eligibility criteria should be uniform from state to state? Why or why not?
7. In the long term, do you believe that managed care will have a positive or negative effect on Medicaid and its recipients? Why?
8. How would you restructure Medicaid to ensure that it best meets the needs of low-income Americans at a reasonable cost?

KEY TOPICS AND TERMS

Assignment
Cost sharing
Federal Medical Assistance Percentage (FMAP)
Managed care
Mandated categorically needy
Medicaid
Medically needy
Medicare
Medicare advantage
Medicare Part A
Medicare Part B
Medicare Part C
Medicare Part D
Medicare Star Ratings
Medicare supplement (Medigap) insurance
Optionally categorically needy
Pay for performance (P4P)
Pharmacy Quality Alliance (PQA)
Temporary Assistance for Needy Families (TANF)
Waiver

REFERENCES

American College of Emergency Physicians. (2015). Medicare's hospital readmission reduction program FAQ. Retrieved from http://www.acep.org/Physician-Resources/Practice-Resources/Administration/Financial-Issues-/-Reimbursement/Medicare-s-Hospital-Readmission-Reduction-Program-FAQ/

Ball, R. M. (1995). What Medicare's architects had in mind. *Health Affairs, 14*(4), 62–72.

Boccuti C., Fields C., Casillas G., & Hamel L. (2015, October 30). Primary care physicians accepting Medicare: A snapshot. Henry J. Kaiser Family Foundation. Retrieved from http://kff.org/medicare/issue-brief/primary-care-physicians-accepting-medicare-a-snapshot/

Centers for Medicare and Medicaid Services. (2003a). *Your Medicare benefits.* Baltimore, MD: U.S. Department of Health and Human Services.

Centers for Medicare and Medicaid Services. (2003b). *Medicaid eligibility.* Baltimore, MD: U.S. Department of Health and Human Services. Retrieved from https://www.medicaid.gov/medicaid-chip-program-information/by-topics/eligibility/eligibility.html

Centers for Medicare and Medicaid Services. (2005a). *Brief summaries of Medicare & Medicaid.* Baltimore, MD: U.S. Department of Health and Human Services. Retrieved from http://www.mindfully.org/Health/2005/Medicare-Medicaid-Summaries1nov05.htm

Centers for Medicare and Medicaid Services. (2005b). *Medicaid at-a-glance 2005.* Baltimore, MD: U.S. Department of Health and Human Services.

Centers for Medicare and Medicaid Services. (2009a). *Brief summaries of Medicare and Medicaid.* Baltimore, MD: U.S. Department of Health and Human Services. Retrieved from https://www.cms.gov/Research-Statistics-Data-and-Systems/Statistics-Trends-and-Reports/MedicareProgramRatesStats/SummaryMedicareMedicaid.html

Centers for Medicare and Medicaid Services. (2009b). *Medicare and Medicaid statistical supplement, 2009.* Baltimore, MD: U.S. Department of Health and Human Services. Retrieved from https://www.cms.gov/Research-Statistics-Data-and-Systems/Statistics-Trends-and-Reports/MedicareMedicaidStatSupp/2009.html

Centers for Medicare and Medicaid Services. (2010). *Medicare & you 2010.* Baltimore, MD: U.S. Department of Health and Human Services. Retrieved from http://www.patientadvocatetraining.com/wp-content/themes/patientadvocate/static/pdf/5_Medicare___You.pdf

Centers for Medicare and Medicaid Services. (2012). *Medicaid/CHIP Affordable Care Act Implementation.* Baltimore, MD: U.S. Department of Health and Human Services. Retrieved from https://www.medicaid.gov/state-resource-center/FAQ-medicaid-and-chip-affordable-care-act-implementation/downloads/Eligibility-Policy-FAQs.pdf

Centers for Medicare and Medicaid Services. (2013). *Brief summaries of Medicare and Medicaid.* Baltimore, MD: U.S. Department of Health and Human Services. Retrieved from http://www.cms.gov/MedicareProgramRatesStats/Downloads/MedicareMedicaidSummaries2013.pdf

Centers for Medicare and Medicaid Services. (2015a). *Medicare Parts A & B Premiums and Deductibles Announced.* Baltimore, MD: U.S. Department of Health and Human Services. Retrieved from https://www.cms.gov/Newsroom/MediaReleaseDatabase/Press-releases/2015-Press-releases-items/2015-11-10.html

Centers for Medicare and Medicaid Services. (2015b). *HHS FY2016 budget in brief.* Baltimore, MD: U.S. Department of Health and Human Services. Retrieved from http://www.hhs.gov/about/budget/budget-in-brief/cms/medicare/index.html

Centers for Medicare and Medicaid Services. (2015c, March). *Report to the Congress: Medicare payment policy* (p. 92). Baltimore, MD: U.S. Department of Health and Human Services. Retrieved from http://www.medpac.gov/documents/reports/chapter-4-physician-and-other-health-professional-services-(march-2015-report).pdf

Centers for Medicare and Medicaid Services. (2016). *Choosing a Medigap policy: A guide to health insurance for people with Medicare.* Baltimore, MD: U.S. Department of Health and Human Services. Retrieved from https://www.medicare.gov/Pubs/pdf/02110-Medicare-Medigap.guide.pdf

Center for the Study of Services. (1995). *Consumers' guide to health plans.* Washington, DC: Center for the Study of Services.

Coleman, T. S. (1990). *Legal aspects of Medicare & Medicaid reimbursement: Payment for hospital and physician services.* Washington, DC: National Health Lawyers Association.

Congressional Budget Office. (2015). March 2015 baseline: Medicare. Retrieved from http://kff.org/medicare/fact-sheet/medicare-spending-and-financing-fact-sheet/

Cubanski, J., Neuman, T., & Jacobson, G. (2014, January 13). *Raising Medicare premiums for higher-income beneficiaries: Assessing the implications.* Menlo Park, CA: Henry J. Kaiser Family Foundation. Retrieved from http://kff.org/medicare/issue-brief/income-relating-medicare-part-b-and-part/

Cubanski, J., Swoope, C., Boccuti, C, Jacobson, G., Casillas, G., Griffin, S., & Neuman, T. (2015, March 20). *A Primer on Medicare: Key facts about the Medicare program and the people it covers.* Menlo Park, CA: Henry J. Kaiser Family Foundation. Retrieved from http://kff.org/medicare/report/a-primer-on-medicare-key-facts-about-the-medicare-program-and-the-people-it-covers/

Davis, M. H., & Burner, S. T. (1995). Three decades of Medicare: What the numbers tell us. *Health Affairs, 14*(4), 231–243.

Department of Health & Human Services. (2014, December 2). *FY2016 federal medical assistance percentages.* Retrieved from https://aspe.hhs.gov/basic-report/fy2016-federal-medical-assistance-percentages

Fein, R. (1989). *Medical care, medical costs* (2nd ed.). Cambridge, MA: Harvard University Press.

Friedman, E. (1987). Medicaid's overload sparks a crisis. *Hospitals, 61*(2), 50–54.

Friedman, E. (1990). Medicare and Medicaid at 25. *Hospitals, 64*(15), 38, 42, 46, 48, 50, 52, 54.

Ginsburg, P. B. (1988). Public insurance programs: Medicare and Medicaid. In H. E. Frech III (Ed.), *Health care in America* (pp. 179–218). San Francisco, CA: Pacific Research Institute for Public Policy.

Health Care Financing Administration. (1996). *Your Medicare handbook, 1996*. Baltimore, MD: U.S. Department of Health and Human Services.

Health Care Financing Administration. (1998). *A profile of Medicare chart book*. Baltimore, MD: U.S. Department of Health and Human Services.

Hellman, S., & Hellman, L. H. (1991). *Medicare and Medigaps: A guide to retirement health insurance*. Newbury Park, CA: Sage.

Henry J. Kaiser Family Foundation. (2003). *Medicare+Choice*. Menlo Park, CA: Henry J. Kaiser Family Foundation.

Henry J. Kaiser Family Foundation. (2005a). *Medicare chart book 2005*. Menlo Park, CA: Henry J. Kaiser Family Foundation.

Henry J. Kaiser Family Foundation. (2005b). *The Medicare prescription drug benefit*. Menlo Park, CA: Henry J. Kaiser Family Foundation.

Henry J. Kaiser Family Foundation. (2009a). *Medicare Part D 2010 data spotlight: Benefit design and cost sharing*. Menlo Park, CA: Henry J. Kaiser Family Foundation.

Henry J. Kaiser Family Foundation. (2009b). *Low-income assistance under the Medicare drug benefit*. Menlo Park, CA: Henry J. Kaiser Family Foundation.

Henry J. Kaiser Family Foundation. (2009c). *The Medicare prescription drug benefit*. Menlo Park, CA: Henry J. Kaiser Family Foundation.

Henry J. Kaiser Family Foundation. (2010a). *Medicare advantage 2010 data spotlight: Benefits and cost sharing*. Menlo Park, CA: Henry J. Kaiser Family Foundation.

Henry J. Kaiser Family Foundation. (2010b). *Explaining health care reform: Questions about Medicaid's role*. Menlo Park, CA: Henry J. Kaiser Family Foundation.

Henry J. Kaiser Family Foundation. (2010c). *Summary of new health reform law*. Menlo Park, CA: Henry J. Kaiser Family Foundation.

Henry J. Kaiser Family Foundation. (2010d). *Medicaid at a glance*. Menlo Park, CA: Henry J. Kaiser Family Foundation.

Henry J. Kaiser Family Foundation. (2011). *Medicare advantage plan star ratings and bonus payments in 2012*. Menlo Park, CA: Henry J. Kaiser Family Foundation. Retrieved from https://kaiserfamilyfoundation.files.wordpress.com/2013/01/8257.pdf

Henry J. Kaiser Family Foundation. (2015a, June 29). *Medicare advantage*. Menlo Park, CA: Henry J. Kaiser Family Foundation. Retrieved from http://kff.org/medicare/fact-sheet/medicare-advantage/

Henry J. Kaiser Family Foundation. (2015b). *The Medicare part D prescription drug benefit*. Menlo Park, CA: Henry J. Kaiser Family Foundation. Retrieved from http://kff.org/medicare/fact-sheet/the-medicare-prescription-drug-benefit-fact-sheet/

Henry J. Kaiser Family Foundation. (2015c, June 22). *Medicaid delivery system and payment reform: A guide to key terms and concepts*. Menlo Park, CA: Henry J. Kaiser Family Foundation. Retrieved from http://kff.org/medicaid/fact-sheet/medicaid-delivery-system-and-payment-reform-a-guide-to-key-terms-and-concepts/

Henry J. Kaiser Family Foundation. (2015d, October 13). *The Medicare part D prescription drug benefit*. Menlo Park, CA: Henry J. Kaiser Family Foundation. Retrieved from http://kff.org/medicare/fact-sheet/the-medicare-prescription-drug-benefit-fact-sheet/

Hutchison, B. (2008, August). Pay for performance in primary care: Proceed with caution, pitfalls ahead. *Healthcare Policy*, *4*(1), 10–15.

Institute of Medicine. (2007). *Rewarding provider performance: Aligning incentives in Medicare*. Washington, DC: The National Academies Press.

Kaiser Commission on the Future of Medicaid. (1995). *Medicaid and managed care: Lessons from the literature*. Washington, DC: Henry J. Kaiser Family Foundation.

Kaiser Commission on Medicaid and the Uninsured. (2008). *Medicaid benefits: Online database*. Retrieved from http://www.kff.org/medicaid/benefits/service.jsp?gr=off&nt=on&so=0&tg=0&yr=4&cat=5&sv=32

Kaiser Commission on Medicaid and the Uninsured. (2009). *Where are states today? Medicaid and state-funded coverage eligibility levels for low-income adults*. Washington, DC: Henry J. Kaiser Family Foundation.

Klees, B. S., Wolfe, C. J., & Curtis, C. A. (2014). *Brief summaries of Medicare & Medicaid*. Retrieved from https://www.cms.gov/Research-Statistics-Data-and-Systems/Statistics-Trends-and-Reports/MedicareProgramRatesStats/Downloads/MedicareMedicaidSummaries2014.pdf

Longest, B. B., Jr. (1994). *Health policymaking in the United States*. Ann Arbor, MI: Association of University Programs in Health Administration Press/Health Administration Press.

Medicare.gov. (2015, December 27). Star ratings. Retrieved from https://www.medicare.gov/find-a-plan/staticpages/rating/planrating-help.aspx?AspxAutoDetectCookieSupport=1

Medicare and Medicaid Statistical Supplement. (1992). *Health Care Financing Review, 14*(suppl).

Medicare and Medicaid Statistical Supplement. (1995). *Health Care Financing Review, 16*(suppl).

Medicare and Medicaid Statistical Supplement. (2001). *Health Care Financing Review, 21*(suppl).

Medicare Payment Advisory Commission. (2009). Report to the Congress: Medicare payment policy. Retrieved from http://medpac.gov/documents/reports/march-2009-report-to-congress-medicare-payment-policy.pdf

Muirhead, G. (1996). More Medicaid programs turning to managed care. *Drug Topics, 140*(8), 50–51.

National Academy for State Health Policy. (2015, December 29). Map: Where states stand on Medicaid expansion decisions. Retrieved from https://www.statereforum.org/Medicaid-Expansion-Decisions-Map

National Center for Health Statistics. (1993). *Health, United States, 1992*. Hyattsville, MD: Public Health Service, U.S. Department of Health and Human Services.

Noel-Miller C. (2015, October). *Medicare Beneficiaries' Out-of-Pocket Spending for Health Care*, American Association of Retired Persons, AARP Policy Institute.

Oberg, C. N., & Polich, C. L. (1988). Medicaid: Entering the third decade. *Health Affairs, 7*(4), 83–96.

O'Neill, T. (2015, June 2). Primer: The Medicare advantage star rating System. *American Action Forum*. Retrieved from http://americanactionforum.org/research/primer-the-medicare-advantage-star-rating-system

Paradise, J. (2015, March 9). *Medicaid moving forward*. Menlo Park, CA: Henry J. Kaiser Family Foundation, Figure 8. Retrieved from http://kff.org/health-reform/issue-brief/medicaid-moving-forward/

Pharmacy Quality Alliance. (2015). PQA measures used by CMS in the star ratings. Retrieved from http://pqaalliance.org/measures/cms.asp

Pharmacy Times. (2006). Medicare offers seniors advice for dealing with Part D glitches. Retrieved from http://www.pharmacytimes.com/article.cfm?ID=3327

Truffer, C. J., Keehan, S., Smith, S., Cylus, J., Sisko, A., Poisal, J. A., … Clemens, M. K. (2010). Health spending projections through 2019: The recession's impact continues. *Health Affairs, 29*(3), 522–529.

Ukens, C. (2006). Medicare Part D off to rocky start. Retrieved from http://www.drugtopics.com/drugtopics/article/articleDetail.jsp?id=283609

Zarabozo, C., Taylor, C., & Hicks, J. (1996). Medicare managed care: Numbers and trends. *Health Care Financing Review, 17*(3), 243–261.

CHAPTER

19

Pharmacoeconomics

Scott K. Griggs, Craig I. Coleman, Taehwan Park, and Kenneth W. Schafermeyer*

Case Scenario

Crohn's disease (CD) is a lifelong, relapsing systemic inflammatory disease that can affect any part of the gastrointestinal tract (Baumgart & Sandborn, 2012) and has a prevalence of about 241 per 100,000 Americans (Kappelman, Moore, Allen, & Cook, 2013). Patients with CD can display an assortment of gastrointestinal symptoms, including weight loss, malaise, abdominal pain, diarrhea (bloody or nonbloody) and fevers, depending on the location of the inflammation. CD can also be complicated by various extraintestinal manifestations and related immune disorders (e.g., mouth ulcers, psoriasis, large joint arthritis, asthma, autoimmune thyroid disease).

CD is associated with markedly elevated healthcare utilization (Baumgart, 2012). Only about 10% of CD patients experience prolonged clinical remission, with one in every five patients requiring hospitalization each year. Moreover, at least 50% of adult patients will require surgery within the 10 years and nearly one-half will experience an intestinal complication within 20 years of diagnosis.

In addition to increased healthcare utilization, CD has detrimental effects on work productivity and health-related quality of life (HrQoL) (Cohen et al., 2014; Lönnfors et al., 2014). Studies suggest as many as 15% of CD sufferers are unable to work within 5 to 10 years following diagnosis. This work disability, along with disease activity, corticosteroid treatment, and need for frequent hospitalization have been shown to have a negative effect on CD patient HrQoL.

In the United States, pharmacologic management of CD generally involves a stepwise approach (Terdiman et al., 2013). Treatment of CD aims to achieve sustained remission and to interrupt the progressive disease course that eventually results in intestinal failure and subsequent complications (Baumgart & Sandborn, 2012). Corticosteroids (systemic and nonabsorbable) are generally reserved for the treatment of acute flares of CD, with 5-aminosalicate drugs (e.g., mesalamine), thiopurines (6-mercaptopurine [6-MP] and azathioprine) and methotrexate used to maintain remission. When these agents fail to maintain disease remission on their own, biologic agents such as infliximab,

(*Continues*)

*The authors wish express appreciation to Emily R. Cox, Ph.D., for her contributions to a previous edition of this chapter.

adalimumab, natalizumab, vedolizumab, and certolizumab pegol are used (often in combination with prior agents). Biologic therapies offer a distinct advantage in CD treatment because their mechanism of action is targeted to particular enzymes and proteins (i.e., tumor necrosis factor [TNF]) that have already been aberrant in people with CD. Biologic agents, however, have an annual cost that far exceeds that of nonbiologic treatments. For example, infliximab is typically administered at a dose of 5 mg/kg at 0, 2, and 6 weeks (induction therapy), then every 8 weeks thereafter (maintenance therapy). With an estimated cost per dose of infliximab of ~$1,900 per 100 mg, an 80-kg patient would get 400 mg per dose at a cost of $7,600 per dose (>$45,000 annually).

A well-done randomized controlled trial is published in a respectable medical journal demonstrating that adding a biologic agent, infliximab, to previous therapy improves outcomes for patients with moderate-to-severe CD (Rutgeerts et al., 1999; Targan et al., 1997). Specifically, a greater proportion of patients taking infliximab 5 mg/kg achieved clinical improvement defined as a 70-point improvement in their CD activity index (CDAI) score compared to those receiving only their prior therapy plus placebo.

Robert, the chairman of a large managed care organization's (Husky Health) pharmacy and therapeutics committee, is asked to consider the economic impact of adding infliximab to the formulary for the "moderate-to-severe CD treatment" indication. He needs to assess the pharmacoeconomic literature or perform his own pharmacoeconomic evaluation to aid him in his decision-making process.

LEARNING OBJECTIVES

Upon completion of this chapter, the reader shall be able to:

- Define pharmacoeconomics and explain how it is used.
- Explain how perspective can affect a pharmacoeconomic study.
- Define and differentiate among cost-minimization analysis (CMA), cost-benefit analysis (CBA), cost-effectiveness analysis (CEA), cost-utility analysis (CUA), cost-of-illness (COI) analysis, and cost-consequence analysis (CCA) (when should each be used, how they differ with regard to measuring costs and outcomes, and so on). Given a case study or a scenario, be able to calculate each and use them to decide among alternatives.
- Define, differentiate, and give examples of inputs, outputs, and outcomes.
- Compare and contrast efficiency, efficacy, and effectiveness.
- Define, differentiate, and give examples of the four types of costs used in pharmacoeconomic analyses.
- Differentiate between a clinical end point and an outcome.
- Critically appraise the conduct and reporting of a pharmacoeconomic study.

CHAPTER QUESTIONS

Begin formulating in your mind how Robert might begin to assess whether he should make this formulary addition.

1. Should Robert recommend infliximab (or other biologic agents) be covered?
2. Upon what criteria should he base his decision?
3. What therapies should be compared to infliximab?
4. What would the impact of adding infliximab be to Husky Health's pharmacy benefits budget?

INTRODUCTION

By 2017, global spending for pharmaceuticals is anticipated to reach $1.2 trillion. The United States ranks first in total pharmaceutical spending, with sales expected to increase by up to 4%, and total spending surpassing $350 billion by 2017 (IMS Institute for Healthcare Informatics, 2014). Pharmaceutical spending increases in high-income countries such as the United States are presently being driven largely by specialty medicines such as biologic agents. It is anticipated that biologic agent spending will continue to outpace overall pharmaceutical spending, eventually representing about 20% of total pharmaceutical sales by 2017. Infliximab, a TNF-alpha blocker agent used to treat moderate-to-severe CD, is one of the top 10 selling drugs in the United States, generating more than $5 billion in sales in 2013 (FiercePharma, 2014). Those most alarmed by rising pharmaceutical (and in particular biologic agent) costs are, of course, those responsible for paying for and managing these costs. Payers of pharmaceuticals include employers, managed care organizations, and a myriad of healthcare institutions such as inpatient hospitals and the Veterans Administration. Those responsible for managing these costs are the individuals within these institutions who, through their own expertise and with the help of outside management organizations, such as pharmacy benefit management companies, attempt to constrain pharmacy costs in the face of limited budgets.

Decision makers charged with managing pharmacy costs have historically focused on the ingredient cost of the product along with its clinical profile in assessing a product's value. This is often referred to as the "silo approach" to evaluating pharmaceuticals. However, this approach does not consider how pharmaceuticals affect other healthcare costs, such as hospitalizations, physician visits, laboratory services, and need for surgery or other procedures. All these are important aspects to consider so as to capture the true value of pharmaceuticals.

Pharmacoeconomics is a term used to describe a compilation of methods that evaluate the economic, clinical, and humanistic outcomes (the ECHO model) of pharmaceutical products and services (Gunter, 1999). More formally, pharmacoeconomics identifies, measures, and compares the costs and consequences of the use of pharmaceutical products and services (Bootman, Townsend, & McGhan, 1996). In its most simplistic form, a pharmacoeconomic evaluation compares the economic resources consumed (inputs) to produce the health and economic consequences of products or services (outcomes). This relationship is presented graphically in **Figure 19-1**.

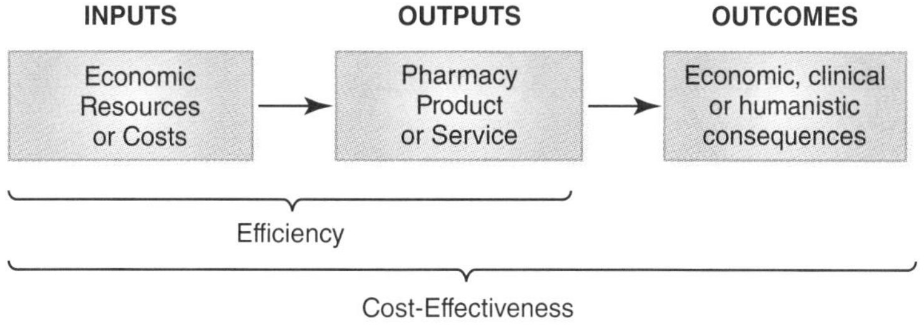

Figure 19-1 Pharmacoeconomic Evaluation of Health Care. Pharmacoeconomic studies compare the economic resources or costs (inputs) associated with provision of pharmacy services or products (outputs) to the outcomes of the product or service. *Efficiency* refers to the lowest cost per unit of output while *cost-effectiveness* refers to the lowest cost to achieve the desired outcome.

The economic evaluation of health care began to take shape in the late 1970s with the writings of Weinstein & Stason (1977). The techniques used were taken from the field of public economics, particularly methods related to CBA. The application of economic evaluation to pharmacy began around the same time. These early writings and studies on the subject did not evaluate pharmaceuticals, but rather pharmacy services (Bootman, McGhan, & Schondelmeyer, 1982; Bootman, Wertheimer, Zaske, & Rowland, 1979). The focus shifted to evaluation of products after the term *pharmacoeconomics* appeared in the literature in 1986 (Townsend, 1986). A tremendous growth in the number of pharmacoeconomic studies appearing in the literature has occurred since that time.

Pharmacoeconomic evaluations have been used as a tool in selecting formulary products, developing treatment guidelines, conducting disease-management programs, establishing prior authorization policies, implementing step-therapy programs, and designing prescription drug benefit programs (Motheral, Grizzle, Armstrong, Cox, & Fairman, 2000). Together with information on a product's clinical efficacy, effectiveness, and safety, pharmacoeconomic information assists decision makers in optimizing the use of prescription therapy.

The economic evaluation of pharmaceuticals and pharmacy services grew out of the need to establish value or to respond to the question of value. Statements of product or service value center on the following two attributes: cost and benefit. From the consumer's perspective, the price paid should reflect the benefit gained from use of the product or service. Several factors have created the need to monitor the value of pharmaceuticals more closely, including increased cost and thus growing concern on the part of payers, increased number of alternatives available to treat illness and disease, growing demand for pharmaceuticals, and the proliferation of high-cost biotechnology products (Hartman et al., 2010).

To conduct pharmacoeconomic evaluations, the following six common methodological approaches are used: (1) CMA, (2) CBA, (3) CEA, (4) CUA, (5) COI analysis, and (6) CCA. This chapter covers each of these methods, including their advantages and disadvantages and their application to pharmaceutical products and services.

First, however, it is important to distinguish between several terms that are often confused with one another: efficiency, efficacy, and effectiveness. Efficiency can refer to a number of economic goals, such as properly allocating resources or increasing production. In our context, efficiency refers to the lowest cost per unit of output (or the biggest bang for the buck). It should be noted that an output is not the same as an outcome. For example, reducing the cost of prescriptions (outputs) may be efficient but it does not necessarily improve health outcomes.

Efficacy and effectiveness address outcomes. Efficacy answers the question, "*Does the product work?*" This question is answered through the clinical trial process, where it is determined whether the product does more good than harm. Effectiveness, however, seeks to determine whether the product works in real-life practice settings. Effectiveness answers the question, "*Does the product work in those individuals it was designed to treat?*"

COMPARING PHARMACOECONOMIC METHODOLOGIES

Table 19-1 shows four basic types of pharmacoeconomic methods (CMA, CBA, CEA, and CUA). Each measures costs in monetary units (e.g., U.S. dollars) but differs in the method that consequences are measured.

In both CMA and CEA, the consequences or outcomes of the intervention being evaluated are measured in natural units of effectiveness. Natural units of effectiveness are typically clinical measures of a product's efficacy or effectiveness, such as mm Hg (for antihypertensives) or blood glucose

Table 19-1 Measurement of Costs and Outcomes Under Four Types of Pharmacoeconomic Methodologies

Methodology	Cost	Outcomes	Application	Calculation	Decision rule
Cost-minimization analysis (CMA)	$	Assumed to be equal	To compare alternative products or services that have equal efficacy and safety (e.g., brand vs. generic substitution, biologic vs. biosimilar)	Cost of A vs. cost of B	Choose the alternative with the lowest total cost.
Cost-benefit analysis (CBA)	$	Monetized to dollars or other monetary unit	To compare programs with different outcomes (e.g., a vaccination program and a colon cancer screening clinic)	Net benefit = Σ benefits − Σ costs	Choose alternatives where the net benefits are positive, or if more than one alternative is being compared and resources are limited, choose the alternative with the greatest net benefit.
				Benefit-to-cost ratio = benefit ÷ cost or Cost-to-benefit ratio = cost ÷ benefit	Choose alternatives with benefit-to-cost ratios >1 or cost-to-benefit ratios <1. If resources are limited, choose the alternative with the highest benefit-to-cost ratio or the lowest cost-to-benefit ratio.
Cost-effectiveness analysis (CEA)	$	Natural units, such as blood glucose, blood pressure, peak flow (clinical indicators), life years gained, or symptom-free life years	To compare alternatives with similar indications or goals measured in the same unit of consequence (e.g., number of intervention with patients achieving >70 point improvement on the CDAI)	Average cost-effectiveness ratio = cost ÷ outcome Average effectiveness-to-cost ratio = outcome ÷ cost	Cost-effectiveness: choose the alternative with the lowest cost per unit of outcome. Effectiveness-to-cost: choose the alternative with the best outcome per dollar of input (i.e., highest "bang for the buck")
				Incremental cost-effectiveness ratio = (cost of A − cost of B) ÷ (outcome of A − outcome of B)	A negative ICER indicates that one treatment is dominant (more effective and less expensive); for a positive ICER, one must consider whether it is worth the additional cost to achieve an additional unit of outcome.

(Continues)

Table 19-1 Measurement of Costs and Outcomes Under Four Types of Pharmacoeconomic Methodologies (continued)

Methodology	Cost	Outcomes	Application	Calculation	Decision rule
Cost-utility analysis (CUA)	$	Quality-adjusted life years (QALYs)	To compare alternatives that results in changes in both quantity and quality of life (e.g., chemotherapy regimen or biologic agent for treatment of moderate-to-severe Crohn's disease)	Cost-utility ratio = cost ÷ QALYs	Choose the alternative with the lowest cost per QALY.
				Incremental cost-utility ratio = (cost of A − cost of B) ÷ (QALYs for A − QALYs for B)	A negative ICUR indicates one of the treatments is dominant (greater QALYs and lower cost); a positive ICUR must be assessed in terms of the decision maker's willingness to pay for a QALY (whether the additional QALYs are worth the additional cost).

CDAI, Crohn's disease activity index; ICER, incremental cost-effectiveness ratio; ICUR, incremental cost-utility ratio; QALY, quality-adjusted life year; Σ, sum.

Table 19-2 Measurement of Costs and Outcomes for Cost-of-Illness and Cost-Consequence Analyses

Methodology	Cost	Outcomes	Application
Cost-of-illness (COI) analysis	$	Not assessed	Determine the total economic burden of a disease on society (e.g., the economic burden of treating Crohn's disease)
Cost-consequence analysis (CCA)	$	Natural units, QALYs	To present all costs and effects in a disaggregated format so that decision makers can choose among those that best fit their perspective

levels (for antidiabetic agents), or in our CD/infliximab scenario, improvement in CDAI. Natural units of effectiveness also include years of life saved (for chemotherapeutic agents), judgments of clinical success (for antibiotics), or cases averted because of an intervention (for influenza vaccination). CBA measures the consequences of the intervention in dollars, whereas CUA (often considered a special type of CEA) measures the consequences of therapy in quality-adjusted life years (QALYs).

Table 19-2 lists two other types of pharmacoeconomic methods—CCA and COI analysis. CCA also measures costs in dollars, but is different from the other methods in that multiple outcome measures are presented to the decision maker. COI analyses do not aim to compare treatment alternatives, but rather estimate the cost burden of a disease in a specific population. Each of these methods will be covered in greater detail later in the chapter.

The remainder of this chapter will not only familiarize readers with the terminology and concepts of pharmacoeconomics, but also present some of the basic guidelines for conducting pharmacoeconomic studies and equip students and practitioners for critical appraisal of the literature.

STEPS FOR CONDUCTING A PHARMACOECONOMIC EVALUATION

Before the specifics of each method are presented, some important points need to be considered. When conducting a pharmacoeconomic evaluation, it is important to (1) define the problem and state the objective; (2) identify the perspective and the alternative interventions to be compared; (3) identify and measure the outcomes of each alternative; and (4) identify, measure, and value the costs of all alternatives. Other important aspects of pharmacoeconomic evaluations to be discussed are discounting and performing sensitivity analysis.

Define the Problem and State the Objective

All pharmacoeconomic evaluations should begin with a clear and concise statement of the problem or question to be addressed. In the chapter-opening case scenario, Robert could evaluate biologic therapy with infliximab compared to no additional therapy in patients getting suboptimal response to their current agents (as evaluated in the original randomized trial), or he could compare infliximab to other available biologic agents which have also been compared to no additional therapy in moderate-to-severe CD patients (perhaps using a network meta-analysis or indirect treatment comparison to compare agents efficacy and safety). Examples of problem statements include "Is the addition of infliximab cost-effective for the treatment of moderate-to-severe CD in patients failing standard non-biologic agents?" and, more broadly, "What is the most cost-effective biologic agent for the treatment of moderate-to-severe CD in patients failing standard non-biologic agents?"

Identify the Perspective

Establishing the perspective of a study is an important step in pharmacoeconomic evaluation. Pharmacoeconomic evaluations can be conducted from several different perspectives, including those of the employer, the patient, the health insurance plan, society, and the government. For example, the perspective of the case scenario could be that of either Husky Health or the managed care organization's major employer group. The study perspective is an important factor in determining the costs considered relevant (i.e., cost of lost productivity is pertinent to the employer's perspective, but not to the healthcare provider's perspective), how costs are valued (i.e., the cost of a drug might be valued at actual acquisition cost from the provider's perspective, but as out-of-pocket costs or copayment amount in the patient's perspective), the choice of outcomes measured (e.g., HrQoL or patient satisfaction is often only included in analyses conducted from the patient or societal perspective), and the time period over which the product or service will be evaluated (in the case of CD, this could be the period of time over which infliximab was studied in its clinical trial or over a patient's lifetime).

An example from the literature highlights the importance of perspective and how it can influence the results of the study. A CBA of a routine varicella (chickenpox) vaccination program for healthy children was conducted from two perspectives—that of society and that of the payer of health services (e.g., a health plan) (Lieu et al., 1994). The study found that from a payer's perspective, the vaccine had a benefit-to-cost ratio that was less than 1:1 (i.e., the benefits were less than the costs). However, when conducted from a societal perspective, the benefit-to-cost ratio was greater than 1:1, suggesting that the program should be implemented. The difference in findings derived from which costs were considered relevant from the different perspectives. From society's perspective, costs related to lost workdays avoided because of the vaccine were relevant and, therefore, were included. From a payer's perspective, these costs were not considered relevant and, therefore, were not included in the analysis.

Identify Alternative Interventions

The decision as to which alternatives should be compared in pharmacoeconomic evaluations is important. A simple question to ask when considering which alternatives to compare is, "*Have all relevant treatment alternatives been considered in addressing the research question?*" In many studies, as in our case scenario, the alternatives involve drug-to-drug comparisons; in other situations, drug therapy is compared to no or nonpharmacologic therapies (or no alternative at all).

As shown in **Figure 19-2**, alternatives need to be analyzed in detail only when one of the alternatives is both more costly and more effective than the other options.

Figure 19-3 represents what is commonly referred to an incremental cost-effectiveness plane, with the horizontal axis representing the difference in effectiveness between alternatives (incremental effectiveness) and the vertical representing the difference in cost (incremental cost). Four scenarios exist when comparing two different therapies (alternatives A and B). Alternative A is either more costly than B or less costly than B. The same relationship applies to the degree of effectiveness. In our case scenario, it is believed that a biologic agent such as infliximab is more effective but also more costly than not adding an agent to ongoing but suboptimal treatment. If alternative A represents the addition of infliximab and alternative B no additional therapy, this scenario would

Cost-Effectiveness of Drug A versus Drug B	Cost Drug A < Cost Drug B	Cost Drug A = Cost Drug B	Cost Drug A > Cost Drug B
Effect Drug A < Effect Drug B	Cost Effectiveness Analysis (ICER)	Prefer Drug B	Prefer Drug B (A Dominated by B)
Effect Drug A = Effect Drug B	Prefer Drug A	Indifferent	Prefer Drug B
Effect Drug A > Effect Drug B	Prefer Drug A (A Dominant over B)	Prefer Drug A	Cost Effectiveness Analysis (ICER)

Figure 19-2 Cost-Effectiveness Grid. To determine if a therapy or service is cost effective, both the cost and the effectiveness should be assessed. If two therapies, Drug A and Drug B are compared, several potential alternatives are possible. If Drug A is both less expensive and more effective (see the bottom left square), then Drug A is dominant over Drug B. Similarly, if Drug A is both more costly and less effective (see top right square), then Drug A is dominated by Drug B; thus Drug B is preferred. The top left and bottom right squares necessitate performing an incremental cost effectiveness ratio to assist the decision maker in determining if the lower cost is worth the lower effectiveness or the extra cost is worth the extra effectiveness.

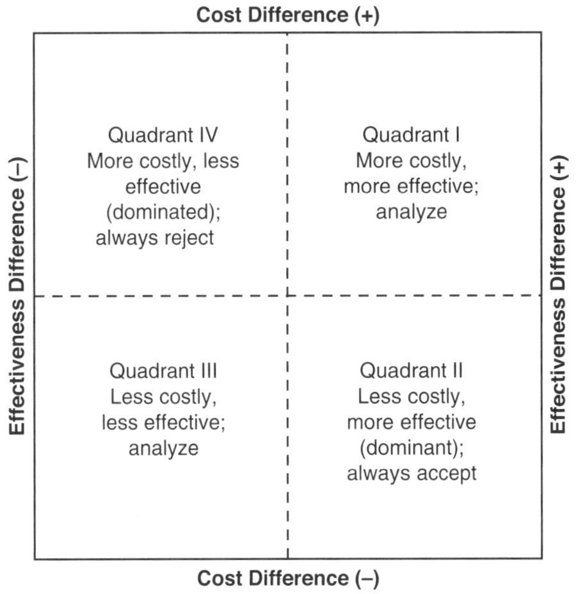

Figure 19-3 Incremental Cost-Effectiveness Plane and the Decision to Conduct a Pharmacoeconomic Evaluation. The incremental cost-effectiveness plane can be broken into four quadrants (I–IV). When comparing two agents, quadrants I and III represent scenarios where pharmacoeconomic analysis is helpful to determine how much additional money needs to be spent to get additional benefit. Quadrant II represents a scenario where one agent is dominant (i.e., less costly and more effective) over the other, whereas quadrant IV represents a scenario where one agent is dominated (i.e., more costly and less effective) by the other. In both cases, analysis would not be necessary.

fall in the upper-right cell (quadrant I). The researcher would then analyze the differences in costs and effects between these two alternatives. The same comparison could also be interpreted as no additional therapy being less costly and less effective (quadrant III). In these scenarios, the question then becomes, *"Is the additional gain in benefit or effectiveness worth the additional cost?"* In those scenarios where one alternative is dominant (i.e., less costly and more effective) over the other, or is dominated (i.e., more costly and less effective) by the other, such as in the lower-right and upper-left quadrants (quadrants II and IV, respectively) of the incremental cost-effectiveness plane, no analysis is necessary, since such analysis would provide little additional information.

Identify and Measure Outcomes of Each Alternative Intervention

When a clinician thinks about evaluating pharmaceutical products, the products' clinical effects immediately come to mind. In general terms, treatment could result in one of several outcomes (listed in order from most desirable to least desirable):

- A cure (health is restored)
- Extended life
- Improved HrQoL
- Decreased incidence of morbidity
- Relief or reduction in symptoms (reduced CDAI score)
- No effect
- Increased morbidity (e.g., drug interactions or adverse drug reactions)
- Death

Some of these outcomes are easier to measure than others. Death, for example, is an objective outcome that is easy to measure. In contrast, measures such as decreased risk of morbidity and improved HrQoL are less exact (more subjective). Moreover, some outcomes may be difficult to measure because of the long follow-up required to determine whether the outcome has been achieved. For example, the desirable outcome for treatment of hypertension would be prevention of strokes or heart attacks (i.e., decreased incidence of morbidity). Achieving a normal blood pressure reading (e.g., diastolic reading < 90 mm Hg) is not, in itself, the desired outcome; it is merely an intermediate or surrogate measure or clinical end point that is a useful, but imperfect, predictor of a health outcome.

Although we would prefer to measure final or terminal outcomes, this process can require years, even decades. However, given that normal blood pressure is correlated with fewer heart attacks and strokes, we often accept intermediate measures (i.e., clinical end points) as surrogate indicators of outcomes. For diabetes, for example, the desirable outcomes are prevention of complications (e.g., retinopathy, neuropathy, nephropathy). Because these outcomes also occur over the long term, we use intermediate measures such as blood glucose and glycosylated hemoglobin (HbA1c) levels as predictors of risk for complications of diabetes. For patients with asthma, we might desire an outcome of fewer complications (e.g., respiratory infections) or fewer emergency department visits or hospitalizations; the clinical indicators correlated with these outcome measures are peak-flow meter readings.

The outcomes discussed in the preceding paragraph were described in clinical terms. In fact, outcomes can also be described in humanistic terms (e.g., patient HrQoL or satisfaction) or in economic terms (cost per day, cost per course of therapy, or cost per member per month). For a patient with asthma, for example, we could measure outcomes not only as the clinical end point of peak-flow rate but also in terms of the patient's HrQoL and cost of treatment over a given period of time. Using economic measurement assumes that a patient who is achieving the desired outcomes will need less intervention and treatment, such as physician visits, medications, emergency department visits, or hospital admissions.

Identify, Measure, and Value Costs

As stated previously, the principles of pharmacoeconomics require one to identify, measure, and compare the costs and consequences of the use of pharmaceutical products and services. From a measurement aspect, two components exist—costs and consequences. Some of the issues related to identifying and measuring consequences or outcomes of therapy have been covered already. Our focus now shifts to the following three considerations that affect the cost side of the equation: identifying, measuring, and placing a value on resources or costs.

Identifying Relevant Costs

The first step in measuring costs is identifying all relevant resources consumed in association with the product or service under evaluation. To determine whether a cost is relevant, consider this question: "*Would this cost have been incurred had the program not been implemented?*"

As a method of identification, costs are often categorized as direct medical, direct nonmedical, indirect, or intangible costs (**Table 19-3**).

Table 19-3 Examples of Types of Costs Included in Pharmacoeconomic Analyses

Direct medical costs
- Services of health professionals
- Hospitalizations and emergency room (ER) visits
- Medications
- Supplies
- Laboratory tests
- Ambulance service

Examples of direct nonmedical costs
- Transportation costs for health care (gas/car, bus, taxi)
- Hotel costs for patient/family for out-of-town health care
- Food costs for out-of-town health care
- Daycare (child care) services
- Nonmedical assistance for condition (housekeeping)

Examples of indirect costs (i.e., opportunity costs)
- Lost productivity for patient
- Lost productivity for caregiver(s)
- Productivity foregone due to premature death

Examples of intangible costs
- Pain
- Suffering
- Anxiety
- Inconvenience
- Fatigue

Direct medical costs are resources consumed for medical services or products that are directly related to the product or service being evaluated. They include physician services, emergency department visits, laboratory and diagnostic testing services, prescribed medications (e.g., infliximab to treat moderate-to-severe CD), hospitalizations, and surgeries. These costs are typically services covered by third-party payers, such as insurance companies, managed care organizations, or the government.

Direct nonmedical costs are those nonmedical resources consumed as the result of providing the product or service. They include transportation to treatment facilities (or infusion centers in the case of infliximab) and additional housing expenses incurred by the patients and their family when traveling to healthcare facilities outside their hometown. Other examples are special diets (often a key component of CD management) and exercise equipment required as a component of treatment or rehabilitation. These costs are not typically covered by third-party payers and are usually the responsibility of the patient.

Indirect costs are those costs indirectly associated with the product or service under evaluation. Illness and disease have an impact on resources outside the medical sector. For example, people who are sick may be unable to work or may be less productive. This loss of productivity is an important cost that should be captured in an evaluation. The inclusion of indirect costs is controversial in the literature, primarily because of the difficulty in measuring lost productivity and establishing causal links between illness and lost productivity. Nevertheless, many pharmacoeconomic studies attempt to measure the impact of morbidity or the ill effects of the treatment or health condition on worker productivity. These costs are often borne by patients, caregivers, employers, the government, and society.

Intangible costs are costs associated with pain and suffering resulting from treatment or the illness itself. Whereas these costs are important aspects of the product or service being evaluated, they can be very difficult to measure or quantify. Nevertheless, from the patient's perspective, these are real costs that the individual must bear.

Different types of costs are borne by different parties, and, consequently, the responsibility for payment of healthcare expenditures is fragmented. Managed care organizations, for example, determine what they will pay for in their statement of benefits; the patient then pays the remaining costs. In some cases, either patients or payers may try to shift costs to each other. When reviewing a pharmacoeconomic study, one should be aware of whether true cost savings have occurred or just cost shifting.

Measuring Costs

Once costs have been identified, the next step is to measure them. Depending on the type of cost, measurement often involves counts of units of resources consumed. These units can be an amount of time or occurrence of certain events, such as hospitalizations or physician visits. For example, the number of office visits, hospitalizations, laboratory services, procedures, or surgeries would be counted per patient over the time period of the evaluation. Measuring the cost of personnel services, whether it is nursing or pharmacist time, involves counts in units of time (often measured in what is commonly referred to as a time-motion study). However, some would argue that personnel time is a fixed cost and would be incurred whether the program was implemented or not. The inclusion of this cost is warranted if the time spent on the program detracts from other required responsibilities.

Valuing Costs

Once costs have been measured, the final step involves placing a dollar value on the resource or service. In a perfectly competitive market, the value of the resource would be based on the market price of the commodity or service. Of course, the price does not reflect the true opportunity cost for many healthcare products or services. Opportunity cost—an important concept in the valuation of resources—is defined as the value of a resource in its next best use.

To illustrate the idea of opportunity cost, consider a pharmacist who owns and operates his own independent pharmacy. The pharmacist has decided to expand the pharmaceutical care services he provides by offering flu vaccines to local senior citizens. As part of the proposal he has developed, he needs to estimate the additional hours he will spend on this service and place a value on these hours. The value of his time would not be based on the wages the pharmacist pays himself (which often vary based on the profitability of the business), but rather would be based on wages he would earn if he was employed elsewhere. In other words, his time should be valued based on the market price he could obtain if he were employed as a pharmacist at another local community pharmacy.

A critical component in the valuation of resources goes back to the issue of perspective. Perspective is important in health care, as in other sectors of the economy, because of the many ways in which the price of a commodity can vary by consumer. Consider the difference in price paid by a teaching hospital and the price paid by an independent pharmacy for the same pharmaceutical product. As discussed earlier, the resource should be valued based on its opportunity costs. However, because opportunity costs are often difficult to infer, researchers often use reference prices or reimbursement rates.

Reference prices are published list prices that serve as a reference for providers of those services or products. For example, a reference price for pharmaceuticals is the average wholesale price (AWP) assigned to products by the manufacturer. Many reference price lists are publicly available for a myriad of healthcare products and services (Else, Armstrong, & Cox, 1997).

Another method of valuing resources is by identifying actual reimbursement rates for services. Actual reimbursement rates are difficult to obtain because they are considered proprietary and thus are not publicly available. Comprehensive sources of healthcare reimbursement rates that are publicly available are those for the Centers for Medicare and Medicaid Services. Through commonly used methods (Tumeh, Moore, Shapiro, & Flowers, 2005), those conducting pharmacoeconomic evaluations can use Healthcare Common Procedure Coding System/Current Procedural Terminology codes, Ambulatory Payment Classifications, International Classification of Disease codes, and Diagnosis Related Groups to assign value to inpatient and outpatient physician, procedure and laboratory test, and inpatient and outpatient healthcare utilization.

What is controversial about using reference price lists or reimbursement rates as a proxy for actual cost is that these costs do not reflect the opportunity costs of using that resource elsewhere. Thus, cost data should be adjusted when they are known to be very different from market prices. This adjustment ensures that costs are a true reflection of the opportunity cost of using those resources. Many methodological issues exist regarding valuation of costs, and readers should be aware of these controversies in conducting any economic evaluation (Copley-Merriman & Lair, 1994).

Sensitivity Analysis

Sensitivity analysis involves testing key outcomes or cost assumptions of an analysis to determine how sensitive the results are to variation or uncertainty in these estimates. In many pharmacoeconomic evaluations, the accuracy with which costs can be identified, measured, or valued will vary. Variation around the measurement of outcomes also exists. In critiquing studies, it is important to determine the key areas of uncertainty within a study and note whether researchers addressed areas of uncertainty through sensitivity analysis.

Numerous methods are available to test the impact of uncertainty within pharmacoeconomic evaluations (Briggs, Sculpher, & Buxton, 1994). Simple deterministic sensitivity analysis is the most commonly used and involves varying study assumptions (either cost or outcome) within the range of plausible values to determine if the original conclusions remain sound. When only one variable is altered at a time, this is called one-way simple sensitivity analysis. For example, the cost for a biologic agent such as infliximab to treat moderate-to-severe CD could range from a lower bound to an upper bound. The lower bound could be the actual price paid by the hospital or even to the price of a lower-priced biosimilar product, if it is available. The upper bound could be the standard reference price, such as AWP. If the pharmacoeconomic evaluation's conclusions remain similar, they could be considered robust (insensitive) to changes in biologic drug cost, and the researcher can more easily defend his or her conclusions. If more than one variable is altered at a time, this is called multiple-way simple sensitivity analysis and is conducted and interpreted in the same fashion as a simple sensitivity analysis.

Analysis of extremes is conducted by reassigning values of both cost and effectiveness variables concurrently to their highest and lowest extremes in order to determine the robustness of the conclusions in the best- and worst-case situations. The best-case scenario is depicted by the highest effectiveness and lowest cost estimates, and the worst-case scenario is the lowest effectiveness and highest costs estimates. In order for this analysis to be useful to decision makers, sufficient detail of the extremes must be provided to determine whether the extremes being evaluated are near their own health plan's resource cost. The usefulness of analysis of extremes is questionable because it is doubtful that all worst-case or best-case findings will occur at the same time.

Threshold sensitivity analysis requires that a single assumption in the analysis be varied until the alternative treatment option has the same outcome and there is no advantage between the treatment options. The value determined by conducting such an analysis is often referred to as a break-even point. This break-even point can then be compared by decision makers to their value to make decisions concerning the validity of the evaluation's results to their institution.

Probabilistic sensitivity analysis allows researchers to assign plausible ranges for variables and an estimate of the distribution of the data points for each variable. The most common type of probabilistic sensitivity analysis is Monte Carlo simulation, which uses computer simulation to generate a large number of possible outcomes by randomly sampling from a probability distribution for each variable.

Adjustment and Discounting

The final step in calculating costs relates to the issue of adjusting and discounting. In those instances where the program or service being evaluated extends more than 1 year into the past (i.e., before the study), adjustment (or standardization) of costs should be made so that the resources used are valued at one point in time. Alternately, future costs must be discounted, that is modified to reflect future dollars in terms of current dollar values.

Table 19-4 Example of Adjustment Using Units Multiplied by Costs

Healthcare resource utilized	Number of resource units	Costs in 2014 dollars (costs/unit)	Total costs in 2014 dollars
Prescription medication	16 capsules	$1.14	$18.24
Hospitalization (includes room and personnel)	2 days	$1,400	$2,800
Laboratory procedures	3 blood samples	$38	$114

One method of standardizing costs, illustrated in **Table 19-4**, uses the current unit cost of the resource (e.g., medication or hospitalization) multiplied by the number of units.

In the event that a pharmacoeconomic analysis assesses the resources utilized over the past several years (e.g., 2012 through 2014), these costs should be adjusted so that they can be compared in a fair and unbiased manner to reflect the fact that costs tend to increase over time. For instance, when a retrospective evaluation is undertaken, the value of both costs and outcomes was likely assigned at the time the resource was consumed or outcome realized. When conducting a study in 2014, the cost of a hospitalization occurring in 2012 (say $10,000) must be adjusted to reflect 2014 dollars. In these situations, the past cost must be adjusted (standardized) to represent present-day value. A second method of standardizing past costs, shown in **Table 19-5**, is to multiply the cost of the resources used in the previous years by the corresponding medical inflation rate, the consumer price index (CPI) for

Table 19-5 Example of Adjustment Using the Medical CPI as an Inflation Rate

Healthcare resource utilized	Approximate cost for healthcare resource	Year that the cost was incurred	Total costs adjusted to 2014 dollars
Prescription medication	$16.42	2012	$17.23*
Hospitalization (includes room and personnel)	$1,900	2013	$1,945.60†
Laboratory procedures	$97	2014	$97

Medical CPI for 2013 = 2.5%; medical CPI for 2014 = 2.4%.

* $16.42 × 1.025 [1 + MCPI for 2013] × 1.024 [1 + MCPI for 2014].

† $1,900 × 1.024 [1 + MCPI for 2014].

Medical Care [MCPI], for that year. The MCPI, which is calculated by the U.S. Bureau of Labor Statistics, represents the percentage change in the prices paid by urban consumers for medical care–related products and services. Thus, the $10,000 hospitalization in 2012 is valued at $10,496 in 2014 dollars ($10,000 × 1.025 [the 2013 MCPI was 2.5%] × 1.024 [the 2014 MCPI was 2.4%]) (Gold et al., 1996).

The purpose of discounting is to determine the present value of future costs and to incorporate society's time preference for money. We all have a preference for when we would like to receive money. Most, if not all, of us would rather receive $10 today than $10 a year from now. Because money can generate interest income, $10 received today is worth more than $10 received 1 year from now. In most, if not all, cases, people prefer to incur costs later and reap benefits earlier. This same time preference applies to healthcare costs. Thus, costs or benefits of alternatives realized at different times should be discounted to a present value to make valid comparisons.

The effects that discounting, or failure to discount, can have on study results are presented in **Table 19-6**. In this example, the total costs of two competing programs, A and B, are the same ($85,000), but the costs occur at different time periods. Assuming that money received today is worth 4% more than money received 1 year later (a 4% discount rate), the present value of costs are $75,022 for program A and $81,318 for program B, a difference of more than $6,000.

The choice of a discount rate is important, as it can significantly affect the results of the evaluation. The U.S. Public Health Service Panel on Cost-Effectiveness in Health and Medicine recommends using a discount rate of 3% (Gold, Siegel, Russell, & Weinstein, 1996). Drummond and colleagues suggest several other factors to consider when discounting (Drummond, O'Brien, Stoddart, & Torrance, 1998), including:

- Presenting results in their undiscounted form so that the reader can evaluate the impact of discounting
- Using sensitivity analysis to vary the discount rate over a range of values
- When discounting affects the results, being clear with readers so that they are aware of its influence on the study's findings.

Table 19-6 Discounted versus Undiscounted Costs

Program	Year					Undiscounted	Discounted at 4%
	0	1	2	5	10	Total	Total
A	$25,000	$15,000	$15,000	$10,000	$20,000	$85,000	$75,022
Discount calculation	$25,000 ÷ $(1.04)^0$	$15,000 ÷ $(1.04)^1$	$15,000 ÷ $(1.04)^2$	$10,000 ÷ $(1.04)^5$	$20,000 ÷ $(1.04)^{10}$		
B	$40,000	$20,000	$15,000	$10,000		$85,000	$81,318
Discount calculation	$40,000 ÷ $(1.04)^0$	$20,000 ÷ $(1.04)^1$	$15,000 ÷ $(1.04)^2$	$10,000 ÷ $(1.04)^5$			

Discount factor = $1/(1 + r)^t$, where t = number of years in the future, and r = rate per year or the discount rate.

PHARMACOECONOMIC METHODOLOGIES

Cost-Minimization Analysis

Cost-minimization analysis (CMA) compares the costs and consequences of two or more therapeutic interventions that are equivalent in terms of their outcomes or consequences. Thus, the purpose of CMA is to choose the least costly alternative among interventions with equivalent outcomes. CMA is often confused with cost analysis, in which only the costs of therapy are evaluated. However, consequences are also evaluated in CMA to show or prove equivalency.

The requirement of equivalent outcomes limits the application of CMA to those situations where equivalency of both effectiveness and safety consequences has been established. They include, but are not limited to, comparisons between branded (or biologics) and generic products (or biosimilars), comparisons of different routes of administration of the same drug, and comparison of different settings for the administration of the same drug therapy—for example, inpatient versus home therapy. In all these instances, the evidence supporting equivalent outcomes should be clearly stated and, where appropriate, statistically confirmed.

Because the consequences of alternatives being compared are shown to be equivalent, CMA focuses on cost differences. These differences in cost can be presented as average cost per patient or average total cost of care if the number of patients is the same under each alternative. When choosing between alternatives, decision makers will then choose the alternative with the lowest total cost.

Cost-Benefit Analysis

Cost-benefit analysis (CBA) was first defined as:

> a way of assessing the desirability of projects, where it is important to take a long view (in the sense of looking at repercussions in the future) and a wide view (in the sense of allowing for side effects of many kinds on many persons, industries, regions, etc.), i.e., it implies the numeration and evaluation of all relevant costs and benefits. (Prest & Turvey, 1965, p. 721)

The two aspects of CBA—taking a long and wide view—have made it most applicable to decisions with a broad societal impact, such as whether to fund immunization programs or whether to implement child safety seat legislation. In evaluating each of these programs, researchers would take a long view (estimating the value of the lives lost in terms of future productivity on the community) and the wide view (estimating not only the direct benefits but also the indirect benefits to the community from reduced risk of illness to those not immunized).

In measuring outcomes in dollars, CBA enjoys an advantage over other economic evaluations. It can compare alternatives that are not measured using the same natural unit of effectiveness. For example, CBA could compare an immunization program to child safety seat regulations to determine which program would yield the highest net benefit (total benefits minus total costs).

One of the methodologically challenging aspects of CBA is measuring and valuing benefits in dollars. Two broad categories of direct benefits can be measured in CBA—personal health benefits and medical resource benefits. The measurement and valuation of medical resource benefits have already been discussed. The measurement of personal health benefits is more challenging. Personal health benefits include the alternative's effects on morbidity or mortality. Changes in morbidity are reflected in the following two ways: changes in medical resource consumption for treatment of illness, and intangible benefits such as reduction in pain and suffering. The impact on mortality is captured as the number of lives saved. Two methods are commonly used to value lives saved: the human capital approach and the willingness-to-pay approach.

The human capital approach measures the value of a life saved in terms of the income that the person could have earned over his or her remaining productive years. The criticism of the human capital approach of valuing human life is that it focuses on the productivity of the individual and not his or her value to family and friends. Also, because of imperfections in the labor market, this method tends to undervalue women, the elderly, the unemployed, and minorities.

Willingness to pay values both the intervention's impact on lives saved and intangible benefits. In measuring willingness-to-pay values, individuals are presented with a hypothetical statement describing the illness or disease and asked to express their willingness to pay to reduce the risk of death, pain, or suffering (Gafni, 1991). The advantage of willingness to pay is that, in theory, it measures the full range of benefits, including productivity and intangible benefits. The disadvantage is that the willingness-to-pay approach is a difficult method to apply and relies on individuals' abilities to comprehend and respond to hypothetical statements regarding small changes in health risks.

Net Benefit

Two methods are most commonly used to present results in CBA; the first is net benefit. The formula for calculating net benefit when costs and benefits do not extend beyond 1 year is presented in **Equation 19-1**. If the project lifetime extends beyond 1 year, the net benefits should be adjusted using an appropriate discount rate, where $1/(1 + r)^t$ is the discount factor (r is the discount rate, and t is the number of years in the future).

$$\text{Net benefit} = \text{Total benefits} - \text{Total costs} \qquad (19\text{-}1)$$

The decision rules for determining net benefit are definite. The decision criteria when results are presented as net benefit, assuming a limited budget, would be to choose the project that provides the greatest net benefit or—if funds allow—to choose those projects that provide a positive (>0) net benefit.

Ratio Analysis

The second method commonly used to present results in CBA is benefit-to-cost or cost-to-benefit ratios. The formulas used in calculating benefit-to-cost ratios are presented in **Equation 19-2**.

$$\text{Benefit-to-cost ratio} = \text{Total benefits} \div \text{Total costs} \qquad (19\text{-}2)$$

The decision rule for choosing among projects when results are presented as ratios would be to choose those projects with a benefit-to-cost ratio greater than one, or inversely where the cost-to-benefit ratio is less than one. Assuming limited resources, the task would then be to select the project or projects with the highest benefit-to-cost ratio or the lowest cost-to-benefit ratio.

How results are presented (net benefit vs. ratios) can influence the decision. As an example, **Table 19-7** presents four hypothetical program options with their benefits and costs. Results are calculated both as net benefit and benefit-to-cost ratios.

Based on the information in Table 19-7 and assuming unlimited resources, the free oral contraceptives, the statewide drug abuse program, and the smoking cessation programs would be considered because their benefits are greater than their costs and the benefit-to-cost ratios are all greater than 1:1. Under conditions of limited resources, if one was to choose the project with the greatest net benefit, the choice would be the drug abuse treatment program. If the decision was based on benefit-to-cost ratio, however, the choice would be the free oral contraception program.

Table 19-7 Presentation of Results in Hypothetical Cost-Benefit Analysis

Option	Benefits ($)	Costs ($)	Net benefit	Benefit-to-cost ratio
Free oral contraceptives at County Health Department	$45,000	$20,000	$25,000	2.25
Statewide drug abuse treatment program	$2 million	$1.5 million	$500,000	1.33
Additional police protection in high-crime neighborhoods	$85,000	$90,000	– $5,000	0.94
Smoking cessation program	$200,000	$100,000	$100,000	2.00

It is generally agreed that presenting results in terms of the net benefit provides decision makers with more information. For example, presenting results as a ratio does not provide information on the magnitude of both costs and benefits. Although the drug abuse treatment program included in Table 19-7 provides the greatest net benefit, it also requires an outlay by the state of $1.5 million.

Summary

CBA remains a unique method of assessing the costs and benefits of programs and therapy interventions. However, it is applicable only when outcomes are easily converted to dollars and is most appropriate in situations where the objectives are broad in scope.

Cost-Effectiveness Analysis

Cost-effectiveness analysis (CEA) is the most commonly used pharmacoeconomic method. Its popularity is attributable in part to the way in which outcomes or consequences are measured (e.g., natural units of effectiveness). CEA is restricted to those situations in which the outcomes of the alternatives are all measured on the same scale, such as mm Hg or serum cholesterol levels. The purpose of CEA is to compare the costs and consequences of two or more alternatives to determine which alternative can achieve the best outcome at the lowest cost.

The term *cost effective* is often misused in the literature. The judgment of whether a product is cost effective is relative and often subjective. It is relative in the sense that when a product or service is deemed cost effective, this distinction is made in comparison to the costs and outcomes of other alternatives. It is subjective in the sense that the decision maker determines whether the additional cost is worth the additional gain in effectiveness. Some guidelines exist to determine under what range of values a product would be considered cost effective (e.g., cost per life year gained). In many other situations, it is left to the decision maker to determine what qualifies as cost effective. Unlike CBA where the decision rules for determining cost benefit are definite, the decision rules in CEA can be subjective.

Incremental CEA

Results of a CEA take the form of a ratio of incremental cost to incremental outcomes, which, as shown in **Equation 19-3**, is the incremental difference in costs divided by the incremental difference in outcomes.

$$\text{ICER} = \Delta \text{ Costs} \div \Delta \text{ Outcomes} \tag{19-3}$$

Table 19-8 presents the average total costs per patient and the average outcome per patient for three therapies used to treat a common toenail fungus. Also shown in the table are the average cost-effectiveness ratios and the incremental cost-effectiveness ratios (ICERs). The outcome is measured simply as number of successful cases. When determining whether an alternative is cost effective, one has to ask, "Are you willing to pay $122, $155, or $187 per successfully treated patient?" The investigator might be willing to pay all three prices, but certainly $122 per successful treatment appears to be the more efficient treatment regimen when compared to doing nothing. In other words, alternative B is an efficient treatment option in that this option is the least costly to get a successful case ($122/successful case) given that willingness to pay per successfully treated case is equal to or greater than $122. Of course, comparing an alternative to doing nothing is not a realistic approach.

ICERs are a more appropriate way to compare product alternatives in a cost-effective analysis. What additional amount must be paid to obtain the additional successfully treated cases? Comparing alternatives A and B (because B is both more costly and more effective), we see the additional cost of $10 would provide an additional gain in the rate of successfully treated cases of 0.23.

Table 19-8 Average and Incremental Cost-Effectiveness Ratios

Alternative	Average cost per patient	Outcome (success rate)	Average cost-effectiveness ratio	Incremental cost-effectiveness ratio (ICER)*
A	$85	0.55	$155/successful case	—
B	$95	0.78	$122/successful case	$43/additional successful case treated
C	$150	0.80	$187/successful case	$260/additional successful case treated

*Referencing common baseline (alternative A).

The cost per additional successfully treated case is $43 ($10 ÷ 0.23). Comparing alternatives A and C shows that the incremental ratio is $260 per additional successfully treated case.

No established guidelines exist to determine which alternative is the most cost effective in this example. However, in this scenario, if decision makers are willing to pay equal to or greater than $260 to get additional successfully treated case, alternative C would be the most favorable option because this treatment option gives the highest success rate (outcome). If their willingness to pay is less than $260, but equal to or greater than $43 per additional successfully treated case, alternative B would be the most preferred option. The decision makers would select alternative C if their willingness to pay is less than $43 to get additional successfully treated case.

Budget Impact Analysis

Budget impact analysis is increasingly being considered an integral companion to a comprehensive CEA (Mauskopf et al., 2007). Budget impact analyses aim to estimate the financial impact of adoption and diffusion of a new healthcare intervention (deemed cost effective in a CEA) within a specific healthcare setting. Specifically, budget impact analyses predict how a change in the formulary mix of drugs used to treat a disease state will affect healthcare spending for that disease state, and therefore, can be used for budget planning. Many managed care organizations in the United States now require pharmaceutical companies to submit budget impact analyses along with cost-effectiveness data to support their requests for formulary inclusion.

Cost-Utility Analysis

While CEA is the most popular pharmacoeconomic methodology, in certain healthcare decision-making situations, CEA may not provide a sufficient or optimal decision to answer the question at hand. For example, suppose a patient with cancer has a choice of two chemotherapy agents. The newer, more expensive chemotherapy agent is expected to increase the patient's life span modestly in comparison to an older and cheaper agent. However, during treatment with the newer agent, the patient is expected to experience greater discomfort than with the older agent, and, as a result, be unable to carry out activities of daily living such as bathing or dressing. Thus, while the newer chemotherapy agent will extend the patient's life, the patient's preference for those extended years of life may be diminished when the quality of those additional years of life is considered.

CUA, often considered a subtype of CEA, measures both the quantity and quality aspects of two or more therapies. Most commonly in CUA, the natural effectiveness units of life years saved are converted to QALYs by multiplying a utility value by life years saved (**Equation 19-4**). Utility is often perceived as preference, and it is measured on a scale of 0.0 to 1.0, where 0 represents death and 1 represents perfect health. Most health states fall somewhere between these extremes. Therefore, one life year multiplied by a utility of 1.0 equals 1.0 QALY, as does two life years with a utility of 0.5 (two life years saved × 0.5 = 1 QALY). Utility scores are elicited from patients through a number of methodologies including visual analog scales, validated questionnaires, and by employing standard gamble or time trade-off game theories. All are similar in that they assume that when given a choice, patients will choose the health state with the highest utility score assigned to it.

$$\text{QALY} = \text{Utility} \times \text{years of life saved} \qquad (19\text{-}4)$$

As in CEA, both average and incremental cost-utility ratios (ICURs) are calculated in CUA. The additional cost of a given treatment is divided by the additional effectiveness, as illustrated by **Equation 19-5**.

$$\text{ICUR} = \Delta\ \text{Costs} \div \Delta\ \text{QALYs} \qquad (19\text{-}5)$$

The only difference is that effectiveness is measured as a QALY rather than in life years alone or other natural units of effectiveness. To continue our example, consider that patients with moderate-to-severe CD and failing standard nonbiologic treatment (the 5-aminosalicylate, mesalamine) could have a biologic agent, say infliximab, added to their regimen or nothing at all. In this scenario, we could use CUA to assess the cost-effectiveness of choosing one treatment strategy over the other. Let us assume that after administering the biologic agent infliximab to patients for 5 years, average total treatment cost for these patients is $48,000. Average total treatment when no additional drug therapy is added is $40,000. Assume further that infliximab results in patients having an average utility value of 0.75 and 6-MP a utility value of 0.70. "*Would infliximab be considered a cost-effective treatment?*", "*Would its use be preferable to no additional treatment?*"

An interactive example demonstrating how a visual analog scale can be used to elicit a utility score is provided in **Exhibit 19-1**.

If we conducted a CUA, the ICUR would be:

Incremental cost utility ratio = Change in costs/change in QALYs

= ($48,000 – $40,000) ÷ (5 years × 0.83 utility) – (5 years × 0.79 utility)]

= $8,000 ÷ (4.15 QALY – 3.95 QALY)

= $8,000 ÷ 0.20 QALY

= $40,000 per additional QALY gained

Although this is somewhat arbitrary, many have concluded that an intervention that results in an ICUR more than $50,000 to $150,000 per QALY gained may not be considered cost effective (Harvard Public Health Review, 2004; Neumann, Cohen, & Weinstein, 2014; Weinstein & Skinner, 2010). The $40,000 additional cost per QALY calculated in the previous scenario is below this threshold and, consequently, suggests that the extra benefits of infliximab to treat moderate-to-severe CD may be considered to be worth the extra cost.

Exhibit 19-1 Visual Analog Scale

Imagine you suffered from moderate-to-severe CD as described below:

You are a 39-year-old man who has failed treatment with oral and rectal mesalamine therapy. You are currently experiencing five to six episodes of bloody diarrhea a day. As a result of your frequent bloody stools, you are anemic and fatigued much of the time. You are also suffering some extraintestinal effects of CD, mainly painful ulcers in your mouth and throat. Although you enjoy being outside, you have started to feel quite emotionally distraught in public places because you are worried about being close to a bathroom. You also lack the energy you had before your CD diagnosis. Recently, you have begun to go to your gastroenterologist's office for infusion therapy with infliximab. Following your first infusion, you have to return 2 weeks later, then 6 weeks after that, and now every other month to receive an intravenous infusion lasting about 2 hours. This treatment course has mostly eliminated your diarrhea (only occurs on occasion); however, you are

(Continues)

still uncomfortable due to hemorrhoids that developed during your recent CD flare-up (and that the infusion is not treating). In addition, you are self-employed and find having to spend time getting the infusions at your gastroenterologist's office problematic. You also worry about the side effects of this new treatment because it predisposes you to serious infections and a very rare but nearly always fatal type of cancer.

If 0.0 represents death and 1.0 represents perfect health (the best health imaginable for a person of your age), please mark on the line the level of health described before and after the infliximab infusion therapy.

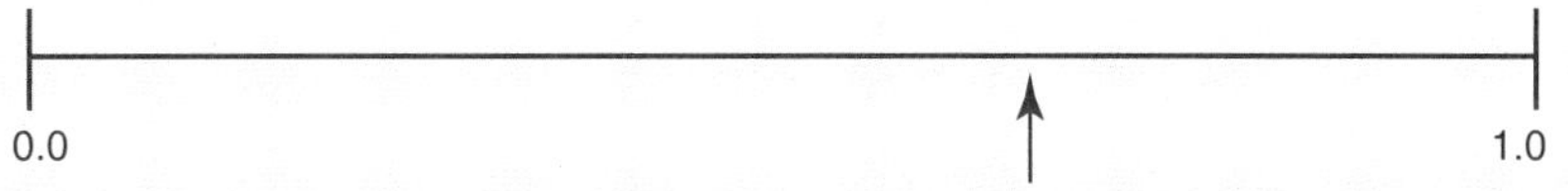

The literature would suggest that the average patient with moderate-to-severe active CD as initially described above would provide a utility score between 0.4 and 0.79 (Marchetti & Liberato, 2014). After successful induction and maintenance therapy with infliximab, a typical utility score might be 0.83 to 0.89 (Marchetti & Liberato, 2014).

If you lived for 2 years with moderate-to-severe active CD as described above and reported a utility value of 0.79 during those years, then you would have accumulated 1.58 QALYs. If you lived 2 years in remission following infliximab induction and maintenance therapy at a utility score of 0.83, then you would have accrued 1.66 QALYs.

Cost-of-Illness Analysis

Cost-of-illness (COI) analyses (also commonly referred to as burden-of-illness analyses) attempt to estimate the magnitude of resources needed for a specific disease state in a defined population. COI analyses include both direct and indirect costs associated with prevention, treatment, and disease-related morbidity and mortality. Such analyses provide a unique benefit to healthcare decision makers because these analyses do not compare competing treatment alternatives but rather provide insight into the value of disease prevention or treatment of an illness. They can also be used to compare the relative economic burden of one disease state compared to another to aid decision makers in allocating limited healthcare resources and research funding monies.

COI analyses have been used to estimate the economic burden of many different chronic diseases in the United States, such as type 2 diabetes mellitus. Related to the CD case scenario at the beginning of this chapter, a COI published in 2008 found the cost of CD (regardless of treatment strategy) to be approximately $18,022 per patient per year in the United States, with indirect (work/productivity) costs accounting for 28% of the cost burden (Yu, Cabanilla, Wu, Mulani, & Chao, 2008).

Cost-Consequence Analysis

Cost-consequence analysis (CCA) has been defined as an analysis that presents all costs and effects in a disaggregated format (Mauskopf, Paul, Grant, & Stergachis, 1998). Costs are listed in

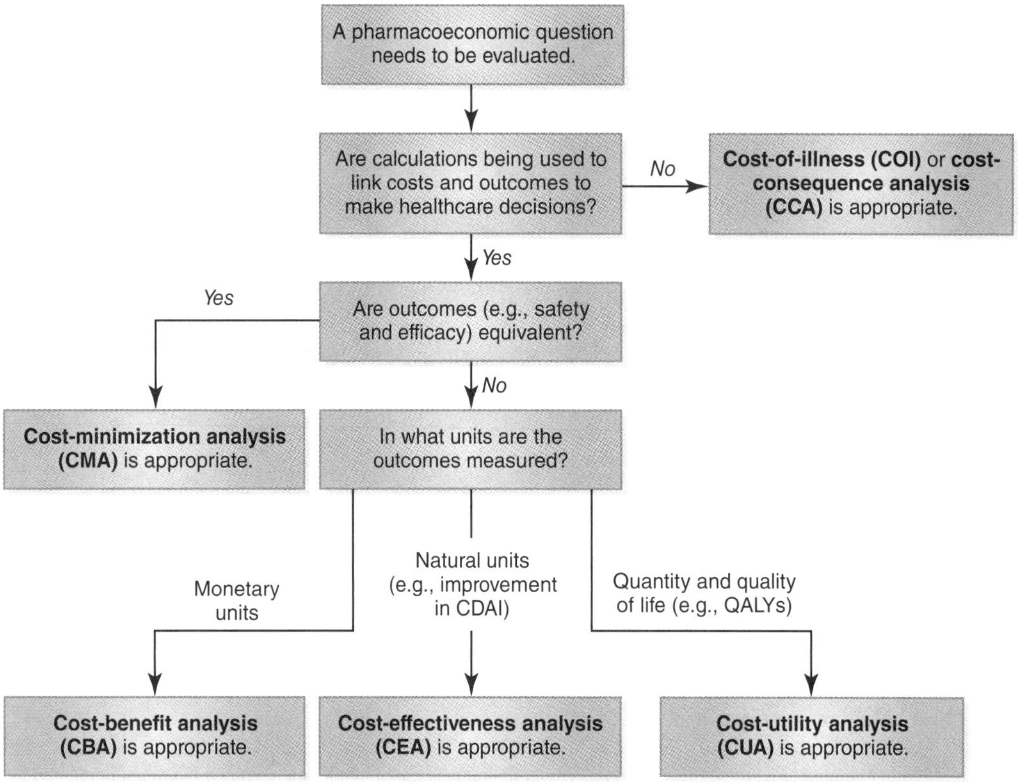

Figure 19-4 Selection of Pharmacoeconomic Methodology.

table format by type of costs (e.g., direct medical, direct nonmedical, indirect costs, and intangible costs) as are outcomes (e.g., clinical intermediaries, dollars, and QALYs). Decision makers can then choose among the costs and outcomes that best fit their perspective. The advantage of CCA lies in its comprehensiveness and transparency for decision makers. The disadvantage of CCA is that the researcher must identify, collect, and value costs and outcomes salient to a variety of perspectives. This burden of analysis, however, far outweighs the potential gain for decision makers.

Selection of Type of Pharmacoeconomic Study

Figure 19-4 depicts a decision algorithm to assist decision makers in selecting the most appropriate pharmacoeconomic methodology. While each type of pharmacoeconomic analysis measures costs in dollars, the way in which the outcomes are measured and calculated varies.

APPROACHES TO CONDUCTING PHARMACOECONOMIC STUDIES

Pharmacoeconomic evaluations can be conducted using several approaches, including randomized controlled trials, naturalistic designs, decision analysis, and retrospective claims analysis.

Randomized Controlled Trials

Randomized controlled trials involve randomly assigning patients to the alternative therapies being considered. A standard protocol is established, and patients are followed over a specified time period. Patients and investigators are blinded as to which alternative they receive. The advantage of this design is that it has strong internal validity—that is, the results are attributable to the intervention and not to other extraneous factors. The disadvantage is that randomized controlled trials can be costly, and the strict adherence to treatment protocols is not reflective of real-world practice settings.

Naturalistic Designs

Naturalistic designs are similar to clinical trials in that patients are randomly assigned to treatment groups, but the patients recruited and the follow-up care delivered would be representative of routine clinical care (Simon, Wagner, & Vonkorff, 1995). Whereas this type of study design does have its advantages, it can be expensive.

Decision Analysis

Decision analysis is a systematic approach to decision making under conditions of uncertainty. Rather than conducting the study prospectively or collecting data on individual patients, decision analysis synthesizes clinical data from the literature with data on resource use to simulate or model the question or problem. The following two modeling types are often used to represent the decision process: decision analysis and Markov models. Decision analysis is employed when direct observation is not feasible or when time or money constraints prohibit collecting data prospectively. The advantage of decision analysis as compared to clinical or naturalistic trial study designs is that results can be obtained in a timely and cost-efficient manner.

The use of decision analytic models (also known as decision trees) is becoming increasingly popular in the literature. **Figure 19-5** depicts a simplified decision tree for the decision of whether to treat a particular disease with drug therapy. The decision node, represented by the square (□), designates the point at which the decision to treat or not to treat is made. If the decision is to treat, the process follows the branch of the tree for drug therapy. The branch then comes upon a chance or probability node, represented by a circle (○), at which point a probability of experiencing a side

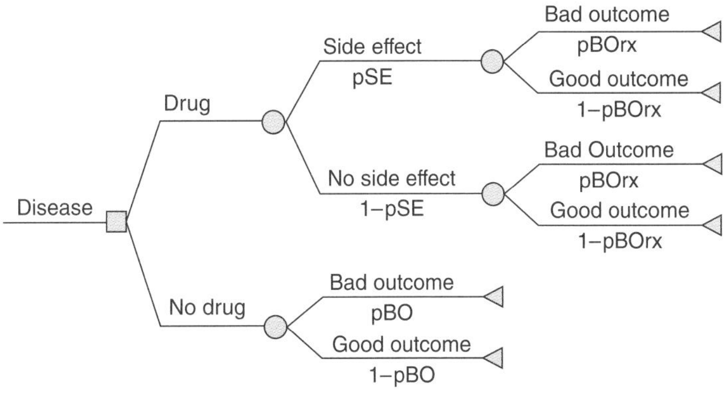

Figure 19-5 Decision Analysis Tree.

effect (pSE) exists. Patients must either experience a side effect or not experience a side effect, so the probability of no side effect is therefore 1 minus the probability of a side effect (1 – pSE). The terminal branch (depicted as a triangle, Δ) for each alternative (drug or no drug) is the chance of a bad outcome (pBOrx) or a good outcome (1 – pBOrx). The probabilities used in the model are derived from the published literature or expert opinion, and resource utilization is inferred from either accepted practice standards or expert opinion.

As an example, assume three antiepileptic medications could be used. Drug A costs $120 per month, Drug B costs $160 per month, and Drug C costs $230 per month. Assume also that Drug A is 60% effective, Drug B is 80% effective, and Drug C is more than 90% effective. The managed care organization has already decided that Drug C should be used only in those cases in which either Drug A or Drug B has been tried unsuccessfully. An unsuccessful trial of either Drug A or B will result in an additional physician office visit costing $30 plus the cost of Drug C. Which drug, A or B, would be more cost effective?

One way to answer this question is to use a decision tree like the one depicted in **Figure 19-6**. For Drug A, the cost of effective treatment is multiplied by the probability of effectiveness (pE), whereas the cost of unsuccessful treatment ($120 for Drug A, plus $30 for the additional office visit, plus $230 for the new Drug C) is multiplied by the probability that Drug A is not effective (1 – pE). The sum of these costs is compared to the sum of the same costs for Drug B. The results show that although Drug B costs more than Drug A, it is actually more cost effective. Therefore, based on this information, Drug B would be preferred. As presented, the assumption is made that the products do not differ substantially in any other aspect, such as their side-effect profiles.

Markov Modeling

Decision trees are difficult to use for modeling chronic disease states in which patients may experience intermittent relapses and remissions. A convenient solution to this problem is to use Markov models. Markov models offer advantages when a problem involves risk that is continuous, when the timing of events is important, and when important events may happen more than once (Sonnenberg & Beck, 1993). The Markov model frames the decision in terms of health states and follows patients as they undergo transition from one state to another.

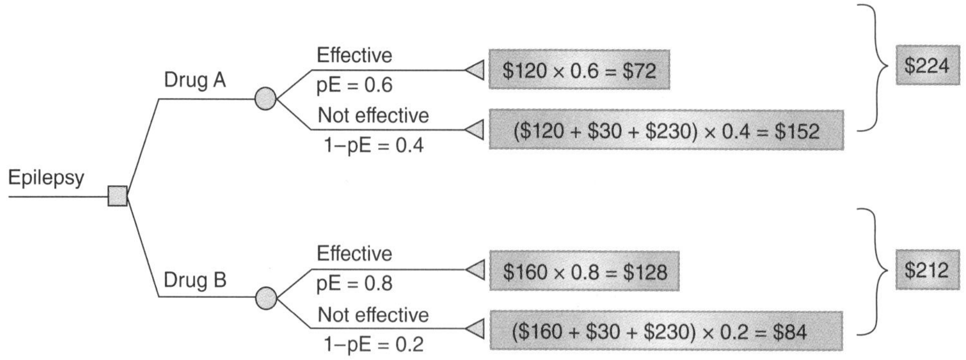

Figure 19-6 Hypothetical Decision Tree for First-Line Epilepsy Treatment.

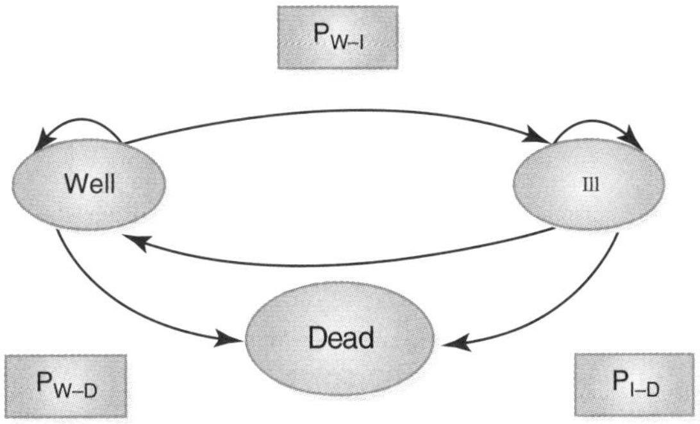

Figure 19-7 Three-State Markov Model.

Source: Sonnenberg, F. A., & Beck, J. R. (1993). Markov models in medical decision making: A practical guide. *Medical Decision Making, 13*(4), 322–338. Reprinted by permission of Sage Publications, Inc.

Figure 19-7 illustrates a three-state Markov model in which the health states are well, ill, or dead. When patients are well, there is a probability that they will become ill, stay symptom free, or die. When they experience symptoms, there is a probability that they could go into remission, stay symptomatic, or die. Of course, when they die, patients cannot change to other health states. In this way, Markov models simulate the natural progression of chronic diseases (Elliott & Payne, 2005).

The probabilities of moving from one state to the other are usually included in Markov models based on data published in the literature. (For example, a researcher could determine from the literature the probability that a patient with CD will either experience an asymptomatic period or die.) More sophisticated analyses may recognize that the probability of illness and death increases according to the duration of the disease, the age of the patient, and other variables. To the extent possible, these factors could also be included to determine probabilities of events. While pharmacoeconomics calculations using Markov models are beyond the scope of a single-chapter overview of pharmacoeconomics, it is useful for students to know that Markov models are a better choice than decision trees for analysis of certain chronic diseases such as multiple sclerosis, osteoporosis, and arthritis.

Retrospective Claims Analysis

Retrospective analysis of claims data (also known as observational data) can also be used to evaluate the costs and consequences of drug therapy. The advantages of using claims data are that they reflect routine clinical care, are comprehensive, and provide a large sample of patients to evaluate. Additionally, the evaluations often involve less time and lower costs than randomized controlled trials or naturalistic designs. However, claims data were developed for billing and reimbursement purposes rather than to monitor and track healthcare costs and outcomes. As a consequence, several limitations apply to their use in pharmacoeconomic research—namely, the lack of information regarding clinical indicators, incompleteness of data, inaccuracies in coding of diagnoses and procedures, and the valuation of healthcare utilization as charges (what the patient paid) and not costs (what the true value of the utilization was). This latter concern can often be overcome by obtaining cost-to-charge ratios from the healthcare provider (Gold et al., 1996). Cost-to-charge ratios, which are simply the ratio of the cost of providing services and the reimbursement obtained for those same services, are used to adjust available charge data to better reflect actual costs.

No particular study design is inherently superior to another. Each design approach has its advantages and disadvantages, and the final choice will depend on many factors. In critiquing a study with respect to study design, it is important to determine whether the disadvantage of a particular method affects the results.

CRITICAL APPRAISAL OF A PHARMACOECONOMIC STUDY

Many articles in the literature claim to study the cost-effectiveness or cost benefit of alternative treatments. Readers should be cautioned, however, that many of these articles are flawed because they do not adequately identify, measure, or value costs and consequences. At least a dozen published guidelines or checklists for the conduct and/or reporting of economic evaluations have been published in the medical literature (Husereau et al., 2013; Ofman et al., 2003; Task Force on Principles for Economic Analysis of Health Care Technology, 1995). More than half of these provide checklists and contain as few as seven or as many as 37 main items or criteria. One of the most recent and perhaps comprehensive reporting tools available for economic studies is the "Consolidated Health Economic Evaluation Reporting Standards" or CHEERS statement. The CHEERS statement was produced by an International Society of Pharmacoeconomics and Outcomes Research (ISPOR) Task Force and consists of a 24-item checklist. The checklist includes items deemed essential for transparent reporting of economic analyses across six domains including: (1) title and abstract, (2) introduction, (3) methods, (4) results, (5) discussion, and (6) other. In addition, an explanation and elaboration document for CHEERS is available that is intended to enhance the use and understanding of the statement, providing meaning and rationale for each checklist item through examples and explanations (Husereau et al., 2013).

CONCLUSION

As a larger number of students of pharmacy and practitioners become familiar with the concepts of pharmacoeconomics, the application of these tools in everyday practice will grow. The potential exists for pharmacoeconomic information to aid greatly in decision making in the ever more cost-conscious and value-minded field of health care.

QUESTIONS FOR FURTHER DISCUSSION

1. Clinicians tend to focus their efforts on the measurement of outcomes of clinical therapy, including measures of clinical effectiveness or side effects. Discuss the importance of measuring the inputs of clinical therapy.
2. Discuss the reasons why a pharmaceutical company might use one methodological approach over another (e.g., decision analysis, naturalistic design, or retrospective analysis) in conducting a pharmacoeconomics evaluation for its product. How might this differ based upon where the product is in its life cycle (e.g., products at market maturity or products yet to be launched)?
3. Discuss how pharmacists in various practice settings (e.g., retail, hospital, or managed care) might apply pharmacoeconomic principles.

4. Discuss why various decision makers might be more inclined to select one pharmacoeconomic method over another. Various decision makers could include managed care organizations, public health officials, pharmacy benefit managers, physicians, hospital pharmacists, or members of a pharmacy and therapeutics committee.

KEY TOPICS AND TERMS

Analysis of extremes
Benefit-to-cost ratio
Break-even point
Budget impact analysis
Clinical end point
Consolidated Health Economic Evaluation Reporting Standards (CHEERS)
Consumer price index (CPI)
Cost-benefit analysis (CBA)
Cost-consequence analysis (CCA)
Cost-effectiveness analysis (CEA)
Cost-minimization analysis (CMA)
Cost-of-illness (COI) analysis
Cost-to-charge ratio
Cost-utility analysis (CUA)
Decision analysis
Decision tree
Direct medical costs
Direct nonmedical costs
Discounting
Effectiveness
Efficacy
Efficiency
Health-related quality of life (HrQoL)
Human capital approach
Incremental cost-effectiveness plane
Incremental cost-effectiveness ratio (ICER)
Incremental cost-utility ratio
Indirect costs
Inflation
Inputs
Intangible costs
International Society of Pharmacoeconomics and Outcomes Research (ISPOR)
Markov model
Naturalistic designs
Net benefit
Net present value
Opportunity cost
Outcome
Perspective
Pharmacoeconomics
Probabilistic sensitivity analysis
Quality-adjusted life year (QALY)
Randomized controlled trials
Retrospective claims analysis
Simple sensitivity analysis
Threshold sensitivity analysis
Utility score
Willingness-to-pay approach

REFERENCES

Baumgart, D. C., & Sandborn, W. J. (2012). Crohn's disease. *Lancet, 380*, 1590–1605.

Bootman, J. L., McGhan, W. F., & Schondelmeyer, S. W. (1982). Application of cost-benefit and cost-effectiveness analysis to clinical practice. *Drug Intelligence and Clinical Pharmacy, 16*, 235–243.

Bootman, J. L., Townsend, R. J., & McGhan, W. F. (1996). *Principles of pharmacoeconomics* (2nd ed.). Cincinnati, OH: Harvey Whitney Books.

Bootman, J. L., Wertheimer, A., Zaske, D., & Rowland, C. (1979). Individualizing gentamicin dosage regimens on burn patients with gram negative septicemia: A cost-benefit analysis. *Journal of Pharmacy Science, 68*, 267–272.

Briggs, A., Sculpher, M., & Buxton, M. (1994). Uncertainty in the economic evaluation of health care technologies: The role of sensitivity analysis. *Health Economics, 3*, 95–104.

Cohen, B. L., Zoéga, H., Shah, S. A., Leleiko, N., Lidofsky, S., Bright, R., ... Sands, B. E. (2014). Fatigue is highly associated with poor health-related quality of life, disability and depression in newly-diagnosed patients with inflammatory bowel disease, independent of disease activity. *Alimentary Pharmacology & Therapeutics, 39*, 811–822.

Copley-Merriman, C., & Lair, T. J. (1994). Valuation of medical resource units collected in health economic studies. *Clinical Therapy, 16*(3), 553–567.

Dao, T. D. (1985). Cost-benefit and cost-effectiveness analysis of drug therapy. *American Journal of Hospital Pharmacy, 42,* 791–802.

Drummond, M. F., O'Brien, B. J., Stoddart, G. L., & Torrance, G. W. (1998). *Methods for the economic evaluation of health care programmes* (2nd ed.). New York, NY: Oxford University Press.

Elliott, R., & Payne, K. (2005). *Essentials of economic evaluation in healthcare* (p. 163). London, England: Pharmaceutical Products Press,.

Else, B. A., Armstrong, E. P., & Cox, E. R. (1997). Data sources for pharmacoeconomic and health services research. *American Journal of Health-Systems Pharmacy, 54,* 2601–2608.

FiercePharma. (2014). Remicade. The 10 best-selling drugs of 2013. Retrieved from http://www.fiercepharma.com/special-reports/remicade-best-selling-drugs-2013

Gafni, A. (1991). Willingness-to-pay as a measure of benefits: Relevant questions in the context of public decision making about health care programs. *Medical Care, 29*(12), 1246–1252.

Gold, M. R., Siegel, J. E., Russell, L. B., & Weinstein, M. C. (Eds.). (1996). *Cost-effectiveness in health and medicine.* New York, NY: Oxford University Press.

Gunter, M. J. (1999). The role of the ECHO model in outcomes research and clinical practice improvement. *American Journal of Managed Care, 5*(4), S217–S224.

Hartman, M., Martin, A., Nuccio, O., Catlin, A.; The National Health Expenditure Accounts Team. (2010). Health spending growth at a historic low in 2008. *Health Affairs, 29,* 147–155.

Harvard Public Health Review. (2004, Winter). *What price health?* Retrieved from http://www.hsph.harvard.edu/review/review_fall_04/risk_pricetxt.html

Husereau, D., Drummond, M., Petrou, S., Carswell, C., Moher, D., Greenberg, D., ... Loder, E.; ISPOR Health Economic Evaluation Publication Guidelines-CHEERS Good Reporting Practices Task Force (2013). Consolidated Health Economic Evaluation Reporting Standards (CHEERS)–explanation and elaboration: A report of the ISPOR Health Economic Evaluation Publication Guidelines Good Reporting Practices Task Force. *Value Health, 16*(2), 231–250.

IMS Institute for Healthcare Informatics. (2014). *The global use of medicines: Outlook through 2017.* Parsippany, NJ.

Institute of Medicine. (2009). Initial national priorities for comparative effectiveness research. Retrieved from http://www.iom.edu/Reports/2009/ComparativeEffectivenessResearchPriorities.aspx

Institute of Medicine Roundtable on Evidence-based Medicine. (2011). Learning what works best: The nation's need for evidence on comparative effectiveness in health care. Retrieved from http://www.ncbi.nlm.nih.gov/books/NBK64784/

Kappelman, M. D., Moore, K. R., Allen, J. K., & Cook, S. F. (2013). Recent trends in the prevalence of Crohn's disease and ulcerative colitis in a commercially insured US population. *Digestive Diseases and Sciences, 58,* 519–525.

Lieu, T. A., Cochi, S. L., Black, S. B., Halloran, M. E., Shinefield, H. R., Holmes, S. J., ... Washington, A. E. (1994). Cost effectiveness of a routine varicella vaccination program for US children. *Journal of the American Medical Association, 271,* 375–381.

Lönnfors, S., Vermeire, S., Greco, M., Hommes, D., Bell, C., & Avedano, L. (2014). IBD and health-related quality of life—discovering the true impact. *Journal of Crohn's and Colitis, 8,* 1281–1286.

Marchetti, M., & Liberato, N.L. (2014). Biological therapies in Crohn's disease: Are they cost-effective? A critical appraisal of model-based analyses. *Expert Review of Pharmacoeconomics & Outcomes Research, 14*(6), 815–824.

Mauskopf, J. A., Paul, J. E., Grant, D. M., & Stergachis, A. (1998). The role of cost-consequence analysis in healthcare decision making. *Pharmacoeconomics, 13*(3), 277–288.

Motheral, B. R., Grizzle, A. J., Armstrong, E. P., Cox, E., & Fairman, K. (2000). Role of pharmacoeconomics in drug benefit decision-making: Results of a survey. *Formulary, 35,* 412–421.

Neumann, P. J., Cohen, J. T., & Weinstein, M. C. (2014). Updating cost-effectiveness—the curious resilience of the $50,000-per-QALY threshold. *New England Journal of Medicine, 371*(9), 796–797.

Ofman, J. J., Sullivan, S. D., Neumann, P. J., Chiou, C. F., Henning, J. M., Wade, S. W., & Hay, J. W. (2003). Examining the value and quality of health economic analyses: Implications of utilizing the QHES. *Journal of Managed Care Pharmacy, 9*(1), 53–61.

Prest, A. R., & Turvey, R. (1965). Cost-benefit analysis: A survey. *Economics Journal, 75*(12), 683–735.

Rutgeerts, P., D'Haens, G., Targan, S., Vasiliauskas, E., Hanauer, S.B., Present, D.H., ... Van Deventer, S. J. (1999). Efficacy and safety of retreatment with anti-tumor necrosis factor antibody (infliximab) to maintain remission in Crohn's disease. *Gastroenterology, 117*(4), 761–769.

Simon, G., Wagner, E., & Vonkorff, M. (1995, March). Cost-effectiveness comparisons using "real world" randomized trials: The case of new antidepressant drugs. *Journal of Clinical Epidemiology, 48*(3), 363–373.

Sonnenberg, F. A., & Beck, J. R. (1993, October–December). Markov models in medical decision making: A practical guide. *Medical Decision Making, 13*(4), 322–338.

Targan, S. R., Hanauer, S. B., van Deventer, S. J., Mayer, L., Present, D. H., Braakman, T., ... Rutgeerts, P. J. (1997). A short-term study of chimeric monoclonal antibody cA2 to tumor necrosis factor alpha for Crohn's disease. Crohn's Disease cA2 Study Group. *New England Journal of Medicine, 337*(15), 1029–1035.

Task Force on Principles for Economic Analysis of Health Care Technology. (1995). Economic analysis of health care technology: A report on principles. *Annals of Internal Medicine, 122*, 61–70.

Terdiman, J. P., Gruss, C. B., Heidelbaugh, J. J., Sultan, S., Falck-Ytter, Y. T.; AGA Institute Clinical Practice and Quality Management Committee. (2013). American Gastroenterological Association Institute guideline on the use of thiopurines, methotrexate, and anti-TNF-α biologic drugs for the induction and maintenance of remission in inflammatory Crohn's disease. *Gastroenterology, 145*(6), 1459–1463.

Townsend, R. J. (1986). Post marketing drug research and development: An industry clinical pharmacist's perspective. *American Journal of Pharmacy Education, 50*, 480–482.

Tumeh, J. W., Moore, S. G., Shapiro, R., & Flowers, C. R. (2005). Practical approach for using Medicare data to estimate costs for cost-effectiveness analysis. *Expert Review of Pharmacoeconomics Outcomes Research, 5*, 153–162.

Weinstein, M. C., & Skinner, J. A. (2010). Comparative effectiveness and health care spending—implications for reform. *New England Journal of Medicine, 362*, 460–465.

Weinstein, M. C., & Stason, B. (1977). Foundations and cost-effectiveness analysis for health and medical practitioners. *New England Journal of Medicine, 296*, 716–721.

Yu, A. P., Cabanilla, L. A., Wu, E. Q., Mulani, P. M., & Chao, J. (2008). The costs of Crohn's disease in the United States and other Western countries: a systematic review. *Current Medical Research and Opinion, 24*(2), 319–328.

CHAPTER

20

International Healthcare Services

Ana C. Quiñones-Boex and Gregory A. Garcia

Case Scenario

Chloe is a pharmacy student who has accepted an internship at the Department of Health and Human Services. Her main task is to research various healthcare systems across the globe and to compare them to the United States healthcare system in light of the recently instituted Patient Protection and Affordable Care Act of 2010 (a.k.a. Obamacare, ACA). The goal of the assignment is to determine how the changes seen thus far compare to countries with unique healthcare systems. Chloe decides to evaluate Canada, Germany, United Kingdom, and Cuba. She has a good understanding of the United States' healthcare system from a course she took in pharmacy school, but this is the first time that Chloe has to learn about the systems of several foreign countries and evaluate their structure, financing, etc.

Background

A student who wants to learn about how other countries provide healthcare services might start by doing a quick online search comparing the United States' healthcare system to that of other countries. A recent article by the Commonwealth Fund, *Mirror, Mirror on the Wall, 2014 Update: How the U.S. Health Care System Compares Internationally,* assesses 11 healthcare systems around the world (The Commonwealth Fund, 2014). All the healthcare systems included in the report belong to wealthy, developed nations. Eighty indicators were grouped to address five dimensions of performance: quality of care, access, efficiency, equity, and healthy lives. Based on all these indicators and dimensions, the United Kingdom ranks first, Germany ranks fifth, Canada ranks tenth, and the United States ranks last. One characteristic of all the countries studied, except for the United States, is that of universal coverage (or universality).

The Commonwealth Fund report included information from two important sources of health systems data: the Organization for Economic Cooperation and Development (OECD) and the World Health Organization (WHO). The OECD systematically collects and summarizes heathcare statistics on its member countries. Canada, Germany, United Kingdom, and United States are amongst the OECD members. OECD Health Statistics 2015 includes information on each country's spending on health, among other healthcare-related data (OECD, 2015). OECD's figures on health spending were included in the *Mirror, Mirror on the Wall, article and they indicate that the United States spends more on health care than any other OECD country.*

(*Continues*)

The WHO collects and disseminates health statistics and World Health Reports relating to all countries on Earth. Thus, it provides information on Canada, Germany, United Kingdom, United States, and Cuba and publishes reports encompassing more countries than those in the OECD publications. Prior to the Commonwealth Fund's *Mirror, Mirror on the Wall report,* WHO's *World Health Report 2000, Health systems: improving performance was routinely quoted when comparing health care systems around the world.* This report compared health systems' ability to achieve their goals based on their: (1) overall level of health or life expectancy; (2) responsiveness of how well people rated performance of their healthcare system; (3) fairness in responsiveness among different groups in the same country; and (4) fairness of financing among different groups, which looked at what proportion of income is devoted to health care (WHO, 2000a, Hilts, 2000).

The *World Health Report 2000* listed among the highest-ranking countries France, Italy, Singapore, Spain, Austria, and Japan (WHO, 2000b). Canada, Germany, and the United Kingdom fared better than the United States in the World Health Report 2000 rankings. The United States outspent all other countries and ranked near the top on average health measures, but failed to deliver good health care to a large proportion of its population and distributes the cost relatively unfairly, leaving it ranked 37th on the WHO list (WHO, 2000b). Cuba received a health systems performance score of 39 and can be considered unique due to its extraordinary health outcomes despite its developing nation status.

LEARNING OBJECTIVES

Upon completion of this chapter, the student shall be able to:

- Describe the differences between the following healthcare models: socialized insurance program, decentralized national health program, and socialized medicine.
- Compare and contrast the healthcare delivery systems of a developing country and a developed country.
- Describe several factors that affect the health of a country's population.
- Describe the main characteristics of the healthcare systems of Canada, Germany, the United Kingdom, and Cuba.
- Describe how the healthcare systems of Canada, Germany, the United Kingdom, and Cuba compare to the healthcare system in the United States.

CHAPTER QUESTIONS

1. What are the general features of the healthcare systems of:
   a. Canada?
   b. Germany?
   c. The United Kingdom?
   d. Cuba?
2. How does the healthcare delivery system of a developing country differ from that of a developed country?
3. Describe several factors that affect the health of a country's population.
4. Compare and contrast the healthcare systems of Canada, Germany, the United Kingdom, Cuba, and the United States.

INTRODUCTION

The failure of the U.S. healthcare system to provide universal access to healthcare services at a reasonable cost has prompted many observers to regularly examine the healthcare systems of other countries for possible solutions. This chapter, therefore, highlights different methods of structuring and financing healthcare services. It provides an overview of the unique features of the healthcare systems of several countries and discusses the characteristics of and issues faced by healthcare systems in both developed and developing countries.

The chapter analyzes the major features of four healthcare systems that illustrate the variety of models of healthcare delivery available—namely, the healthcare systems of Canada, the United Kingdom, Germany, and Cuba. The discussion of each of these systems includes a brief description of the history of each country's healthcare system, the system's main features, the health status of the population, the structure of the healthcare system (e.g., healthcare facilities and workforce, with a focus on hospitals, physicians, and pharmaceuticals), health education, healthcare financing (i.e., how the system is funded and what contributions are rendered by the government, citizens, and employers), and current issues that appear to present concerns for each system. **Table 20-1** summarizes the key aspects of these systems, comparing them to the features of the U.S. healthcare system.

Healthcare systems for different countries can be classified as belonging to four broad models:

1. The Beveridge model, also known as socialized medicine, in which health care is both financed by and provided by the government. The government employs healthcare practitioners, owns healthcare facilities, and administers the healthcare system. The health systems of Cuba and the United Kingdom are examples of the Beveridge model, which is named after the British social reformer who inspired the United Kingdom's National Health Service (Reid, 2009a).
2. The Bismark model, also referred to as a decentralized national health program, in which employers and employees are required to obtain private health insurance, usually provided by nongovernment insurance companies. Hospitals and clinics are privately owned. Germany created the first decentralized national health program (Reid, 2009a). Other countries with similar models include Japan and Switzerland.
3. The national health insurance model, also known as a socialized insurance model, in which a single, government-run insurance program finances healthcare services that are provided by private payers with negotiated reimbursement. Canada and, more recently, Taiwan are examples of countries with a socialized insurance model.
4. The out-of-pocket model is common in developing countries in which there is a lack of private health insurance and no government-sponsored healthcare system. This lack of private or government health insurance is usually accompanied by shortages of healthcare facilities, low expenditures, and poor health outcomes.

"DEVELOPED" AND "DEVELOPING" COUNTRIES

Based on per capita income, the world can be divided into low-income, middle-income, and high-income economies. Low- and middle-income economies are also referred to as "developing" countries, a term "used for convenience; it is not intended to imply that all economies in the group are experiencing similar development or that other economies have reached a preferred or

Table 20-1 Summary of Healthcare Delivery Systems' Key Aspects

	United States	Canada	Germany	United Kingdom	Cuba
Total population (2013)	320,051,000	35,182,000	82,727,000	63,136,000	11,266,000
% of GDP devoted to health (2013)	17.1%	10.9%	11.3%	9.1%	8.8%
Total health expenditure per capita (2013)	$9,146	$4,759	$4,812	$3,311	$1,828
Life expectancy at birth (years, 2013)	Males: 76 Females: 81	Males: 80 Females: 84	Males: 79 Females: 83	Males: 79 Females: 83	Males: 77 Females: 80
Infant mortality rate per 1,000 (2013)	5.9	4.6	3.2	3.9	5
Universal coverage?	No	Yes	Yes	Yes	Yes
Hospital beds per 10,000 (2009)	30	32	82	33	59 (2010)
Physicians per 10,000 (2011)	24.52	20.68	38.89 (2012)	28.09 (2013)	67.23 (2010)
Licensed pharmacists per 10,000 (2012)	27.5	3.5	7.8	5.1	1.4 (2003)
Public health expenditure as % of health spending (2012)	47%	70.1%	76.7%	84%	94.2%
Hospital payment	Contracted prospective DRGs; per diem; and discounted fee-for-services	Global budget; and activity based funding (varies by province)	Cost-per-case prospective budget; DRGs	HRGs	National Budget
Physician payment	Mix of fee-for-service and capitation	Fee-for-service; and some capitation (varies by province)	Fee-for-service	Mix of fee-for-service, capitation, and performance-related scheme	Salary

Table 20-1 Summary of Healthcare Delivery Systems' Key Aspects (continued)

	United States	Canada	Germany	United Kingdom	Cuba
Drugs	Coverage by Medicare, Medicaid, and most private insurance; high cost-sharing requirements	Limited coverage; varies by province; some employer coverage	Coverage through sickness funds (copayments required)	Through NHS	Full coverage

DRG = Diagnosis related group; HRG = Healthcare resource group; NHS = National Health Service.

Data from: The World Health Organization (2015b), the 2012 FIP Global Pharmacy Workforce Report, and the OECD iLibrary.

final stage of development (World Bank, 2015)." "Developed" nations (i.e., high-income, mostly capitalistic and social democratic societies in industrialized countries) have per capita incomes of more than $12,476 (World Bank, 2015) and tend to have strong health infrastructures and positive healthcare outcomes. Developing nations account for 85% of the world's population but only 12% of global health expenditures.

The income and health expenditures gap between developing and developed countries underscores the enormous difference in terms of capacities and types of health services that can be provided. This translates into large differences in the health infrastructure and the health outcomes of populations in developing countries. A limiting factor for developing countries is the large portion of their budgets required to finance the most basic of primary healthcare services.

Lack of resources, poor administrative capacity, and the competing needs for other social and economic programs have a profound effect on the burden of disease in developing countries (Schieber & Maeda, 1999). Worldwide, one death in every three is attributable to largely preventable communicable diseases such as infectious disease, maternal and perinatal conditions, and nutritional deficiencies. Communicable diseases that are mainly preventable remain the leading causes of death in developing countries; indeed, almost all deaths from communicable diseases occur in developing countries (WHO, 2009). Approximately 1 in every 500 women in developing countries dies from complications related to pregnancy and childbirth, compared with only 1 in 6,300 women in the established market economies (WHO, 2014).

In the coming decades, important demographic and epidemiologic changes are expected to occur in developing countries. These changes will alter the demand for health services and increase the pressure to make new investments in their healthcare systems (Harvard School of Public Health, 2000; Schieber & Maeda, 1999). Life expectancy at birth is expected to increase for women in all regions. Men are not expected to do as well on the longevity front, partly because of the effects of tobacco use on their life expectancy (Harvard School of Public Health, 2000).

Although overall deaths from communicable diseases are expected to decline, a steep increase is expected in the number of deaths resulting from noncommunicable diseases (e.g., heart disease, stroke, cancer, diabetes) as well as the number of deaths from injuries. In part, the projected reduction in deaths from communicable diseases reflects increased income, education, and technological progress in the development of antimicrobials and vaccines. The expected increase in deaths from noncommunicable diseases and injury is largely driven by aging of the population as well as exposure to tobacco. In the future, health systems in developing countries will need to change their health systems to focus on treatment and prevention of noncommunicable diseases instead of the more cost-effective and lower cost interventions targeted toward communicable diseases—a trend that will further strain these already fragile health systems (Schieber & Maeda, 1999).

The health of a population or country is also influenced by a number of socioeconomic variables, such as the distribution of resources within a country, income per capita, the number of years of schooling in adults, and—to some extent—the ability to adopt new health technologies. Studies have also found the educational level and status of women to be indicators of the health outcomes in a household. Women are often the primary caregivers for the health and nutritional needs of other family members. As a consequence, greater educational attainment in women can contribute to improved understanding of disease prevention and better nutritional health within a household. When girls are offered educational opportunities, their value within the household increases. Thus the allocation of resources such as food and medicine within a household tends to be more equitable when parents place equal value on their children regardless of their gender.

A strong inverse relationship exists between per capita income and child mortality under 5 years of age. That is, as per capita income increases, infant mortality rates tend to decrease. However, variability exists among countries, indicating that social and cultural factors strongly influence these mortality rates, as do differences in the use of maternal and child health programs and the extent to which they achieve equity and efficiency in the delivery of health services (Schieber & Maeda, 1999). The distribution of limited health resources is also affected by whether services are administered through a public or private system. A strong direct relationship exists between an economy's health spending and its per capita gross domestic product (GDP—a measure of the value of the final goods and services produced in a given country). On a worldwide basis, for every 10% increase in per capita GDP, health spending increases by 13% (Schieber & Maeda, 1999).

Public health expenditures tend to be more responsive to income differences than private health expenditures. Thus, as countries' incomes increase, a larger share of total health spending tends to come from public sources. Public health expenditures account for 40% of health spending in low-income countries, 56% in middle-income countries, and 61% in high-income countries (WHO, 2013). These differing rates may be attributable to the relatively greater ability to tax and generate revenue in higher-income countries as well as governments' decisions to address health sector and health insurance market failures through public rather than private financing. The fact that such a large portion of health expenditures is privately financed in developing countries has important implications for both equity and efficiency in health care, because governments need to focus on efficient allocation of combined public and private resources (Schieber & Maeda, 1999). Typically, those countries with a higher proportion of publicly financed healthcare systems have also achieved better and more equitable health outcomes primarily through a more equitable distribution of scarce health resources. For this reason, certain socialist economic systems, even in developing countries, have achieved health outcomes that are comparable to those found in many industrialized countries.

Other factors—for example, public health improvements in drinking water, access to prenatal and perinatal care, population planning, immunizations, and the allocation of food supplies—also directly affect the health of a population. Rational and efficient investments in primary healthcare services could afford most developing countries a cost-effective package of basic primary care and emergency services, although data reveal that a disproportionate share of limited public health spending is allocated to tertiary care instead of primary care (Schieber & Maeda, 1999). In most developing countries, individuals in the highest income brackets can still enjoy access to health services (either within their country or by traveling outside the country) that is comparable to the best healthcare services available in higher-income countries. Nevertheless, the majority of people living in developing countries lack access to even basic primary healthcare services.

HEALTHCARE DELIVERY SYSTEMS IN SELECTED NATIONS

Canada's Healthcare System

The origins of Canada's current healthcare system date back to the 1940s, when the first government-financed insurance was established for hospital services in Saskatchewan (OECD, 1994). In 1957, the Hospital Insurance and Diagnostic Service Act established public insurance that provided inpatient hospital care coverage for all Canadians. In 1966, the Medical Care Act established the main principles of Canada's current healthcare system, which include:

1. Portability of benefits: Coverage is kept, even when the individual is absent from the province.
2. Comprehensiveness: All necessary physician and hospital services are covered.
3. Universality: All citizens of a province are entitled to the same services.
4. Accessibility: Reasonable access to services is assured.
5. Public administration: A nonprofit, public organization accountable to the provincial government runs the plan (Rozek & Mulhern, 1994).

This legislation was implemented on a province-by-province basis. By 1972, Canada's 10 provinces and two territories had implemented medical insurance measures, realizing the goal of national health insurance for the country. In 1984, the Canada Health Act aggregated the provisions of the Medical Care Act and Hospital Insurance and Diagnostic Service Act into one updated piece of legislation.

As a consequence of these measures, Canada has 13 different health insurance plans (a new territory was created in 1999). These plans are kept consistent through adherence to the five main principles of portability, comprehensiveness, universality, accessibility, and public administration. Failure to ensure that these principles are maintained would prevent a province from qualifying for federal subsidies (Rozek & Mulhern, 1994).

The Canadian system has been successful in providing universal access to care regardless of patients' ability to pay, and the services covered are extensive. As a result, the health status of the Canadian population is good. In 2013, life expectancy at birth was 80 years for men and 84 years for women—about 3 years longer than in the United States. That same year, infant mortality was 4.6 deaths per 1,000 births—compared to about 5.9 deaths per 1,000 births in the United States (WHO, 2015a). Canada's success in providing universal access and caring for the less fortunate has been a great source of pride for its citizens, who view it as presenting a striking contrast to the U.S. system that has left a significant portion of the population uninsured. However, recent polls indicate that public confidence in the system is eroding as long waiting times continue and availability of physicians and services becomes more limited.

Structure: Healthcare Facilities and Workforce

Since Canada has socialized health insurance, healthcare delivery systems in the country are mostly private. Hospitals are primarily nonprofit community and teaching hospitals, although 4% of hospitals belong to the federal government. Provinces set the standards for hospital facilities and staffing.

The Canada Medical Care Act explicitly prohibited private hospitals or insurance companies from providing or financing core medical services provided by the Canada Medical Care Act. However, a 2005 Canadian Supreme Court ruling struck down a Quebec law banning private medical insurance and private medical clinics (Marchildon, 2013). The court ruled that waiting lists at publicly financed hospitals had become so long that "the prohibition on obtaining private health insurance is not constitutional where the public system fails to deliver reasonable services" (Krauss, 2005). Supporters of the publicly financed system fear that the introduction of privately financed services will encourage physicians and private clinics to leave the publicly financed system for higher reimbursement—a system that favors better access to treatments for individuals with higher incomes (Canadian-healthcare, 2006).

The national health insurance program, called Medicare, covers physician care and the following hospital services: room and meals, nursing services, diagnostic procedures, and medications prescribed for inpatient use. Private insurance is available only as a supplement to the national health insurance. Until the 2005 court decision regarding private insurance, private policies provided coverage only for private or semiprivate rooms in a hospital and other services not covered through Medicare, such as cosmetic surgery, dental services, and outpatient medications for those not covered under provincial law (Rozek & Mulhern, 1994). Most Canadians have supplemental private insurance. Delivery systems other than hospitals are available to Canadians, but these options vary from province to province. These systems, which include community health centers and long-term care, aim to provide preventive care and other services for which an acute care hospital setting is not necessary (Rozek & Mulhern, 1994).

Under the Canada Health Act, primary care doctors, specialists, and dental surgery are all covered by provincial policies. In 2012, approximately half of all Canadian physicians were primary care doctors (e.g., general practitioners or family physicians) (The Commonwealth Fund, 2015). Primary care physicians function as gatekeepers, serving as the initial point of contact for patients at the forefront of Canadian health care. Patients have free choice of physicians. Typically, patients are referred to specialists by their primary care physicians.

The distribution of physicians across Canada is not homogeneous, and there is an undersupply in rural areas. A decrease in the supply of physicians is one of the latest concerns to arise regarding the country's healthcare resources (Iglehart, 2000). The government statistical agency estimates that more than 9% of the population does not have a primary care physician (Canadian Institute for Health Information, 2009). This compares to an estimated 20% of U.S. residents who do not have or have difficulty accessing a primary care physician (NACHC, 2014).

Medicare covers outpatient prescription drugs for senior citizens, individuals with low incomes, and patients with specific disease states. Each of the provinces and territories has their own form of a publicly funded outpatient prescription program (Morgan et al., 2015). In Quebec, it is mandatory by law for employers to provide a private prescription drug program (Morgan et al., 2015). Canada is the only developed country with universal health care that does not have universal coverage for prescription medications (Morgan et al., 2015). Most of the population relies on private insurance for outpatient prescription drug coverage, but subscribing to such supplemental coverage is often dependent on income. Coverage gaps exist in other areas of health care, such as nonsurgical dental care, which are also filled by private health insurance (Marchildon, 2013).

Health Education

Requirements for medical schools in Canada are similar to those in the United States. Applicants are required to have a bachelor's degree, in which they have completed a set amount of credits relating to science courses and general education courses (Med School Admissions, 2015; University of Toronto, 2015a). Six of the seventeen medical schools in Canada do not require applicants to take the Medical College Admission Test (MCAT) (Ivy Global, 2015). Medical schools in Canada are 4-year programs except for the University of Calgary and McMaster University, both of which are 3-year programs (Ivy Global, 2015). The medical school programs are split into pre-clerkship and clerkship. The pre-clerkship is based on lectures and focuses on anatomy while the clerkship is based on applying knowledge in medical facilities (University of Calgary, 2015; Dalhousie University, 2015). In the 2010–2011 school year, the price of tuition for first-year students at McMaster University was less than $14,300, the most expensive of all the medical schools in Canada (Maclean's, 2010), compared to an average tuition of $21,276 for first-year students attending an American public medical school in the state in which they had residence (AAMC, 2015).

There are 10 pharmacy schools in Canada. Completion of one of these programs is required to become a practicing pharmacist in Canada (Canadian Pharmacists Association, 2015). In the last decade, most pharmacy programs have transitioned from baccalaureate programs to entry-level Doctor of Pharmacy degrees (Smith, 2104). Most schools in Canada offer curriculums similar to schools in the United States in which the first 3 years are devoted to lectures and the fourth year is devoted to rotations/internships (University of Toronto, 2015b; Canadian Pharmacists Association, 2015).

Financing

The Canadian system is not one centralized plan, but rather 13 separate systems that are controlled by the provinces and territories. The universal insurance is paid for by personal and corporate taxes and distributed to each province according to budgets established on both national and provincial levels. Provinces may obtain additional funds from other sources such as lottery proceeds and sales taxes. The provinces of Alberta, British Columbia, and Ontario also charge health premiums to supplement health spending (Canadian-healthcare, 2006).

The provincial governments carefully plan how to allocate resources within their budgets. Because the government is the only insurer, administrative overhead is tightly controlled in Canada. In 2011, health administrative costs in Canada were less than half of the costs in the United States (Himmelstein, 2014). The additional administrative costs in the U.S. system can be attributed to the nature of a pluralistic insurance system that has complex billing and reimbursement procedures that vary considerably among payers.

Costs are controlled through set fees for medical services. Every year, the government publishes a list of the fees that physicians are permitted to charge the government for treating patients. Physicians are then paid directly by the provincial government on a fee-for-service basis. Canada's physicians are paid lower salaries than their U.S. counterparts, with the average salary for a Canadian physician being about half that for a U.S. physician (PayScale, 2014; U.S. News, 2013). Even so, physicians are amongst the highest-paid professionals in Canada. Their salaries are higher than those of Japanese physicians and similar to those of British physicians (Healthcare Salaries, 2015). In 2011, there were approximately 2 physicians for every 1,000 residents in Canada—slightly less than in the United States (WHO, 2015a).

Hospitals in Canada work on a budget that cannot be exceeded, which not surprisingly results in some strain on the system. Many hospitals have closed or merged, causing a shrinking hospital sector (Naylor, 1999). Because most hospitals are run at capacity in Canada, waiting lists are commonplace. For example, a study in 2010 discovered that the waiting period for a coronary artery bypass graft surgery in Nova Scotia averaged 109 days (Légaré et al., 2010). Another study found that 25% of patients in Canada waited longer than 4 months for an elective surgery, compared to only seven percent of patients in the United States (Schoen et al., 2014).

While all inpatient prescription expenses are covered under the Canada Health Act, each province may offer varying levels of coverage for drugs prescribed on an outpatient basis. The publicly funded drug programs are generally established based on patients' age, income, and medical condition (Health Canada, 2006a). Only those medications listed on the Medicare formularies are covered. In recent years, drug spending has been increasing and has become the second largest category of healthcare-related expenditures in Canada, after hospital services.

Although drug prices are set at the federal level, purchasing takes place at the provincial level. Provinces, therefore, face the responsibility of controlling increasing drug expenditures without having direct control over pricing (Anis, 2000).

Current Status

Over the years, Canada has struggled with waiting times for diagnostic tests, hip and knee replacements, cancer treatments, and elective surgeries, among other things. Canada is ranked inferior to the United States in terms of patient waiting time for primary care and nonemergency procedures (Marchildon, 2013). In addition to the difficulties attributable to the misdistribution of physicians and long waiting lists for certain services, the federal government has decreased its contribution to provincial plans significantly (The Commonwealth Fund, 2015). Moreover, the single-payer structure prevents the system from rapidly responding to local changes in the healthcare environment. Dissatisfaction with the current waiting lists for services and the shortage of primary care physicians in some areas has grown sharply as well.

In 2003, the First Ministers' Accord on Health Care Renewal was adopted. This accord consisted of an agreement on a vision, principles, and action plan for renewal of the Canadian health system (Health Canada, 2006b). It incorporated an agreement on the value of a publicly funded health system, the need for reform, and the priorities for reform. The priorities established included additional investments in primary health care, home care, and catastrophic drug coverage to create a long-term, sustainable public healthcare system in Canada (Health Canada, 2006b). The federal government agreed to establish a health reform fund by 2004 to be used toward reform objectives by the provinces and territories (The Commonwealth Fund, 2015).

Since the Supreme Court in Quebec ruled in favor of allowing private insurance, the Québécois government has agreed to pay for certain procedures such as cancer and heart surgeries performed in private institutions to help reduce patient wait times (Starfield, 2010; Marchildon, 2013). Other provinces are considering similar modifications (Starfield, 2010). However, the current healthcare system has generally been strongly supported by most of the public, and most Canadian citizens identify with it as part of the Canadian national character (Krauss, 2005). Additional attempts to reduce wait times in Canada include programs such as the Wait Time Reduction Fund. This program allocated $4.5 billion over 10 years to reduce surgical and diagnostic wait times in priority areas. The result of the program significantly reduced wait times in certain procedures (The Commonwealth Fund, 2015). Additionally, the government has recommendations on how long patients should wait from the time they schedule the procedure to the time they undergo the procedure (Canadian Institute of Health Information, 2014). Over the past few years, Canadian patients have been undergoing medical procedures at higher rates than previously. However, the wait times of these procedures has not increased (Canadian Institute for Health Information, 2014). Other procedures, such as radiation therapy, are meeting the government recommended wait time at high percentages and joint replacement wait times have improved (Canadian Institute for Health Information, 2014).

Coverage gaps exist in dental care and prescription drugs. In these areas, some provincial governments offer additional coverage to certain demographics such as the elderly or Canadians may purchase private. (Marchildon, 2013). Canada has some problems with equitable health with the use of private insurance decreasing wait times and providing additional health care benefits, (Marchildon, 2013).

Canada's three largest provinces have approved healthcare reform measures in order to control rising healthcare costs (Newman, 2010). Quebec has proposed to charge a $25 copayment per doctor visit, while British Columbia is considering changing hospital global budgets to a payment scheme based on the procedures each hospital performs. In 2010, British Columbia introduced a payment scheme based on procedures (The Commonwealth Fund, 2015). However, the organization that was responsible for executing the new payment scheme closed in 2013 (The Commonwealth Fund, 2015). In 2012, Ontario introduced a similar payment scheme to be fully implemented by 2016 (The Commonwealth Fund, 2015). The goal is to have a global budget, prospective population-based model, and activity based payment account for 30%, 40%, and 30% of the total hospital funding, respectively (The Commonwealth Fund, 2015). Additionally, there has been a trend toward centralization for certain health services due to provincial governments reducing the number of Regional Health Authorities. The goal is to modify the system to decrease costs (Marchildon, 2013).

In 2012, public funding and out of pocket expenses accounted for approximately 70% and 15% of total health expenditures, respectively. The remaining expenses come from private insurance coverage. Most out-of-pocket expenses were related to prescription drugs and long-term care (The Commonwealth Fund, 2015). When compared to Americans, Canadians spend less out of pocket on prescription drugs and use fewer drugs (Starfield, 2010). The Patented Medicine Prices Review Board (PMPRB) is "quasi-judicial body" that regulates the prices of newly patented medications (The Commonwealth Fund, 2015). Prices of patented medications are frequently reviewed to determine if prices are too excessive. If the PMPRB deems that prices are too high, they can intervene to regulate the price (The Commonwealth Fund, 2015). Additionally, the Pan-Canadian Pricing Alliance was given authority in 2010 to negotiate prices of brand name medications (The Commonwealth Fund, 2015).

Recently, the focus on healthcare reform has been to create an interdisciplinary primary care team that will be able to provide broader healthcare services around the clock (Marchildon, 2013). Provincial and territorial governments have been working together to improve access to multidisciplinary primary care teams under the 10-Year Plan to Strengthen Health Care. The federal government has also contributed $647 million over a 6-year period via the Primary Care Transition Fund to improve the utilization and quality of primary care (The Commonwealth Fund, 2015). With focus of reform shifting toward interdisciplinary teams, Canadians should expect a decrease in wait times, increase in quality care, and improved management of chronic conditions. It remains to be seen whether Canada's reform efforts will enable it to continue to achieve the health outcomes it has experienced in the past.

Germany's Healthcare System

Germany's current healthcare system has its roots in the statutory health insurance (SHI) system (sickness funds) for manual industrial workers instituted by Chancellor Bismarck in 1883 (Beske, 1988). It constitutes the world's oldest national healthcare system (Reid, 2009b). This law, in conjunction with the accident insurance law of 1884 and the disability and old-age pension insurance law of 1889, remains the backbone of Germany's social security system. Although sickness funds started as coverage for certain occupations, they evolved to accept all qualified persons whose place of work fell within the geographical boundaries covered by the fund. During the 1990s, occupational and geographical limits on most of the sickness funds were lifted (Jackson, 1997). Today, only funds for small farmers remain closed (Busse and Blümel, 2014). Moreover, potential enrollees cannot be discriminated against based on their age, gender, or other risk factors.

Thus Germany has no comprehensive national health plan. Instead, German citizens are covered by either the health insurance system (Krankenkassen, or sickness funds) or the social welfare program for the unemployed. Additionally, Germans can utilize substitutive private health insurance (The Commonwealth Fund, 2015). The sickness funds are considered self-governing, non-profit, quasi-public corporations. Simply stated, they are corporations under public law (Busse & Blümel, 2014), so the statutory system is decentralized. In 2003, 319 sickness funds were in charge of the healthcare insurance of the individuals they covered (Busse, 2004). Due to recent mergers, the number of sickness funds has decreased to 131 as of July 2014 (The Commonwealth Fund, 2015). Although insured individuals are allowed to change sickness funds at any time, when they do, they have to stay with their new fund for the next 18 months.

Sickness funds can be classified in six types all of which provide a guaranteed healthcare package of comprehensive services. In 2014, 11 regional funds insured 35% of the population, 6 substitute sickness funds insured 37% of the population, and 107 company-based sickness funds insured 17% of the population; the rest of the population was insured by guild, miner/sailor, or agricultural sickness funds (Busse & Blümel, 2014). The Statutory Health Insurance Modernization Act of 2004 was passed, allowing sickness funds to offer complementary and supplementary policies (Busse & Blümel, 2014). Each year, more Germans purchase these insurance policies, which grant them better access to services such as ambulatory and dental care.

In 2012, 70 million Germans, or 85% of the population, were covered by a sickness fund (Busse & Blümel, 2014). The remaining portion of the population had either private insurance (11%), or received free medical services (4%) (Busse & Blümel, 2014). The police, members of the armed forces, prisoners, immigrants seeking asylum and welfare recipients all qualify for free medical care (Busse & Blümel, 2014). Germans who earn more than a certain level of income have a choice of private insurance or voluntary membership in the sickness funds. As of 2014, coverage via SHI was mandatory for employed citizens earning less than $68,336 per year (The Commonwealth Fund, 2015). Approximately 9% of the population covered through sickness funds joined voluntarily on this basis (Busse & Blümel, 2014). Persons who elect to purchase private insurance, however, cannot switch back to a sickness fund (Jackson, 1997). Since 2009, private insurers must offer the same benefits as sickness funds at a premium that is not higher than the average maximum contribution rate (Busse & Blümel, 2014).

Three main values underlie the German healthcare system:

1. Self-governance: The system is administered by a self-managing organization (e.g., the sickness funds).
2. Social partnership: Both the employer and the employee have a share in the system.
3. Social solidarity: Ensuring equality in health care through some members of society subsidizing other members' healthcare costs (Hoffmeyer, 1994). A strong commitment to social solidarity exists in Germany (Jackson, 1997).

Germany's decentralized system appears to be successful in keeping its population healthy. The country's infant mortality rate was 3.2 deaths per 1,000 live births in 2013—almost half of the rate in the United States (5.9 per 1,000) (WHO, 2015a). In 2013, life expectancy was 79 years for men and 83 years for women in Germany (WHO, 2015a). These and other health status indicators are similar to those associated with other industrialized countries, but significantly better than the indicators for the United States.

Structure: Healthcare Facilities and Workforce

In 2012, Germany had a ratio of 6.2 hospital beds per 1,000 persons; this figure has been decreasing since the 1990s (Busse & Blümel, 2014). This ratio is higher than any other country in the European Union and the United States. In recent years, there has been a trend of decreasing beds in public and nonprofit institutions (Busse & Blümel, 2014). Germany has a mix of public, private nonprofit, and private for-profit hospitals (Busse & Blümel, 2014). Government and nonprofit organizations own the majority of German hospitals, although the number of private, for-profit hospitals has been increasing (The Commonwealth Fund, 2015).

There were nearly 39 physicians for every 10,000 people in Germany in 2012—a significantly higher rate than in the United States and about twice the rate of Canada (WHO, 2015a). This ratio indicates that there may currently be an oversupply of physicians that could eventually lead to increased healthcare costs. Physicians working in office-based practices act as gatekeepers for institutionalized care. If they wish to be reimbursed by sickness funds, physicians have to qualify and apply for accreditation with a regional association of physicians. Germans have freedom of choice of physicians. If a patient wants to switch physicians, however, he or she has to wait three months before selecting another office-based physician.

Germany has a well-developed pharmaceutical industry, with significant drug development occurring in the country (Spivey, Wertheimer, & Rucker, 1992). In 2008, Germany was the world's fourth largest producer of pharmaceuticals (The Pharmaceutical Industry in Germany, 2011). Medications are covered through the sickness funds and are available from both hospital and retail pharmacies. Retail pharmacies in Germany have to be owned by pharmacists. Originally, pharmacists were only allowed to own one retail pharmacy. Since 2004, pharmacists may own up to four pharmacies. The three pharmacies that have been branched from the original must be in the same county or a neighboring county (Busse & Blümel, 2014).

Health Education

German medical school admissions have some similarities to American schools. In Germany, applicants must have an *Abitur*, which can be compared to an associate's degree, in order to apply to medical schools (Chenot, 2009). The Central Office for the Allocation of Places in Higher Education (ZVS) is a federal institution responsible for applications (Chenot, 2009). Education programs typically exceed 6 years; the average medical student in Germany completes the program in 6.8 years (Chenot, 2009). The curriculum is broken down into three sections: basic science, clinical science, and clinical year (Chenot, 2009). Basic science is usually about 2 years comprising anatomy, physiology, and other sciences (Chenot, 2009). Clinical science is about 3 years and includes physical examinations, pharmacology, and microbiology (Chenot, 2009). The clinical year is about 1 year long and is devoted to rotations that can be completed in hospitals and ambulatory care settings (Chenot, 2009). Attending medical school used to be free of charge to students until recently (Chenot, 2009). In 2009, most of the medical schools in Germany had tuition prices of $570 (Chenot, 2009).

In Germany, pharmacy schools do not require students to have an undergraduate degree and programs typically are 4 years in duration (Global Knowledge Exchange Network, 2009). After completion of the program, pharmacy students earn a Bachelor of Pharmacy (Global Knowledge Exchange Network, 2009). The curriculum in Germany consists of "coursework, clinical practice, a 12-month practical year, and a three-part state examination with written and oral components" (Global Knowledge Exchange Network, 2009). Interestingly, pharmacists are not required to participate in continuing education in Germany as they are in the United States; however, there are opportunities for continuing education, which pharmacists volunteer to attend (Global Knowledge Exchange Network, 2009).

Financing

The statutory health system is financed primarily through payroll taxes; employers and employees make equal contributions to this system. The contributions represent a percentage of the employees' income up to a certain threshold. Sickness funds are financed to a lesser extent by pension funds, local unemployment offices, and welfare organizations (Hoffmeyer, 1994). In 2009, a uniform contribution rate was set by the government and then became federal law in 2011 (The Commonwealth Fund, 2015). The rate was set at 15.5% in 2011 and 2012 (Busse & Blümel, 2014). The sum of the contribution rate was split amongst employees and/or pensioners at a rate of 8.2% and the employer and/or pension fund at a rate of 7.3% (The Commonwealth Fund, 2015). The sickness funds collect the contributions and distribute them into the newly created Central Reallocation Pool, which then redistributes the collections back to the sickness funds based on risk (Busse & Blümel, 2014).

Hospitals and most physicians negotiate their fees with the sickness funds. Physicians working in hospitals, however, are salaried employees. Payment for office-based physicians follows a fee-for-service system that is based on negotiations between the sickness funds and physicians. Additional copayments for adults 18 years and older were introduced in 2004 for ambulatory visits, including dentist visits. They were eventually removed in 2013; copayments for outpatient prescriptions continue to exist (The Commonwealth Fund, 2015). Each state has a union of physicians that provides services to the sickness funds that are in charge of negotiating budgets (Jost, 1998). Hospital payments are based on diagnosis-related groups and are revised annually (The Commonwealth Fund, 2015). Patients are charged a copayment for some hospital procedures, but the majority of services are free at the point of delivery (The Commonwealth Fund, 2015).

Sickness funds also provide reimbursement for approved medications. Individual SHI and pharmaceutical manufacturers negotiate prices (The Commonwealth Fund, 2015). Reference pricing, whereby drugs with similar properties would be reimbursed at the same level, was introduced in 1989. Beginning in 2011, manufacturers were required to submit dossiers that provide evidence of additional therapeutic benefits when compared to its appropriate comparator (Henschke, Sundmacher, & Busse, 2012). The Federal Association of SHI Funds determines the reference prices, which can then be reimbursed. This reimbursement applies to the sickness funds and private health insurance. Sickness funds are allowed to negotiate contracts with individual manufacturers to modify or complement the price. Patients typically pay copayments for medications; they can also save money through generic substitution (Busse & Blümel, 2014).

Current Status

The Health Fund, a key component of the country's 2007 healthcare reform, has become the new central entity in charge of collecting and allocating a nationwide uniform contribution fee from all sickness funds since 2009 (The Commonwealth Fund, 2015). The government also contributes a subsidy to the fund. The payments are allocated based on a risk structure compensation scheme that adjusts for age, gender, and well-defined morbidities for each sickness fund member. "This ensures a fairer allocation of financial resources with respect to the risk-structure of the sickness funds" (Zander et al., 2009, p. 4). After Germany's 2009 election, the new governing coalition agreed to fundamental health reform aimed at adjusting the Health Fund (Facts about Germany, 2011; Zander, Kimmerle, Sundmacher, & Bäumler, 2009).

Prior to 2009, contribution rates used to be set by sickness funds. In 2011, German lawmakers agreed to set a contribution rate that would remain the same in coming years. (Göpffarth & Henke, 2012). Contribution rates are not to be increased with future increases in health expenditures. However, if the funds provided to the sickness funds are insufficient, then additional premiums may be utilized by the sickness funds (Göpffarth & Henke, 2012). In 2012, all but one of the sickness funds abolished or consolidated the additional premiums (Göpffarth & Henke, 2012) The Central Health Fund (CHF) distributes funds based on predictions of revenue allocated to the CHF (Göpffarth & Henke, 2012). In 2011, revenue was greater than predicted due to increased market performance, thus creating a surplus; the surplus is then allocated into reserves to be used for any future losses (Göpffarth & Henke, 2012).

In 2009, SHI members were allowed to opt out and receive private health insurance if their income exceeded the threshold for three calendar years (Busse & Blümel, 2014). However, with the passing of the Health Financing Act of 2011, SHI members can now choose to opt out if their income exceeds the threshold for one calendar year (Bäumler, Sundmacher, & Zander, 2010).

In 2011, it was estimated that 0.17% of the population did not have health insurance. The goal was to reduce that percentage with the institution of mandatory SHI or private insurance coverage in 2009 (Busse & Blümel, 2014). In 2013, out-of-pocket expenses accounted for nearly 13% of total health spending (The Commonwealth Fund, 2015). According to WHO, Germany devoted 11.3% of their GDP to health expenditures (WHO, 2015a). The expenditure per capita is high compared to other most countries, but growth has been moderate since the 2000s (Busse & Blümel, 2014).

About 90% of physicians with private practice use electronic health records. Likewise, hospitals have implemented them with varying degrees. The use of a universal electronic health record is an area that is in need of improvement (The Commonwealth Fund, 2015). In October 2011, a policy was implemented to create an electronic medical chip card. The card would contain details such as name, address, date of birth, and sickness fund. There is hope to expand the use of these electronic devices to include more information and allow patients control over the information stored (The Commonwealth Fund, 2015).

Multiple studies and surveys draw similar conclusions that Germany is one of the best when it comes to access to medical care (Busse & Blümel, 2014). Furthermore, Germany ranks superior in even distribution of physicians when compared to most other OECD countries (Busse & Blümel, 2014). However, cost-related problems do exist. Germany ranked 10th among 11 OECD countries in regards to patients forgoing physician visits for medical treatment due to costs (Busse & Blümel, 2014). In addition, problems lie with access to medical care due to different payment structures between SHI and private health insurance (Busse & Blümel, 2014). This has caused some patients in sickness funds to feel less involved in health care decisions and receive shorter consultation times with physicians when compared to privately insured patients (Busse & Blümel, 2014).

The United Kingdom's Healthcare System

The movement toward the United Kingdom's current healthcare system started after World War I (Harrison, 1988). In 1939, only half of the nation's population had insurance coverage (Allen, 1984), and people were concerned about creating a more rational and comprehensive health service. Planning for a comprehensive healthcare delivery system continued during World War II, although major disagreement existed between different players regarding the system administration, funding, and physicians' roles in the system.

The National Health Service Act was finally passed in 1946 (Harrison, 1988). The National Health Service (NHS) presented the following three innovations: (1) universal comprehensive service,

(2) financing through general taxation with little or no charge at point of service, and (3) nationalization of the country's hospitals (Allen, 1984). This system can be defined as socialized medicine whereby most of the services are provided by practitioners who work for the government.

Since the implementation of the NHS, the United Kingdom has experienced longer life expectancy rates and concomitant changes in disease patterns. In 2013, life expectancy was 79 years for men and 83 years for women (WHO, 2015a). Infant mortality was less than 4 deaths per 1,000 live births in the same year (WHO, 2015a).

Structure: Healthcare Facilities and Workforce

The United Kingdom's healthcare system includes the following three major components: hospitals, community services, and primary medical and dental care (Harrison, 1988). All of these services are available to the entire population, and only hospital care requires referral from a primary care physician. Primary care is delivered by a wide range of health professionals, including family practitioners, nurses, dentists, pharmacists, and opticians.

In the United Kingdom, primary care usually consists of physicians who work outside of a hospital setting (Boyle, 2011). General practitioners (GPs) are in charge of primary care and act as the gatekeepers for hospital and specialty care. Additionally, a variety of healthcare professionals can provide primary care such as pharmacists and nurses (Boyle, 2011). Patients have to register with a GP practice but are allowed to change GPs whenever they like. Usually, patients end up scheduling appointments with a GP that is available (Boyle, 2011). Most GPs receive a General Medical Services contract. GPs contracts for 2014–2015 required practices to assign patients over 75 years old "a named accountable general practitioner" (The Commonwealth Fund, 2015).

In 2002, physicians were organized into approximately 300 primary care trusts (PCTs) (Bindman & Weiner, 2000).These groups include about 50 GPs each and are in charge of managing primary health services budgets for their patients (Enthoven, 2000). In 2006, physicians were reorganized into approximately 152 primary care trusts (PCTs) (Boyle, 2011). As a result of the NHS Health and Social Care Act of 2012, PCTs were converted into Clinical Commissioning Groups (CCGs) in 2013 (NHS Choices, 2015a). Additionally, the Health and Social Care Act created a new government entity, the NHS Commissioning Board (now called NHS England), to handle the day-to-day activities of the NHS such as the NHS budget and overseeing the CCGs (The Commonwealth Fund, 2015). In 2013, there were 211 CCGs (NHS England, 2015). The CCGs are in charge of self-governing their resources for the populations they serve (The Commonwealth Fund, 2015).

CCGs control about 60% of the total NHS budget (NHS Choices, 2015a). Given that providers are paid based on quality incentives rather than the quantity of care provided, physicians in PCTs have incentives to work as part of a primary care team along with other healthcare providers, including nurses, midwives, and pharmacists. Pharmacists, although limited, are currently being trained to prescribe some medications and/or approve patient refills and other primary care roles (APhA, 2014).

Community trusts are in charge of those community services not provided by GPs, such as specialized mental health services (The Commonwealth Fund, 2015). Additional trusts have been established to provide specialized or specific services. For example, mental health trusts serve people with mental health problems, care trusts combine social care and healthcare services, and ambulance trusts respond to life-threatening emergencies. All trusts operate within an annual budget allocated by the federal budget and based on the region and the size of the population they serve (The Commonwealth Fund, 2015).

Secondary and tertiary care is delivered by specialists ("consultants"), provided mainly in hospitals (Boyle, 2011). Secondary care includes maternity care, pathology, radiology, and emergency care. Tertiary care deals with highly specialized services such as organ transplants and treatments for rare diseases. Physicians who work in NHS hospitals are salaried employees.

Patients are not charged for their visits to health providers who work as part of the NHS system (NHS Choices, 2015b). Patients can also choose to receive care from private providers, but these services are not reimbursed by the NHS (The Commonwealth Fund, 2015).

Non-European visitors and illegal immigrants are entitled to treatment in emergency departments and for specific infectious diseases (The Commonwealth Fund 2015). The 2014 Immigration Act removes the right from patients outside of the Economic European Area (EEA) from receiving free NHS services (Poduval et al., 2015). Additionally, this law levies a surcharge of about $275 "payable on the issuance of a visa" for utilizing an NHS service (Poduval et al., 2015). There are growing concerns that this will increase disparities in the healthcare system and place a financial strain on the NHS (Poduval et al., 2015). Patients with a European Health Insurance Card may receive free healthcare services in the United Kingdom (The Commonwealth Fund, 2015).

All drugs available through the NHS are reviewed by the National Institute for Clinical Excellence, which confirms the drugs' clinical efficacy and cost-effectiveness (Morgan et al., 2006). The NHS creates a negative formulary that lists drugs that are excluded from coverage and then determines which drugs it will provide on a subsidized basis to the regional populations commissioning groups (Morgan et al., 2006). In 2009, almost 83% of the medications prescribed in the United Kingdom were generics (Boyle, 2011). Medications prescribed in NHS hospitals are dispensed at no cost. However, there is a copayment approximately $12 per prescription dispensed in an outpatient setting (The Commonwealth Fund, 2015). In 2013, nearly 90% of all prescriptions were dispensed free of charge (The Commonwealth Fund, 2015). Patient groups exempt from copayments for prescription drugs include children under the age of 16, adults over the age of 60, pregnant women, and those with low incomes (The Commonwealth Fund, 2015). Interestingly, the United Kingdom offers quarterly and yearly payment plans to help patients purchase outpatient prescription drugs, which saves the patient money (NHS Choices, 2015c). Prices for pharmaceutical products are negotiated by NHS and drug manufacturers (Jacobzone, 2000). Drug development in the United Kingdom is significant, and the U.K. drug industry continues to be one of the largest producers of pharmaceutical products worldwide, ranking in the top five in 2008 (The Pharmaceutical Industry in Germany, 2011).

Health Education

There has been an increasing number of students that are accepted into medical schools in the United Kingdom (NHS Careers, 2015b). Programs, on average, are 4 to 6 years in duration (Royal College of Obstetricians & Gynaecologists, 2015). The maximum tuition price that schools can charge students is around $14,200, although one school in Scotland offers free education (British Medical Association, 2015). Interestingly, "tuition fee loans [are not] payable until [students] start earning over [$32,960]" and they are "wiped after 30 years" (British Medical Association, 2015). Upon completion of the program, students earn a Bachelor of Medicine and Surgery (NHS Careers, 2015c).

Pharmacy students in the United Kingdom must complete a 4-year Masters of Pharmacy program, "followed by the compulsory 1-year work program prior to application for registration as a pharmacist" (Sosabowski & Gard, 2009). Similar to Germany, students do not need a bachelor's degree upon the acceptance into a program (Global Knowledge Exchange Network, 2009). In 2007, the government suggested that pharmacists undergo revalidation (Global Knowledge Exchange Network, 2009; Pharmaceutical Society of Northern Ireland, 2015); the goal being to "require pharmacists to demonstrate continued fitness to practice" (Global Knowledge Exchange Network, 2009).

Financing

All health care through the NHS is free at the point of delivery to anyone who is a U.K. resident. All taxpayers, employees, and employers contribute to the system. Approximately 84% of the cost of health services is paid by the government (The Commonwealth Fund, 2015). Employers and employees pay most of the rest through premiums (KaiserEDU.org, 2011). Out-of-pocket expenses accounted for 9% of total expenditures, most of which were spent on outpatient medications and medical equipment (The Commonwealth Fund, 2015). Transportation expenses to and from providers are covered through the NHS for low-income patients (The Commonwealth Fund, 2015).

GPs are contracted to provide services to their patients. Most GPs receive a General Medical Services contract. The contract stipulates a capitation payment—based on patient demographics—for essential services, optional fee-for-service for services such as vaccines, and an optional performance-related payment scheme (The Commonwealth Fund, 2015). Performance bonuses can account for up to 25% of income; however, bonuses are expected to decrease in the coming years (The Commonwealth Fund, 2015). General practices are reimbursed monthly on the services they provide patients, which are recorded electronically. Patient demographics are used to determine capitation and are reviewed quarterly (The Commonwealth Fund, 2015). According to the NHS, GPs are paid on a range scale. The salary maximum for GPs is less than what U.S. physicians make, on average (U.S. News, 2013; NHS Careers, 2015a).

Specialists working full-time, however, in the past, were allowed to hold contracts for private practice that account for as much as 10% of their gross income (Booer, 1994). In 2003, a new payment scheme was agreed upon which consisted of basic pay, additional programmed activities, on-call supplements, clinical excellence awards payments, and other fees and allowances (Boyle, 2011). Additionally, there was no longer a restriction on earnings from private practice (Boyle, 2011). The new contracts led to an increase of 8% per year in specialist salaries from 2002 to 2006 (Boyle, 2011).

Public hospitals are divided into two groups: NHS trusts and foundation trusts. NHS trusts rely on heavier control from the central government and foundation trusts are somewhat independent. The government hopes that all hospitals will soon become foundation trusts. The hospitals contract with CCGs that are then reimbursed based on its own form of DRGs, called healthcare resource groups (HRG). NHS England and Monitor, which is an economic regulator of public and private providers, determine the rates of the HRGs (The Commonwealth Fund, 2015).

Current Status

In 2000, the NHS released The NHS Plan, a 10-year plan intended to increase the efficiencies of its services. This plan was followed by two documents, The NHS Improvement Plan and Creating a Patient-led NHS, which outlined the goals of giving patients more choice about their providers and health, increasing the country's health spending, increasing preventive care, expanding patient education for chronic conditions, creating new urgent care strategies, making healthcare services more convenient, and improving coordination of social and healthcare services (Partnership

Development Team, 2011). Other reforms included the establishment of NHS Direct, a free nursing phone line, and future online appointment services through NHSnet, a computer-based network linking NHS organizations (Dobson, 1999). NHSnet has been replaced by N3 (N3, 2011). The United Kingdom has also implemented maximum waiting times for cancer treatments, emergency room treatment, and some elective procedures (Commonwealth Fund, 2015).

Perhaps, one of the most significant changes to the NHS recently was the abolishment of PCTs and the creation of CCGs due to the Health and Social Care Act of 2012. The goal was to allow these groups to better manage resources and have more control over purchasing health care for their local populations (The Commonwealth Fund, 2015). The same Act created NHS England, which would oversee CCGs. Additionally, NHS England has the duty to bestow those involved in the daily operations of the NHS more independence from the government (The Commonwealth Fund, 2015). NHS England was given the responsibility to manage the budget ("budgetary control") and to set rates for HRGs (The Commonwealth Fund, 2015). With the abolishment of PCTs and the creation of the new organizations, about 10,000 staff members lost their job due to redundancies in the system (The Commonwealth Fund, 2015).

The NHS is facing severe budget constraints, and it is feared that the program will prove inadequate to respond to increased technological advances and the aging of the U.K. population. Health care expenditures fell in United Kingdom in 2011, but have since risen (The Commonwealth Fund, 2015). Initiatives have been instituted with the hope of saving funds to help with the rising demand and costs of health care. Goals have been met in terms of the amount saved; however, there is still major concerns due to 65 hospital trusts reporting deficits in 2014 and increasing patient waiting times (The Commonwealth Fund, 2015). Although a guaranteed healthcare package exists, it is not properly codified and differences remain in various parts of the country. As a result, the CCGs are attempting to address these disparities (The Commonwealth Fund, 2015).

Long-term care payments from the NHS have been reducing dramatically (The Commonwealth Fund, 2015). Usually, long-term care is provided by the local authorities or private sector; however, this may present a problem because social care funded from the local authorities is not universal (The Commonwealth Fund, 2015). Additionally, there are strict eligibility criteria to receive full support from a local authority (The Commonwealth Fund, 2015). There are intentions to decrease long-term care costs. The goal of the Care Act of 2014 is to place a cap on long-term care expenses; it will take effect until 2016 and there are concerns as to how much this will alleviate increasing expenditures (The Commonwealth Fund, 2015).

There is a target of treatment within 18 weeks of diagnosis in the United Kingdom, but lack of facilities has resulted in 2015 attaining the highest level of waiting times in 7 years (Siddique, 2015). Maximum wait times are set for cancer and emergency treatments (The Commonwealth Fund, 2015). In 2012, private insurance was utilized by nearly 11% of the population to help alleviate patient waiting times (The Commonwealth Fund, 2015).

Although there is general dissatisfaction with waiting lists and restricted access to certain services, the United Kingdom has been able to achieve health outcomes that exceed those found in the United States (WHO, 2015a). However, when faced with long waiting lists in their own country, many British individuals travel to foreign countries, such as India and other parts of Europe, to seek treatment if they can afford to do so (Rai, 2005). Overall health spending is set by the British Parliament, which has defined efficient use of resources as a policy goal.

A survey of healthcare systems of 11 nations (Australia, Canada, France, Germany, Netherlands, New Zealand, Norway, Sweden, Switzerland, United Kingdom, and United States) was performed in 2013 and found that the United Kingdom had the best overall health care while the United States ranked last. Additionally, the United Kingdom had the best-rated health care in terms of quality and only scored poorly in "healthy lives." (The Commonwealth Fund, 2015; the Commonwealth Fund, 2014). Interestingly, the United Kingdom was placed third in "Timeliness of Care" even though there are growing concerns of patient waiting times. The government's current financial commitment to the existing U.K. system may mean that the country will continue to achieve high health outcomes at a fraction of what the United States spends on health care. In 2013, the government began the Better Care Fund which allocated $5.5 billion for integration projects aimed at improving coordination of health services; the projects will begin in 2016 (The Commonwealth Fund, 2015).

In 2011, a private health care company, Circle, took over the management of a failing NHS hospital (Porter, 2011). In January 2015, Circle decided to pull out of its contract of managing the hospital due to budget constraints (Williams, 2015). The company stated that they could not afford to operate the hospital due to increased demand on emergency services and decreased funding (Williams, 2015).

Currently, certain areas are developing the concept of "years of service," which is a fee for the total cost of care a chronically managed patient receives over 12 months (The Commonwealth Fund, 2015).

Cuba's Healthcare System

Cuba's current healthcare system is the product of the socialist transformations that have occurred in this island nation since the revolution of 1959. This system can be classified as socialized medicine. Cuba's healthcare system is ruled by the following five basic principles:

1. Health care is a right.
2. Health care is the responsibility of the state.
3. Preventive and curative services are integrated.
4. Everyone participates in the function of the healthcare system.
5. Healthcare activities are integrated with economic and social development (Santana, 1987).

Additionally, Cuba has a principle stating global health cooperation being an obligation of the system and its professionals (Keck & Reed, 2012). Two main programs have been instrumental in achieving Cuba's basic healthcare principles: the Medicine in the Community program (1975) and the Family Physician program (1985) (Santana, 1987).

By the end of the 1960s, Cuba's healthcare resources had been aggregated into a single system. The Cuban Ministry of Public Health was established in conjunction with polyclinics (discussed in detail in the next section) that provided primary care services at the local level. The Medicine in the Community program was proposed in 1975 to promote, maintain, and improve individual and community health through individuals' participation in the functioning, organizing, and use of the system. The polyclinics were restructured to become responsible for the total health services of a geographic area and population, as well as teaching and research activities. However, the polyclinics' staffs were not able to integrate fully with the communities they served. Moreover, the number of persons assigned to a community team was sometimes too high, and continuity of care was not easy to achieve (Santana, 1987). The healthcare reform that Cuba underwent was particularly beneficial for rural areas. Prior to the revolution, Cuba only had one rural hospital and infant mortality rate was 100 per 1,000 births (Keck and Reed, 2012). By 1970, the number of rural hospitals increased to 53 (Keck and Reed, 2012). This has dramatically reduced health disparities in Cuba and has likely been a driving force in the country's improved health outcomes.

The Family Physician program of 1985 changed the way primary care was delivered by increasing the number of family physicians and changing the role of the polyclinic. Under this program, a physician–nurse team works in a small office in charge of the medical and public health needs of a geographical area consisting of roughly 1500 persons (Keck and Reed, 2012). In 1990, 50% of the population was covered by the Family Physician program (Roemer, 1993). The program now claims to have enough family physicians to cover almost every neighborhood on the island (Sanchez, 2009). This goal proved difficult to reach, however, given Cuba's economic crisis, which continues to this day.

The restructuring of Cuba's healthcare system after the Cuban revolution of 1959 clearly improved the health of the nation's population. Cuba's health indicators are better than those of all other countries except those with industrial capitalist economies (Nayeri, 1995). In 2012, life expectancy was 77 years for men and 80 years for women in Cuba (WHO, 2015a). From the 1980s to the turn of the century, in the Western Hemisphere, only the United States and Canada have ranked better than Cuba in terms of infant and child mortality indicators (Susser, 1993). Since the early 2000s, Cuba surpassed the United States with greater infant mortality indicators (WHO, 2015a). The health profile of the majority of Cubans resembles that of their counterparts in developed societies; the leading health problems are chronic and degenerative diseases, including heart disease, cancer, and diabetes (Pan American Health Organization, 2012).

Structure: Healthcare Facilities and Workforce

The Family Physician program (Médico de Familia) currently constitutes the backbone of Cuba's healthcare delivery system. Family physicians and nurses are assigned to an office-consultation room (consultorio) in a given community. Living quarters either in the same building or nearby are provided for these caregivers (Ramers, 2001). Family physicians hold office hours during the mornings. In the afternoons, they follow patients in the hospital, make visits, and inspect community facilities such as food stores, pharmacies, and day care centers (Santana, 1987). Thus the family physician is in charge of the complete well-being of the whole community rather than just the health of a given number of patients.

An integral part of the well-being of the community is the concept of prevention. Preventive medicine is a large component of the Cuban health system (Pan American Health Organization, 2012; Keck & Reed, 2012). An example of this can be noted with Cuba's vaccination record. It has been reported that Cuba has vaccinated 98% of infants against 13 diseases (Keck & Reed, 2012). Additionally, Cuba has stressed the importance of HIV/AIDS prevention and reducing transmission strategies (Pan American Health Organization, 2012; Keck & Reed, 2012).

Cuba places a great emphasis on maternal care leading to and after birth. In Cuba, pregnancy is a public health issue, while in other parts of the globe, it is a condition requiring medical care (Bragg et al., 2012). Pregnant women in Cuba are admitted into maternal homes based on risk factors, usually around the 20th week of pregnancy (Bragg et al., 2012), (Otiniano Verissimo et al., 2013).

Patients in need of additional services are generally referred to a polyclinic (policlínico). The polyclinic has evolved into an ancillary facility that provides laboratory and emergency services as well as specialty consultations. In addition, it serves as a setting for physician residency training. Each polyclinic serves 20 to 40 consultorios providing care for 30,000–60,000 people (Atun et al., 2015). Hospital services are also available, but they focus on tertiary care. In 2012, there were 488 polyclinics and 265 hospitals in Cuba (Keck and Reed, 2012).

Cuba prides itself on the advances it has achieved in medically related scientific endeavors. Resources have been allocated to training for primary care and to improving research into and knowledge of new diagnostic and treatment techniques (Santana, 1987). For example, computed tomography scans, organ transplants, and other high-technology facilities are all available in Cuba (Nayeri, 1995).

The healthcare workforce in Cuba has grown dramatically to fulfill the goals of the Family Physician program. Cuba had 76,506 physicians in 2010 (Pan American Health Organization, 2012). Cuba has one of the highest physician per capita ratios in the world (WHO, 2015a).

Health Education

A physician trained through the Family Physician program spends 6 years learning medicine with a preventive, prophylactic, and epidemiologic view. More than half (59%) of family physicians and medical students in Cuba are women (Pan American Health Organization, 2012). However, physicians' salaries remain modest (Santana, 1987).

A unique feature of Cuba's healthcare workforce is its internationalist focus. A number of Cuban physicians participate in a program that sends them abroad for 2 years of service to another country in Latin America, the Caribbean, Africa, the Middle East, or Asia (Nayeri, 1995). Cuba is also involved with the education of foreign doctors. The Escuela Latinoamerciana de Medicina (Latin American School of Medicine), which is sponsored by the Cuban government, was originally established to train doctors of poor origins from Latin American countries affected by Hurricanes George and Mitch in 1998. It has about 9,000 students from 29 countries, including those from Asia, African, and the United States (MEDICC, 2015). U.S. students in the program are exempted from the U.S. government's ban on travel to Cuba (Mullan, 2004).

Financing

The government controls health care in Cuba, so financing for health care is entirely public. Even providers' medical education is paid for by the state, which provides additional financial aid to students with dependents (Nayeri, 1995). National budgets established for healthcare services are an important part of the country's expenditures. Private health care in Cuba is illegal (Atun et al., 2015). Out-of-pocket payments account for around 10% of total health expenditures (Atun et al., 2015).

Current Status

Cuba has been facing an economic crisis originally driven by the following two external factors: the fall of the Soviet bloc and the U.S. economic embargo (Nayeri & Lopez-Pardo, 2005; Nayeri, 1995). Before the Cuban revolution, most of the country's pharmaceutical products were imported; more than 80% came from the United States. Importation of goods, including drugs, shifted to the Soviet Union and Soviet bloc nations before the dissolution of this Soviet alliance in 1991. With the downfall of the Soviet bloc, Cuba lost the main supplier of its basic needs.

Cuba's situation is unique, in that a trade embargo imposed by the United States has influenced Cuba's healthcare system by affecting the flow of medical supplies and related materials to Cuba. This embargo has been in place since the 1960s and is one of the world's few sanctions that explicitly includes both food and medical supplies (Williams, 1997). The embargo was strengthened in the United States by passage of the Cuban Democracy Act of 1992, which prohibited foreign subsidiaries of U.S. companies from trading with Cuba (Barry, 2000). This measure effectively banned Cuba from purchasing half of the new world-class drugs available on the market (Barry, 2000; Williams, 1997). The lack of medical supplies and equipment has also reduced surgical rates in Cuba as well as the country's use of laboratory and radiologic services such as mammography and other diagnostic tools (Williams, 1997).

The Cuban government has tried to preserve both education and healthcare services, despite the ongoing economic crisis. For example, the use of alternative medicine (called traditional medicine in Cuba) has increased (Dresang et al., 2005; Quick, 1997). The Family Physician program has not appeared to be affected by the economic pressures so far (Nayeri & Lopez-Pardo, 2005; Nayeri, 1995). Interestingly, only half of the family physicians live in the geographic area they serve due to a housing shortage (Nayeri & Lopez-Pardo, 2005). Interviews suggest that Cuban patients are generally satisfied with their family physicians and have easy access to them and the polyclinic (Nayeri & Lopez-Pardo, 2005). Some health problems may be related to the scarcity of food supplies. Nevertheless, the infant mortality rate has remained low, at 5 deaths per 1,000 live births in 2013, which is lower than the rate in the United States (5.9 deaths per 1,000) (WHO, 2015a). Restrictions relating to the U.S. embargo on Cuba were further tightened in 2004 (Garfield, 2004); however, the Obama administration favors a different policy toward Cuba (Drain & Barry, 2010). In December 2014, President Obama and President Raúl Castro each announced the restoration of the U.S.–Cuban relationship (Renwick & Lee, 2015). The U.S. has loosened its travel regulations on Americans travelling to Cuba (Renwick & Lee, 2015). In May 2015, President Obama announced that the United States would remove Cuba from the list of State Sponsors of Terrorism, which would allow it to access financial markets (Archibold & Davis, 2015), (BBC News, 2015). After 50 years of no diplomatic relations, the United States and Cuba reopened their embassies in each other's capital, in July 2015 (Renwick & Lee, 2015), (Archibold & Davis, 2015). Even though the trade embargo has not been lifted, these recent changes suggest a positive turn for Cuba's international relations, its economy, and its health care system. It will be interesting to see how the Cuban economy and health care respond to these rapid changes.

INTERNATIONAL HEALTHCARE SYSTEMS: IMPLICATIONS FOR THE UNITED STATES

The United States has a fragmented, multiple-payer healthcare system that makes it difficult to reduce inefficiencies and inappropriate spending (Keeler, 2006). Interestingly, the United States does not have a single health system model; it actually has elements of all four healthcare models—different models for different segments of the population, including:

1. Working Americans who receive insurance benefits through their employment characterize a Bismarck model.
2. Veterans, the military, and Native Americans receive health care through systems that resemble the Beveridge model.
3. The elderly and disabled participating in Medicare and the medically indigent covered by Medicaid are participating in a national health insurance model.
4. Uninsured Americans exemplify the out-of-pocket model representative of most developing nations (Reid, 2009a).

After discussing the health-related issues of developed and developing nations and the major features of four healthcare systems representing a variety of models of healthcare delivery, Chloe (introduced in the case scenario at the beginning of this chapter) has been able to extract several lessons. The same pattern is evident in each of the countries examined—namely, a cycle of unsustainable spending growth, followed by implementation of numerous cost-containment strategies (Anderson et al., 2005).

Policymakers continue to try to determine whether prices, technology, aging, waste, inefficiency, the legal system, new disease patterns, corporate consolidation, or too many consumers and providers are to blame for rising costs (Anderson et al., 2005). In the United States, past cost-containment strategies have focused on increased cost-sharing requirements in an effort to decrease demand for services, albeit so far with negligible results. In comparison, both the United Kingdom and Canada have sought to limit the supply of services, resulting in waiting lists/times for elective procedures.

In 2012, the United States spent $8,845 per capita on health expenditures, whereas Germany spent $4,635 per capita, Canada spent $4,610 per capita, and the United Kingdom spent $3,235 per capita for health care (WHO, 2015a). The United States continues to pay more per capita for health care than any other country. While one might expect the dollar amount spent on health care to be higher in the United States because of higher incomes, the United States still has the highest expenditures when looking at healthcare costs as a percentage of total gross domestic product (GDP)—the total value of all final goods and services produced in a country during a given year. For the United States, the percentage of GDP devoted to health care in 2012 was 17%, which was 50% greater than healthcare expenditures in Canada (10.9%) or Germany (11.3%), and almost twice that of the United Kingdom (9.3%) or Cuba (8.6%) (WHO, 2015a).

Some important lessons can be learned by comparing how health services are structured in the various countries. Both Canada and the United Kingdom set annual budgets that restrict reimbursement and tend to limit supply of certain services, especially elective procedures. By contrast, both the United States and Germany have a plentiful supply of physicians, technology, and health resources. While this ready supply has been cited as a cost driver for these systems, it has also meant that many U.S. residents cannot afford basic medical services. In the United States, resources are distributed in a decidedly nonegalitarian fashion. People who have the ability to pay for services, either through income or insurance, can enjoy the best possible health care in the world. Even after the Patient Protection and Affordable Care Act (commonly known as Affordable Care Act or ACA) provided public or private insurance coverage to many previously uninsured Americans, a significant number of individuals remains uninsured and lack access to even the most basic primary care services. This system stands in contrast to the U.K. system, where approximately 80% of the annual healthcare budget is spent on primary care services, but spending on heroic end-of-life technology is limited.

Another interesting component in the comparisons of systems is the role played by government in financing the systems of care. In this regard, the United States is unique in its reliance on private systems and funding for health care. Generally, as most countries achieve a high per capita income, the government assumes a greater role in financing healthcare services through public expenditures. In the United States, expenditures on health care represented about 47% of total public spending in 2012, compared with about 84% of total public expenditures in the United Kingdom, 70.1% of total public expenditures in Canada, and 76.7% of total public expenditures in Germany. These contrasts in public funding reflect a strong ethos in the United States that emphasizes the private sector's role and responsibility in the healthcare delivery system. This is reflected in the ACA's creation of the Health Insurance Marketplace, "a resource where individuals, families, and small businesses can: learn about their health coverage options; compare health insurance plans based on costs, benefits, and other important features; choose a plan; and enroll in coverage" (Healthcare.gov, 2015). The Marketplace provides private insurance options for previously uninsured Americans but does not change the United States pluralistic, fragmented delivery system and its unique opportunities to shift costs between public and private payers.

While a high per capita income is generally associated with improved health outcomes, both the United States and Cuba, in their own ways, demonstrate that increased expenditures alone cannot improve health outcomes. In Cuba, which has a low per capita income, health outcomes are comparable to those achieved in many developed countries. In contrast, in the United States, having a high per capita income and health care expenditures that exceed those in all other countries has not improved health outcomes considerably. Clearly, how fairly and equitably health resources are distributed is an important consideration when comparing health systems.

CONCLUSION

Although healthcare systems may differ from nation to nation, they enable us to compare and contrast those characteristics that move a system toward the goals of providing affordable, accessible, and equitable health care for all populations. As pointed out by the case scenario at the beginning of the chapter, lessons can be learned from both industrialized and developing countries. Healthcare systems constantly evolve and change. Many factors—including consumer activism, political change, and public and private financing efforts—influence these complex processes. The distribution of healthcare resources both globally and within a particular country has a profound impact on how healthcare services will be delivered and used.

The need for health personnel in a healthcare system, in terms of both the number of providers and the mix of skills, is directed by policy decisions within a particular country. If policies direct greater involvement of pharmacists or other allied health professionals, then significant resource planning must be undertaken to ensure the availability of appropriately trained personnel. Appropriately trained personnel may be among the many constraints that planners face when developing healthcare policies. The disparities in the distribution of healthcare resources will continue to strain all healthcare systems, but particularly those in developing countries where competing social and economic programs are equally justified for funding.

QUESTIONS FOR FURTHER DISCUSSION

1. Is a ranking of a country's healthcare system based on the amount of money spent per capita on health care a fair measurement of how a healthcare system performs?
2. Are there components or features of the healthcare delivery systems discussed in this chapter that could be adopted to improve healthcare delivery in the United States?

KEY TOPICS AND TERMS

Beveridge model
Bismark model
Decentralized national health program
Developed nation
Developing nation
Gross domestic product (GDP)
Infant mortality rate
Life expectancy
National health insurance model
Out-of-pocket model
Portability
Sickness funds
Social partnership
Social solidarity
Socialized health insurance
Socialized medicine
Universality

REFERENCES

Allen, D. (1984). Health services in England. In M. W. Raffel (Ed.), *Comparative health systems* (pp. 197–257). University Park, PA: Pennsylvania State University Press.

American Pharmacist Association (APhA). (2014). A tale of two countries: The path to pharmacist prescribing in the United Kingdom and Canada. *Pharmacy Today*. Retrieved from http://www.pharmacist.com/tale-two-countries-path-pharmacist-prescribing-united-kingdom-and-canada

Anderson, G., Hussey, P., Krogner, B., & Waters, H. (2005). Health spending in the United States and the rest of the industrialized world. *Health Affairs*, *24*(4), 903–914.

Anis, A. H. (2000). Pharmaceutical policies in Canada: Another example of federal–provincial discord. *Canadian Medical Association Journal*, *162*(4), 523–526.

Archibold, R. C., and Davis, J. H. (2015). Cuba to be removed from U.S. list of nations that sponsor terrorism. *The New York Times*. Retrieved from http://www.nytimes.com/2015/04/15/world/americas/obama-cuba-remove-from-state-terror-list.html?_r=0

Association of American Medical Colleges (AAMC). (2015). Tuition and student fees reports. Table 1: U.S. medical school schools tuition and student fees - first year students 2010–2011 and 2009–2010. Retrieved form https://services.aamc.org/tsfreports/report_median.cfm?year_of_study=2011

Atun, R., Monteiro de Andrade, L. O., Almeida, G., et al. (2015). Health-system reform and universal health coverage in Latin America. *The Lancet, 385*, 1230–1247.

Barry, M. (2000). Effect of the U.S. embargo and economic decline on health in Cuba. *Annals of Internal Medicine, 132*(2), 151–154.

Bäumler, M., Sundmacher, L., and Zander, B. (2010) Major reform of German SHI contributions. *Health Policy Monitor*. Retrieved from http://www.hpm.org/survey/de/a16/2

BBC News. (2015). *US removes Cuba from list of state sponsors of terrorism*. Retrieved from http://www.bbc.com/news/world-us-canada-32926821

Beske, F. (1988). Federal Republic of Germany. In R. B. Saltman (Ed.), *The international handbook of health-care systems* (pp. 93–106). Westport, CT: Greenwood Press.

Bindman, A. B., & Weiner, J. P. (2000). The modern NHS: An underfunded model of efficiency and integration. *Health Affairs, 19*(30), 120–122.

Booer, T. (1994). The health care systems in the United Kingdom. In U. K. Hoffmeyer & T. R. McCarthy (Eds.), *Financing health care* (pp. 1071–1145). Dordrecht, Netherlands: Kluwer.

Boyle, S. (2011). United Kingdom (England): Health system review. *Health Systems in Transition, 13*(1), 1–514.

Bragg, M., Salke, T. R., Cotton, C. P., & Jones, D. A. (2012). No child or mother left behind; implications for the US from Cuba's maternity homes. *Health Promotion Perspectives, 2*(1), 09–19.

British Medical Association. (2015). *Applying to medical school. What you need to know*. Retrieved from http://bma.org.uk/developing-your-career/medical-student/how-to-become-a-doctor/applying-to-medical-school

Busse, R. (2004). Disease management programs in Germany's statutory health insurance system. *Health Affairs, 23*(3), 56–67.

Busse, R., & Blümel, M. (2014). Germany health system review. *Health Systems in Transition, 16*(2), 1–296.

Canadian-healthcare. (2006). *Canadian health care*. Retrieved from http://www.canadian-healthcare.org

Canadian Institute for Health Information. (2009). *Experiences with primary health care in Canada*. Retrieved from https://secure.cihi.ca/estore/productFamily.htm?pf=PFC1332&lang=fr&media=0

Canadian Institute for Health Information. (2014). *Wait times for priority procedures in Canada, 2014*. Retrieved from https://secure.cihi.ca/free_products/2014_WaitTimesAiB_EN.pdf

Canadian Pharmacists Association. (2015). *Pharmacy in Canada. Becoming a pharmacist in Canada*. Retrieved from http://www.pharmacists.ca/index.cfm/pharmacy-in-canada/becoming-a-pharmacist-in-canada/

Chenot, J. F. (2009). Undergraduate medical education in Germany. *German Medical Science*, 7:Doc02. doi: 10.3205/000061. Retrieved from http://www.egms.de/static/en/journals/gms/2009-7/000061.shtml

The Commonwealth Fund. (2015). *International profiles of health care systems, 2014*. Retrieved from http://www.commonwealthfund.org/~/media/files/publications/fund-report/2015/jan/1802_mossialos_intl_profiles_2014_v7.pdf

The Commonwealth Fund. (2014). *Mirror, mirror, on the wall, 2014 update: How the U.S. health care system compares internationally*. Retrieved from http://www.commonwealthfund.org/publications/fund-reports/2014/jun/mirror-mirror

Dalhousie University. (2015). Undergraduate medical education. *MD program*. Retrieved from http://medicine.dal.ca/departments/core-units/undergraduate/program.html

Demers V., Melo M., Jackevicius C., Cox J., Kalavrouziotis, D., Rinfret, S., Humphries, K., et al. (2008). Comparison of provincial prescription drug plans and the impact on patients' annual drug expenditures. *Canadian Medical Association Journal, 178*(4), 405–409.

Dobson, F. (1999). Modernizing Britain's national health services. *Health Affairs, 18*(3), 40–41.

Dresang, L. T., Brebrick, L., Murray, D., Shallue, A., & Sullivan-Vedder, L. (2005). Family medicine in Cuba: Community-oriented primary care and complementary and alternative medicine. *Journal of the American Board of Family Practice, 18*, 297–303.

Drain, P. K., & Barry, M. (2010). Fifty years of U.S. embargo: Cuba's health outcomes and lessons. *Science, 328*, 572–573.

Enthoven, A. C. (2000). In pursuit of an improving national health service. *Health Affairs, 19*(3), 102–119.

Facts about Germany. (2011). *Medical care for everyone*. Retrieved from http://www.tatsachen-ueber-deutschland.de/en/society/main-content-08/medical-care-for-everyone.html

Garfield, R. (2004). Health care in Cuba and the manipulation of humanitarian imperatives. *Lancet, 364*, 1007.

Global Knowledge Exchange Network. (2009). *An overview of education and training requirements for global healthcare professionals: Pharmacists*. Retrieved from http://www.gken.org/Docs/Workforce/Pharmacy%20Education%20FINAL%20102609.pdf

Göpffarth, D., & Henke, K-D. (2012). The German Central Health Fund – recent developments in health care financing in Germany. *Health Policy, 109*(3), 246–252.

Harrison, S. (1988). Great Britain. In R. B. Saltman (Ed.), *The international handbook of health-care systems* (pp. 123–143). Westport, CT: Greenwood Press.

Harvard School of Public Health. (2000). *Burden of disease unit*. Retrieved from http://www.hsph.harvard.edu/organizations/bdu/index/htm

Health Canada. (2006a). *Access to insurance coverage for prescription medicines*. Retrieved from http://www.hc-sc.gc.ca/hcs-sss/pharma/acces/index-eng.php

Health Canada. (2006b). *2003 First Ministers' Accord on health care renewal*. Retrieved from http://www.hc-sc.gc.ca/hcs-sss/delivery-prestation/fptcollab/2003accord/index-eng.php

Healthcare.gov. (2015). *Health insurance marketplace*. Retrieved from https://www.healthcare.gov/glossary/health-insurance-marketplace-glossary/

Healthcare Salaries. (2015). *Physician salary based on geographic location*. Retrieved from http://www.healthcare-salaries.com/physicians/physician-salary-based-on-geographic-location

Henschke, C., Sundmacher, L., & Busse, R. (2012). Structural changes in the German pharmaceutical market: Price setting mechanisms based on the early benefit evaluation. *Health Policy, 109*(3), 263–269.

Hilts, P. J. (2000, June 21). Europeans perform highest in ranking of world health. *The New York Times*, p. 9.

Himmelstein, D. U., Jun, M., Busse R., et al. (2014, September). A comparison of hospital administrative costs in eight nations: U.S. costs exceed all others by far." *Health Affairs, 33*(9), 1586–1594.

Hoffmeyer, U. (1994). The health care system in Germany. In U. K. Hoffmeyer & T. R. McCarthy (Eds.), *Financing health care* (pp. 419–512). Dordrecht, Netherlands: Kluwer.

Iglehart, J. K. (2000). Revisiting the Canadian health care system. *New England Journal of Medicine, 342*(26), 2007–2012.

International Pharmaceutical Federation. (2012). *2012 FIP global pharmacy workforce report*. Retrieved from http://www.fip.org/files/members/library/FIP_workforce_Report_2012.pdf

Jackson, J. (1997). The German health system: Lessons for reform in the United States. *Archives of Internal Medicine, 157*(2), 155–161.

Jacobzone, S. (2000). *Pharmaceutical policies in OECD countries: Reconciling social and industrial goals* (Vol. *40*, pp. 1–98). Paris, France: Organization for Economic Cooperation and Development.

Jost, T. (1998). German health care reform: The next steps. *Journal of Health Politics, Policy and Law, 23*(4), 697–711.

KaiserEDU.org (2011). *International Health Systems–UK*. Retrieved from http://www.kaiseredu.org/Issue-Modules/International-Health-Systems/UK.aspx

Keck, C. W., & Reed, G. A. (2012). The curious case of Cuba. *American Journal of Public Health*. Vol. *102*, No. 8.

Keeler, E. (2006). Can we say no? The challenge of rationing health care. *The New England Journal of Medicine, 354*(12), 1327–1328.

Krauss, C. (2005, June 10). *In blow to Canada's health system, Quebec law is voided*. Retrieved from http://www.nytimes.com/2005/06/10/international/americas/10canada.html

Légaré, J. -F., Li, D., & Buth, K. J. (2010). How established wait time benchmarks significantly underestimate total wait times for cardiac surgery. *The Canadian Journal of Cardiology, 26*(1), e17–e21.

Maclean's. (2010). *How much does medical school cost?* Retrieved from http://www.macleans.ca/news/canada/how-much-they-pay-for-it/

Marchildon, G. (2013). Canada health system review. *Health Systems in Transition, 15*(1)

Med School Admissions. (2015). *Admission requirements*. Retrieved from http://medschooladmissions.com/admissions/admissions-requirements

Medical Education Cooperation with Cuba (MEDICC). (2015). *Mentors welcome: MEDICC launches program for US students & grads of Latin American medical school*. Retrieved from http://medicc.org/ns/?p=244

Morgan, S. G., Martin, D., Gagnon, M. A., Mintzes, B., Daw, J. R., & Lexchin, J. (2015). The future of drug coverage in Canada. *Pharmacare 2020*.

Morgan, S., McMahon, M., Mitton, C., Roughead, E., Kirk, R., Kanavos, P., & Menon, D. (2006). Centralized drug review processes in Australia, Canada, New Zealand, and the United Kingdom. *Health Affairs, 25*(2), 337–348.

Mullan, F. (2004). Affirmative action, Cuban style. *New England Journal of Medicine, 351*(26), 2680–2682.

N3. (2011). *The N3 Story*. Retrieved from http://n3.nhs.uk/n3scotland/TheN3Story/TheN3Story.cfm

National Association of Community Health Centers (NACHC). (2014). *Access is the answer: Community health center, primary care & the future of American health care*. Retrieved from http://www.nachc.com/client/PIBrief14.pdf

Nayeri, K. (1995). The Cuban health care system and factors currently undermining it. *Journal of Community Health, 20*(4), 321–334.

Nayeri, K., & Lopez-Pardo, C.M. (2005). Economic crisis and access to care: Cuba's health care system since the collapse of the Soviet Union. *International Journal of Health Services, 35*(4), 797–816.

Naylor, C. D. (1999). Health care in Canada: Incrementalism under fiscal duress. *Health Affairs, 18*(3), 9–26.

Newman, D. (2010). Health-care reform, Canadian-style. *CBC news*. Retrieved from http://www.cbc.ca/canada/story/2010/04/15/f-vp-newman.html

NHS Careers. (2015a). *Pay for doctors*. Retrieved from http://www.nhscareers.nhs.uk/explore-by-career/doctors/pay-for-doctors/

NHS Careers. (2015b). *Undergraduate medical education*. Retrieved from http://www.nhscareers.nhs.uk/explore-by-career/doctors/training-to-become-a-doctor/undergraduate-medical-education/

NHS Careers. (2015c). *Entry requirements for medical school*. Retrieved from http://www.nhscareers.nhs.uk/explore-by-career/doctors/training-to-become-a-doctor/undergraduate-medical-education/entry-requirements-for-medical-school/

NHS Choices. (2015a). *The NHS in England. The NHS structure explained*. Retrieved from http://www.nhs.uk/NHSEngland/thenhs/about/Pages/nhsstructure.aspx

NHS Choices. (2015b). *The NHS in England. About the National Health Service (NHS)*. Retrieved from http://www.nhs.uk/NHSEngland/thenhs/about/Pages/overview.aspx

NHS Choices. (2015c). *Help with health costs. Get help with prescription costs*. Retrieved from http://www.nhs.uk/NHSEngland/Healthcosts/Pages/Prescriptioncosts.aspx

NHS England (2015). *News: Bulletin for CCGs Issue 31, 28 March 2013*. Retrieved from http://www.england.nhs.uk/2013/03/28/ccg-bulletin-issue-31/#authorised

Organization for Economic Cooperation and Development (OECD). (1994). *The reform of health care systems*. Paris, France: Organization for Economic Cooperation and Development.

OECD iLibrary. (2009). *Health at a Glance 2009: OECD indicators. Health workforce: Pharmacists*. Retrieved from http://www.oecd-ilibrary.org/sites/health_glance-2009-en/03/13/index.html?contentType=&itemId=%2Fcontent%2Fchapter%2Fhealth_glance-2009-35-en&mimeType=text%-2Fhtml&containerItemId=%2Fcontent%2Fchapter%2Fhealth_glance-2009-35-en&accessItemIds=)&_csp_=5c9679a1d4ee0a51898d11a5169f9d20

OECD. (2015). *Health Statistics*. Retrieved from http://www.oecd.org/els/health-systems/health-statistics.htm

Otiniano Verissimo, A.D., Currie, D., & the 2010 APHA Delegation to Cuba. (2013). Continuing the dialogue on health: Insights from the 2010 APHA delegation to Cuba. American Journal of Public Health. 103(7), 1168–1171.

Partnership Development Team. (2011). *Latest information and useful resources*. Retrieved from http://www.pdteam.org.uk/news/nhsimprovementplan.htm

Pan American Health Organization. (2012). *Health in the Americas: Cuba*. Retrieved from http://www.paho.org/saludenlasamericas/index.php?option=com_docman&task=doc_view&gid=125&Itemid=

PayScale. (2014). *Family physician/doctor salary (Canada)*. Retrieved from http://www.payscale.com/research/CA/Job=Family_Physician_%2F_Doctor/Salary

The Pharmaceutical Industry in Germany. (2011). *Germany Trade and Invest.* Issue 2011.

Poduval, S., Howard, N., Jones, L., Murwill, P., McKee, M., Legido-Quigley, H. (2015). Experiences among undocumented migrants accessing primary care in the United Kingdom: A qualitative study. *International Journal of Health, 45*(2), 320–333.

Porter, A. (2011). Private company to take over "failing" NHS hospital. *The Telegraph.* Retrieved from http://www.telegraph.co.uk/news/health/news/8880225/Private-company-to-take-over-failing-NHS-hospital.html

Pharmaceutical Society of Northern Ireland. (2015). *Revalidation/Continuing fitness to practise.* Retrieved from http://www.psni.org.uk/cpd/revalidation/

Quick, R. (1997). A health care revolution. *Nursing Times, 93*(29), 17.

Rai, S. (2005, April 7). *Low costs lure foreigners to India for medical care.* Retrieved from http://www.nytimes.com/2005/04/07/business/worldbusiness/low-costs-lure-foreigners-to-india-for-medical-care.html

Ramers, C. (2001). Medicina Cubana: A fresh perspective. *The Western Journal of Medicine, 175*(2), 129.

Reid, T. R. (2009a). Different models, common principles. In *The healing of America; a global quest for better, cheaper and fairer health care* (pp. 16–27). New York, NY: The Penguin Press.

Reid, T. R. (2009b). Germany: Applied Christianity. In *The healing of America; a global quest for better, cheaper and fairer health care* (pp. 16–27). New York, NY: The Penguin Press.

Renwick, D. & Lee, B. (2015). *U.S.-Cuba relations. Council on foreign relations.* Retrieved from http://www.cfr.org/cuba/us-cuba-relations/p11113

Roemer, M. I. (1993). Primary health care and hospitalization: California and Cuba. *American Journal of Public Health, 83*(3), 317–318.

Royal College of Obstetricians and Gynaecologists. (2015). *Medical education in the UK: An overview.* Retrieved from https://www.rcog.org.uk/en/careers-training/considering-a-career-in-og/medical-education-in-the-uk-an-overview/

Rozek, R., & Mulhern, C. (1994). The health care system in Canada. In U. K. Hoffmeyer & T. R. McCarthy (Eds.), *Financing health care* (pp. 255–344). Dordrecht, Netherlands: Kluwer.

Sanchez, R. (2009). Army of Cuban doctors hunt for possible swine flu carriers. *Sun Sentinel.com.* Retrieved from http://www.sun-sentinel.com/news/nationworld/sfl-cuba-swine-flu-051309-story.html

Santana, S. M. (1987). The Cuban health care system: Responsiveness to changing population needs and demands. *World Development, 15*(1), 113–125.

Schieber, G., & Maeda, A. (1999). Health care financing and delivery in developing countries. *Health Affairs, 18*, 193–205.

Schoen, C., Osborn, R., Squires, D., Doty, M. M., Pierson, R., & Applebaum, S. (2010). How health insurance design affects access to care and costs, by income, in eleven countries. *Health affairs. 29*(12), 2323–2334.

Siddique, H. (2015). NHS hospital waiting time figures worst in seven years. *The Guardian.* Retrieved from http://www.theguardian.com/society/2015/apr/09/nhs-hospital-waiting-time-figures.

Smith, A. (2014). Postbaccalaureate PharmD Programs for Canadian Pharmacists: Options and Considerations. *The Canadian Journal of Hospital Pharmacy, 67*(4), 313–314.

Sosabowski, M. H., & Gard, P. R. (2008). Pharmacy education in the United Kingdom. *American Journal of Pharmaceutical Education, 72*(6), 130.

Spivey, R. N., Wertheimer, A. I., & Rucker, T. D. (1992). *International pharmaceutical services: Drug industry and pharmacy practice in 23 major countries of the world.* New York, NY: Haworth Press.

Starfield B. (2010). Reinventing primary care: Lessons from Canada for the United States. *Health Affairs, 29*(5),1030–1036.

Susser, M. (1993). Health as a human right: An epidemiologist's perspective on the public health. *American Journal of Public Health, 83*(3), 418–426.

University of Toronto. (2015a). *Undergraduate medical education. Frequently asked questions.* Retrieved from http://www.md.utoronto.ca/admissions/information/faq.htm#prerequ

University of Toronto. (2015b). *PharmD. Current students.* Retrieved from http://pharmacy.utoronto.ca/pharmd/current-students

University of Calgary. (2015). *Introduction to the curriculum. Year 3 (Clerkship).* Retrieved from http://www.ucalgary.ca/mdprogram/current-student/introduction-curriculum/year-3-clerkship

U.S. News. (2013). *Physician salary.* Retrieved from http://money.usnews.com/careers/best-jobs/physician/salary

Williams, C. (2015). First private operator of NHS pulls out amid cuts. *The Telegraph*. Retrieved from http://www.telegraph.co.uk/finance/newsbysector/supportservices/11334622/Private-operator-of-Hinchingbooke-Hospital-pulls-out.html

Williams, R. (1997). In the shadow of plenty: Cuba copes with a crippled health care system. *Canadian Medical Association*, *157*(3), 291–293.

World Bank. (2015). *Updated income classifications*. Retrieved from http://data.worldbank.org/news/2015-country-classifications

World Bank. (2015). *Hospital beds (per 1,000 people)*. Retrieved from http://data.worldbank.org/indicator/SH.MED.BEDS.ZS?page=1&order=wbapi_data_value_2011%20wbapi_data_value&sort=asc

World Health Organization. (2000a). *The world health report 2000, health systems: Improving performance*. Geneva, Switzerland: WHO.

World Health Organization. (2000b, June 21). France, Italy provide best healthcare. *Reuters*.

World Health Organization. (2009). *World health statistics: Table 2 cause-specific mortality and morbidity*. Retrieved from http://www.who.int/whosis/whostat/EN_WHS09_Table2.pdf

World Health Organization. (2014). *Maternal mortality*. Retrieved from http://www.who.int/mediacentre/factsheets/fs348/en/

World Health Organization. (2015a). *World health statistics*. Retrieved from http://www.who.int/gho/publications/world_health_statistics/2015/en/

World Health Organization. (2015b). *World Health Statistics, 2015–Part II: Global Health Indicators*. Retrieved from http://www.who.int/gho/publications/world_health_statistics/EN_WHS2015_Part2.pdf?ua=1

Zander, B., Kimmerle, J., Sundmacher, L., Bäumler, M. (2009). Health policy in Germany after the election. *Health Policy Monitor*. Retrieved from http://www.hpm.org/en/Surveys/TU_Berlin_-_D/14/Health_Policy_in_Germany_after_the_election.html

CHAPTER

21

Healthcare Reform

Catherine N. Otto and Thomas E. Buckley*

LEARNING OBJECTIVES

Upon completion of this chapter, the student shall be able to:

- Describe the effects of lack of access to health care in the United States.
- Compare and contrast demand and need with respect to healthcare delivery.
- Identify potential outcomes of proposals addressing the insolvency of the Medicare program.
- Discuss the federal government's provisions to support health care as a right: Kerr-Mills Act, Medicare, Medicaid, and Patient Protection and Affordable Care Act (ACA).
- Summarize the key components of federally proposed cost-containment methods for health care.
- Explain the key concepts of uncompensated care pools, employer mandates, and Medicaid waivers.
- Discuss methods to increase access to health insurance in Massachusetts and Vermont.
- Define employer and employee mandates, health savings accounts (HSA), and portability of health insurance coverage.

CHAPTER QUESTIONS

1. Why is healthcare reform an issue in the United States?
2. What state and federal healthcare reform efforts have been introduced in the past?
3. What solutions have been proposed in the healthcare reform debate?
4. How can pharmacists influence healthcare reform? What responsibility do pharmacists have? Why is pharmacist participation in the healthcare reform debate important?

*The authors acknowledge the contributions of Craig A. Pedersen to this chapter in previous editions of this text.

INTRODUCTION

An in-depth discussion of the topics covered in this chapter could fill an entire book. In many ways, this chapter integrates material from other chapters of this text as well as information on history, politics, financing, and the structure of the U.S. healthcare system. It discusses the problems of the U.S. healthcare system, the politics of healthcare reform, past landmark efforts to reform the U.S. healthcare system, current reform efforts, and pharmacy's role in reform efforts. This chapter can serve as an introductory guide to this textbook or as a capstone to the information provided elsewhere in this text.

This chapter does not endorse any particular side on any of the controversial issues, nor does it hold the answers to the complex problems the United States faces today regarding health care for its citizens. Instead, this chapter seeks to outline the issues, suggest questions for debate, and stimulate readers to look deep within themselves and their core values to come to a reasonable and rational opinion on these issues. Finally, it suggests that pharmacists have the opportunity and responsibility to work proactively to ensure that the profession of pharmacy plays an integral part in the future of health care in the United States.

IDENTIFICATION OF THE PROBLEM

The people and the government of the United States are unique in their approach to health and health care. The United States is the only developed country that does not ensure access to health care through guaranteed coverage. This structural uniqueness of the U.S. healthcare system fragments the financing system and makes it difficult for the poor and the sick to seek preventive care. Thus, expensive safety nets that drive up costs and aggravate the problem of cost shifting are required.

As discussed in the chapter about international healthcare systems, the United States spends more of its gross domestic product on health care and has higher per capita expenditures on health care than any other industrialized nation (Anderson & Poullier, 1999; OECD Health Statistics, 2015). The cost of health care in the United States has been increasing since the early 1960s. This rise can be attributed to multiple factors, including an aging population, patient demand for the best care available, technological advancements, increasing therapeutic options, and general and healthcare inflation.

Yet, although the U.S. levels of spending exceed those of other industrialized nations and cost increases outstrip the growth of other components of the U.S. economy, researchers report that Americans are generally dissatisfied with the healthcare system (Donelan, Blendon, Schoen, Davis, & Binns, 1999; Smith, Altman, Leitman, Moloney, & Taylor, 1992). This dissatisfaction is rooted in the high cost of health care, lack of universal access, and lack of demonstrated gains in life expectancy. Life expectancy at birth for female Americans was 81.2 years in 2013. The United States ranked below the Organization for Economic Cooperation and Development (OECD) median of 83.0 years for women, and behind Japan (86.6 years), France (85.6 years), Sweden (83.8 years), Germany (83.2 years), and Canada (83.6 years). At birth, males have considerably shorter life expectancies of 76.4 years in the United States, compared with the Organization for Economic Cooperation and Development median of 77.8 years (OECD Health Statistics, 2015). Meanwhile, the United States has spent a considerably larger percentage of its gross domestic product on health care than these other countries, 16.4% of its GDP in 2013 compared to the median of 8.9% for OECD countries (OECD Health Statistics, 2015). Clearly, the United States has not gained in life expectancy from the additional money spent. Therefore, a crisis appears to exist in U.S. health care.

AN ISSUE OF ACCESS

Although the purpose of the ACA was to increase accessibility to health care; access to health care in the United States continues to be determined by age, economic status, and race/ethnicity. The enactment of Medicare and Medicaid in 1965 addressed some of the access issues for the elderly and the indigent. Even so, the number of uninsured Americans has increased from 27 million in 1977 to about 46 million in 2008, 17.3% of the population (Kaiser Commission on Medicaid and the Uninsured, 2009b). The percentage of nonelderly uninsured individuals peaked at 18.2% in 2010 and dropped to 16.7% in 2013 prior to the implementation of the ACA (Kaiser Commission on Medicaid and the Uninsured, 2015).

Thirty-two million nonelderly individuals were uninsured in 2014, the first year of implementation of the ACA (Kaiser Commission on Medicaid and the Uninsured, 2015). Of those who are uninsured, approximately 80% have incomes below 400% of the poverty level and more than 50% are people of color (Kaiser Commission on Medicaid and the Uninsured, 2015). Uninsured individuals are more likely to live in states that did not expand their Medicaid programs during the implementation of the ACA, live in the southern states, and to have been uninsured for more than 5 years (Kaiser Commission on Medicaid and the Uninsured, 2015).

Lack of access to health care in the United States is a high-profile issue for several reasons. First, health insurance coverage is an important determinant of access to care. Second, lack of adequate health coverage puts individuals at risk for high medical expenses. Third, everyone ends up paying for costs shifted because of uncompensated care (Brown & Wyn, 1996).

THE BEST HEALTH CARE?

Does the United States have the best healthcare system in the world? Many say yes—we are the leaders. We have the latest and best treatment available anywhere in the world. Fuchs (1992) agrees that the United States is the leader in technological advances related to medicine. Physicians come from around the world to receive the most advanced training. Very wealthy patients come from around the world to receive care in the United States. At the same time, Fuchs suggests other dimensions in which the United States may not be the best: public health, service, efficiency, and distribution equity.

The United States ranks below average among developed countries in most public health measures. Frequently, access to providers is limited, and many providers lack the caring nature that patients desire. If the U.S. healthcare system were efficient, it seems that we should be able to spend amounts comparable to those spent by other countries to achieve the same level of public health. Also, the distribution of health care in the United States is clearly not equal. The large number of uninsured and underinsured Americans is evidence of this fact. Thus, Fuchs suggests, for the United States to claim to have the best healthcare system, improvements in efficiency (controlling the high cost of care), distributional equity (providing universal coverage), service, and public health are necessary (Fuchs, 1992).

The United States clearly has made judgments about the nature of access to its healthcare system. Structurally, health care is a privilege in the United States and not a right. Nevertheless, many question the wisdom of not providing universal health coverage for all Americans.

DEMAND VERSUS NEED

In the late 1960s, economists began analyzing demand versus need—an important component to understanding access to medical care in the United States. Needs are normative judgments concerning the quantity of medical services that ought to be consumed (Jeffers, Bognanno, & Bartlett, 1971). Frequently, needs are fixed by policy makers. An example is the need for prenatal care.

Society and policy makers believe that every pregnant woman needs prenatal care. It is difficult to object to this position because, without such care, the health of the unborn infant can be at risk.

Need is often criticized by economists as being too mechanical, as denying the individuality and autonomy of the patient, and as characterizing the human body as a machine that needs fuel in the form of food and repairs in the form of medication or surgery. Demand, by comparison, implies patient autonomy, choice, and tailoring inputs to individual preferences (Blue Boulding, 1996). Demand, therefore, is the quantity of medical services that patients think they ought to consume based on their perceptions of their healthcare needs (Jeffers, Bognanno, & Bartlett, 1971). Individual tastes and preferences determine utilization.

HEALTHCARE REFORM EFFORTS BY THE FEDERAL GOVERNMENT

In an effort to eliminate some of the economic barriers to medical care for the elderly and medically indigent, the federal government has addressed the notion of health care as a right and not a privilege, at least for some people in the United States. Enactment of the Kerr-Mills Act and establishment of the Medicare and Medicaid programs in the 1960s paved the way for health care to be perceived as a basic human right.

Kerr-Mills Act

Amendments to the Social Security Act (SSA) in 1960 provided healthcare coverage to elderly indigent individuals. This landmark legislation, known as the Kerr-Mills Act, was the first to provide health care to elderly or indigent persons on a broad scale. Many critics were concerned that the states would not implement this legislation in a timely manner. These predictions were confirmed. Many states had failed to adopt Kerr-Mills by 1963, when 90% of the funds were received by the five largest industrialized states (Starr, 1982).

Kerr-Mills did not provide healthcare coverage to the nonindigent elderly or the indigent nonelderly. These groups were not covered until amendments to the SSA in 1965 established Medicare coverage for elderly persons (regardless of income) and Medicaid coverage for the poor.

Medicare and Medicaid

Medicare and Medicaid were significant healthcare reform programs. Before 1960, many elderly people in the United States lacked any kind of health insurance coverage. The Kerr-Mills Act and its successor, Medicare, addressed this need. Medicare Part A covers hospitalization, and Medicare Part B covers outpatient and physician bills. The third layer of reform was Medicaid, which covers indigent persons.

These programs reflected contrasting traditions. Medicare had popular support, and Social Security had made it acceptable for the elderly to receive government retirement benefits. Medicaid, however, was burdened by the stigma of public assistance (Starr, 1982). Medicare had uniform national criteria for eligibility, whereas Medicaid allowed states to determine the breadth of their programs. These differences persist today.

The Cost-Containment Era

By the early 1970s, Americans understood that their healthcare system was in a financial crisis. One survey in 1970 found that approximately three fourths of heads of households agreed with the statement, "There is a crisis in health care in the United States" (Starr, 1982). Terms used to describe costs included *skyrocketing* and *runaway inflation*. Medical care had become very expensive, and costs were exceeding inflation at an alarming rate. Coupled with worries about high prices for medical care were concerns about access, such as the diminishing number of primary care practitioners and patients' inability to obtain care from a physician on the weekends or in the evenings (Starr, 1982).

During this era, cost containment became a primary concern. Several strategies were implemented to control rising costs. They included voluntary hospital planning, wage and price freezes, changes in the amounts and methods of reimbursement for services, development of more cost-effective healthcare delivery systems, and regulatory programs such as utilization review and controls on hospital capital expenditures. Ultimately, most of those strategies proved unsuccessful in controlling costs.

Another significant healthcare reform effort was the 1972 amendments to the SSA, which established professional standards review organizations. Professional standards review organizations were a national network of utilization review programs that had dual responsibility for medical cost containment and quality assurance. This program did not work, however, and it was replaced in 1983 by peer review organizations with a local focus.

Yet another cost-containment program was Section 1122 of the 1972 amendments to the SSA, which required states to review proposed capital improvement expenditures of healthcare organizations and to provide authorization through a certificate of need at the state level. The certificate-of-need program was intended to reduce unnecessary duplication of services but was unsuccessful in meeting this goal. Some states have since eliminated the certificate-of-need requirements for capital improvements.

In 1973, President Richard Nixon signed the Health Maintenance Organization (HMO) Act. The HMO Act encouraged the use of these lower-cost healthcare delivery systems and provided financial assistance for the development of nonprofit HMOs. This act constituted the federal government's first effort to develop an alternative to fee-for-service medicine (Iglehart, 1982). Healthcare reimbursement would be forever changed by this act.

Diagnosis-Related Groups

These cost-containment efforts did not appreciably restrain the growth of healthcare costs in the United States. By contrast, the 1983 implementation of diagnosis-related groups (DRGs)—a type of prospective payment system for hospital services—was a landmark effort to control hospital reimbursement under Medicare. Medicare established a fixed schedule of fees to be paid to hospitals, where the fee varied for each diagnosis. If the actual cost to the hospital is less than the set fee, the hospital keeps the difference; if the service costs more than the set fee, the hospital absorbs the loss.

The objective of DRGs is to promote rational use of healthcare dollars and to stimulate competition among hospitals. Under this system, hospitals are reimbursed on an episode-of-care rather than a fee-for-service basis, placing the hospital at risk for inpatient healthcare costs.

DRG-based reimbursement has substantially slowed the growth of hospital expenditures, but physician expenditures, which are not uniformly subject to prospective payment incentives, continue to grow. Concern also exists about hospitals dumping patients and discharging patients early (Epstein, Bogen, Dreyer, & Thorpe, 1991). Inappropriate use of these mechanisms without proper controls has the potential to hurt quality of care.

Portability of Coverage

The Health Insurance Portability and Accountability Act (HIPAA) of 1996 addressed the following three issues in the healthcare reform debate: (1) preexisting condition exclusions, (2) elimination of health discrimination applications to eligibility rules, and (3) guaranteed renewability for plans that cover more than one employee. Later, HIPAA was expanded to address patient confidentiality issues.

Under HIPAA, individuals cannot be denied coverage because they have a preexisting medical condition if they agree to an exclusionary period (also known as an elimination period) for that condition, which cannot exceed 1 year. After a year, the policy holder can no longer be denied coverage for the preexisting condition. As long as the policyholder remains continuously enrolled in a plan, with breaks no longer than 63 days, the exclusion period cannot be reimposed. In short, HIPAA guarantees that policies and benefits available to a specific group cannot be withheld if an exclusionary period has already been met.

The second part of the act addresses the discriminatory practice of eliminating individuals and groups from the insurance market based on risk, preexisting conditions, or utilization history. In the past, the practice of "cherry-picking," or selecting the healthiest groups, was commonplace in the insurance industry. Now, however, insurance companies are required to sell coverage to small employer groups and individuals who lose coverage without regard to their health history. This issue is especially important to employers with fewer than 50 employees. Previously, one employee with a high risk factor could jeopardize the coverage of all members of the small group (Cantor, Long, & Marquis, 1995). A significant component missing here is controls on insurance prices for these small groups and individuals.

The third component of HIPAA is that insurers must renew policies they sell to groups and individuals. Previously, insurance companies were allowed to eliminate costly individuals or groups from their policies by denying renewal of coverage.

Health Savings Accounts

The Medicare Prescription Drug, Improvement, and Modernization Act of 2003 included a provision creating health savings accounts (HSA) (Remler & Giled, 2006). HSAs are a type of medical savings account (MSA)—a pilot project Congress created in 1996 for self-employed individuals and employers with fewer than 50 employees as a method of paying for medical care expenses. Under the Medicare Prescription Drug, Improvement, and Modernization Act, an employer of any size may offer an HSA as a health insurance option to its employees (Minicozzi, 2006). Like MSAs, HSAs are tax-free savings accounts that are used for the out-of-pocket medical expenses for those individuals who select a high-deductible health insurance plan (in 2016, a minimum deductible of $1,300 per individual or $2,600 per family) (HSA Center.com, 2015). Contributions from pre-tax income are limited to the amount of the deductible ($3,350 for an individual or $6,750 for a family) and may be made by either the employer or the employee. Total out-of-pocket spending is capped at $6,650 for an individual and $13,100 for a family; after this point, the health insurance will cover all healthcare expenses. Balances in HSAs do not expire, but rather accumulate over time, even if a person is no longer covered by a high-deductible health insurance plan (HSA Center.com, 2015).

MSAs and HSAs are designed to create price sensitivity among healthcare consumers. Patients with traditional health insurance coverage are largely unaware of the cost of medical care services. Economists suggest that this lack of knowledge is one of the reasons why healthcare costs have risen so dramatically over the years (American College of Physicians, 1996). Unlike most health insurance plans, MSAs and HSAs do not shield the consumer from the cost of medical care. The consumer becomes directly responsible for dollars spent on health care (up to the amount of the deductible) and thus becomes more price sensitive. Consumers are at partial risk for expenditures, because a significant portion of the money comes from their MSAs or HSAs to pay for care. As a consequence, they have an incentive to avoid medical care that is not worth the cost (Goodman &

Pauly, 1995). Proponents of MSAs and HSAs have suggested that these accounts will reduce wasteful utilization of resources and hold down healthcare cost inflation rates (Hsiao, 1995).

Critics of MSAs and HSAs remain concerned about the prospect of adverse selection with these accounts. As discussed in previously, adverse selection occurs when insured individuals can accurately predict their future need for health insurance coverage (Folland, Goodman, & Stano, 1997). With these types of plans, the fear is that healthy individuals would drop their low-deductible health insurance in favor of MSAs combined with high-deductible plans. Premiums in the low-deductible plan would then skyrocket because only the sick would participate in the plan (Gardner, 1995).

Since the implementation of the ACA, employers have dramatically increased their offerings of high-deductible plans eligible for an HSA, from less than 15% of employers offering an HSA to 41% in 2014 (Greene, 2015). This has resulted in a corresponding increase of HSA accounts, covering 19.7 million people in January 2015, compared to 5.7 million in 2010 (AHIP, 2015).

Although access to health care in the United States may not be significantly altered by either MSAs or HSAs, the growth of healthcare spending may be slowed by their adoption. However, consumers may be unwilling or unable to determine the appropriateness, quality, and cost of healthcare services given the specialized nature of healthcare delivery and thus do little to decrease spending. Also, consumers who have limited resources may forgo necessary care, potentially resulting in increased spending to compensate for their delays in seeking treatment.

HSAs represent a radical change in healthcare reform—moving away from the concept of collective responsibility and toward the notion of individual accountability (Robinson, 2005). Their consequences—intended and unintended—to healthcare delivery systems, employer health insurance costs, and individual health outcomes are unknown.

Patient Protection and Affordable Care Act

The Patient Protection and Affordable Care Act, P.L. 111-148 (referred to as the ACA), was signed into law by President Obama on March 23, 2010. The ACA is the most comprehensive healthcare legislation since Medicare and Medicaid were created in 1965. A number of programs, reforms, and requirements took place in the first year (Kaiser Family Foundation, 2010b); however, due to vast changes and infrastructure that needed to be developed prior to implementation, a majority of the provisions began in 2014. When the law is fully implemented in 2019, it is predicted that 32 million previously uninsured individuals will have health insurance (Kaiser Family Foundation, 2010c).

The purpose of the ACA was to expand access to healthcare services using an individual mandate requiring U.S. citizens and legal residents to obtain health insurance. Individuals who do not enroll in a health insurance plan are assessed a tax penalty. However, this is balanced with premium credits (a subsidy) based upon the individual's income for those who do not have access to an employer-based plan and subsequently purchase health insurance on their own (Kaiser Family Foundation, 2010c).

Coupled with mandating individuals to enroll in health insurance plans are requirements placed on employers. The incentive for employers to offer health insurance is balanced with the risk of paying penalties for failing to offer this benefit. Requirements and penalties placed upon employers are determined according to its number of employees. Large employers—those with more than 200 employees—are required to automatically enroll employees into health insurance plans. Most large employers currently offer health insurance, thus this requirement will appear seamless to these employees. Employers with 50 or more employees who do not offer health insurance to their employees and who have at least one full-time employee who receives a tax credit for purchasing health insurance will be assessed a $2,000 fee per full-time employee after exempting the first 30 employees (Kaiser Family Foundation, 2010c).

ACA expands the health insurance infrastructure by authorizing the development of state-based insurance exchanges and nonprofit health insurance companies. Individuals and small businesses that have 100 employees or fewer may purchase health insurance through state-based health benefit exchanges and small business health options programs (Kaiser Family Foundation, 2010c). These exchanges are administered by a nonprofit organization or government agency. Opportunities to purchase health insurance plans are further expanded by the creation of a consumer-operated and oriented plan to develop nonprofit, member-run health insurance companies in each state. Current health insurance companies were ineligible to create a consumer-operated and oriented plan (Kaiser Family Foundation, 2010c).

Medicaid was expanded to non-Medicare eligible individuals under age 65 with incomes up to 138% of the federal poverty level, (Kaiser Family Foundation, 2010a). It was estimated that half of the newly insured under ACA would receive their coverage from Medicaid and the Children's Health Insurance Program because ACA has essentially changed the eligibility requirements for the Medicaid program (Rosenbaum, 2010). To assist with the increased cost, states received 100% federal funding for the expansion of the Medicaid program beginning in 2014. By 2020, federal support will be reduced to 90% (Kaiser Family Foundation, 2010a). Some states refused to expand their Medicaid programs for political reasons even though such expansion would have decreased the costs incurred for uncompensated care by hospitals and other providers and increased health insurance premiums if Medicaid is not expanded in their state.

Insurance companies will have to comply with a number of new regulations. Access to health insurance was improved in the first year of implementation for two populations—adult children until age 26 and individuals with preexisting health conditions (Kaiser Family Foundation, 2010c). Health insurance companies must provide dependent coverage for adult children up to age 26 for individual and group policies. This will be of great benefit to recent college graduates having difficulty finding jobs. For individuals with a preexisting medical condition who have been uninsured for at least 6 months, a temporary national high-risk pool was created to provide health insurance (Kaiser Family Foundation, 2010c).

Multiple funding sources were created to finance increased access to health insurance through ACA. In addition to employer and individual tax penalties, some of the provisions to pay for increased access include imposing an excise tax on insurers of employer-sponsored health plans with high costs, reducing the amount allowed for contributions to flexible medical spending accounts, increasing the threshold for itemized deductions for unreimbursed medical expenses, imposing a tax on nonprofit hospitals for failing to comply with new requirements, and annual fees on both pharmaceutical manufacturing and health insurance sectors (Kaiser Family Foundation, 2010c).

Modifications and adjustments to Medicare focus primarily on changes in reimbursement mechanisms. In an effort to slow the growth of Medicare spending and to reward the provision of quality care, payments to hospitals were reduced for preventable hospital readmissions and for hospital-acquired conditions. Once a hospital value-based purchasing program is developed, hospitals will be paid based on performance on quality measures (Kaiser Family Foundation, 2010c). Value-based purchasing programs are also expected to be developed for ambulatory surgical centers, skilled nursing facilities, and home health agencies. An independent payment advisory board will be established to make annual recommendations for reducing the growth rate of Medicare spending (Kaiser Family Foundation, 2010c). These recommendations will be nonbinding, as Congress has final authority for appropriating funds for federal programs (Jost, 2010).

Improving healthcare quality was an important focus of ACA by establishing a national quality improvement strategy and the nonprofit, independent Patient-Centered Outcomes Research Institute. The quality improvement strategy will identify processes to develop and use quality measures to improve healthcare delivery, patient health outcomes, and population health (Kaiser Family Foundation, 2010c). The Patient-Centered Outcomes Research Institute is expected to identify and conduct comparative clinical effectiveness research of medical treatments. Both of these provisions will incorporate input from stakeholders including that of patients.

Provisions specific to pharmacy practice and Medicare reimbursement policies for the Medicare Part D coverage gap include its gradual elimination by 2020, a phase-in of federal subsidies for generic prescriptions filled, and the requirement for pharmaceutical manufacturers to provide a 50% discount on brand name prescriptions provided (Kaiser Family Foundation, 2010c).

Virginia's Attorney General filed a suit in federal court challenging the constitutionality of the ACA based upon a bill passed by its General Assembly stating that its residents were not required to obtain individual health insurance (Helderman, 2010). Arguments in support of constitutionality are based upon the notion that ACA is not a mandate, but it is a tax (Balkin, 2010). On June 28, 2012, the Supreme Court upheld the constitutionality of the ACA's two major provisions: individual mandate and Medicaid expansion. The individual mandate was upheld under Congress' authority to impose taxes and spend their revenues. The decision on the Medicaid expansion was more complex. The Court allowed expansion of Medicare provided that the Secretary of Health and Human Services could not withhold a state's existing Medicaid funding for failure to comply with the required Medicaid expansion (Kaiser Family Foundation, 2012b). The individual mandate went into effect in 2014, and Medicaid expansion remained optional for each state. In mid-2015, 29 states (including the District of Columbia) have adopted Medicaid expansions. An individual living in a state without a Medicaid expansion program who has been denied Medicaid coverage is exempt from the mandate to purchase health insurance and will not owe a tax (Kaiser Family Foundation, 2015a). By mid-2015, there were 14 state-based health insurance marketplaces and 37 states had some combination of a federally supported or federally managed health insurance marketplace (Kaiser Family Foundation, 2015b).

The ACA survived a subsequent challenge in June 2015 when the Supreme Court examined the language authorizing tax credits for those who buy insurance in marketplaces "established by the state." The Court determined that the tax credits applied to all states, not just in those states that fund and manage their own health insurance exchanges. The Court determined that, even though the legislative language was problematic, the intent of Congress was clear in that the only way the ACA would work is if the subsidy to purchase health insurance was available in all states (Barnes, 2015).

Although the full impact of the ACA will not be felt for more than a decade, there are implications that the law has already made an impact on access to care, and in some cases cost and quality of care. By March 2015, approximately 16.4 million uninsured people gained health insurance coverage. This included 14.1 million adults, reducing the uninsured rate from 20.3% in October 2013 to 13.2% in March 2015 (a 35% decline). It also included 2.3 million young adults (age 19–25) who gained coverage due to the provision allowing young adults to remain on a parent's plan until age 26. Since the first enrollment period in October 2013, there has been a greater decline in the uninsured rate among African Americans and Latinos than among Caucasians. Among Caucasians, the uninsured rate decreased by 5.3% to 9%, while the African American uninsured rate decreased by 9.2% to 13% and the Latino uninsured rate decreased by 12.3% to 29.5%. Health insurance coverage gains were especially strong in states that expanded Medicaid and were concentrated in low- and middle-income population groups in all states. Additionally, there was a greater decline in the uninsured rate among females than males in all states (Office of the Assistant Secretary for Planning and Evaluation, U.S. HHS, 2015a).

An estimated 16.9 million people were newly insured as a result of the ACA through Medicaid expansions, employer-sponsored health plans and state insurance exchanges (RAND Corporation, 2015). The RAND Corporation study estimated that 125.2 million Americans—about 80% of the nonelderly population that had insurance in September 2013—experienced no change in the source of insurance during the period (RAND Corporation, 2015).

Cost savings attributed to the ACA have been examined in states that have expanded their Medicaid programs. Kentucky and Arkansas, two states with previously high uninsured rates, have benefited significantly from Medicaid expansions. Kentucky estimated cost savings of $820 million from 2014 to 2021, while Arkansas estimated cost savings of $370 for the same time period (The State Health Reform Assistance Network, 2015). Historically, many states support programs and services for uninsured adults with general fund dollars. Under Medicaid expansion programs, virtually all beneficiaries of these programs and services can secure coverage as new adults, which means that states can fund these services with federal, not state, dollars. Kentucky saved $9 million in 2014 for enrollees in behavioral and mental health programs who were fully covered by Medicaid (The State Health Reform Assistance Network, 2015). Other states reported higher than expected savings for their budgets due simplification and streamlining of the Medicaid enrollment process (Kaiser Family Foundation, 2015c).

There has been a reduction in "uncompensated care" in hospital settings due to fewer uninsured patients and increases to insurance premium have decreased. An estimated reduction of $7.4 million in uncompensated care costs occurred in 2014 for all hospitals, representing a 21% reduction in uncompensated care spending (Office of the Assistant Secretary for Planning and Evaluation, U.S. HHS, 2015a). Health insurance premiums increased 26% for the 5-year period since ACA implementation, but rose to 36% in the previous 5-year period, and 72% in the period of 1999 to 2004. Total healthcare expenditures increased approximately 4% per year between 2009 and 2013; the lowest increases since the Centers for Medicare & Medicaid Services started compiling the National Health Expenditure Accounts data in 1960 (Robertson, 2015).

Long-term studies need to be completed to determine whether improvements in individual and population health have been achieved. Increased access to healthcare services implies that more Americans will receive preventive and primary care services. The ACA requires private plans to cover the following four broad categories of services for adults and children: evidence-based screenings and counseling, routine immunizations, preventive services for children and youth, and preventive services for women. Approximately 137 million people (55.6 million women, 53.5 million men, and 28.5 million children) have received no-cost coverage for preventive services since the ACA went into effect (Office of the Assistant Secretary for Planning and Evaluation, U.S. HHS, 2015b). While the number of individuals who have gained coverage for no-cost preventive services is large, public awareness of the preventive services requirement is relatively low. In March 2014, 4 years after the ACA was passed by Congress, less than half the population (43%) reported they were aware that the new law eliminated out-of-pocket expenses for preventive services (Kaiser Family Foundation, 2015d). The ACA provides increased access to preventive services without financial barriers, yet questions remain as to whether use of these services will increase, and if so, whether this provision will improve the population's health and reduce overall healthcare costs.

HEALTHCARE REFORM EFFORTS BY THE STATES

Reforms at the state level have primarily consisted of adjustments to the financing of healthcare delivery. A number of states, however, have developed unique approaches intended to expand access to health care for their citizens. These approaches include uncompensated care pools subsidized by taxes on acute care services, employer mandates to provide health insurance for employees, and a federal waiver allowing states to expand access to the Medicaid program.

Uncompensated Care Pools

The American Hospital Association estimates that U.S. hospitals provide more than $16 billion of uncompensated care each year (Weissman, 1996). States have set up uncompensated care pools, also referred to as free care pools, to reimburse hospitals for a portion of these uncompensated services delivered to uninsured and underinsured individuals who meet some means test, usually based on level of income. Uncompensated care pools are primarily financed by placing a tax on the hospital bills of individuals who have health insurance, but they may also be supported by funds from general tax revenues. Hospitals apply to the pool for reimbursement for those patients who are unable to pay for their hospital care.

Unlike the expansion of Medicaid programs, uncompensated care pools do not directly increase access to healthcare services. These programs simply finance acute care received in a hospital setting. However, the existence of an uncompensated care pool creates an incentive for hospitals to offer care to the uninsured. In the current competitive market, without the availability of an uncompensated care pool, many public hospitals may close or reduce the care offered to indigent individuals (Weissman, 1996). An uncompensated care pool is only one aspect of financing health care for a state's citizens. It is most effective when used in conjunction with other state programs that increase access to primary care services.

Employer Mandates

In 1974, long before there was a national debate about universal access to health care, Hawaii passed the Prepaid Health Care Act, a type of legislation referred to as an employer mandate (Budde, Patrick, & Budde, 1995; Lewin & Sybinsky, 1993). The Prepaid Health Care Act requires all employers to provide a standard, state-established health insurance package for their employees who work 20 or more hours per week. The program requires both employers and employees to share in the cost of the health insurance package. The employers pay at least 50% of the cost of the insurance. Employees pay up to 1.5% of their monthly salaries toward the monthly health insurance premium (Lewin & Sybinsky, 1993).

The Prepaid Health Care Act mandates a minimum set of basic services: hospitalization, emergency treatment, surgical services, physician office visits, laboratory tests, radiology services, and maternity services (Lewin & Sybinsky, 1993). Within the state, the options for health insurance include fee-for-service and managed care plans.

Considering that the cost of living in Hawaii is significantly higher than in most of the United States, one might expect that the cost of health insurance would also be higher. However, health insurance in Hawaii is less expensive than it is in the states on the mainland. There are two explanations for this phenomenon (Lewin & Sybinsky, 1993). First, because the employer mandate requires all employers to provide health insurance, there is less need to subsidize health care for uninsured individuals; this allows health insurance companies to use community rating rather than experience rating, which is frequently used when insuring small businesses. Thus, small businesses and large employers are offered similar rates. Second, because Hawaii has experienced a lower rate of hospitalization and a subsequent higher rate of outpatient physician visits than the rest of the country, health insurance premiums can be reduced.

Health outcomes for Hawaiian citizens have been better than those for the rest of the U.S. population with respect to extended longevity, low infant mortality, and low premature morbidity and mortality for cancer, cardiovascular disease, and pulmonary disease (Lewin & Sybinsky, 1993). One might think that the environment—the sunshine—and perhaps a healthy lifestyle cause these outcomes. In reality, these factors do not appear to significantly affect health outcomes in Hawaii. Although Hawaiians exhibit health risk behaviors common to all Americans, their commitment to outpatient care and prevention—instead of hospitalization—has improved health outcomes and decreased costs. Hawaiians visit their physicians twice as often and are hospitalized half as often as the national average (Lewin & Sybinsky, 1993). With less costly outpatient care and the use of preventive measures, expensive hospitalizations are used less frequently; this allows health insurance to remain at a lower rate than in other states.

From Hawaii's experience, it appears that an employer mandate could eliminate the largest percentage of uninsured individuals in the United States. However, since Hawaii's Prepaid Health Care Act was passed in 1974, several other states have passed employer mandate legislation. These states have been unable to implement their laws because of the Employee Retirement Income Security Act (ERISA), which restricts the types of mandates that states can impose on the benefits that employers offer their employees. Because Hawaii's Prepaid Health Care Act was enacted before ERISA was passed in 1974, it was not initially affected by ERISA. Yet, since ERISA has been enacted, no amendments have been made to Hawaii's Prepaid Health Care Act. Changes that might improve Hawaii's program, such as requiring coverage of dependents or adjusting the employer and employee contributions to the health insurance premiums, cannot be implemented because they would violate ERISA.

The intent of ERISA is to protect employees' retirement plans. Under ERISA, the federal government is solely responsible for regulating employee benefit plans, with its authority superseding any state laws (Gostin & Widiss, 1993). ERISA does not apply to the regulation of insurance. However, one-half to two-thirds of employers provide healthcare benefits for their employees with self-insurance. Self-insurance, also referred to as self-funded arrangements, involves setting aside money specifically to pay for employees' medical expenses rather than purchasing an insurance policy to protect them against financial loss. Employers who use self-insurance for their employees' health benefits are exempt from state employer mandates under ERISA.

Employer versus Employee Mandates

Frequently, discussion about federal healthcare reform turns into a debate over employer versus employee mandates. Employer mandates place the burden for financing on the employer. Employee mandates place the burden on the employee.

Economists argue that benefits are a component of reimbursement. Direct payments and benefits are both considered employee compensation. For example, the Medicare tax for employees and employers is set at 1.45% each. If the employer did not have to pay this Medicare tax, he or she could afford to provide a higher wage to the employee. Either way, the employee pays the tax—whether directly through taxes or indirectly through lower compensation.

Thus, the distinction between employer and employee mandates matters in the sense of the wage a worker receives, although total compensation remains constant. When the employee is forced to participate through payroll deduction, he or she is more likely to realize the true cost of the mandate. However, employer mandates shield the employee from the true cost. This price sensitivity is at the core of theory behind cost sharing. For this reason, increasing patient cost sharing is usually a component of healthcare reform.

Medicaid and State Requests for Waiver

Medicaid program costs have increased annually since the program went into effect in 1966. They are now the fastest-growing state expenditures, often limiting the ability of states to support higher education and other social programs. The increasing proportion of state budgets—as much as 20%—devoted to Medicaid has prompted states to look at methods to limit the growth of this spending (Holahan, Coughlin, Ku, Lipson, & Rajan, 1995). The federal government allows states to enroll Medicaid patients into managed care plans and to experiment with other cost-containment programs through a Medicaid waiver procedure (see Chapter 18 for further information).

Other State Initiatives to Increase Access to Health Insurance

Legislation to provide universal access had not been attempted since the late 1980s, but two states—Massachusetts and Vermont—passed sweeping legislation intended to increase access to health insurance in 2006. Both accomplished this feat with bipartisan support from Republican governors and Democratic-controlled legislatures. The primary focus of these reforms was a requirement that individuals purchase health insurance policies. Both states also require employers to pay an assessment to help finance the programs.

Massachusetts

Massachusetts passed an individual health insurance mandate in April 2006, requiring all residents 18 years and older to purchase a minimum level of health insurance by July 1, 2007 (Steinbrook, 2006). Failure to comply with the law results in a fine of 50% of the cost of an affordable insurance premium. Although this program is not an employer mandate, it does have an employer financing component, requiring businesses with 11 or more full-time employees who do not provide or contribute to health insurance to pay a fee of $295 per employee per year. The state subsidizes premium payments for families who earn less than 300% of the federal poverty level. The law also expanded Medicaid to include the children of families who earn up to 300% of the federal poverty level (Steinbrook, 2006).

Since implementation began in 2006, it is estimated that 439,000 previously uninsured people have insurance coverage, and that 96.9% of Massachusetts residents are insured (Blue Cross Blue Shield of Massachusetts Foundation, 2014). Other key features of the Massachusetts program include the creation of the Massachusetts Health Connector to administer the insurance components of the law. This organization serves as a clearinghouse to link individuals and businesses with fewer than 50 employees with insurance products. Health insurance is portable for individuals who purchase health insurance through the Massachusetts Health Connector (Steinbrook, 2006). By December 2008, 57% of the newly insured were enrolled in public coverage, and the remaining 43% were enrolled in private coverage through the Commonwealth Connector (Kaiser Commission on Medicaid and the Uninsured, 2009a).

As part of the state's cost containment efforts, the legislature created a Special Commission on the Health Care Payment System. In July 2009, the Commission recommended that the state shift from a fee-for-service system in which healthcare providers are paid per encounter to a system where providers work together to share responsibility for the patient's care. These accountable care organizations receive a global payment for all services patients receive (Kaiser Commission on Medicaid and the Uninsured, 2009a). To address increased healthcare costs during the implementation of universal health insurance coverage, Chapter 224 was enacted in 2012 (Massachusetts Health Policy Commission, 2015). Chapter 224 sets a benchmark for the growth of healthcare costs, 3.6% for 2013–2015 (Center for Health Information and Analysis, 2015; Massachusetts Health Policy Commission, 2015). Nine years after enacting comprehensive healthcare reform, Massachusetts has been successful in expanding coverage to the uninsured through a public-private approach. Nearly half of the newly insured have enrolled in private coverage through their employer or purchased an individual plan. As a result of the employer role in health reform, Massachusetts experienced an increase in employer-based coverage. The state's experience demonstrates the viability of an individual mandate (required insurance coverage), when combined with affordable health coverage options, as a method to reduce the number of uninsured. The Massachusetts initiatives of mandated insurance coverage and payment system options (accountable care organizations) were the basis of many recommendations for federal healthcare reform (Blue Cross Blue Shield of Massachusetts Foundation, 2014; Robert Wood Johnson Foundation State Health Access Reform Evaluation, 2009). Since 2000, Massachusetts has had the lowest rate of uninsured in the country (Blue Cross Blue Shield of Massachusetts Foundation, 2014). When health reform was enacted in 2006, its uninsured rate was 6.4% compared to the 15.2% for the country (Blue Cross Blue Shield of Massachusetts Foundation, 2014). Those who remain uninsured after implementation of Massachusetts' Chapter 58 and the ACA are more likely to be between 18 and 64 years, low income (<150% federal poverty level), and Hispanic (Blue Cross Blue Shield of Massachusetts Foundation, 2014). The success in decreasing the number of uninsured individuals has the potential to limit affordability for some individuals now and others in the future because healthcare costs are expected to double by 2020 if no efforts are made to contain costs (Blue Cross Blue Shield of Massachusetts Foundation, 2014; Kaiser Family Foundation, 2012a). Recognizing that healthcare costs and healthcare spending in Massachusetts are the highest in the nation (Kaiser Family Foundation, 2012a), Massachusetts has identified a benchmark for growth in spending of 3.6% for 2013 to 2015 (Massachusetts Health Policy Commission, 2015). Healthcare spending increased by 2.3% in 2013 and 4.8% in 2014 attributable to the implementation of the ACA and increased prescription drug costs (Massachusetts Health Policy Commission, 2015).

Vermont

Vermont's legislature has passed many progressive healthcare reform bills. In May 2006, Vermont passed the 2006 Health Care Affordability Act, which created Catamount Health. It is available to anyone who has been uninsured for the previous 12 months effective October 1, 2007 (Vermont, State of, 2006). Premiums were subsidized based on income for persons with incomes at or below 300% of the federal poverty level, both for those who enroll in Catamount Health and for those employed with comparable employer-sponsored health insurance (Vermont, State of, 2006). Vermont's Health Care Affordability Act also created a chronic disease management plan called Blueprint for Health, which incorporated early disease screening, promoted patient self-management tools, and financially rewarded healthcare providers for using proactive chronic-care management tools (Vermont, State of, 2006).

In April 2010, the Vermont legislature passed a bill directing the State Health Care Reform Commission to prepare three financing options and implementation plans for three new healthcare financing systems (Cheney, 2010). The bill required the three options to include a single-payer option, a public option, and an option based upon that created by the ACA (Cheney, 2010).

Act 48, "An Act Relating to a Universal and Unified Health System," was signed by Governor Shumlin creating Green Mountain Care in May 2011 (Fox & Blanchet, 2015). The Act also prepared the state for implementation of the ACA, by creating the Vermont Benefit Exchange (Fox & Blanchet, 2015). Three financial projections were completed in 2011, 2013, and 2014 by Harvard researchers, University of Massachusetts researchers, and the State of Vermont, respectively, to examine the costs and savings of a single-payer health plan (McDonough, 2015). New taxes were estimated to be 9.4% of payroll for employers in 2011 and 11.5% in 2014 (McDonough, 2015). Estimated costs to employees were 3.1% of income in 2011 and a sliding scale up to 9.5% in 2014 (McDonough, 2015). The 2014 report estimated that the state would need to fund Green Mountain Care $2.5 billion in order to implement Green Mountain Care (McDonough, 2015).

Green Mountain Care, Vermont's single-payer health insurance program, was abandoned in December 2014 (McDonough, 2015). Green Mountain Care was projected to cost $4.3 billion, an addition to the $4.9 state budget that the governor determined was too great a risk for the state (Fitzgerald, 2015) even though taxes to pay for Green Mountain Care would have been similar to the amount employers and employees would pay for health premiums (Fox & Blanchet, 2015).

The Pharmacy Profession and Information Technology

Prior to the historic health reform act of 2010, the following two laws were enacted in 2009: the Children's Health Insurance Program Reauthorization Act and the American Recovery and Reinvestment Act. The Children's Health Insurance Program Reauthorization Act was expected to provide access for 4 million children by 2013, while the American Recovery and Reinvestment Act provided an unprecedented level of healthcare spending on health information technology, comparative effectiveness research, and wellness and prevention activities (Reynolds, 2009).

The American Recovery and Reinvestment Act contained $1.1 billion in funding for comparative effectiveness research (Steinbrook, 2009), an amount nearly 37 times the annual federal spending on comparative effectiveness research (Schumock & Pickard, 2009). The Congressional Budget Office defined comparative effectiveness research as "a rigorous evaluation of the impact of different options that are available for treating a given medical condition for a particular set of patients" (Bertagna, 2009). Its goal is to provide patients, healthcare professionals, and payers with evidence to support treatment decisions.

Combining investments in health information technology for implementing electronic health records in more hospitals and physician offices, comparative effectiveness research has the potential to provide clinical decision support tools for clinicians. Comparative effectiveness research will impact policy decisions for formularies and provide opportunities to implement evidence-based decisions in pharmacy practice.

The $1 billion spending provision from the American Recovery and Reinvestment Act in wellness and prevention may also impact pharmacist services and represents the largest allocation of funding to prevention activities in American history (Steinbrook, 2009). With substantial new spending on clinical and community-based prevention activities toward chronic disease, immunizations for low-income communities, and initiatives to reduce healthcare-associated infections, pharmacists are well positioned to play a more active role in coordinated care activities.

The Pharmacy Profession and the Patient Protection and Affordable Care Act

Several provisions included in the Patient Protection and ACA were designed to promote coordination among healthcare providers and will improve the quality of pharmacy practice. The Patient-Centered Outcomes Research Institute provides pharmacists with opportunities to apply for grants for medication therapy management (MTM) services to chronically ill patients. Under the newly created Innovation Center within the Centers for Medicare and Medicaid Services, pharmacists may participate in pilot projects to examine and evaluate payment mechanisms to reduce expenditures and quality improvement protocols to enhance healthcare quality (Kaiser Family Foundation, 2010c). Working with community health teams to provide transition care, pharmacists may work with other members of the healthcare team to provide medication reconciliation and discharge planning with MTM services.

Expanding payment for pharmacist-provided MTM services has been a key objective of pharmacy organizations' lobbying efforts for many years prior to ACA enactment. The MTM grant program through the newly created Patient-Centered Outcomes Research Institute will provide grants to pharmacists employed by organizations that are involved with collaborative, multidisciplinary care of chronically ill patients.

In anticipation of this provision, pharmacists in many states advocated for collaborative drug therapy management legislation to be applicable in any practice setting in their state. The combination of protocol-driven therapy through collaborative drug therapy management authority and MTM provides a new paradigm of pharmacy practice. Hospitals, through their MTM subsidiary, could provide pharmacist-driven MTM services to a local public health agency or a health insurance company, or to patients discharged home after an acute-care episode. Initially, MTM services would be reimbursed as part of the grant, with the opportunity for the development of new payment mechanisms from health insurance companies or public health agencies.

The statutory definition of pharmacist-driven MTM services is ground breaking, because prior to the enactment of the ACA, MTM services were loosely defined and no specifications for pharmacist oversight were delineated. Identification of the true value of pharmaceutical care services may be identified because MTM programs will be required to evaluate their clinical effectiveness. Although Congress acknowledged the potential benefit of MTM services by incorporating them into the law, an annual funding authorization was not defined. Therefore, funding of the program will be determined by future appropriations bills.

Additional MTM opportunities are available through the ACA requirement of an annual pharmacist review of medications for patients receiving Medicare Part D. While Medicare beneficiaries are allowed to opt out of the service, the annual review would provide a foundation for follow-up services for covered patients. Pharmacists may also provide MTM services in demonstration projects that include medical home models, a Medicaid health home, and a community transition program for high-risk Medicare patients who are discharged from the hospital, all components of ACA.

The 2009 American Recovery and Reinvestment Act and 2010 ACA provided vast opportunities for pharmacists to incorporate comprehensive pharmaceutical care services into the healthcare delivery system, work collaboratively with other healthcare providers, and demonstrate improved patient outcomes.

THE PHARMACY PROFESSION AND HEALTHCARE REFORM: A CALL FOR ACTION

The pharmacy profession is in a unique position to influence healthcare reform efforts. Pharmacists have more contact with the general public than do other healthcare professionals. Community pharmacists have ample opportunities to interact with patients who receive a prescription or who are visiting the pharmacy to pick up an over-the-counter drug product or other products stocked on pharmacy shelves. Whether dispensing a prescription to a patient or helping a customer in the store, pharmacists have direct and frequent contact with the public.

Although insurance coverage for prescription drugs has broadened in recent years, it still lags behind coverage for other components of medical care. Consumers are less sheltered from the burden of paying for prescription medications than from the burden of paying for other medical care services because of the higher utilization of prescription services coupled with the higher percentages of cost sharing they are forced to bear. Pharmacists are in the position to understand the patient's perspective, and they also have the opportunity to manage reimbursement from the third-party payer's perspective.

Reforms for reimbursement of pharmacist MTM services have progressed in numerous areas in the past 10 years and more opportunities appear on the horizon from both state and federal legislative initiatives. Buoyed by collaborative practice laws, some states have enacted provider recognition laws to include pharmacists as providers of healthcare services. This has paved the way for reimbursement of medication management services from state payers such as Medicaid, some commercial payers, and potentially through innovative shared savings programs proposed through the ACA. However, pharmacists and pharmacists' patient care services are not included in key sections of the SSA, which determines eligibility for Medicare Part B. Omission of pharmacists as listed providers limits Medicare beneficiaries' access to pharmacists' services in the outpatient setting. Many state and private health plans cite the omission from Medicare Part B as rationale for omitting coverage for beneficiaries or lack of compensation of pharmacists for providing comprehensive, patient-centered care. Omission from Medicare Part B results in a barrier to optimizing the use of pharmacists' patient care services in emerging integrated care delivery models promoted by the ACA, such as medical homes and accountable care organizations.

Pharmaceutical care offers members of the pharmacy profession an opportunity to move from providing a product to providing true service and securing a more important role in the changing healthcare marketplace. A pharmacist who becomes a disease state manager, for example, will be better able to influence public policy and healthcare system change. Pharmacists should get involved in their professional associations, in community groups, and in insurance plans. They should understand the perspectives of different players so that they can address the concerns of others as well as promote their own perspective.

Healthcare system reform should not frighten pharmacists. It should provide a challenge and an opportunity to carve out a niche in tomorrow's healthcare system.

CONCLUSION

Reform of the healthcare delivery system has been accomplished in many ways, such as requiring a certificate of need prior to building a new hospital, creating the Medicare and Medicaid programs, requiring Medicaid patients to receive their care in a managed care setting, and requiring that all citizens obtain health insurance either through their employer or purchased themselves. Ideally, these reforms would balance access with cost containment and improved quality and effectiveness of care. At the core of healthcare reform is people's willingness to pay for changes to the healthcare system.

Healthcare reform is far from being completed. Provisions and requirements delineated in the ACA require many years for implementation. Stakeholders will continue to voice their opinions and concerns to impact these processes.

QUESTIONS FOR FURTHER DISCUSSION

1. Which healthcare reform solutions are most viable?
2. What should be done to save Medicare?
3. Should the United States move toward a basic health benefit for all?
4. What are the intended and unintended consequences of the individual and employer requirements under the Patient Protection and ACA?

KEY TOPICS AND TERMS

Affordable Care Act (ACA)
American Recovery and Reinvestment Act (ARRA)
Children's Health Insurance Program (CHIP)
Comparative effectiveness research
Cost containment
Diagnosis-related group (DRG)
Employee mandate

- Employee Retirement Income Security Act (ERISA)
- Employer mandate
- Health Insurance Portability and Accountability Act (HIPAA)
- Health savings account (HSA)
- Kerr-Mills Act
- Managed care
- Medicaid
- Medicaid waiver
- Medical Savings Account (MSA)
- Medicare
- Medication therapy management (MTM) services
- Patient Protection and Affordable Care Act (PPACA)
- Social Security
- Uncompensated care pool

REFERENCES

AHIP. (2015). Health savings accounts and consumer-directed plans. Retrieved from https://www.ahip.org/Issues/Health-Savings-Accounts-and-Consumer-Directed-Plans.aspx

American College of Physicians. (1996). Position paper: Medical savings accounts. *Annals of Internal Medicine*, *125*, 333–340.

Anderson, G. F., & Poullier, J. P. (1999). Health spending, access, and outcomes: Trends in industrialized countries. *Health Affairs*, *18*, 178–192.

Balkin, J. J. (2010). The constitutionality of the individual mandate for health insurance. *New England Journal of Medicine*, *362*, 482–483.

Barnes, R. (2015, June 25). Affordable Care Act survives Supreme Court challenge. *Washington Post.* Retrieved from http://www.washingtonpost.com/politics/courts_law/obamacare-survives-supreme-court-challenge/2015/06/25/af87608e-188a-11e5-93b7-5eddc056ad8a_story.html

Bertagna, L. M., & Dreyer, N. (2009). Comparative effectiveness research: Coming soon? Retrieved from http://pharmexec.findpharma.com/pharmexec/Regulatory/Comparative-Effectiveness-Research-Coming-Soon/ArticleStandard/Article/detail/589172?ref=25

Blue Boulding, K. E. (1996, October). The concept of need for health services. *Milbank Memorial Fund Quarterly*, *44*, 202–223.

Blue Cross Blue Shield of Massachusetts Foundation. (2014, March). Health reform in Massachusetts, expanding access to health insurance coverage, assessing the results. Retrieved from http://bluecrossfoundation.org/publication/updated-health-reform-massachusetts-assessing-results

Brown, E. R., & Wyn, R. (1996). Public policies to extend health care coverage. In R. J. Anderson, T. H. Rice, & G. F. Kominski (Eds.), *Changing the U.S. health care system: Key issues in health services, policy, and management* (pp. 41–61). San Francisco, CA: Jossey-Bass.

Budde, J. C., Patrick, W. K., & Budde, M. T. (1995). Hawaii HealthQUEST: A managed care demonstration project. *Hawaii Medical Journal*, *54*, 720–722.

Cantor, J. C., Long, S. H., & Marquis, M. S. (1995). Private employment-based health insurance in ten states. *Health Affairs*, *14*, 199–234.

Center for Health Information and Analysis. (2015). Performance of the Massachusetts health care system annual report. Retrieved from http://www.chiamass.gov/assets/2015-annual-report/2015-Annual-Report.pdf

Cheney, T. (2010, April 23). Vermont house passes comprehensive health care reform bill. *Vtdigger*. Retrieved from http://vtdigger.org/2010/04/23/vermont-house-passes-comprehensive-health-care-reform-bill/

Donelan, K., Blendon, R. J., Schoen, C., Davis, K., & Binns, K. (1999). The cost of health system change: Public discontent in five nations. *Health Affairs*, *18*, 206–216.

Epstein, A. Z. M., Bogen, J., Dreyer, P., & Thorpe, K. E. (1991). Trends in lengths of stay and rates of readmission in Massachusetts: Implications for monitoring quality of care. *Inquiry*, *28*, 19–28.

Fitzgerald, J. (2015, January 25). Costs derail Vermont's dream of a single-payer health plan. *The Boston Globe.* Retrieved from https://www.bostonglobe.com/business/2015/01/25/costs-derail-vermont-single-payer-health-plan/VTAEZFGpWvTen0QFahW0pO/story.html

Folland, S., Goodman, A. C., & Stano, M. (1997). *The economics of health and health care* (2nd ed.). Englewood Cliffs, NJ: Prentice-Hall.

Fox, A. M., & Blanchet, N. J. (2015, June). The little state that couldn't could? The politics of "single payer" health coverage in Vermont. *Journal of Health Politics, Policy and Law, 40*(3), 447–485.

Fuchs, V. R. (1992). The best health care system in the world? *Journal of the American Medical Association, 268*, 916–917.

Gardner, J. (1995). Medical savings accounts make waves. *Modern Healthcare, 25*(9), 57.

Goodman, J. C., & Pauly, M. V. (1995). Tax credits for health insurance and medical savings accounts. *Health Affairs, 14*, 126–139.

Gostin, L. O., & Widiss, A. I. (1993). What's wrong with the ERISA vacuum? *Journal of the American Medical Association, 269*, 2527–2532.

Greene, J. (2015, July). HSAs surge, leaving HRAs in a niche. *Managed Care*. Retrieved from http://www.managedcaremag.com/archives/2015/7/hsas-surge-leaving-hras-niche

Helderman, R. S. (2010, May 25). Obama administration asks judge to dismiss Virginia suit against health-care law. *The Washington Post*. Retrieved from http://www.washingtonpost.com/wp-dyn/content/article/2010/05/24/AR20105240473.html

Holahan, J., Coughlin, T., Ku, L., Lipson, D. J., & Rajan, S. (1995). Insuring the poor through Section 1115 waivers. *Health Affairs, 14*(1), 199–216.

HSA center.com. (2015). 2016 HSA contribution limits, deductibles, and out-of-pocket expenses. Retrieved from http://www.hsacenter.com/2016-hsa-contribution-limits.html

Hsiao, W. C. (1995). Medical savings accounts: Lessons from Singapore. *Health Affairs, 14*, 260–266.

Iglehart, J. K. (1982). The future of HMOs. *New England Journal of Medicine, 307*, 451–456.

Jeffers, J. R., Bognanno, M. E., & Bartlett, J. C. (1971). On the demand versus need for medical services and the concept of "shortage." *American Journal of Public Health, 61*, 46–63.

Jost, T. S. (2010). The independent payment advisory board. *New England Journal of Medicine, 363*, 103–105.

Kaiser Commission on Medicaid and the Uninsured. (2009a). Massachusetts health care reform: Three years later. Publication no. 7777-02. Retrieved from http://www.kff.org/uninsured/7777.cfm

Kaiser Commission on Medicaid and the Uninsured. (2009b, October). The uninsured: A primer, key facts about Americans without health insurance. Report no. 7451-05. Retrieved from http://www.kff.org/uninsured/7451.cfm

Kaiser Family Foundation. (2010a, May). Financing new Medicaid coverage under health reform: The role of the federal government and states. Publication no. 8072. Retrieved from http://www.kff.org/healthreform/8072.cfm

Kaiser Family Foundation. (2010b). Focus on health care reform: Health care reform implementation timeline. Publication no. 8060. Retrieved from http://www.kff.org/healthreform/8060.cfm

Kaiser Family Foundation. (2010c). Focus on health care reform: Summary of new health reform law. Publication no. 8061. Retrieved from http://www.kff.org/healthreform/upload/8061.pdf

Kaiser Family Foundation. (2012a, May). Focus on health reform: Massachusetts health care reform: Six years later. Retrieved from http://kff.org/health-costs/issue-brief/massachusetts-health-care-reform-six-years-later/

Kaiser Family Foundation. (2012b, July). A guide to the Supreme Court's Affordable Care Act decision. Retrieved from https://kaiserfamilyfoundation.files.wordpress.com/2013/01/8332.pdf

Kaiser Commission on Medicaid and the Uninsured. (2015, October 5). Key facts about the uninsured population. Retrieved from http://kff.org/uninsured/fact-sheet/key-facts-about-the-uninsured-population/

Kaiser Family Foundation. (2015a). Status of state action on the Medicaid expansion decision. Retrieved from http://kff.org/health-reform/state-indicator/state-activity-around-expanding-medicaid-under-the-affordable-care-act/

Kaiser Family Foundation. (2015b). State health insurance marketplace types, 2015. Retrieved from http://kff.org/health-reform/state-indicator/state-health-insurance-marketplace-types/

Kaiser Family Foundation. (2015c). The effects of the Medicaid expansion on state budgets: An early look in select states. Retrieved from http://files.kff.org/attachment/issue-brief-the-effects-of-the-medicaid-expansion-on-state-budgets-an-early-look-in-select-states

Kaiser Family Foundation. (2015d). Preventive services covered by private health plans under the Affordable Care Act. Retrieved from http://kff.org/health-reform/fact-sheet/preventive-services-covered-by-private-health-plans/

Lewin, J. C., & Sybinsky, P. A. (1993). Hawaii's employer mandate and its contribution to universal access. *Journal of the American Medical Association, 269*, 2538–2543.

Massachusetts Health Policy Commission. (2015). Health care cost growth benchmark. Retrieved from http://www.mass.gov/anf/budget-taxes-and-procurement/oversight-agencies/health-policy-commission/

McDonough, J. E. (2015, April). The demise of Vermont's single-payer plan. *New England Journal of Medicine, 372*, 1584–1585.

Minicozzi, A. (2006). Medical savings accounts: What do the data tell? *Health Affairs, 25*, 256–267.

OECD Health Statistics. (2015). Paris, France: Organisation for Economic Cooperation and Development. Retrieved from http://www.oecd.org/health/health-data.htm. https://stats.oecd.org/index.aspx

Office of the Assistant Secretary for Planning and Evaluation, U.S. HHS. (2015a, March 23). Insurance expansion, hospital uncompensated care, and the Affordable Care Act. Retrieved from http://aspe.hhs.gov/health/reports/2015/MedicaidExpansion/ib_UncompensatedCare.pdf

Office of the Assistant Secretary for Planning and Evaluation, U.S. HHS. (2015b, May 5). Health insurance coverage and the Affordable Care Act. Retrieved from http://aspe.hhs.gov/health/reports/2015/uninsured_change/ib_uninsured_change.pdf

RAND Corporation. (2015, May 6). Health coverage grows under Affordable Care Act. Retrieved from http://www.rand.org/news/press/2015/05/06.html

Remler, D. K., & Giled, S. A. (2006). How much more cost sharing will health savings accounts bring? *Health Affairs, 25*(4), 1070–1078.

Reynolds, S. (2009). Obama's crusade to make U.S. healthcare work efficiently and effectively. Retrieved from http://about.datamonitor.com/media/archives/1893

Robert Wood Johnson Foundation State Health Access Reform Evaluation. (2009). The secrets of Massachusetts' success: Why 97 percent of state residents have health coverage. Retrieved from http://www.shadac.org/files/shadac/publications/SecretsOfMassSuccessLongPaper.pdf

Robertson, L. (2015). Slower premium growth under Obama. FactCheck.org. Retrieved from http://www.factcheck.org/2015/02/slower-premium-growth-under-obama/

Robinson, J. C. (2005). Health savings accounts—the ownership society in health care. *New England Journal of Medicine, 353*(12), 1199–1201.

Rosenbaum, S. (2010). A "customary and necessary" program—Medicaid and health care reform. *New England Journal of Medicine, 362*(21), 1952–1955.

Schumock, G. T., & Pickard, A. S. (2009). Comparative effectiveness research: Relevance and application to pharmacy. *American Journal of Health-Systems Pharmacists, 66*, e2–e10.

Smith, M. D., Altman, D. E., Leitman, R., Moloney, T. W., & Taylor, H. (1992). Taking the public's pulse on health system reform. *Health Affairs, 11*, 125–133.

Starr, P. (1982). *The social transformation of American medicine.* New York, NY: Basic Books.

Steinbrook, R. (2006). Health care reform in Massachusetts: A work in progress. *New England Journal of Medicine, 354*(20), 2095–2098.

Steinbrook, R. (2009). Health care and the American Recovery and Reinvestment Act. *New England Journal of Medicine, 360*(11), 1057–1060.

The State Health Reform Assistance Network, RWJ Foundation. (2015, March 4). Medicaid expansion states see significant budget savings and revenue gains. Retrieved from http://statenetwork.org/resource/state-network-medicaid-expansion-states-see-significant-budget-savings-and-revenue-gains/

Vermont, State of. (2006). A summary of the 2006 Health Care Affordability Act. Retrieved from http://www.csgeast.org/Annual_Meeting/2006/healthchen2.pdf

Weissman, J. (1996). Uncompensated hospital care: Will it be there if we need it? *Journal of the American Medical Association, 276*, 823–828.

Glossary

Academic detailing (counterdetailing): as a follow-up to physician profiling, some health plans and PBMs provide counterdetailing.

Accrediting agency: independent organization authorized to grant accreditation based on pre-determined standards.

Activities of daily living: activities that are performed during the course of a normal day, such as bathing, toileting, dressing, and eating.

Activity–passivity model of patient care: as described by Szasz and Hollender, practitioner–patient communication in which the patient is passive. This interaction can be compared to a parent–infant relationship.

Actual acquisition cost (AAC): the price that pharmacies pay for drug products after subtracting all discounts.

Actuary: an insurance company employee who conducts a statistical analysis of an insured population to estimate the income (premiums) that must be earned to cover the estimated expenses, usually expressed as cost per member per month.

Adherence: refers to patients taking medications as prescribed.

Adjudication: the process of reviewing or screening claims to determine payment.

Administration on Aging: a DHHS agency that works to provide services that enable elders to live independently—especially those who are disadvantaged.

Administrative agencies: units of executive branch that promulgate and enforce regulations needed to implement laws.

Adverse drug events: any untoward medical occurrence causing harm that may present during treatment with a pharmaceutical product, but which does not necessarily have a causal relationship with this treatment.

Adverse drug reaction: an undesirable or harmful reaction to a drug that occurs at doses normally used for the treatment, prevention, or diagnosis of a disease.

Adverse selection: a situation in which individuals or companies purchase insurance only when they expect a loss.

Affordable Care Act (ACA): See "Patient Protection and Affordable Care Act."

Agency for Healthcare Research and Quality: DHHS agency that supports research regarding the organization, financing, delivery, quality assessment, and improvement of the health delivery in the United States.

Aging-in-place: a concept where older adults do not have to move from their present residence in order to secure necessary support services in response to changing needs.

Ambulatory patient groups (APGs): a type of prospective payment for outpatient services that is based on diagnosis.

American Hospital Association: a national organization composed of hospitals, healthcare organizations, and individual members. It provides education to the public and its members and advocates for and represents its membership in legislative and regulatory issues.

American Recovery and Reinvestment Act (ARRA): also known as the "Stimulus Act of 2009," it was enacted by Congress with the intention to create jobs and to promote investment and consumer spending during the recession.

Analysis of extremes: a sensitivity analysis method conducted by reassigning values of both cost and effectiveness variables concurrently to their highest and lowest extremes in order to determine the robustness of the conclusions in the best and worst case situations.

Assignment: the payment of a healthcare service directly to the provider rather than the beneficiary; usually requires a participating provider agreement between the health plan and the provider.

Average manufacturer's price (AMP): a proposed method for estimating pharmacy acquisition costs that is based on actual costs charged by manufacturers rather than the wholesale list price.

Average wholesale price (AWP): the list price established by the manufacturer. AWP is higher than the actual acquisition cost (AAC) that pharmacies pay for drug products and is discounted by the payer to arrive at the estimated acquisition cost (EAC).

Balanced Budget Act: law enacted in 1997 that required the implementation of a prospective payment system (PPS) for home health services, reductions in reimbursement rates for home medical equipment, and implementation of competitive bidding processes. Under a PPS, a home health agency is paid a flat rate to care for a Medicare recipient.

Behavioral health: an umbrella term which encompasses mental illnesses, addictive disorders, and developmental disorders.

Benchmarking: enables organizations to use measures to answer key questions, such as: (1) Where are we now in this particular patient care process? and (2) Where do we want to be or what should our goal be?, as well as make comparisons to other organizations.

Benefit-to-cost ratio: a method of representing outcomes in a cost-benefit analysis whereby total benefits are divided by total costs.

Beveridge model: socialized medicine program developed in United Kingdom. Named after the British social reformer who inspired United Kingdom's National Health Service.

Biologics: a complex drug that is designed to mimic a human protein or is a monoclonal antibody.

Biosimilar: a copy of a biologic drug.

Bismark model: decentralized national health program developed in Germany. Named after the German Chancellor who instituted this social health insurance system.

Blue Cross and Blue Shield: originally a non-profit health insurance established in 1929 offering comprehensive plans. Most Blue Cross and Blue Shield plans switched to for-profit status in the 1990s.

Break-even point: the point found in a threshold sensitivity analysis where two alternative treatment options have the same outcome and there is no advantage between the treatment options. The break-even point is determined by varying a single assumption in the threshold sensitivity analysis until the outcomes are the same for both options.

Budget impact analysis: an estimation of the financial impact of adoption and diffusion of a new healthcare intervention within a specific healthcare setting. For example, budget impact analyses can predict how a change in the formulary mix of drugs used to treat a disease state will affect healthcare spending for that disease state, and therefore, can be used for budget planning.

Capitation: a type of prospective payment in which providers are paid a fixed amount each month for each enrolled patient, regardless of the number of healthcare services actually provided.

Catastrophic hazard: a situation in which an insurance company incurs excessive losses due to widespread and catastrophic events such as hurricanes, acts of war, and earthquakes. Companies that provide casualty insurance limit their exposure for catastrophic events by trying to avoid insuring large numbers of policy holders in the same geographic area.

Centers for Disease Control and Prevention (CDC): a DHHS agency that works to prevent and control infectious and chronic diseases, injuries, workplace hazards, disabilities, and environmental health threats.

Centers for Medicare and Medicaid Services (CMS): a DHHS agency that oversees Medicare, state Medicaid programs, and the Children's Health Insurance Program (CHIP), and regulates self-insured employers.

Centralized pharmacy services: pharmacy services that are provided from a single location within the hospital.

Chain pharmacy: a retail pharmacy that serves the general public and that is owned by a larger corporation (e.g., Walgreens, CVS, Rite-Aid).

Changes in demand: a shift in an entire demand curve such that the quantity demanded changes even though price remains constant. An increase in demand is represented by a rightward shift of the demand curve; a decrease in demand is illustrated by a leftward shift of the demand curve.

Change in quantity demanded: a movement along a given demand curve caused by a change in price. The demand schedule shows that as the price charged increases, the quantity demanded decreases. Therefore, a change in quantity demanded is caused solely by a change in the price charged to customers.

Change in quantity supplied: a movement along a given supply curve caused by a change in price. The supply schedule shows that, as the price that customers are willing to pay increases, the quantity supplied increases. Therefore, a change in quantity supplied is caused solely by a change in the price charged to customers.

Change in supply: a shift in an entire supply curve such that the quantity supplied changes even though the price customers are willing to pay remains constant. An increase in supply is represented by a rightward shift of the supply curve; a decrease in supply is illustrated by a leftward shift of the supply curve.

Charitable hospitals: medical care facilities in the 19th century that housed impoverished patients who had no friends or relatives to care for them. These institutions provided patients with only the bare necessities. The public generally perceived these institutions as places to die; professionals saw them as places to develop clinical experience.

Children's Health Insurance Program (CHIP): a medical coverage source for individuals under 19 whose parents earn too much income to qualify for Medicaid but not enough to pay for private coverage.

Children's Health Insurance Program Reauthorization Act: in 2009, the Children's Health Insurance Program was extended by Congress with the passage of the Children's Health Insurance Program Reauthorization Act. Funding through the Act assists states in insuring children who otherwise would not have health insurance.

Chronic diseases or noncommunicable diseases (NCDs): illness that lasts a long time, affecting patients either continuously or episodically. Chronic illnesses such as heart disease and cancer began to appear with greater frequency in the early 20th century.

Clinical end point: refers to the occurrence of a disease, symptom, sign or laboratory abnormality that constitutes one of the target outcomes of a trial.

Clinical trial: study conducted to evaluate potential new drugs.

Coinsurance: a form of patient cost sharing that requires patients to pay a specified percentage (usually 20%) of the cost of covered services; the plan pays the remainder.

Collaborative working relationships: the process by which pharmacists can establish effective and productive working relationships with other health professionals.

Community health centers: federally supported health center that provides primary care services (e.g., physicians, physician extenders, laboratory services, dental services, social services, and pharmaceutical services) to underserved areas in urban and rural areas of the United States.

Community pharmacy: any independent, chain, or supermarket-based pharmacy that provides pharmaceutical products and services to ambulatory patients.

Community rating: a method of setting insurance premiums based on the insurance company's overall expenses for a specific geographic area during the previous year.

Community-based health care: healthcare services provided for individuals within a community who need healthcare assistance at home.

Comparative effectiveness research (CER): designed to inform healthcare decisions by providing evidence on the effectiveness, benefits, and harms of different treatment options. The evidence is generated from research studies that compare drugs, medical devices, tests, surgeries, or ways to deliver health care.

Complements: product that tends to influence the purchase of other related products, such that an increase in the price of one good can cause a decrease in the demand for another good.

Compliance: refers to the patient following a health professional's recommendations, or in other words, the patient complies with what a health professional tells him to do.

Consolidated Health Economic Evaluation Reporting Standards (CHEERS): a 24-item checklist developed by the International Society of Pharmacoeconomic and Outcomes Research designed to promote transparent reporting of economic analyses of medications.

Consultant pharmacist: a pharmacist who provides advice on individual medication use, institutional-based medication use, and/or institutional pharmacy services.

Consumer drug use: the act of using medications by the general public.

Consumer model of care: a practitioner–patient model of care in which patients have a greater autonomy in decision making and are somewhat skeptical buyers of medical care.

Consumer price index (CPI): an economic indicator published by the Bureau of Labor Statistics that measures increases in the price level (i.e., inflation) of a set of goods and services purchased by consumers. Data can be used to determine inflation rates for many types of consumer goods and services such as medical care or prescription drugs.

Consumer-driven health plan (CDHP): refers to a health insurance plan which combines high-deductible insurance coverage with a personal health savings account such as a health savings account (HSA) or a health reimbursement arrangement (HRA).

Continuing care retirement community: a retirement community that provides a continuum of independent living, assisted living, and skilled nursing care on a single campus.

Continuity of care: refers to a process to systematically evaluate and improve care or services provided to patients.

Continuous quality improvement: a structured, organizational process for involving personnel in planning and executing a continuous flow of improvements to provide quality health care that meets or exceeds expectations.

Coordination of benefits: a provision in insurance contracts that is designed to prevent duplicate payments by more than one insurance plan for the same medical care by limiting total reimbursement from all insurance plans for the same event to the amount of the actual loss. Health insurance policies usually pay after automobile, homeowners', or workers' compensation insurance policies have paid their portion.

Copayment: under a copayment system, patients pay a specified dollar amount every time a service is received (e.g., $50 per hospital admission or $5 per prescription).

Cost containment: concept considered to either decrease healthcare spending or restrain the growth of healthcare spending. It has become the focus of much of healthcare reform since the 1970s.

Cost sharing: a provision in managed care plans requiring patients to share in the cost of services received. Cost sharing attempts to optimize utilization of health services by making patients more cost conscious. It can take many forms, including co-payments, coinsurance, deductibles, out-of-pocket limits, or maximum benefits.

Cost-benefit analysis (CBA): a method used to evaluate two or more alternatives where the input and outcomes are measured in dollars.

Cost-consequence analysis (CCA): a method used to evaluate two or more alternatives where the inputs are measured in dollars and the outcome is measured using a variety of methods, including natural units of effectiveness, quality-adjusted life years (QALYs), or dollars.

Cost-effectiveness analysis (CEA): a method used to evaluate two or more alternatives where the inputs are measured in dollars and the outcome is measured in natural units of effectiveness.

Cost-minimization analysis (CMA): a method used to evaluate two or more alternatives where the inputs are measured in dollars and the consequences or outcomes of the alternatives are identical.

Cost-of-illness (COI) analysis: a type of pharmacoeconomic analysis that estimates the magnitude of resources needed for a specific disease state in a defined population. The resources needed include both direct and indirect costs associated with prevention, treatment, and disease-related morbidity and mortality. This type of analysis can provide insight into the value of disease prevention or treatment of an illness or to compare the relative economic burden of one disease state compared to another to aid decision makers in allocating limited healthcare resources and research funding monies. Also commonly referred to as *burden-of-illness analysis*.

Cost-to-charge ratio: the ratio of the cost of providing services and the reimbursement obtained for those same services. This calculation is sometimes used in retrospective claims analysis to adjust available charge data to better reflect actual costs.

Cost-utility analysis (CUA): a method used to evaluate two or more alternatives where the input is measured in dollars and the outcome is measured as life years saved or patient-preference weighted outcome.

Counterfeit drugs: fraudulently created medical product passed off as the real thing.

Critical pathways: comprehensive management plans that aim to optimize and streamline patient care.

Culture: is a shared system of values, beliefs, and learned patterns of behavior that specifies acceptable and nonacceptable behaviors and offers individuals guidance on dealing with aspects of life.

Culture of safety: a belief among individuals working in a healthcare system dedicated to providing safe patient care.

Data exclusivity period: period of time when a generic or biosimilar manufacturer cannot rely upon the clinical trial data of the drug they are copying.

Decentralized national health program: a type of healthcare system where the administration of healthcare delivery is divided among various groups, usually the government and private agencies.

Decentralized pharmacy services: pharmacy services that are provided from satellite locations in patient care areas, or specialized areas, such as the operating room or emergency department.

Decision analysis: a systematic approach to decision making under conditions of uncertainty. This approach uses existing data and models the outcomes based on the best available data.

Decision tree: a type of decision analysis whereby all possible consequences of a decision are mapped in a branching or tree shape.

Deductible: a form of patient cost sharing that requires patients to pay their own healthcare expenses until a specified dollar amount has been paid out of pocket during a given period of time, usually a year.

Demand: the ability and willingness of a consumer to pay for a good or service.

Demand curve: a graphic representation of a demand schedule.

Demand schedule: a table or chart that shows the amounts of a commodity consumers are willing and able to purchase at each specific price charged in a set of possible prices during some specified period of time. The following two variables exist: (1) the price charged by the supplier (independent variable) and (2) the quantity demanded by the consumer at each given price (dependent variable). It is assumed, for the sake of simplicity, that all other variables are held constant.

Department of Health and Human Services (DHHS): a cabinet-level federal agency with numerous branches that are engaged in the delivery of health services and directly involved in the formation of health policy. Some DHHS offices and agencies provide social services or deliver administrative and support functions. DHHS also assumes a significant role in the research and development activities of the healthcare system, by conducting and sponsoring fundamental research, assuring the safety of food and drugs, and monitoring the adoption of information technology.

Developed nation: any country with a high standard of living that is characterized by high per capita incomes, strong health infrastructures, and positive healthcare outcomes. Also known as an industrialized country.

Developing nation: any country with a low standard of living that is characterized by low per capita incomes, weak health infrastructures, and poor healthcare outcomes.

Diagnosis-related group (DRG): a categorization of diseases or conditions created initially by the federal government as a means to reimburse hospitals prospectively for services provided to patients.

Direct medical cost: the medical input or resource consumed that is directly related to the product or service being evaluated.

Direct nonmedical cost: a consumed nonmedical resource that is directly related to the product or service being evaluated.

Disability-adjusted life years: a measure developed by the WHO that represents the loss of 1 year of full health.

Discounted fee-for-service: a retrospective reimbursement rate in which healthcare providers are paid a negotiated fee each time a service is provided. The agreed-upon rate is lower than the providers' usual and customary charges to cash-paying patients.

Discounting: the process of converting dollars, either paid out or received over time periods of more than 1 year, to their present value. The purpose is to incorporate the time preference for money into the analysis.

Disease state management: a continuous and coordinated process that seeks to manage and improve the health status of a patient population over the course of a disease.

Dispensary: separate, freestanding institutions in urban neighborhoods designed to provide medical care for the poor, usually employing a physician and/or pharmacist.

Dispense as written (DAW): a provision in the participating pharmacy agreement that allows full reimbursement for the higher cost multiple-source drug product if the pharmacy indicates on the prescription claim that the prescriber demanded a brand-name product instead of its generic equivalent.

Dispenser: points of distribution for medications through the pharmaceutical supply chain (e.g., manufacturer, wholesaler, pharmacy).

Drug therapy monitoring: verifying drug, dose, and route of administration and monitoring for medication-related problems to optimize drug therapy.

Drug utilization evaluation (DUE): an evaluation of the use of one or more drugs prescribed for one or more diseases or conditions within the context of quality assurance and risk management procedures.

Drug utilization review (DUR): the review of physician prescribing, pharmacist dispensing, and patient use of drugs with the goal of ensuring that drugs are used appropriately, safely, and effectively. A DUR may be conducted prospectively or retrospectively.

Drug wholesaler: a company that buys pharmaceuticals directly from manufacturers and then resells those drugs to individual pharmacies.

Duration of treatment: a measure of how long patients continue receiving treatment. For hospitals, this means length of stay; for physicians, the episode of care; and for pharmacies, the number of prescription refills.

Earned discount: the difference between the average wholesale price and the pharmacy's actual acquisition cost.

Economic resources: land, including all natural resources; labor; and capital, including physical resources produced by labor. Economists refer to these three basic economic resources as factors of production because they are used to produce those things that people desire (commodities).

Economics: the study of how individuals and societies allocate their limited resources in attempts to satisfy their unlimited wants.

Effectiveness: the ability of a product to produce an effect in real-world practice, typically outside of the well-controlled setting of clinical trials.

Efficacy: the ability of a product to produce an effect, typically demonstrated in randomized controlled clinical trials.

Efficiency: the goal of producing the greatest output for the lowest net cost.

Elastic demand: a situation in which consumers are relatively sensitive to price changes, such that an increase in price will result in a decrease in total revenue.

Elasticity: an economic concept that measures the responsiveness of consumer demands to a change in price.

Elimination period: a restriction found in group insurance policies that is aimed at reducing adverse selection by restricting coverage for preexisting health problems until after the policy holder has been covered for a given period of time. Expenses related to pregnancy and childbirth, for example, may not be covered for the first 9 months of a new policy. Elimination periods are often waived when new employees are hired and during open enrollment periods.

Emergency services: a wide range of emergent and urgent services provided in hospital emergency rooms to emergency medical services (e.g., 9-1-1, emergency medical vans, paramedics, trauma centers, and emergi-centers).

Employee mandate: a requirement usually set by a state law requiring all employees to purchase health insurance.

Employee Retirement Income Security Act (ERISA): a federal law designed to protect employees' benefits, including health insurance and retirement plans. Self-insured plans are exempt from state employer mandates under ERISA.

Employer mandate: proposal that would require employers to provide health insurance for all their workers or pay a tax that would create an insurance pool for the uninsured.

Epidemiology: the study of the factors that determine the frequency and distribution of disease in human populations.

Equilibrium point: the point where a demand curve intersects the supply curve. The coordinates for the equilibrium point are the equilibrium price and the equilibrium quantity.

Equilibrium price: the price corresponding to the point where the demand curve and the supply curve intersect; the price where the market can rest without a natural tendency to increase or decrease price.

Equilibrium quantity: the quantity corresponding to the point where the demand curve and the supply curve intersect; the quantity where the market can rest without a natural tendency to increase or decrease the quantity supplied or demanded.

Error reporting: a process used for healthcare providers in reporting errors that occur in the provision of patient care.

Estimated acquisition cost: the amount paid by a pharmacy benefit manager for drug ingredient costs, calculated as a percentage of the average wholesale price.

Experience rating: a method of setting insurance premiums based on the insurance company's overall expenses for a specific subset of insured individuals—usually an employer group—based on the group's experience from the previous year.

Failure mode effects analysis (FMEA): systematic approach to identify failures in a process.

Federal Medical Assistance Percentage (FMAP): the portion of Medicaid program costs that is paid by the federal government for provider services. Each state's portion is determined annually through the use of a formula that compares a given state's average per capita income to the national average. By law, the percentage can be no greater than 83% and no less than 50% for any given state. States that are wealthier in terms of average per capita income have a smaller share of their Medicaid costs paid by the federal government than do relatively poorer states. There are some exceptions that limit the portion of a state's administrative costs that are paid by the federal government and other exceptions that allow the federal government to reimburse states at a higher rate for family planning services and for healthcare services provided through Indian Health Service facilities.

Federal public health agencies: includes Agency for Healthcare Research and Quality, Administration for Community Living, Centers for Disease Control and Prevention, Centers for Medicare and Medicaid Services, Food and Drug Administration, Health Resources and Services Administration, Indian Health Service, National Institutes of Health, Substance Abuse and Mental Health Services Administration, Environmental Protection Agency, and Veterans Administration.

Fee-for-service (FFS): reimbursement in which a fee is paid to a provider for each service performed. FFS was the predominant reimbursement mechanism before managed care; some managed care organization contracts still allow a discounted FFS. FFS provides incentives to increase the quantity of services provided.

Fellowship program: is a post-graduate program more focused on developing one to be an independent investigator as compared to residency.

First-dollar coverage: a reimbursement mechanism in which there is no provision for patient cost sharing.

Fiscal intermediary: an organization that facilitates exchanges between healthcare payers and healthcare providers by underwriting and/or administering healthcare benefit programs.

Flat of the curve: a point where additional healthcare expenditures produce relatively little incremental benefit to the patient.

Flexner report: a report on the state of medical education in the United States sponsored by the Carnegie Foundation and prepared by Abraham Flexner in 1910. The report examined such factors as entrance requirements, teaching, labs, financing, and clinical status. Recommendations of the report resulted in closure of inadequate medical schools and new emphasis on scientific, lab-based medical education.

Floor-stock distribution: a drug distribution system that involves supplying the nursing staff units with a predetermined number of dosage forms, which are stored in a separate drug room on each patient care area. Nurses dispense the medications to any number of patients from this supply, and then they reorder from the pharmacy as needed.

Food and Drug Administration (FDA): the federal agency responsible for ensuring the safety and effectiveness of drugs and medical devices and the purity of food products.

Formulary: a list of medications compiled by a hospital or pharmacy benefit manager that contain either those drugs approved for use within the hospital or for reimbursement by the pharmacy benefit manager. Medications are included based on the relative clinical benefit and cost of the medication as compared to other agents within a similar therapeutic class.

Gatekeeper: a central component of most health maintenance organizations in which primary care physicians must coordinate and authorize all medical services, including laboratory services, specialty referrals, and hospitalizations. In many gatekeeper systems, a patient must receive a referral from his or her primary care physician to receive coverage for a specialist's care. The rationale underlying this approach is that it avoids unnecessary and often expensive referrals to specialists. The gatekeeper may be financially at risk—not only for the services that he or she provides, but also for the medical services provided by specialists to whom a patient is referred.

Generic drug: a drug product manufactured by a company other than the one that originally developed the product, after the original product's patent has expired.

Government Accountability Office (GAO): the investigative arm of Congress charged with evaluating federal programs and activities, examining the use of public funds, and providing analyses, options, and recommendations to Congress.

Gross domestic product (GDP): the market value of all final goods and services produced within a country within a given period of time.

Gross margin: the difference between the selling price and the cost to the pharmacy for the product that was sold.

Group policies: insurance plans sponsored by employer groups for employees and their dependents. Group policies are usually less expensive than individual policies because they are less subject to adverse selection and because they are less expensive to sell and administer.

Group-model HMO: a type of HMO characterized by contracts with large, multispecialty medical groups offering services exclusively to the HMO on a capitated basis.

Guidance–cooperation model of patient care: as described by Szasz and Hollender; practitioner–patient communication in which the patient is active in the interaction, but defers to medical expertise. This interaction can be compared to a parent–adolescent relationship.

Health: a state of physical and mental well-being, not merely the absence of disease or infirmity.

Health behavior models: includes variables that are used to explain and predict human behavior in regards to choices related to health.

Health belief model: a health behavior theory that describes the likelihood an individual will take action to change a behavior. Components of this theory include susceptibility and severity of disease, perceived benefits and barriers, cues to action, self-efficacy, and demographic, sociopsychological, and structural variables.

Health department: a public health agency at the federal, state, or local level that is established to identify and manage health problems that affect individuals and population groups (e.g., environmental sanitation, communicable diseases, chronic diseases, immunizations, maternal and child health clinics, and prevention services).

Health disparities: differences in the overall rate of disease incidence, prevalence, morbidity, mortality, or survival rates.

Health information technology: information technology applied to health and health care to improve quality by increasing adherence to guidelines, enhancing disease surveillance, and decreasing medication errors.

Health insurance: a situation in which individuals or employers buy a plan from a company to assist them in paying for healthcare costs incurred. Insurance coverage varies but often includes physician visits, hospitalizations, laboratory tests, and other medical expenses.

Health Insurance Portability and Accountability Act (HIPAA): a law enacted by Congress in 1996 that limits the amount of time a preexisting condition may be excluded from coverage to 1 year, requires insurance companies to sell health insurance policies to small employers and individuals who lose coverage without regard to their health history, requires insurance companies to renew policies they sell to groups and individuals, and outlines standards for patient confidentiality.

Health literacy: refers to a patient's ability to understand, comprehend, and act upon health information.

Health Maintenance Organization (HMO): a type of managed care organization that shares risk with a network of healthcare providers by requiring that the providers assume some risk, either directly or indirectly, and that generally does not provide coverage for medical care that is received outside the network. The risk arrangement can take many forms, such as capitation or risk pools. The gatekeeper is a central component of most HMOs. The four basic types of HMO models are staff models, group models, network models, and independent practice associations.

Health Maintenance Organization Act: a federal law enacted in 1973 that set standards and provided start-up funds for health maintenance organizations—specialized insurance plans that involve restrictive provider networks and primary care gatekeepers that are responsible for referrals to other healthcare services and risk sharing with providers. This act also required employers with more than 25 employees to offer an HMO plan.

Health savings account (HSA): a provision of the Medicare Prescription Drug, Improvement, and Modernization Act that established tax-free savings accounts to be used for out-of-pocket medical expenses for those individuals who select a high-deductible health insurance plan.

Health status disparities: refers to the differences in the incident of diseases and disabilities based upon socioeconomic and/or geographically defined population groups.

Healthcare disparities: refer to differences in access to or availability of health services or institutions.

Healthcare Effectiveness Data and Information Set (HEDIS): a group of measures that gives plan sponsors objective information that they can use to evaluate MCOs.

Health-related quality of life (HrQoL): a measure of an individual's well being; often used to determine how an individual's well being is affected over time by a given health condition or by treatment of that condition.

Heroic medical therapy: an aggressive type of patient care that used depletive and strengthening measures to return the patient's diseased body to equilibrium. Methods used included leeches, tonics, medical instruments, and medicines to bleed, purge, puke, or sweat patients.

Hill-Burton Act (The Hospital Survey and Construction Act of 1946): is credited with expanding the infrastructure of the healthcare delivery system by creating federal funding sources to build new hospitals, expand and renovate facilities, increase bed capacity, and add emerging technology.

History of pharmacy: the practice of pharmacy and the delivery of pharmacy services developed over time.

Home care: provision of healthcare services in a patient's home that are intended to restore and maintain the patient's optimal level of well-being in a familiar environment.

Home care standards for pharmacists: standards established by the American Society of Health-System Pharmacists that apply to activities pertaining to home care pharmacy practice. These standards establish a minimum level of pharmacy services within this component of pharmacy practice.

Home health services: services usually associated with nursing care provided through a home health agency. They may also include speech and physical therapy or other types of rehabilitation therapies, homemaker services, social services, and hospice care.

Home infusion therapy: the parenteral administration of drugs, solutions, and nutrition to patients in their homes.

Horizontal integration: integration of two or more similar entities, such as hospitals, often through acquisition or merger.

Hospice: care provided for individuals who are terminally ill or close to death.

Hospital clinics: ambulatory care clinics in hospitals that range from family practice and internal medicine (e.g., general medicine, cardiology, dermatology) to surgical clinics (e.g., general surgery, urology, orthopedics, plastic surgery).

Human capital approach: a method used to value lives saved in terms of the income that the person could have earned the remaining productive years of his or her life.

Humoralism: Galen's second-century concept that saw the human body as interrelated and in natural balance. Health equaled a human body in balance; disease meant the body's system was in disequilibrium.

Incidence: the rate of new cases of diseases occurring in a population over a specific time period.

Incremental cost-effectiveness plane: a chart that illustrates the decisions to be made when two alternative treatments are compared when one treatment is both more expensive and more effective than the other.

Incremental cost-effectiveness ratio (ICER): a ratio comparing the additional cost incurred to the additional benefit provided by one alternative relative to another option.

Incremental cost-utility ratio: a ratio comparing the additional cost incurred to the additional quality-adjusted life years provided by one alternative to another option.

Incremental healthcare reform: step-by-step, slow passage of individual pieces of health legislation.

Indemnity: a form of insurance that traditionally required patients to submit claims for reimbursement. Today the term is often used to refer to any health insurance plan with fee-for-service reimbursement and few cost controls.

Independent pharmacy: a retail pharmacy that serves the general public and that is independently owned, usually by a pharmacist.

Independent practice association (IPA)-model HMO: a type of HMO in which physicians form a separate legal entity, usually a corporation or partnership, that then contracts with the managed care organization. The IPA usually shares risk with the managed care organization and individual providers are paid by the IPA for services provided to enrolled patients for a negotiated fee. The IPA may reimburse physicians on a discounted FFS basis or may share some risk with them. These physicians typically have their own private practices and are allowed to provide services to patients enrolled in other managed care organizations.

Indian Health Service (IHS): managed by the U.S. Public Health Service, the system of hospitals and ambulatory care centers that provides health care and pharmacy services to nearly 1.5 million American Indians and Alaska natives living on or near reservations.

Indirect costs: those costs indirectly associated with the product or service under evaluation. Examples of indirect costs include the cost of lost productivity associated with an illness and the costs borne by caregivers.

Induced demand: the increased demand for healthcare services that is created by the availability of insurance payment. Healthcare providers, especially physicians, can increase utilization of health services by creating more demand for the services they provide.

Infant mortality rate: the number of children younger than 1 year of age who die during a particular year divided by the number of live births during the same year.

Infectious diseases: communicable, contagious diseases that historically killed large numbers of people. These diseases are always present (endemic) or appear occasionally with great intensity (epidemic). They include pneumonia, gastritis, measles, smallpox, and scarlet fever.

Inflation: an increase in the price level of specified goods or services over time; often measured by the Bureau of Labor Statistics (BLS) as the Consumer Price Index (CPI).

Informal care or caregiving: care provided by family or friends to an individual.

Inpatient Prospective Payment System (IPPS): the reimbursement or payment mechanism used for Medicare beneficiaries receiving hospital care. Payment is based on the patient's diagnosis and is determined prior to the patient receiving care. Also referred to as the DRG payment method.

Inputs: as related to pharmaceuticals, all resources—including but not limited to human capital and supplies—that are needed to produce optimal outcomes.

Instrumental activities of daily living: activities that are required for independent living but are not necessarily performed on a daily basis, such as meal preparation, housework, balancing a checkbook, driving, and using a telephone.

Insurable hazard: a type of pure risk that can lead to specific, measurable, and substantial losses that are unanticipated for an individual, but that are anticipated and relatively predictable for the group as a whole.

Insurable interest: a situation in which the individual who will receive payment for an insurance claim actually experiences a loss when an insurable hazard occurs.

Intangible costs: those costs that cannot be measured or tracked easily or are not associated with a medical or nonmedical resource. Intangible costs are often associated with the pain and suffering due to illness or disease.

Intellectual property rights (IPRs): regulations that allow for innovators to have market exclusivity in order to recoup development costs.

Intensity of services: a measure of the types and numbers of services provided. It includes the service mix (types of services), the quantity (per capita use), and the quality of services.

Interdisciplinary: involving those professionals who work together for the patient's good and who also communicate effectively among themselves and with the patient.

Interdisciplinary care: involving those professionals who work together for the patient's good and who also communicate effectively among themselves and with the patient.

International Society of Pharmacoeconomics and Outcomes Research (ISPOR): the professional society that promotes pharmacoeconomic and outcomes research.

Internet pharmacy: a retail entity in which consumers can purchase pharmaceuticals via an Internet website. Also known as a cyberpharmacy.

Investigational new drug: a chemical entity that shows promise as a potential new drug and has been approved by the FDA for clinical testing.

Iron Triangle: a model that demonstrates the reciprocal trade-offs among the three variables: access, cost, and quality; in the United States, the relationship among Congress, the bureaucracy, and interest groups.

The Joint Commission: a nonprofit organization that sets standards of practice for, evaluates, and accredits more than 15,000 healthcare organizations and programs in the United States. Formerly known as the Joint Commission on the Accreditation of Healthcare Organizations.

Kerr-Mills Act: a 1960 amendment to the Social Security Act that provided healthcare coverage to poor, elderly individuals.

***King v. Burwell* (2015):** upheld that subsidies to help individuals or small business purchase insurance could be obtained through federal or state operated health insurance exchanges or marketplaces.

Law of demand: an economic principle that states that, as the price charged for a product or service falls, the corresponding quantity demanded rises; alternatively, as the price charged increases, the corresponding quantity demanded falls. In short, an inverse relationship exists between the price charged and the quantity demanded.

Law of diminishing marginal utility: an economic principle that states that the value of any additional goods declines as one consumes more of it. In other words, the more we have of a good, the less we desire it.

Law of large numbers: an insurance principle that states that the larger the number of insured persons, the more accurate the predictions regarding losses. With losses being more predictable, the risk of this loss actually decreases.

Law of supply: an economic principle that states that, as the price customers are willing to pay falls, the corresponding quantity supplied falls; alternatively, as the price customers are willing to pay increases, the corresponding quantity supplied increases. In short, a direct relationship exists between the price customers are willing to pay and the quantity supplied.

Lean: a method that focuses on the value of a particular process and seeks to maximize the uninterrupted flow of that value to the end customer.

Length of stay: the amount of time a patient stays in the hospital, calculated from admission to discharge.

Life expectancy: average number of years remaining for a person of a given age to live.

Long-term care services: a set of services—whether health, personal, or social— that is provided over a period of time to individuals who have lost some aspect of functioning.

Look-alike sound-alike medications: refers to medications and medication names that either look alike or sound alike.

Mail-order pharmacy: the practice of pharmacy in which consumers mail in their prescriptions to a pharmacy to be filled and mailed back.

Major medical insurance: a type of insurance policy designed to help offset expenses incurred by catastrophic illness or injury. These policies usually have high deductibles and are not designed to cover minor expenses.

Managed care: the application of cost and quality controls to health care by controlling patient demand and provider supply. The defining feature of managed care is the use of provider networks through a contractual arrangement specifying the types of services to be provided and the reimbursement to be received in return.

Managed care organization (MCO): an organization designed to manage the cost and quality of a health insurance program. The differentiating feature of managed care plans versus fee-for-service plans is the use of a provider network. MCOs are categorized according to their degrees of (1) risk sharing, (2) provider exclusivity, (3) out-of-network coverage, and (4) physician autonomy and organization.

Mandated categorically needy: groups of Medicaid recipients that the federal government requires state Medicaid programs to cover as a condition for receiving matching federal funding. The groups included are individuals who meet the eligibility criteria for Aid to Families with Dependent Children (AFDC), those receiving government cash assistance through the Supplemental Security program, pregnant women and children under the age of 6 in families with incomes of less than 133% of the federal poverty level, children under the age of 19 in families with income less than the federal poverty level, and certain groups of low-income Medicare recipients.

Marginal utility: the additional utility received from consuming one additional unit of a particular good or service.

Market structure: the categorization of firms based on attributes such as the numbers of buyers and sellers, product differentiation, pricing behavior, and so on. The four types of market structures are perfect competition, monopolistic competition, monopoly, and oligopoly.

Markov model: a type of decision analysis suited for those situations in which the patient may transition from one state to another. The simplest example of a Markov model features a three-state transition—from well to ill to dead.

Maximum allowable cost: the amount paid by a pharmacy benefit manager for the drug ingredient cost for a multiple-source drug. The maximum allowable cost is usually set at the price of a low-cost generic product without regard to whether a brandname or generic product was actually dispensed.

Measuring safety: data measurement, collection, reporting, and analysis are vital to an organization's continuous quality improvement efforts.

Medicaid: Title XIX of the Social Security Act; a joint program between the federal and state governments that pays for medical care for individuals who receive case assistance through the Supplemental Security Income program and certain low-income pregnant women, children, and other vulnerable groups.

Medicaid waiver: a provision established by the Omnibus Budget Reconciliation Act of 1981 that allows states to apply for exceptions to federal Medicaid guidelines for the purpose of either establishing Medicaid managed care plans or creating new initiatives to curb costs or improve delivery of Medicaid services.

Medical Home (or Patient-Centered Medical Home): a team-based healthcare delivery model led by a healthcare provider that is intended to provide comprehensive and continuous medical care to patients with the goal of obtaining maximized health outcomes.

Medical Savings Account (MSA): a provision that allows self-employed individuals and employers with fewer than 50 employees to make tax-deferred deposits to an account that is available to cover future medical expenses. Withdrawals from MSAs are tax free if used for qualified medical expenses.

Medicalization: redefining or relabeling of a personal or social problem as a medical condition, thus necessitating treatment for it in the healthcare system.

Medically needy: a group of individuals who would be eligible for Medicaid under one of the mandated or optional groups except for the fact that their income and/or assets are higher than allowed by the state. Such individuals become Medicaid eligible under the medically needy provision if their medical expenses reduce their net income to the Medicaid eligibility threshold or less. Thus, the medically needy consist of families and children, or elderly, blind, or disabled individuals, who spend down to Medicaid eligibility by incurring high out-of-pocket medical expenses. States may elect to cover these individuals and may qualify for federal matching funds.

Medicare advantage: Medicare Part C (formerly known as "Medicare + Choice"), which expanded Medicare beneficiaries' ability to participate in a wide variety of private health plans, including health maintenance organizations and preferred provider organizations.

Medicare: Title XVIII of the Social Security Act; a federal social health insurance program for individuals 65 years of age and older, individuals who receive disability benefits from Social Security or the Railroad Retirement Board, or individuals with end-stage renal disease requiring dialysis or kidney transplantation.

Medicare Part A: the component of Medicare that pays for inpatient hospital, skilled nursing facilities, and home health care, and is financed by a payroll tax levied on employees and employers. Also called Hospital Insurance.

Medicare Part B: the component of Medicare that pays for physicians' services, outpatient hospital care, and a variety of other medical services not covered under Part A. Financed through premiums and patient cost sharing. Also called Supplemental Medical Insurance.

Medicare Part C: originally known as the Medicare + Choice program, but now is called Medicare Advantage. It expanded beneficiaries' ability to participate in a wide variety of private health plans, including health maintenance organizations (HMOs) and preferred provider organizations (PPOs).

Medicare Part D: a provision that created a new voluntary outpatient prescription drug benefit for Medicare recipients; it became available in 2006.

Medicare Prescription Drug, Improvement, and Modernization Act: the largest revision of Medicare in its 38-year history, was passed in 2003. Its most important provision was Medicare Part D.

Medicare star ratings: a performance standard for pharmacies similar to product ratings by *Consumer Reports*; measures how well prescription programs under Medicare Part D and Medicare Advantage plans perform on a scale of one to five stars, with one being the lowest and five being the highest.

Medicare supplement (Medigap) insurance: insurance available to Medicare recipients that is designed to cover the cost for healthcare services not covered by Medicare.

Medication adherence: refers to patients taking medications as prescribed. Similar to compliance, adherence implies a level of patient decision-making.

Medication errors: any *preventable event* that may cause or lead to inappropriate medication use or patient harm while the medication is in the control of the healthcare professional, patient, or consumer.

Medication regimen review (MRR): a thorough evaluation of the medication regimen of a resident with the goal of promoting positive outcomes and minimizing adverse consequences associated with medication. The review includes preventing, identifying, reporting, and resolving medication-related problems, medication errors, or other irregularities, and collaborating with other members of the interdisciplinary team.

Medication therapy management (MTM) : a broad range of activities within the scope of practice of pharmacists and other qualified healthcare providers intended to ensure that patients with multiple diseases and on many medications get the greatest benefit possible from their medication regimen.

Medication use process: the medication use process is broadly identified as the complete network of interactions spanning acquisition of the medications to be used to the monitoring and follow up after administering them.

Medication-utilization evaluation (MUE): an interprofessional quality assurance program that was incorporated into the Joint Commission's standards in 1992.

Mental health: functioning at a satisfactory level of physical, mental, and social wellbeing; a harmonious balance between the individual, his or her social group, and the larger environment context.

Monopolistic competition: a market structure similar to perfect competition except that it does not have standardized and interchangeable products.

Monopoly: a market structure that has only one seller of a product for which there are no close substitutes.

Monopsony: a market structure that has only one buyer, but several competing suppliers.

Moral hazard: a situation in which patients with insurance coverage overconsume healthcare services to the extent that the additional health benefits achieved from consuming additional health services are not really worth their full costs. Nevertheless, because the enrollees are paying only a fraction of the costs, they still want to use the services. Overconsumption of health services owing to moral hazard increases total health expenditures and insurance premiums.

Morbidity: rates that report the number of instances of a particular disease in an area per year.

Mortality rate: rates that report the number of deaths in an area per year.

Motivational interviewing: is a patient-centered approach to facilitate behavior change through engaging intrinsic motivation.

Multidisciplinary care: refers to many different professionals working for the good of the patient, albeit somewhat independently.

Mutual participation model of patient care: as described by Szasz and Hollender, a practitioner–patient communication in which the patient assumes an active role and is equally powerful to the practitioner. This model is most commonly seen with patients who have chronic diseases and can be compared to a parent–adult child relationship.

National Committee for Quality Assurance (NCQA): an independent, nongovernment agency that promotes performance standards, quality assurance, review standards, and accreditation for health maintenance organizations.

***National Federation of Independent Business v. Sebelius* (2012):** in the 2012 case, *National*

Federation of Independent Business v. Sebelius, the PPACA was found to be constitutional with a 5-4 majority vote.

National health insurance model: any healthcare system characterized by a socialized health insurance plan.

National Institutes of Health (NIH): a DHHS agency that supports health research, especially in cases where economic incentives are lacking or risky.

Naturalistic designs: an approach to pharmacoeconomic analyses in which patients are recruited and randomly assigned to treatment groups with follow up care being representative of routine clinical care.

Net benefit: a method used to represent outcomes in a cost-benefit analysis where the time frame of the analysis is less than or equal to 1 year.

Net present value: a method used to represent outcomes in a cost-benefit analysis where the time frame of the analysis goes beyond 1 year.

Network: a defined group of providers, typically linked through contractual arrangements, who supply a full range of primary and acute healthcare services. Managed care enrollees who use providers outside the network may receive reduced coverage or even no coverage.

Network-model HMO: a type of HMO characterized by nonexclusive contracts with large medical groups. While networks typically bear risk, the nonexclusivity of the arrangement reduces the influence of the risk on the physician's behavior.

New drug application (NDA): the application submitted by a pharmaceutical manufacturer to the FDA for approval of a drug product that has completed the FDA's clinical testing requirements.

Nonprescription (over the counter, nonlegend): pharmaceutical products that can be purchased without a prescription.

Office of Management and Budget (OMB): the agency within the Executive Office of the President that advises the President on the costs and outcomes associated with federal agency activities.

Office of the Inspector General: a DHHS agency that conducts nationwide audits, investigations, and inspections, reports to both the secretary of the DHHS and Congress about program and management problems, and makes recommendations for improvements.

Off-label drug use: use of drugs for an indication for which they do not have formal approval from the FDA.

Older adults: individuals who are at least 65 years of age.

Oligopoly: a market structure that consists of a few sellers and many buyers. Firms in oligopolies are often interdependent, and a dominant firm can exert influence through price leadership.

Oligopsony: a market structure that consists of only a few buyers but several competing suppliers.

Open enrollment period: a short period of time when employees are allowed to join the employer's health insurance plan. Open enrollment, without restrictions for preexisting conditions, is usually available to new employees immediately upon being hired and to incumbent employees during a short period of time (i.e., approximately 2 weeks) each year.

Opportunity cost: the value of a resource based on its highest valued alternative use or market value.

Optionally categorically needy: groups of needy individuals who do not meet the requirements for mandated coverage but may be covered at the option of a state Medicaid program, which then receives federal matching funds. Many of those considered optionally eligible are children or pregnant women.

Orphan diseases: disease that affects very few people every year, typically less than 200,000 per year.

Orthodox physicians: physician who possessed some didactic medical education and underwent apprenticeship to develop his or her clinical skills. He or she practiced heroic medicine.

Outcome: the impact or effect of drug therapy.

Out-of-pocket model: any healthcare system characterized by no insurance coverage.

Pandemics: widespread epidemics of infectious or contagious diseases that affect one or more countries or continents contemporaneously.

Participating pharmacy agreement: a contract between a pharmacy and a pharmacy benefit manager that specifies the rights and duties of each party with regard to prescription drug coverage.

Patent medicines: cheap concoction in tonic or pill form that was widely advertised in newspapers and popular magazines and sold in pharmacies or by traveling tradesmen.

Patent: the right for an innovator to be the exclusive producer for a period of time.

Patient cost sharing: a provision in health insurance plans that provides financial incentives for patients to avoid using unnecessary healthcare services by making them pay a portion of the cost of the service. Patient cost-sharing methods include copayments, coinsurance, deductibles, out-of-pocket limits, and maximum benefit limits.

Patient Protection and Affordable Care Act (PPACA): Signed into law by President Obama in 2010 with the purpose of expanding access to health care services using an individual mandate requiring U.S. citizens and legal residents to obtain health insurance. The law expands Medicaid to cover more individuals, expands access through the creation of state based insurance exchanges and non-profit insurance companies, and creates a Patient-Centered Outcomes Research Institute.

Patient-centered model of care (or Patient-centered care): orientation shifts the focus from just the body to the person as a whole. Practitioners who adopt this model are encouraged to view the illness through the patient's eyes.

Patient-focused care (or Patient-centered care): respects individual patient preferences, needs, and values, and ensures that patient values guide all clinical decisions.

Patient-induced demand: an increase in the quantity of services demanded resulting from insurance coverage that lowers patients' out-of-pocket expenses. By isolating patients from the true cost of healthcare services, health insurance has encouraged patients to consume more healthcare services than they would if they were bearing the full cost of the product or service themselves.

Pay for performance (P4P): (also known as "P4P,") a payment model that rewards healthcare providers or managed care organizations for meeting quality and efficiency performance measures as an incentive for improving quality of care.

Per diem: a type of prospective reimbursement in which hospitals are paid a flat rate for each day of hospital care provided to covered individuals without regard to the actual costs incurred.

Perfect competition: market structure characterized by (1) many buyers and sellers, (2) freedom of entry and exit, (3) standardized products, (4) full and free information, and (5) no collusion.

Personalized medicine: treatments for diseases that are tailored to each individual based on genetic and diagnostic test results.

Perspective: the point of reference (typically the decision maker) from which a pharmacoeconomic analysis will be conducted.

Pharmaceutical care: the responsible provision of drug therapy for achieving specific outcomes that improve a patient's quality of life. A pharmacy's mission is taking responsibility for patients' medication-related outcomes.

Pharmaceutical manufacturer: a company that participates in the manufacturing of drug products.

Pharmaceutical marketing: techniques used to publicize pharmaceutical products to prescribers and users of those products.

Pharmaceutical research and development: the process through which a pharmaceutical company discovers and develops new drug entities.

Pharmacists' patient-centered care: incorporating individual patient preferences, needs, and values when providing pharmacy services.

Pharmacoeconomics: the evaluation of the inputs and outcomes associated with pharmaceuticals or pharmacy services.

Pharmacy benefit manager (PBM): a specialized company that adjudicates prescription drug claims and manages the prescription drug coverage for a third-party payer by containing costs and influencing the quality of services provided.

Pharmacy Quality Alliance (PQA): a consensus-based, multi-stakeholder membership organization committed to improving healthcare quality and patient safety with a focus on the appropriate use of medications.

Pharmacy technician: an assistant to a pharmacist whose roles and functions include medication preparation, customer service, and other activities as deemed appropriate by the employer within the context of state law.

Pharmacy workforce: the number of pharmacists and support personnel available in the United States as measured in terms of the number of full-time equivalent (FTE) employees.

Pharmakon: the Greek term for *drug*, meaning remedy, poison, or magical charm.

Plan-Do-Study-Act (PDSA): which is used as process for continuous quality improvement.

Point-of-service (POS) plan: a type of managed care organization that is a hybrid of a health maintenance organization and a preferred provider organization. As with a PPO, when care is received from a provider outside the network, partial coverage is provided. As with a health maintenance organization, physicians may be at risk or contract exclusively with the plan.

Population effects: a measure of the number of patients and the mix of various demographic factors within the group (e.g., gender, age, socioeconomic status, and other factors) that affect utilization. For hospitals, this means the number of hospital admissions; for physicians, the number of new patients; and for pharmacies, the number of new prescriptions.

Portability: a characteristic whereby healthcare benefits are readily transportable when individuals change their jobs or place of residence.

Postmarketing surveillance: the act of collecting information about a drug's use after it has been on the market for some time and is used more widely in the population.

Preferred provider organization (PPO): a type of managed care organization that creates a network of providers who agree to discount their charges for services delivered to enrolled beneficiaries. Beneficiaries are free to see any provider they choose, but have a financial incentive (i.e., lower out-of-pocket expenses) to receive care from providers in the preferred network.

Prescriber: a healthcare professional who is licensed to prescribe medications.

Prescription: an order written by a prescriber for a patient that describes therapy that a patient should receive.

Prevalence: is the total number of cases in a population who have a specific disease during a defined time period.

Prevention: in a public health model, there are three successive stages to prevent pathologies, to initiate therapy, and to assist in the social reintegration of patients. Primary prevention covers all activities designed to reduce the instances of an illness in a population and to reduce the risk of new cases. Secondary prevention covers activities aimed at reducing the prevalence of an illness in a population and its duration. Tertiary prevention tries to reduce the incidence of chronic incapacity or recurrences of a disease.

Preventive health care: performance of activities or behaviors for the purpose of avoiding or deterring disease and maintaining health.

Primary care: ambulatory services for common ailments provided by primary care (first-order or gatekeeper) providers, who include physicians (e.g., those in family practice, internal medicine, pediatrics, obstetrics, and gynecology), nurse practitioners, and physician assistants.

Primary prevention: refers to the avoidance of disease occurrence as well as actions taken prior to disease onset.

Prior authorization (PA): requires a prescriber to request coverage of nonpreferred or noncovered medications when they are needed for a particular patient.

Probabilistic sensitivity analysis: a type of sensitivity analysis in which researchers assign plausible ranges for variables and an estimate of the distribution of the data points for each variable. The most common type of probabilistic sensitivity analysis is Monte Carlo simulation, which uses computer simulation to randomly assign values from inputted variable ranges and estimating outcomes from models with large numbers of hypothetical patients.

Profession: the characteristics of a profession include a specialized knowledge, confidential relationship, public obligation, common heritage, public interest and an ethical code.

Professional: a person who possesses specialized technical knowledge, is licensed to practice, and is motivated by a desire to be of service to others.

Professional pharmacy organizations: include the American Pharmacists Association, American Society of Health-System Pharmacists, National Community Pharmacists Association, and American Society of Consultant Pharmacists, as well as state affiliates.

Prospective drug utilization review: review of patients' medication records at the time that pharmacists or pharmacy technicians are entering new prescription data in to the online claims system so that potential problems are identified before the prescription is dispensed.

Psychiatric clinical pharmacist: a pharmacist trained in clinical aspects of psychiatric patient care and certified as a Board Certified Psychiatric Pharmacist (BCPP) who is responsible for optimizing drug treatment and patient care, recognizing drug-induced problems, and recommending appropriate treatment plans.

Public health: the practice of preventing disease and promoting health in communities of people. Public health professionals rely on policy and research strategies to understand issues such as substance abuse and chronic disease in particular populations.

Pure risk: type of risk in which there is a possibility of a loss but no possibility of a gain. This type of risk is insurable.

Quackery: false medical knowledge or credentials used to defraud the public; manufacture or sale of nontherapeutic nostrums or medical devices that generally cause harm.

Quality measures: to improve patient outcomes and safety and/or to maintain compliance with various federal and state payment and accreditation programs, organizations are required to collect and report various quality metrics.

Quality of care: optimal sequencing and timing of interventions by healthcare professionals for a particular diagnosis or procedure, designed to minimize delays and resource utilization and maximize the quality of care.

Quality-adjusted life year (QALY): an outcome measured as life years gained adjusted for patient preference or another means of weighting/adjusted gains in life years.

Randomized controlled trials: a research design model in which the unit of analysis (typically a patient) is randomized to one of multiple study arms (typically treatment and control or placebo).

Rebates: payment received by a pharmacy benefit manager from a pharmaceutical manufacturer in return for putting a specific drug on the pharmacy benefit manufacturer's formulary or giving the drug preferred status. The amount of a rebate may be based on performance (e.g., a certain level of prescribing) or market share (i.e., the percentage of all prescriptions within a given therapeutic class that are dispensed for the company's product).

Regulatory agency: a federal or state agency that regulates components of the healthcare industry, such as the Department of Public Health, the Drug Enforcement Administration, or the Food and Drug Administration.

Reinsurance: a type of insurance that protects insurance companies from extraordinary, unexpected losses. Insurance companies are willing to accept some risk of having claims exceed income, but obtain reinsurance to protect them from catastrophic losses. The reinsurance company pools the risks faced by many insurance companies together.

Report cards: a periodic report sent by a managed care organization to inform providers about how their general performance and compliance with plan guidelines compared with the same characteristics for their colleagues or to the managed care organization's standards. Typical information on report cards includes cost per patient per month, number of prescriptions per patient per month, percentage of brand-name versus generic prescriptions, compliance with formulary guidelines, and prescribing patterns for selected prescription drugs.

Residency program: an organized, directed, post-graduate training program designed to develop competencies in a defined area of pharmacy practice.

Retrospective claims analysis: analysis that relies on paid administrative pharmacy or medical claims data. It is retrospective in the sense that researchers are typically evaluating events or measuring associations that have occurred in the past.

Retrospective drug utilization review: review of prescription claims data after prescriptions are dispensed to study physicians' prescribing, pharmacists' dispensing, and patients' use of medications with the aim of improving future prescribing, dispensing, and usage patterns.

Risk bearing: the amount of risk borne by the providers, which can range from full risk to no risk. Physicians typically accept risk in the form of capitation and risk pools; hospitals accept capitation as well as per diem and diagnosis-related group reimbursement.

Risk pool: an arrangement in which a health maintenance organization places a portion of payments in a pool as a source for any subsequent claims that exceed projections, with thc provider and the health maintenance organization sharing in the surplus (or loss) from the risk pool at the end of the year.

Roemer's law: reflects the historical tendency for healthcare providers to increase hospital admissions and the use of healthcare technology when excess capacity exists.

Root cause analysis (RCA): is utilized to obtain a complete understanding of why errors occur.

Secondary prevention: refers to the early diagnosis (detection) and prompt treatment (early intervention) of disease and the avoidance of disability.

Sectarians: rivals to orthodox physicians who sought education or training outside the orthodox medical educational system. They represented various beliefs, therapies, or medical systems that competed with the orthodox practice of medicine and included homeopaths and eclectics.

Self-dosing: do-it-yourself medicine. It uses traditional practices, family recipes, and folk and herbal medicines to treat oneself and one's family.

Service benefit: a form of health insurance plan in which healthcare providers submit claims and are paid directly by the insurance plan.

Shortage: a situation that occurs when the market price is below the equilibrium price, resulting in a quantity supplied that is less than the quantity demanded.

Sickness funds: the common name for the quasipublic, third-party payers characterizing Germany's healthcare system.

Simple sensitivity analysis: a pharmacoeconomic analysis that involves varying study assumptions (either cost or outcome) within the range of plausible values to determine if the original conclusions remain sound. A one-way simple sensitivity analysis allows only one variable to be changed at a time while a multiple-way simple sensitivity analysis allows more than one variable to be changed at a time.

Six Sigma: a data-driven method that focuses on customer satisfaction and defect (error) reduction.

Skilled nursing facility: a facility that provides basic medical and nursing care, as well as additional services or therapies, that can include restorative, physical, and occupational therapies.

Social determinants of health: health is more than simply the absence of disease, and is influenced by income and social status; social support networks; education; employment/working conditions; social environments; physical environments; personal health practices and coping skills; healthy child development; gender; and culture.

Social healers: usually female healers who treated friends and neighbors in rural and small-town communities in the 18th and 19th centuries. Patients sought simple medicines and treatments for boils or wounds as well as advice. Social healers were often also midwives.

Social partnership: characteristic whereby both the employer and the employee contribute funds to the healthcare system.

Social security: a program created by the Social Security Act of 1935 that provides a minimum level of income for qualified individuals who are 65 years of age or older or who are disabled.

Social solidarity: a characteristic whereby some members of a country subsidize other members' healthcare costs.

Socialized health insurance: a type of healthcare system where the government provides health insurance to all citizens. Healthcare providers and facilities are private.

Socialized medicine: a type of healthcare system where the government participates in or enforces participation in the country's healthcare system, employs healthcare practitioners, owns healthcare facilities, and administers the healthcare system.

Speculative risk: a type of risk in which there is the possibility of either a gain or a loss. Business ventures and gambling are examples of activities in which there is speculative risk. This type of risk is not insurable.

Staff-model HMO: a type of health maintenance organization characterized by direct ownership of healthcare facilities and direct-employment physicians. Physicians in a staff-model health maintenance organization typically bear no direct risk, but the health maintenance organization can influence the physician through utilization review (the review of the necessity and efficiency of patients' utilization patterns).

Subrogation: the process in which an insurance company enforces a coordination of benefits provision by determining which insurance company is required to pay first if a particular patient has duplicate coverage.

Substance abuse disorders: disorders related to the use and abuse of various substances, both legal and illegal. Also referred to as addictive disorders and chemical disorders.

Substitutes: related products that may be interchanged by consumers. When the price of one good increases, the quantity demanded for that good decreases and the demand for its substitute increases.

Supplier-induced demand: an increase in demand created by the service provider. Physicians may induce demand for their own services by ordering follow-up care or referring patients to physician-owned laboratory, pharmacy, radiology, or other diagnostic or treatment services.

Supply: the ability and willingness of a supplier to provide a good or service.

Supply curve: a graphic representation of a supply schedule.

Supply schedule: a table or chart that shows the amount of a commodity suppliers are willing and able to supply at each specific price that customers are willing to pay in a set of possible prices during a specified period of time.

Surplus: situation in which the market price exceeds the equilibrium price, resulting in a quantity supplied that is greater than the quantity demanded.

Tall man lettering: a method to reduce errors from look-alike and sound-alike drug names involving the use of capital letters to emphasize and distinguish different parts of similar looking drug names.

Technology: the technical means that a person uses to improve his or her surroundings by extending user capabilities and performing repetitive tasks.

Temporary Assistance for Needy Families (TANF): a federal government program that provides block grants to states to be used for time-limited cash assistance. TANF generally allows a family to receive cash welfare (income maintenance) benefits for no more than 5 years and allows states to impose other requirements related to employment.

Tertiary prevention: refers to the limitation or reduction of disability when disease has already occurred, through rehabilitation designed to encourage recovery and prevent further problems.

Theory of Human Error: a foundational patient safety concept, which notes that when humans work in a system there is always a risk for error and mistakes.

Threshold sensitivity analysis: a type of sensitivity analysis in which a single assumption in the analysis is varied until the alternative treatment option has the same outcome and there is no advantage between the treatment options. The value determined by conducting such an analysis is often referred to as a break-even point.

Tiered copayments: a type of patient cost sharing that specifies multiple copayment levels that are designed to encourage the use of preferred drug products, such as generics and lower cost brand-name drugs.

TriCare: an agency of the Department of Defense that provides medical services to active-duty members and retired personnel of the armed forces, their dependents, and their survivors.

U.S. drug approval process: the process identified by the Food and Drug Administration and by which pharmaceutical manufacturers must abide, for products to be approved for use in the United States.

U.S. drug development process: the process of creating and testing new drugs according to regulations set by the FDA in the U.S.

Unapproved abbreviations: abbreviations that have been identified by safety organizations that are prone to errors and should be avoided.

Uncompensated care pool: an account financed by a tax on hospital bills or general tax revenue that establishes a pool of money used to reimburse hospitals for a portion of the cost of providing medical care to underinsured and uninsured patients.

Underwriting: the process of insuring. Underwriters attempt to calculate the amount of financial risk that they assume for insurable events, estimate losses and administrative expenses (with the aid of actuaries), and set the level of premiums needed to cover expenditures and provide for a reasonable profit.

Unit-dose distribution: a drug distribution system in which each dose of medication is separately packaged and labeled with the drug name, strength, lot number, and expiration date in a ready-to-administer form.

Universality: characteristic whereby all healthcare benefits are provided for all citizens of a given country.

Utility score: a measure of patient preferences elicited from patients by a variety of means, such as analog scales, validated questionnaires, or standard gamble or time trade-off game theories. Scales typically range from zero to 1.0 with the assumption that patients will prefer those health states with higher utility scores.

Utility: the satisfaction obtained from purchasing a particular good or service.

Value-Based Purchasing Program (VBP Program): hospitals are beginning to change processes of care as a result of incentives created by the Hospital Value-Based Purchasing Program.

Vertical integration: the provision of a continuum of healthcare services. For hospitals, it entails expanding healthcare services beyond traditional acute medical care to include nursing home care, home health care, and outpatient and rehabilitation services.

Veterans administration: Department of Defense agency that provides clinics and hospitals that treat injuries and provide rehabilitation services for disabilities resulting from military service, as well as care to veterans with low incomes or special healthcare needs.

Waiver: permission given by CMS to allow states to operate outside of federal guidelines in order to experiment with benefit design and reimbursement alternatives to determine whether they reduce costs or improve quality of care.

Wholesale acquisition cost (WAC): the manufacturer's list price for drug products sold to wholesalers or direct purchasers as reported in wholesale price guides or other publications of drug pricing data. WAC prices are used as one method of calculating reimbursement of drug ingredient costs by some states' Medicaid programs.

Willingness-to-pay approach: a method used to value lives saved and/or the intangible benefits and health risks associated with a product or service, whereby individuals express their willingness to pay to reduce a health risk.

Index

Note: Italicized page locators indicate a figure; tables are noted with a *t*.

A

B

D

E

F

G

H

J

M

N

O

P

S

T

U

V

W

X

Y

Z